PROVIDING YOUR STUDENTS
with **INTERACTIVE TOOLS** to SUCCEED
in **FITNESS** and **WELLNESS**

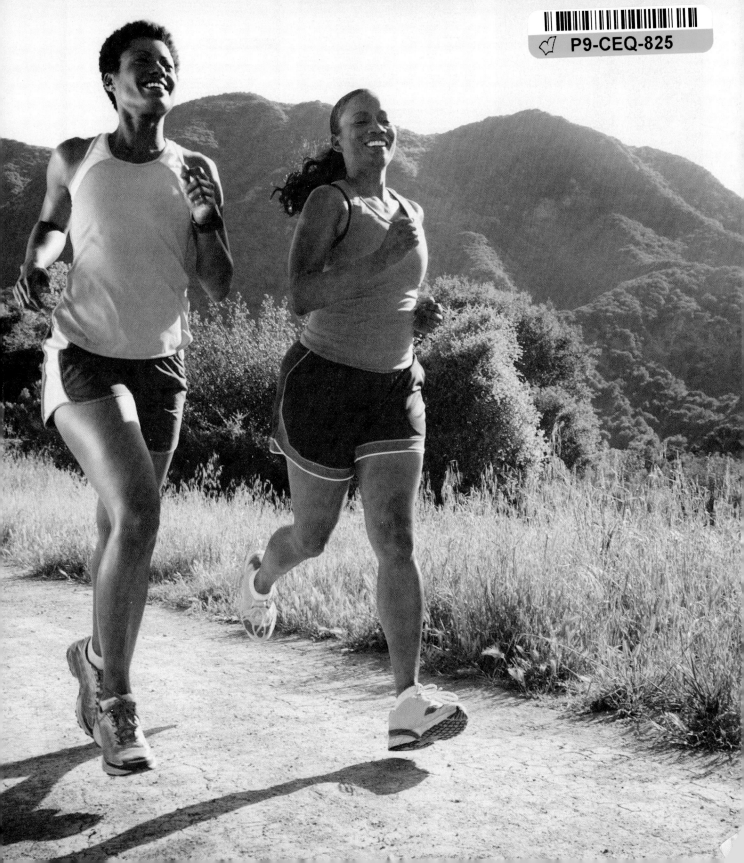

STEP BY STEP **TO STUDENT SUCCESS**

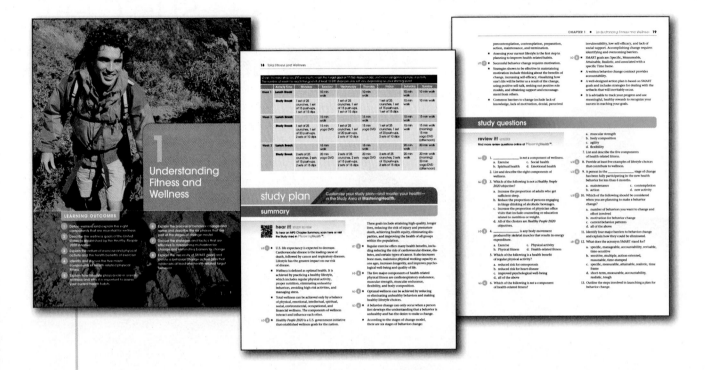

NEW! Study Plan tied to Learning Outcomes

Numbered learning outcomes now introduce every chapter, giving students a roadmap for their reading. Each chapter concludes with a Study Plan, which summarizes key points of the chapter and provides review questions to check understanding, all tied to the chapter's learning outcomes and assignable in MasteringHealth.

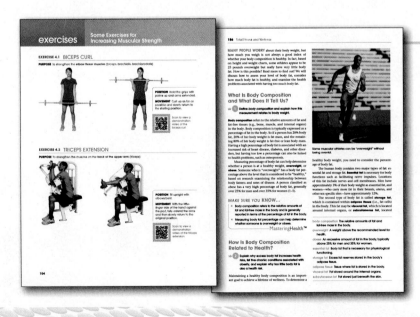

NEW! New book design makes student navigation of the text simple

The book's design and layout have been thoroughly revitalized for today's students. In addition to new photos and figures, the end-of-chapter labs and sample exercise prescription programs have been redesigned to make them easier to use. In addition, the book's table of contents has been streamlined, with information on fitness considerations for special populations (formerly Chapter 12) covered in the relevant sections of the book.

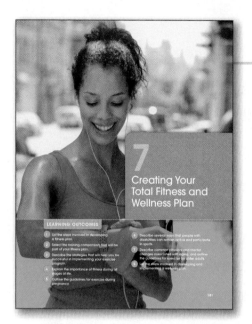

NEW! Chapter reorganization and revision makes planning a fitness program easy

Chapter 7, Creating Your Total Fitness and Wellness Plan, has been thoroughly revised and reorganized to help students develop plans that work for them. The chapter now includes information on fitness apps, a new figure applying the FITT principle to each component of health-related physical fitness, sample training logs, a new lab on writing SMART goals, and more.

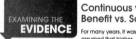

Continuous vs. Interval Training: Benefit vs. Safety?

For many years, it was assumed that higher-intensity levels of training meant a higher probability for injuries. Thus, most professionals have guided fitness enthusiasts away from high-intensity workouts. It was also thought that high-intensity work resulted in a shorter total workout time and, therefore, less benefit than long, slow, distance workouts.

However, an accumulation of recent evidence suggests that we need to reexamine that concept. One study (19) concluded that high-intensity interval training (HIIT) results in cardiovascular adaptations that equal or exceed those found with continuous training. It was also shown that skeletal muscle aerobic adaptations to HIIT are equal to those seen with continuous training.

One of the most controversial aspects of the differences in these training methods has been the metabolic adaptations. While it has long been known that continuous training results in an increased ability to metabolize fats during exercise, it was thought that HIIT primarily worked to increase anaerobic energy

stores. Over the last decade, with more studies done on interval training, we now realize that HIIT also results in aerobic metabolic changes similar to those seen with continuous training (20). In fact, it has been shown that metabolism is significantly increased for a prolonged period after HIIT!

Although there is the continued concern for increased possibility of injury with more intense exercise, if integrated slowly into your continuous, endurance exercise routine, it appears that it can be done with no increase in injury rate. Kuzy and Zielinski (19) also examined sprinters and long-distance runners and found no difference in injury to Achilles and patellar tendons between the groups. Thus, it appears that HIIT can be safely incorporated into the exercise routine of most individuals.

Interestingly, according to a recent survey of fitness professionals (21), the #1 exercise trend in the United States in 2014 was the use of HIIT as a substitute for or complement to continuous/endurance training.

NEW! Examining the Evidence feature boxes

This new research-based feature presents findings from recent studies on various health and fitness topics, such as health hazards of prolonged sitting, the effectiveness of CrossFit training, the effect of yoga on fitness levels, and a comparison of organic and conventional foods.

NEW! *ABC News* Lecture Launchers

New videos from *ABC News* bring health and fitness to life and spark discussion with up-to-date hot topics such as stress among millennials, hate crimes, and rates of heroin use. Assignable multiple-choice questions available in MasteringHealth provide wrong-answer feedback to redirect students to the correct answer.

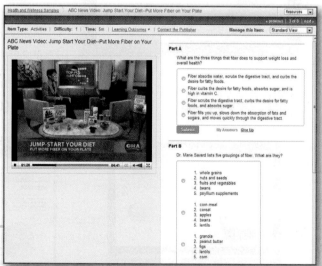

GET YOUR **STUDENTS GOING**
WITH MasteringHealth™

Mastering is the most effective and widely used online homework, tutorial and assessment system for the sciences and now includes content specifically for fitness and wellness courses. Mastering delivers self-paced tutorials that focus on your course objectives, provides individualized coaching, and responds to each student's progress.

BEFORE CLASS — Dynamic Study Modules and eText 2.0 provide students with a preview of what's to come.

NEW! **Dynamic Study Modules** help students study effectively on their own by continuously assessing their activity and performance in real time. Students complete a set of questions with a unique answer format that also asks them to indicate their confidence level. Questions repeat until the student can answer them all correctly and confidently. Once completed, Dynamic Study Modules explain the concept using materials from the text.

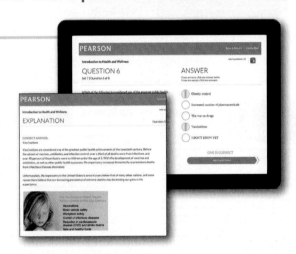

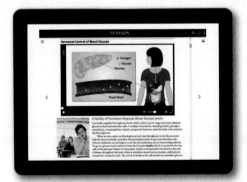

NEW! **Interactive eText 2.0,** complete with embedded media, is mobile friendly and ADA accessible.

- Now available on smartphones and tablets.
- Seamlessly integrated videos and other rich media.
- Accessible (screen-reader ready).
- Configurable reading settings, including resizable type and night reading mode.
- Instructor and student note-taking, highlighting, bookmarking, and search.

DURING CLASS — Engage students with Learning Catalytics

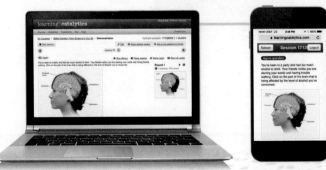
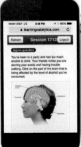

Learning Catalytics, a "bring your own device" student engagement, assessment, and classroom intelligence system, allows students to use their smartphone, tablet, or laptop to respond to questions in class.

AFTER CLASS

Easy-to-Assign, Customizable, and Automatically Graded Assignments

The breadth and depth of content available to you to assign in MasteringHealth is unparalleled, allowing you to quickly and easily assign homework to reinforce key concepts.

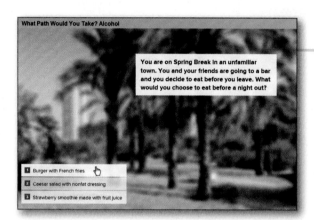

NEW! **Interactive Behavior Change Activities—Which Path Would You Take?** allow students to explore various health choices through an engaging, interactive, low-stakes, and anonymous experience.

In activities covering topics such as nutrition, fitness, and alcohol, students receive specific feedback on the choices they make today and the possible consequences on their future health.

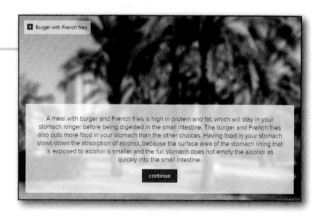

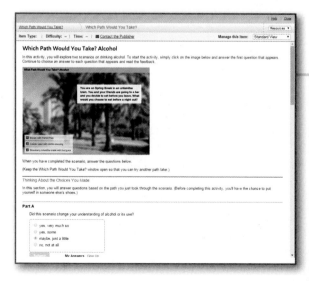

These activities are available in MasteringHealth and made assignable in Mastering with follow-up questions.

AFTER CLASS

Other Automatically Graded Health and Fitness Activities Include . . .

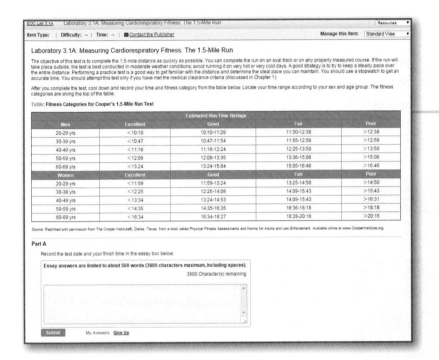

NEW! **Assignable Labs**
25 of the most popularly assigned labs are now available as auto-graded, assignable labs within MasteringHealth.

NEW! **Study Plans** tie all end-of-chapter material (including chapter summary and review questions) to specific numbered Learning Outcomes and Mastering assets. Assignable study plan items contain at least one multiple choice question per Learning Outcome and wrong-answer feedback.

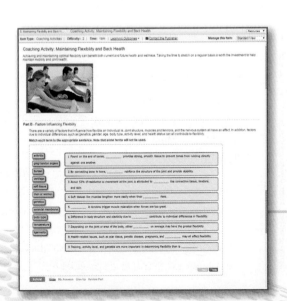

NEW! **Coaching activities** guide students through key health and fitness concepts with interactive mini-lessons that provide hints and feedback.

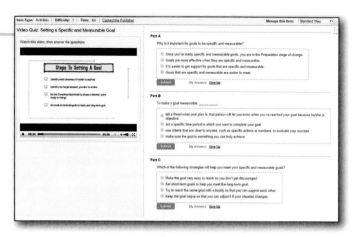

NEW! **Behavior Change Videos** are concise whiteboard-style videos that help students with the steps of behavior change, covering topics such as setting SMART goals, identifying and overcoming barriers to change, planning realistic timelines, and more. Additional videos review key fitness concepts such as determining target heart rate range for exercise. All videos include assessment activities and are assignable in MasteringHealth.

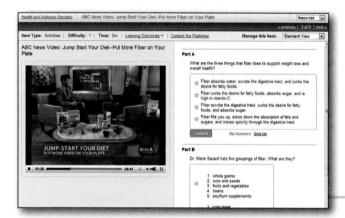

NEW! *ABC News* Lecture Launcher videos bring health and fitness to life and spark discussion with up-to-date hot topics such as do's and don'ts of stretching, potential workout mistakes, low carb and low fat diets, and stress among millennials. Activities tied to the videos include multiple choice questions that provide wrong-answer feedback to redirect students to the correct answer.

UPDATED! **NutriTools Coaching Activities** in the nutrition chapter allow students to combine and experiment with different food options and learn firsthand how to build healthier meals.

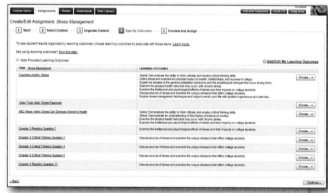

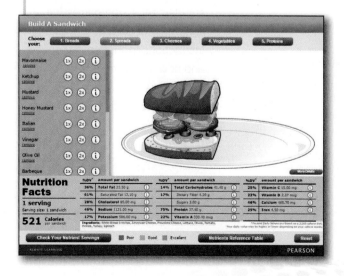

NEW! **Learning Outcomes** All of the MasteringHealth assignable content is tagged to book content and to Bloom's Taxonomy. You also have the ability to add your own outcomes, helping you track student performance against your learning outcomes. You can view class performance against the specified learning outcomes and share those results quickly and easily by exporting to a spreadsheet.

EVERYTHING YOU NEED TO TEACH **IN ONE PLACE**

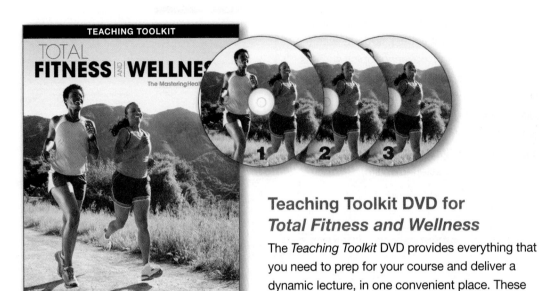

Teaching Toolkit DVD for
Total Fitness and Wellness

The *Teaching Toolkit* DVD provides everything that you need to prep for your course and deliver a dynamic lecture, in one convenient place. These valuable resources are included on three disks:

DISK 1
Robust Media Assets for Each Chapter

- *ABC News* Lecture Launcher videos
- Behavior Change videos
- PowerPoint Lecture Outlines
- PowerPoint clicker questions and Jeopardy-style quiz show questions
- Files for all illustrations and tables and selected photos from the text

DISK 2
Comprehensive Test Bank

- Test Bank in Microsoft Word, PDF, and RTF formats
- Computerized Test Bank, which includes all the questions from the printed test bank in a format that allows you to easily and intuitively build exams and quizzes

DISK 3
Additional Innovative Supplements for Instructors and Students

For Instructors
- Instructor Resource and Support Manual in Microsoft Word and PDF formats
- Step-by-step MasteringHealth tutorials
- Video introduction to Learning Catalytics™
- *Great Ideas in Teaching Health & Wellness*
- *Teaching with Student Learning Outcomes*
- *Teaching with Web 2.0*

For Students
- *Behavior Change Log Book and Wellness Journal*
- *Live Right! Beating Stress in College and Beyond*
- *Eat Right! Healthy Eating in College and Beyond*
- *Food Composition Table*

User's Quick Guide for
Total Fitness and Wellness
This easy-to-use printed supplement accompanies the Teaching Toolkit and offers easy instructions for both experienced and new faculty members to get started with the rich Toolkit content and MasteringHealth.

TOTAL
FITNESS
AND WELLNESS

The MasteringHealth Edition

Seventh Edition

Scott K. Powers
University of Florida

Stephen L. Dodd
University of Florida

PEARSON

Senior Acquisitions Editor: Michelle Cadden
Project Manager: Laura Perry
Program Manager: Susan Malloy
Development Editor: Tanya Martin
Senior Content Producer: Aimee Pavy
Editorial Assistant: Heidi Arndt
Development Manager: Cathy Murphy
Program Management Team Lead: Michael Early
Project Management Team Lead: Nancy Tabor
Production Management: Integra Software Services, Inc.
Compositor: Integra Software Services, Inc.
Design Manager: Mark Ong

Interior Designer: Elise Lansdon Design
Cover Designer: Elise Landson Design
Printer/Binder: Donnelley Menasha
Illustrators: Lumina Datamatics
Rights & Permissions Project Manager: William Opulach
Photo Researcher: Melody English
Manufacturing Buyer: Stacey Weinberger
Executive Product Marketing Manager: Neena Bali
Senior Field Marketing Manager: Mary Salzman
Cover Photo Credit: Blend Images—Erik Isakson/ Getty Images

Library of Congress Cataloging-in-Publication Data

Powers, Scott K. (Scott Kline)
  Total fitness & wellness/Scott K. Powers, University of Florida, Stephen L. Dodd,
  University of Florida,—Seventh edition.
    pages cm
  ISBN 978-0-13-416760-2 (alk. paper)—ISBN 0-13-416760-0 (alk. paper)   1. Physical fitness—
  Textbooks.   2. Health—Textbooks.   I. Dodd, Stephen L.   II. Title.
  III. Title: Total fitness and wellness.
  RA781.P66 2016
  613.7—dc23
                                                                    2015027776

2   16

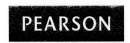
www.pearsonhighered.com

ISBN 10:   0-13-416760-0 (Student Edition)
ISBN 13: 978-0-13-416760-2 (Student Edition)
ISBN 10:   0-13-429714-8 (Instructor's Review Copy)
ISBN 13: 978-0-13-429714-9 (Instructor's Review Copy)

To Jen, Haney, and Will. Your love and encouragement have always meant more than you will ever know.

—Stephen L. Dodd

To my wife Lou and to my mother, who encouraged me to pursue academic endeavors.

—Scott K. Powers

brief contents

contents

1   Understanding Fitness and Wellness 1

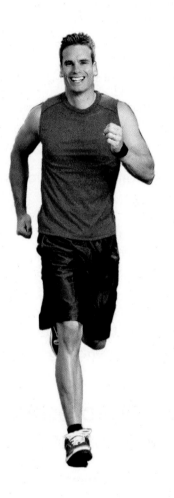

2 General Principles of Exercise for Health and Fitness 35

3 Cardiorespiratory Endurance: Assessment and Prescription 53

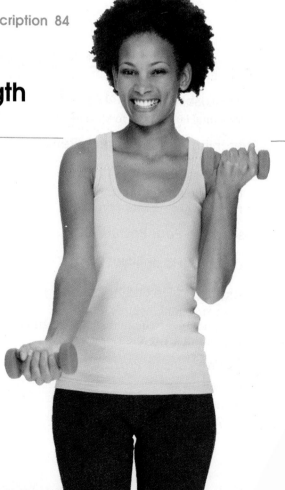

4 Improving Muscular Strength and Endurance 85

5   Improving Flexibility 125

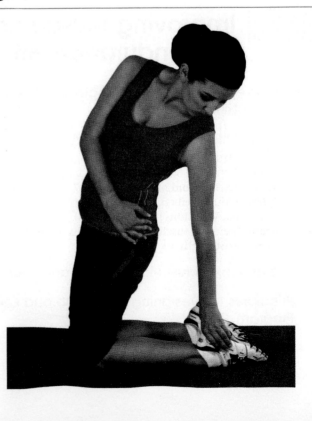

6 Body Composition 155

What Is Body Composition and What Does It Tell Us? 156

How Is Body Composition Related to Health? 156

Overweight and Obesity in the United States 158
Chronic Conditions Associated with Overweight and Obesity 161
Mental and Physical Benefits of a Healthy Weight 161
Health Effects of Too Little Body Fat 162

Assessing Body Composition 164

Field Methods 164
Laboratory Measures 166

Using Body Composition to Determine Your Ideal Weight 168

Behavior Change: Set Goals and Get Regular Assessments 170

Study Plan 170
Summary 170
Study Questions 171
Suggested Reading 172
Helpful Weblinks 172

7 Creating Your Total Fitness and Wellness Plan 181

Steps to Develop a Personal Fitness Plan 182

Step 1. Set Your Goals 182
Step 2. Select Exercises for Your Fitness Program 184
Step 3. Plan Your Weekly Fitness Routine 184
Step 4. Monitor Your Progress 185

Combining Fitness Training Components 185

Putting Your Plan into Action 187

Fitness Is a Lifelong Process 188

Changes in Physical Activity Levels 189

Fitness During Pregnancy 190

8 Nutrition, Health, and Fitness 211

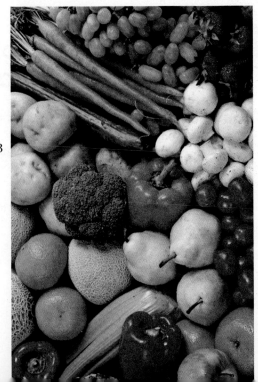

9 Achieving Optimal Body Weight 251

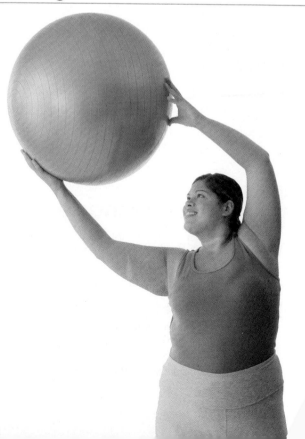

10 Preventing Cardiovascular Disease 275

11 Stress Management 295

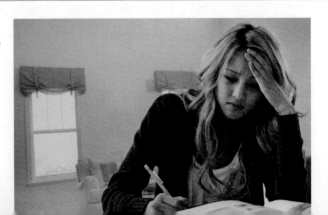

12 Special Considerations Related to Exercise and Injury Prevention 319

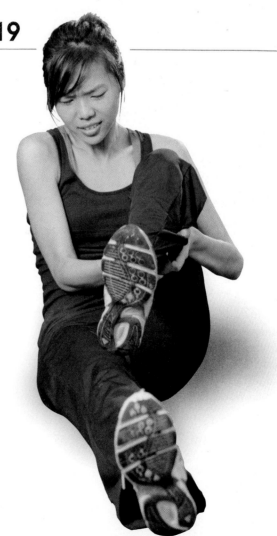

13 Cancer 349

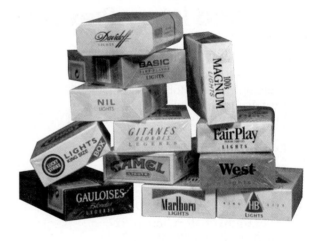

14 Sexually Transmitted Infections 371

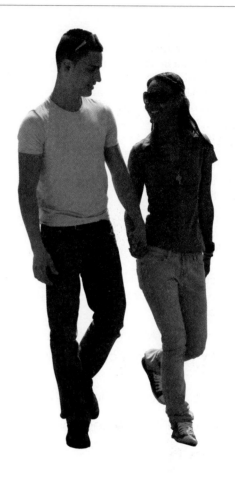

15 Addiction and Substance Abuse 389

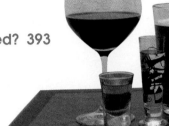

feature boxes

CONSUMER CORNER

labs and programs

SAMPLE PROGRAMS

videos with QR codes

EXERCISE AND ASSESSMENT VIDEOS WITH QR CODES

preface

Good health is our most precious possession. Although we tend to appreciate it only in times of illness or injury, more and more of us are realizing that good health is not simply the absence of disease. Indeed, there are degrees of health, or wellness, and lifestyle can have a major impact on many of its components.

Intended for an introductory college course, *Total Fitness and Wellness* focuses on helping students effect positive changes in their lifestyles, most notably in exercise and diet. The interaction of exercise and diet and the essential role of regular exercise and good nutrition in achieving total fitness and wellness are major themes of the text.

Total Fitness and Wellness, the MasteringHealth Edition, was built on a strong foundation of both exercise physiology and nutrition. The text provides clear, objective, research-based information to college students during their first course in physical fitness and wellness. By offering a research-based text, we hope to dispel many myths associated with exercise, nutrition, weight loss, and wellness. In particular, we show students how to evaluate their own wellness level with respect to various wellness components, such as fitness level and nutritional status. Indeed, the title of the book reflects our goals.

Numerous physical fitness and wellness texts are available today. Our motivation in writing *Total Fitness and Wellness* was to create a unique, well-balanced physical fitness and wellness text that covers primary concepts of physical fitness and wellness and also addresses other important issues such as behavior change, exercise-related injuries, exercise and the environment, and prevention of cardiovascular disease.

New to This Edition

Total Fitness and Wellness, the MasteringHealth Edition, maintains many features that the text has become known for, while incorporating several major revisions, exciting new features, and a more explicit connection between the text and multimedia resources in MasteringHealth. **MasteringHealth** is an online homework, tutorial, and assessment product designed to improve results by helping students quickly master concepts. Students benefit from self-paced tutorials that feature immediate wrong-answer feedback and hints that emulate the office-hour experience to help keep students on track. With a wide range of interactive, engaging, and assignable activities, students are encouraged to actively learn and retain tough course concepts.

The multimedia created for the MasteringHealth Edition is more innovative and interactive than ever and a tighter text/MasteringHealth integration provides students the opportunity to master course content using a variety of resources on and off the page, reflecting the manner in which students study today.

The most noteworthy changes to the text and multimedia as a whole include the following:

- **Numbered learning outcomes** now introduce every chapter, giving students a roadmap for their reading. Each chapter concludes with a **Study Plan,** which summarizes key points of the chapter and provides review questions to check understanding, all tied to the chapter's learning outcomes and assignable in MasteringHealth.

- **Streamlined organization** presents material in 15 chapters (versus 16 in the last edition) by incorporating coverage of environmental factors and special populations (formerly Chapter 12) into the chapters on creating a fitness and wellness plan (Chapter 7) and preventing injuries (Chapter 12).

- **Examining the Evidence** feature boxes give the reader insight into special topics such as the effects of caffeine, the search for a cure for AIDS, road rage, muscle cramps, and anabolic steroid use.

- **Creating Your Total Fitness and Wellness Plan (Chapter 7)** provides students with practical, step-by-step instructions on developing and putting fitness and wellness plans into action. This chapter includes new information, sample exercise programs, and new labs.

- **MP3 Chapter Reviews** are now accessible via QR codes in the book, and are assignable in Mastering.

- **The book's design and layout** have been thoroughly revitalized for today's students. In addition to new photos and figures, the end-of-chapter labs and sample exercise prescription programs have been redesigned to make them easier to use.

- **Suggested Readings** have been moved from the back of book and integrated into the end-of-chapter content to be more visible and useful for students.

- **ABC News Videos**, all referenced in the book with See It! callouts, bring fitness and wellness to life and spark discussion with up-to-date hot topics from 2012–2015. MasteringHealth activities tied to the videos include multiple choice questions that provide wrong-answer feedback to redirect students to the correct answer.

- **eText 2.0** complete with embedded ABC News videos, is mobile friendly and ADA accessible.

  - Now available on smartphones and tablets.
  - Seamlessly integrated videos.
  - Accessible (screen-reader ready).
  - Configurable reading settings, including resizable type and night reading mode.
  - Instructor and student note-taking, highlighting, bookmarking, and search.

Chapter-by-Chapter Revisions

The MasteringHealth Edition has been thoroughly updated to provide students with the most current information and references for further exploration and includes a tighter integration between the text and multimedia resources in MasteringHealth. Learning outcomes are now explicitly tied to chapter sections and the end of chapter Study Plan to create a clear learning path for students. Portions of chapters have been reorganized to improve the flow of topics, and figures, tables, feature boxes, and photos have all been added, improved on, and updated. Throughout the text, all data, statistics, and references have been updated to the most recent possible. The following is a chapter-by-chapter listing of some of the most noteworthy changes, updates, and additions.

Chapter 1:

- This chapter underwent major revision to improve both content and student understanding.
- Includes expanded coverage of wellness to incorporate eight components: physical, intellectual, emotional, spiritual, social, environmental, occupational, and financial.
- Includes new content on life expectancy and how health-related lifestyle choices affect longevity.
- Contains new content on the wellness continuum and lifestyle management for wellness.
- Expanded coverage of behavior change includes effective methods, maintaining motivation, and identifying and eliminating barriers to change.
- New feature: Examining the Evidence: Health Hazards of Prolonged Sitting.
- New lab: Laboratory 1.1: Wellness Evaluation (encompassing all 8 components of wellness).

Chapter 2:

- New and improved figures illustrating the FITT Principle and the physical activity pyramid
- New information added on the negative impact of prolonged sitting on health

Chapter 3:

- New Coaching Corner feature on how smartphone use affects fitness levels.
- New Coaching Corner feature on bodyweight training.
- New feature: Examining the Evidence: Continuous vs. Interval Training: Benefit vs. Safety?
- New feature: Examining the Evidence: What is CrossFit and Does It Work?

Chapter 4:

- Updated with clearer explanations of muscle fiber types and updated Table 4.1 on properties of skeletal muscle fiber types.

- New feature: Examining the Evidence: Does Creatine Supplementation Increase Muscle Size and Strength?
- New Coaching Corner feature on using the 5-point contact principle for injury prevention.

Chapter 5:

- New feature: Examining the Evidence: Can Yoga Improve Your Fitness Levels?
- Updated Coaching Corner feature on effective stretching.

Chapter 6:

- Includes expanded information on creeping obesity.
- New Consumer Corner feature compares various methods of determining body composition.
- Updated Figure 6.3 on U.S. obesity rates.

Chapter 7:

- New table provides overview of selected fitness apps.
- New sections added on lifelong fitness and fitness for special populations (pregnant women, people with disabilities, and older adults).
- Sample fitness programs include plans for beginner, intermediate, and advanced levels plus a plan for healthy older adults.
- New lab: Laboratory 7.1: Developing SMART Goals.

Chapter 8:

- This chapter underwent major revision to improve both content and student learning.
- New and expanded coverage of macro- and micronutrients.
- Updated coverage of healthy diet guidelines.
- New Consumer Corner feature on choosing safe seafood.
- New section on food allergies and intolerances.
- New Examining the Evidence feature on gluten in the diet.
- New sections on specific nutritional needs of athletes and others who exercise.
- New section on protein requirements for active individuals.
- New discussion of the importance of fluid intake to maintain body water balance.
- New table on carbohydrate needs in relation to level of exercise training.
- Updated coverage of dietary supplements and their regulation and labeling.
- New feature: Examining the Evidence: Are Organic Foods Healthier than Conventional Foods?

Chapter 9:

- New and expanded coverage of energy balance.
- New and state-of-the-art coverage of how and why we gain fat.
- New and expanded discussion of how to design a successful weight-loss program to achieve lifetime weight management includes new Coaching Corner feature.
- Addition of up-to-date discussion of popular diet plans.
- Includes 4 new figures to illustrate important concepts.

Chapter 10:

- New feature: Examining the Evidence: What additional factors contribute to atherosclerosis and heart attacks?
- New and updated information on how you can reduce your risk of heart disease.
- New Coaching Corner feature on exercising to reduce risk for CV disease.

Chapter 11:

- New feature: Examining the Evidence: Bullying on College Campuses.
- New table provides overview of selected stress management apps (sleep and meditation aids).
- New multifaceted sample program for stress management.

Chapter 12:

- This chapter, Special Considerations Related to Exercise and Injury Prevention, presents a comprehensive discussion of injury prevention, including environmental concerns related to exercise, other types of exercise-related injuries, and unintentional injuries.
- Includes updated table on leading causes of death of young adults.

Chapter 13:

- New feature: Examining the Evidence: New Cancer Screening Tests on the Horizon.
- Updated coverage of skin cancer.
- New section on obesity and cancer risk.
- Expanded discussion of how to reduce your risk for cancer.
- Includes new figures on major risk factors for cancer and on race and cancer risk.

Chapter 14:

- Includes new figures on the incidence of new cases of sexually transmitted infections.
- New Examining the Evidence feature on the search for a cure for AIDS.

Chapter 15:

- New and expanded discussion of addictive behavior and the awareness that addiction can involve a substance or behavior.
- New feature: Examining the Evidence: Is Marijuana Medicine?
- New feature: Examining the Evidence: Are E-Cigarettes Safe?
- New discussion on strategies to prevent drug abuse.

Text Features and Learning Aids

In addition to the new and revised features described above, continuing features and learning aids in the book that contribute to student success include:

- **Lab exercises** allow students to apply textual information to practical issues, encouraging the immediate development of healthy lifestyle choices and a core fitness plan.
- **Sample fitness and wellness programs** offer easy-to-follow instructions for implementing successful fitness and wellness programs.
- **Coaching Corner** boxes represent the "teacher's voice" throughout the text, offering helpful hints and strategies to overcome fitness and wellness obstacles.
- **Examining the Evidence** boxes give the reader insight into special topics such as the effects of caffeine, the search for a cure for AIDS, road rage, muscle cramps, and anabolic steroid use.
- **Consumer Corner** boxes teach students to be informed and discerning health and fitness consumers, guiding them to make the best fitness and wellness decisions in a market full of fads, gimmicks, and gadgets.
- **Appreciating Diversity** boxes present current health research, covering issues such as how the risk of cancer varies across the United States and how the incidence of drug abuse varies across populations.
- **Steps for Behavior Change** boxes focus students on evaluating their own behaviors (e.g., Are you a fast food junkie? Are you reluctant to strength train? Do you protect your skin from UV light?). New timelines present students with practical steps they can take to make meaningful behavior change.
- **Consider This!** grabs students' attention with surprising statistics and information, prompting them to pause and consider the long-term consequences of specific health behaviors.

Instructor Supplements

A full resource package accompanies *Total Fitness and Wellness* to assist the instructor with classroom preparation and presentation.

- **MasteringHealth** (www.masteringhealthandnutrition .com or www.pearsonmastering.com). Mastering-Health coaches students through the toughest fitness and wellness topics. Instructors can assign engaging tools to help students visualize, practice, and understand crucial content, from the basics of fitness to the fundamentals of behavior change. **Coaching Activities** guide students through key health concepts with interactive mini-lessons, complete with hints and wrong-answer feedback. **Reading Quizzes** (20 questions per chapter) ensure students have completed the assigned reading before class. **ABC News Videos** stimulate classroom discussions and include multiple-choice questions with feedback for students. **NutriTools Coaching Activities** in the nutrition chapter allow students to combine and experiment with different food options and learn firsthand how to build healthier meals. **MP3s** relate to chapter content and come with multiple-choice questions that provide wrong-answer feedback. **Learning Catalytics** provides open-ended questions students can answer in real time. Through targeted assessments, Learning Catalytics helps students develop the critical thinking skills they need for lasting behavior change. For students, the **Study Area** is broken down into learning areas and includes videos, MP3s, practice quizzing, and much more.

- **Teaching Toolkit DVD.** The Teaching Toolkit DVD includes everything an instructor needs to prepare for their course and deliver a dynamic lecture in one convenient place. Resources include: *ABC News* videos, exercise videos, clicker questions, Quiz Show questions, PowerPoint lecture outlines, all figures and tables from the text, PDF and and Microsoft Word files of the *Instructor Resource and Support Manual,* PDF, RTF, and Microsoft Word files of the Test Bank, the Computerized Test Bank, the User's Quick Guide, *Teaching with Student Learning Outcomes, Teaching with Web 2.0, Great Ideas! Active Ways to Teach Health and Wellness, Behavior Change Log Book and Wellness Journal, Eat Right!, Live Right!,* and *Take Charge of Your Health* worksheets.

  - **ABC News Videos and Video Tutors.** New *ABC News* videos, each 3 to 8 minutes long, help instructors stimulate critical discussion in the classroom. Videos are embedded within PowerPoint lectures and are also available separately in large-screen format with optional closed captioning on the Teaching Toolkit DVD and through MasteringHealth.

  - **Instructor Resource and Support Manual.** This teaching tool provides chapter summaries, outlines, integrated *ABC News* video discussion questions, in-class discussion questions, and more.

  - **Test Bank.** The Test Bank incorporates Bloom's Taxonomy, or the higher order of learning, to help instructors create exams that encourage students to think analytically and critically, rather than simply to regurgitate information. Test Bank questions are tagged to global and book-specific student learning outcomes.

  - **User's Quick Guide.** Newly redesigned to be even more useful, this valuable supplement acts as your road map to the Teaching Toolkit DVD.

  - **Teaching with Student Learning Outcomes.** This publication contains essays from 11 instructors who are teaching using student learning outcomes. They share their goals in using outcomes, the processes that they follow to develop and refine the outcomes, and provide many useful suggestions and examples for successfully incorporating outcomes into a personal health course.

  - **Teaching with Web 2.0.** From Facebook to Twitter to blogs, students are using and interacting with Web 2.0 technologies. This handbook provides an introduction to these popular online tools and offers ideas for incorporating them into your personal health course. Written by personal health and health education instructors, each chapter examines the basics about each technology and ways to make it work for you and your students.

  - **Great Ideas! Active Ways to Teach Health & Wellness.** This manual provides ideas for classroom activities related to specific health and wellness topics, as well as suggestions for activities that can be adapted to various topics and class sizes.

  - **Behavior Change Log Book and Wellness Journal.** This assessment tool helps students track daily exercise and nutritional intake and create a long-term nutritional and fitness prescription plan. It also includes a Behavior Change Contract and topics for journal-based activities.

Student Supplements

MasteringHealth

The Study Area of MasteringHealth is organized by learning areas. The *Read It* section contains the Learning Outcomes and up-to-date health news. *See It* includes *ABC News* videos on important health topics and the Behavior Change videos. More than 100 exercise videos demonstrate strength training and flexibility exercises with resistance bands, stability balls, free weights, and gym machines. The exercise videos are also available for download onto iPods or media players. *Hear It* contains MP3 Study Tutor files and audio case studies. *Do It* contains the choose-your-own-adventure-style Interactive Behavior Change Activities—Which Path Would You Take?, interactive NutriTools activities, and Web links. Also here is a pre-course/post-course assessment lets students evaluate their own fitness and wellness status both before and after taking the course. New interactive labs are also available online to students, allowing them to assess their levels of fitness and wellness, learn core skills, and develop behavior change plans to track their progress. Students can easily complete the labs and e-mail them to you directly—eliminating the need for paper entirely.

Review It contains Practice Quizzes for each chapter, Flashcards, and Glossary. *Live It* will help jump-start students' behavior-change projects with interactive Assess Yourself Worksheets and resources to plan change; students can fill out a Behavior Change Contract, journal and log behaviors, and prepare a reflection piece.

eText 2.0, included within MasteringHealth, contains embedded *ABC News* videos and other rich media, is mobile friendly and ADA accessible, available on smartphones and tablets, and includes instructor and student note-taking, highlighting, bookmarking, and search functions.

Behavior Change Log Book and Wellness Journal, found within the Live It section in MasteringHealth, helps students track daily exercise and nutritional intake and create a long-term nutrition and fitness prescription plan. It includes Behavior Change Contracts and topics for journal-based activities.

Additional Student Supplements

- **Digital 5-Step Pedometer** Take strides to better health with this pedometer, which measures steps, distance (miles), activity time, and calories, and provides a time clock.

- **MyDietAnalysis** (www.mydietanalysis.com). Powered by ESHA Research, Inc., MyDietAnalysis features a database of nearly 20,000 foods and multiple reports. It allows students to track their diet and activity using up to three profiles and to generate and submit reports electronically.

Acknowledgments

First and foremost, this edition of *Total Fitness and Wellness* reflects the valuable feedback provided by many people throughout the country. As always, this edition could not have been completed without the work of an enormous number of people at Pearson. From the campus sales representatives to the president of the company, they are truly first rate, and our interaction with them is always delightful.

There were several key people in the process. Our Acquisitions Editor, Michelle Cadden, has been the primary force behind assembling the team and directing the process, and her input has been invaluable. Several new additions to the team have been important in both the revisions of the text and the production process. In particular, the authors would like to thank Laura Perry for significant contributions to this seventh edition. Moreover, special thanks go to Susan Malloy, who offered valuable input during the revision process, to Tanya Martin, for her careful developmental editing, and to Nancy Tabor, who served as the Project Team Leader. Other specific duties were expertly handled by the following professionals; we offer them our utmost appreciation for their efforts: Neena Bali, Executive Product Marketing Manager; Aimee Pavy, Senior Content Producer; Heidi Arndt, Editorial Assistant; William Opulach, Rights and Permissions Project Manager. Denise Wright (Southern Editorial), Tanya Martin, and Aaron Morton (University of Florida) have made major contributions to the ancillaries, and Aaron Morton also made major contributions to the book content.

Finally, there is a long list of professionals whose reviews of the text's content and style or participation in a fitness and wellness forum have helped to shape this book. We owe these individuals a tremendous debt of gratitude:

Ezzeldin Aly, *Grraceland University*
George Abboud, *Salem State University*
Chris Ecklund, *Westmont College*
Amy Howton, *Kennesaw State University*
Ben Meyer, *Shippensburg University*
Peter Morano, *Central Connecticut State University*
Timothy O'Brien, *Mayville State University*
Jennifer Spry-Knutson, *Des Moines Area Community College*

Many thanks to all!

Scott K. Powers
University of Florida

Stephen L. Dodd
University of Florida

TOTAL
FITNESS
AND WELLNESS

The MasteringHealth Edition

Seventh Edition

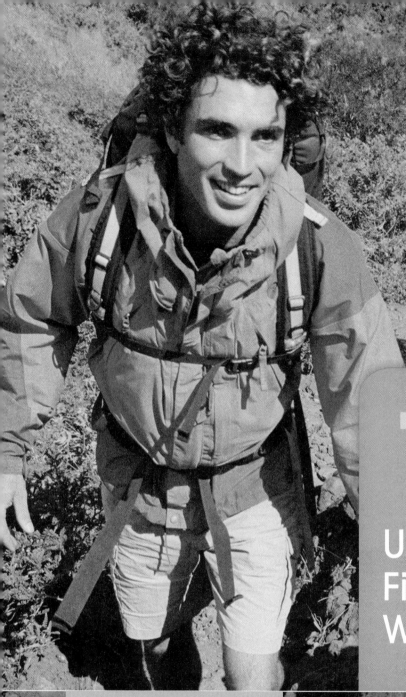

1

Understanding Fitness and Wellness

LIFESTYLE DECISIONS HAVE a major impact on your overall health and well-being. In this book, you will learn about lifestyle factors (behaviors) that can reduce your risk of disease and put you on the path to physical fitness and optimal wellness.

Life Expectancy and Wellness

 LO 1 Define *wellness* and explain the eight components that are essential for wellness.

The current average life expectancy in the United States is 77.4 years for men and 82.2 years for women. Life expectancy for Americans has increased over the past 20 years, but our nation ranks 36th in the world. Experts now predict that life expectancy in the United States will actually *decrease* during the next decade due to the burden caused by several major diseases.

In the United States, cardiovascular disease remains the number 1 cause of death, followed by cancer and respiratory diseases. Deaths due to diabetes are on the rise, as well. A healthy lifestyle can reduce your risk of disease; for example, eating a nutritionally balanced diet, exercising regularly, and maintaining a healthy body weight reduce your risk of cardiovascular disease, diabetes, and several types of cancer. Not smoking and avoiding secondhand cigarette smoke reduce your risk of developing both cardiovascular and respiratory diseases.

According to the Surgeon General, the four major factors that influence health and longevity are lifestyle, the environment, genetics, and health care. Of these factors, *lifestyle has the greatest impact on disease risk,* as 53% of all diseases are lifestyle-related. Approximately 21% of diseases are related to the environment, and only 16% are linked to genetics. Failure to receive adequate health care contributes to approximately 10% of diseases (**FIGURE 1.1**). These statistics reveal that we control as much as 84% of our vulnerability to disease, so the actions we take to safeguard our health and create wellness can have a huge impact.

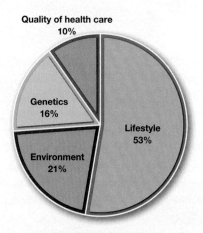

FIGURE 1.1 The four major factors that contribute to health and longevity.

What Is Wellness?

Good health was once defined as the absence of disease. In the 1970s, many exercise scientists and health educators became dissatisfied with this limited definition. These visionary health professionals believed that health includes physical fitness and emotional and spiritual health as well. Their revised concept of good health is called **wellness** (1). Wellness can be defined as *optimal health*, which encompasses all the dimensions of well-being. You can achieve a state of wellness by practicing a healthy lifestyle that includes regular physical activity, proper nutrition, emotional/spiritual balance, and eliminating unhealthy behaviors. Wellness involves a number of components that we will explore in more depth.

Eight Components of Wellness

Wellness consists of eight interrelated components (**FIGURE 1.2**):

- Physical wellness
- Emotional wellness
- Intellectual wellness
- Spiritual wellness
- Social wellness
- Environmental wellness
- Occupational wellness
- Financial wellness

Physical Wellness   Physical wellness refers to all the behaviors that keep your body healthy. Two key aspects are maintaining a healthy body weight and achieving physical fitness. Maintaining a healthy body weight is important because a high percentage of body fat increases your risk of developing type 2 diabetes and heart disease. Physical fitness can have a positive effect on your health by reducing your risk of disease and improving your

consider this! ////////////////

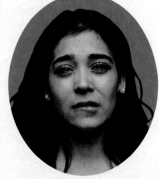

In a given year, approximately one in four adults between the ages of 18 and 44 has a diagnosable mental disorder.

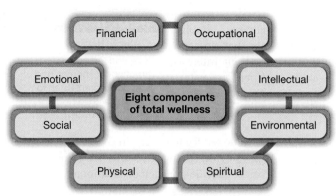

FIGURE 1.2 Total wellness consists of eight interrelated components. Optimal well-being occurs when all components of wellness are working together toward holistic health.

quality of life. Eating a healthy diet, obtaining regular medical exams, and practicing personal safety are other important physical health behaviors.

Emotional Wellness Emotions play an important role in how you feel about yourself and others. Emotional wellness (mental health) includes your social skills and interpersonal relationships. Your level of self-esteem and your ability to cope with the routine stress of daily living are also aspects of emotional wellness.

Emotional stability refers to how well you deal with day-to-day stressors. Most people are well equipped to handle life's ups and downs, but inability to handle everyday situations can lead to poor emotional health or conditions such as depression and anxiety disorders. In fact, mental disorders are the leading cause of disability for people between the ages of 15–44 years (2). Emotional wellness means being able to respond to life situations in an appropriate manner, therefore avoiding prolonged periods of an extremely high or low emotional state.

Intellectual Wellness You can maintain intellectual wellness by keeping your mind active through life-long learning. College life is ideal for developing this component. Attending lectures, reading, and engaging in thoughtful discussions with friends and teachers all promote intellectual health. Your ability to define and solve problems continues to grow, and continuous learning can provide you with a sense of fulfillment. Take advantage of opportunities to broaden your mind. Listen to audio books, keep up with current events, and engage in thoughtful discussions with others.

Spiritual Wellness The term *spiritual* means different things to different people. Most definitions of spiritual wellness include having a sense of meaning and purpose. Many people define spiritual wellness based on religious beliefs, but it is not limited to religion. People find meaning in helping others, being altruistic, enjoying the beauty of nature, or through prayer. However you

define spiritual health, it is an important aspect of wellness because it is closely linked to emotional health (3).

Optimal spiritual wellness includes the ability to understand your basic purpose in life; to experience love, joy, pain, peace, and sorrow; and to care for and respect all living things. Anyone who has experienced a beautiful sunset or smelled the first scents of spring can appreciate the pleasure of maintaining optimal spiritual health.

Social Wellness Social wellness is the development and maintenance of meaningful interpersonal relationships; this results in a support network of friends and family. Good social health helps you feel confident in social interactions and provides you with emotional security. It is not necessarily the number of people in your support network, but the quality of those relationships that is important. Developing good communication skills is crucial for maintaining a strong social network.

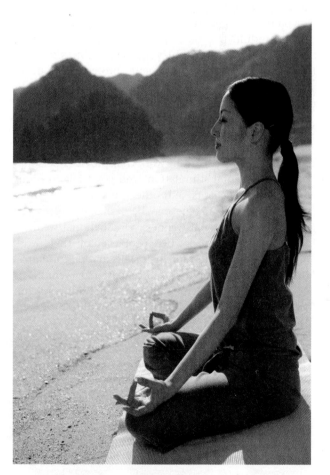

Meditating or spending time outdoors can help you improve spiritual health.

---

wellness A state of optimal health that encompasses all the dimensions of well-being. Consists of eight major components: physical, emotional, intellectual, spiritual, social, environmental, occupational, and financial wellness.

Environmental Wellness Environmental wellness includes the influence of the environment on your health, as well as your behaviors that affect the environment. Our environment can have a positive or negative impact on our total wellness. For example, air pollution and water contamination are environmental factors that can harm physical health. Breathing polluted air can lead to a variety of respiratory disorders. Drinking water contaminated with harmful bacteria can lead to infection, and drinking water that contains carcinogens increases the risk of certain types of cancers.

Your environment can also have a positive influence on wellness. For example, a safe environment evokes feelings of comfort and security, enhancing your emotional health. If your environment is safe, you are more likely to spend time outside being active and improving your physical health.

Our relationship with our environment is a two-way street. How do our behaviors influence the environment? Do you recycle regularly, or does much of your trash end up in a landfill? Do you carpool or take public transportation when you can? Achieving total wellness requires learning about the environment, protecting yourself against environmental hazards, and being responsible in regard to your impact on the environment.

Occupational Wellness Occupational wellness is achieved by a high level of satisfaction in your job or chosen career. This stems from work that provides personal fulfillment, mental stimulation, and good relationships with coworkers, clients, and others in your professional life. While a high income may be desirable, it does not guarantee occupational wellness. Occupational wellness is most often achieved when people enjoy their work and receive recognition for their skills and performance. Like the other components, occupational wellness is not an independent element but an important contributor to emotional, intellectual, and social wellness.

To achieve occupational wellness, establish career goals that are consistent with your interests, skills, and personal values. For instance, a career in health care or military service can be a good choice for people who value service to others. In contrast, those who place a high value on financial security may find a higher-paying career essential for their occupational wellness.

Financial Wellness Financial wellness refers to the ability to live comfortably on your income and have the means to save for financial emergencies and goals such as education and retirement. Financial wellness involves your ability to manage your money in a responsible way. It can provide you with peace of mind and contribute to your emotional, social, and occupational wellness.

hear it!

CASE STUDY

How can Omar connect his physical, mental, and spiritual health? Listen to the online case study at MasteringHealth™.

Interaction of Wellness Components and the Wellness Continuum

None of the components of wellness works in isolation; all eight work closely together. For example, people with an anxiety or depressive disorder who also have a chronic physical illness report more physical symptoms than those who do not have a mental health disorder (4). Strong spirituality is associated with lower rates of mental disorders, better immune function, and greater participation in health-promoting behaviors (3, 5). Total wellness is achieved through a balance of all aspects of wellness....

It is clear that wellness is a dynamic process. The choices you make each day move you along a *continuum* of wellness. At one end of the continuum is total well-being, which is realized by achieving all eight components of wellness simultaneously (**FIGURE 1.3**). At the opposite end of the continuum is a low level of well-being, which results

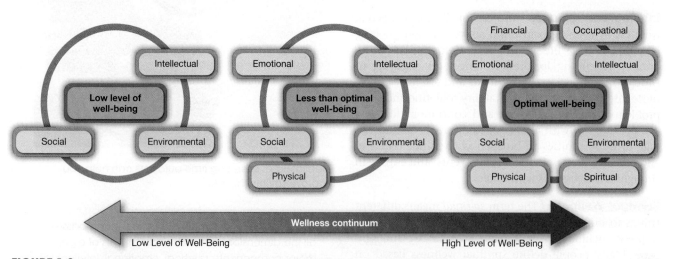

FIGURE 1.3 A person's state of wellness moves along a continuum. Accomplishing optimal well-being (right) requires realizing all eight components of wellness. A low level of well-being (left) results when an individual has successfully addressed only a limited number of wellness components.

APPRECIATING DIVERSITY | Wellness Issues Across the Population

While your behaviors have a significant impact on your health, other factors also influence your risk for certain chronic diseases. Ethnicity, sex, age, family history, and socioeconomic status affect your risk of developing diabetes, cancer, cardiovascular disease, obesity, and other conditions.

For example, black Americans have a higher risk of hypertension (high blood pressure) compared to the U.S. population as a whole. Similarly, diabetes is more common in Native Americans and Latinos than in people from other ethnic backgrounds. Men and women differ in their risk for heart disease, osteoporosis, and certain types of cancer.

Aging also plays a role. The risk of chronic diseases such as heart disease and cancer increases with age. And people of low socioeconomic status often have less access to quality health care and experience higher

rates of obesity, heart disease, and drug abuse. Our goal is to achieve optimal wellness, but individual and demographic differences can present special challenges.

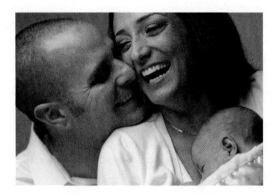

---

live it!

ASSESS YOURSELF

Assess your behavior with the *Health Behavior Self-Assessment* Take Charge Of Your Health! Worksheet online at MasteringHealth™.

from achieving only a few wellness components. You can move toward optimal well-being by eliminating unhealthy behaviors and making healthy habits part of your regular routine. Complete Laboratory 1.1 to determine your overall wellness level.

MAKE SURE YOU KNOW...

- *Wellness* is defined as optimal health, which encompasses all dimensions of well-being. It is a dynamic process that moves along a continuum.
- There are eight interacting components of wellness: physical, emotional, intellectual, spiritual, social, environmental, occupational, and financial wellness.

—— MasteringHealth™

Wellness Goals for the Nation

LO **2** Describe the wellness goals of the United States as established by the *Healthy People 2020* initiative.

A nation of unhealthy people drains resources by reducing worker productivity and increasing government spending on health care. To improve the overall well-being of Americans, the U.S. government established a set of wellness goals known as the *Healthy People* initiative. These goals were first presented in 1980 and have since been

revised every 10 years based on progress toward meeting the objectives. *Healthy People 2020* is the current set of goals aimed at attaining high-quality, longer lives and reducing the risk of injury and premature death. Other goals are to achieve health equity, eliminate disparities, and improve the health of all groups. For more details, see the Examining the Evidence box on the next page and visit www.healthypeople.gov.

live it!

ASSESS YOURSELF

Assess your health with the *Multidimensional Health Locus of Control* Take Charge Of Your Health! Worksheet online at MasteringHealth™.

MAKE SURE YOU KNOW...

- *Healthy People 2020* is a set of wellness goals established by the U.S. government. Goals include attaining high-quality, longer lives, reducing the risk of injury and premature death, achieving health equity, eliminating disparities, and improving the health of all groups.

—— MasteringHealth™

What Is Exercise and Why Should I Do It?

LO **3** Explain the nature of exercise and physical activity and the health benefits of exercise.

When you hear the word *exercise,* do you picture someone running on a treadmill? Or do you imagine hiking up a scenic mountain with a group of friends? Actually, both

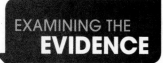

Understanding *Healthy People 2020*

Government agencies and public health professionals developed the *Healthy People 2020* goals. The overall vision of this initiative is to achieve a society in which all people live long and healthy lives. Specific objectives include:

- Reduce the proportion of adults who engage in no leisure-time activity.
- Reduce the death rates due to breast cancer, prostate cancer, and melanoma.
- Increase the proportion of physician office visits that include counseling or education related to nutrition or weight.
- Increase the number of states with nutrition standards for foods and beverages provided to preschool-age children in child care.

- Increase the proportion of adolescents who are connected to a parent or other positive adult caregiver.
- Reduce the proportion of adolescents who engage in disordered eating behaviors in an attempt to control their weight.
- Reduce the proportion of persons engaging in binge drinking of alcoholic beverages.
- Increase the proportion of older adults who are up to date on a core set of clinical preventive services.
- Increase the proportion of adults who get sufficient sleep.

Source: U.S. Department of Health and Human Services, Office of Disease Prevention and Health Promotion, www.healthypeople.gov.

---

activities are forms of exercise that are good for your health. There are numerous fun and interesting ways to exercise, so if going to the gym is not your thing, there are many other ways to be active. One part of designing your personal fitness program is to find out what works best for *you*.

Exercise Is One Type of Physical Activity

Physical activity and *exercise* do not mean the same thing. **Physical activity** includes all physical movement, regardless of the level of energy expenditure or the reason you do it (6). Physical activity can be occupational (done as part of your job), lifestyle, or leisure time. Lifestyle activity includes housework, walking to class, and climbing stairs. Leisure-time physical activity is any activity you choose to do in your free time.

Exercise is a type of leisure-time physical activity (6). Virtually all fitness/conditioning activities and sports are considered exercise because they are planned and help maintain or improve physical fitness. Exercise often involves relatively high-intensity activities (such as running or swimming) and is performed with the goal of achieving health and fitness. Although you can gain health benefits from all types of physical activity, exercise produces the greatest benefits.

Health Benefits of Exercise and Physical Activity

A recent report from the U.S. Centers for Disease Control and Prevention (CDC) reveals that fewer than half of American adults engage in the recommended amount

of exercise to promote health. Most of us are aware that there are many health benefits gained from regular exercise and physical activity. In addition to improving muscle tone and reducing body fat, regular exercise improves our fitness levels and ability to perform everyday tasks. Perhaps even more important, it can help you achieve total wellness (2, 7–15).

The importance of regular exercise and physical activity is emphasized in the U.S. Surgeon General's report on physical activity and health (16). This report concludes that lack of physical activity is a major public health problem and that all Americans can improve their health by engaging in as little as 30 minutes of light-to moderate-intensity physical activity most days of the week. This report recognizes numerous health benefits of physical activity and exercise (**FIGURE 1.4**). Keep in mind that different levels of physical activity or exercise are needed for different health benefits.

Reduced Risk of Heart Disease **Cardiovascular disease (CVD)** (disease of the heart and blood vessels) is a major cause of death in the United States. In fact, one in three Americans dies of CVD (17). Regular physical activity and exercise can significantly reduce your risk of developing CVD (1, 7, 8, 10, 11, 17–21), and strong evidence suggests that regular physical activity reduces the risk of dying during a heart attack (**FIGURE 1.5**) (22–25). Note from Figure 1.5 that exercise training can reduce the magnitude of cardiac injury during a heart attack by more than 60% (23, 24). Many preventive medicine specialists argue that these facts alone are reason enough for engaging in regular physical activity and exercise (7, 18, 26).

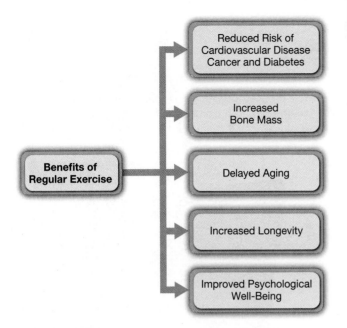

FIGURE 1.4 Regular exercise can produce numerous health benefits.

coaching
corner

What is my wellness level?

Take time to notice how your levels of wellness change from day to day. Revisit this activity throughout the semester for a better understanding of how your well-being changes.

- On a scale of 1 to 10 (10 being completely well), how do you rank yourself in regard to each wellness component?
- Identify people, tasks, obligations, and desires that affect your wellness.
- Create a list of things that add to your stress level and another list of things that motivate you to adopt a healthy lifestyle.
- Identify actions you take each day that positively affect your well-being.

Reduced Risk of Diabetes **Diabetes** is a disease characterized by high blood sugar (glucose) levels. Poorly managed diabetes can result in numerous health problems, including blindness, heart disease, and kidney dysfunction. Regular physical activity and exercise can reduce the risk of type 2 diabetes by improving skeletal muscle health and the regulation of blood glucose (9, 27, 28).

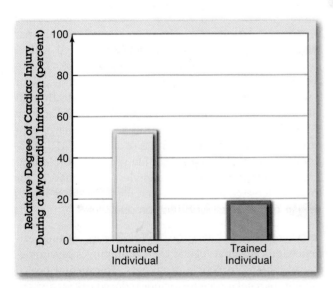

FIGURE 1.5 Regular endurance exercise protects the heart against injury during heart attack. During a myocardial infarction (heart attack), exercise-trained individuals suffer less cardiac injury compared to untrained individuals.

Source: Borges J.P.,et al., Delta Opioid Receptors: The Link between Exercise and Cardio protection. PLoS ONE 9(11): e113541.doi:10.1371/journal.pone.0113541, 2014.

Lower Risk of Cancer Cancer is a major cause of disease and death worldwide. The primary risk factors for cancer are environmental (exposure to cancer-causing agents) and lifestyle (45). One lifestyle factor associated with increased cancer risk is inactivity. Convincing evidence indicates that a sedentary lifestyle increases the risk of colon cancer (45), and growing evidence suggests that regular exercise can reduce the risk of breast and endometrial cancer in women (45). At present, it is unclear if regular exercise can reduce the risk of other forms of cancer.

Increased Bone Mass The bones of the skeleton provide a mechanical lever system to permit movement and protect internal organs. Loss of bone mass and strength is called **osteoporosis**, and it increases the risk

physical activity Movement of the body produced by a skeletal muscle that results in energy expenditure, especially through movement of large muscle groups (i.e., legs).

exercise Planned, structured, and repetitive bodily movement done to improve or maintain one or more components of fitness.

cardiovascular disease (CVD) Disease of the heart and blood vessels.

diabetes Metabolic disorder characterized by high blood glucose levels.

osteoporosis Condition that involves the loss of bone mass.

of bone fractures. Therefore, it is important to maintain strong, healthy bones. Although osteoporosis can occur in men and women of all ages, it is most common in older women.

Exercise can improve bone health by strengthening your bones. Mechanical force applied by muscular activity is a key factor in regulating bone mass and strength. Numerous studies have demonstrated that regular exercise increases bone mass, density, and strength in young adults (29–31). In particular, weight-bearing activities, such as running, walking, and resistance training, are important for bone health. Research on osteoporosis suggests that regular exercise can prevent bone loss in older adults and is also useful in treating osteoporosis (29).

Delayed Aging As we age, we gradually lose our physical capacity to do work, and therefore our ability to perform strenuous activities progressively declines. Although this decline may begin as early as the 20s, the most dramatic changes occur after about age 60 (32–34). Importantly, regular exercise can delay the age-related decline in physical working capacity (32, 35, 36). Indeed, note the differences in physical working capacity among highly trained, moderately trained, and inactive individuals in **FIGURE 1.6**. Although physical working capacity declines with age, regular exercise can maintain your ability to perform various types of physical activities,

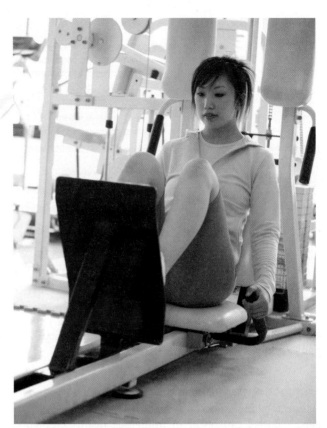

Regular weight-bearing exercise can prevent loss of bone mass.

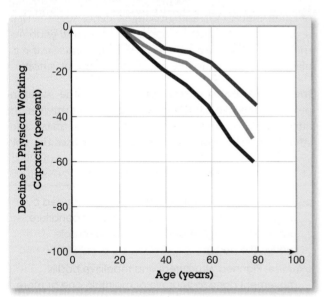

Key

■■■ Highly Trained
(60 min of exercise a day)
■■■ Moderately Trained
(30 min of exercise a day)
■■■ Untrained (sedentary)

FIGURE 1.6 Regular exercise can reduce the natural decline in working capacity that occurs as we age.

increasing your ability to enjoy a lifetime of physical recreation and an improved quality of life.

Increased Longevity Abundant research reveals that regular physical activity and exercise (combined with a healthy lifestyle) can increase longevity (7, 8, 25, 37–39). A classic study of Harvard alumni concluded that men with a sedentary lifestyle have a 31% greater risk of death from all causes than men who engage in regular physical activity (8). Similarly, compared to physically active women, sedentary women also have a higher risk of death (40, 41). These findings translate into a longer life span for people who exercise and have more active lifestyles. The primary factor for this increased longevity is that regular exercise lowers the risk of both heart attack and cancer (7, 8).

Improved Psychological Well-Being Strong evidence indicates that regular exercise improves psychological well-being in people of all ages. The mental health benefits of regular exercise include reduced risk for anxiety disorders and depression (42). Also, people report feeling less anxious and stressed after exercise, even up to 8 hours afterward. These benefits lead to an improved sense of well-being in the physically active individual.

see it!

ABC VIDEO

Exercise May Build Brain Power! Watch an ABC Video at MasteringHealth™.

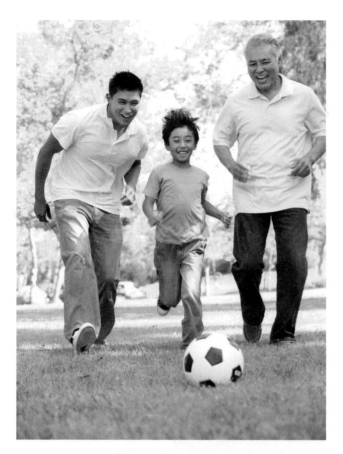

Regular physical activity can help you live longer.

MAKE SURE YOU **KNOW...**

- Regular physical activity and exercise reduce the risk of heart disease, diabetes, and certain types of cancer.
- Exercise increases bone mass in young people and strengthens bone in older adults.
- Regular exercise maintains physical working capacity as a person ages, increases longevity, and improves quality of life.
- Exercise promotes psychological well-being and reduces risk of depressive and anxiety disorders.

MasteringHealth™

Exercise and Activity for Health-Related Fitness

LO **4** Identify and discuss the five major components of health-related physical fitness.

Exercise training programs can be divided into two broad categories: *health-related physical fitness* and *skill-related physical fitness*. This book focuses on health-related fitness. The overall goal of a health-related physical fitness

program is to optimize the quality of life (1, 42). The specific goals of this type of fitness program are to reduce the risk of disease and to improve total physical fitness. In contrast, the goal of sport- and skill-related fitness is to improve physical performance in a specific sport or activity.

Most fitness experts agree that there are five major components of health-related physical fitness:

- Cardiorespiratory endurance
- Muscular strength
- Muscular endurance
- Flexibility
- Body composition

Some fitness experts include motor skill performance as a sixth component. Motor skills are movement qualities such as agility and coordination. Although motor skills are important for sport performance, they are not directly linked to improving health in young adults and are therefore not considered a major component of health-related physical fitness. However, these motor skills may increase in importance as people age, because good balance, coordination, and agility help reduce the risk of falls in older adults.

Cardiorespiratory Endurance

Cardiorespiratory endurance (sometimes called *aerobic fitness* or *cardiorespiratory fitness*) is often considered the key component of health-related physical fitness. It is a measure of the heart's ability to pump oxygen-rich blood to the working muscles during exercise and of the muscles' ability to take up and use the oxygen. Oxygen delivered to the muscles is used to produce the energy needed for prolonged exercise. In practical terms, cardiorespiratory endurance is the ability to perform exercises such as distance running, cycling, and swimming. Someone who has achieved a high level of cardiorespiratory endurance is generally capable of performing 30–60 minutes of vigorous exercise without undue fatigue.

Muscular Strength

Muscular strength is evaluated by how much force a muscle or muscle group can generate during a single

---

cardiorespiratory endurance Measure of the heart's ability to pump oxygen-rich blood to the working muscles during exercise and of the muscles' ability to take up and use the oxygen.

muscular strength Maximal ability of a muscle to generate force.

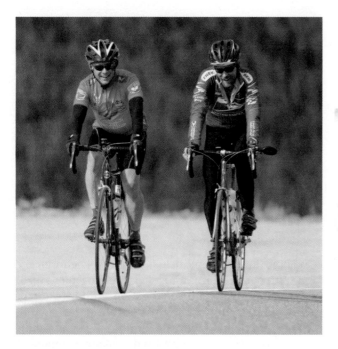

Cyclists who bike for long distances exhibit strong cardiorespiratory endurance.

maximal contraction (how much weight an individual can lift during one maximal effort). Muscular strength is important in almost all sports. Even nonathletes require some degree of muscular strength to function in everyday life. Routine tasks such as lifting bags of groceries and moving furniture require muscular strength. Even modest amounts of resistance exercise can improve muscular strength.

Muscular Endurance

Muscular endurance is the ability of a muscle to generate a submaximal force over and over again. Although muscular strength and muscular endurance are related, they are not the same. A person lifting a 150-pound barbell during one maximal muscular effort demonstrates high muscular strength. If he/she lifts a 75-pound barbell a dozen times, he/she demonstrates muscular endurance. As one develops muscular strength, endurance typically improves. However, muscular strength does not generally improve with endurance exercise training.

Most sports require muscular endurance. For instance, tennis players, who must run and repeatedly swing their racquets during a match, require a high level of muscular endurance. Many everyday activities (such as carrying your backpack all day) also require some level of muscular endurance.

Flexibility

Flexibility is the ability to move joints freely through their full range of motion. Flexible individuals can bend and twist with ease. Without routine stretching, muscles and tendons shorten, reducing the range of motion around joints and impairing flexibility.

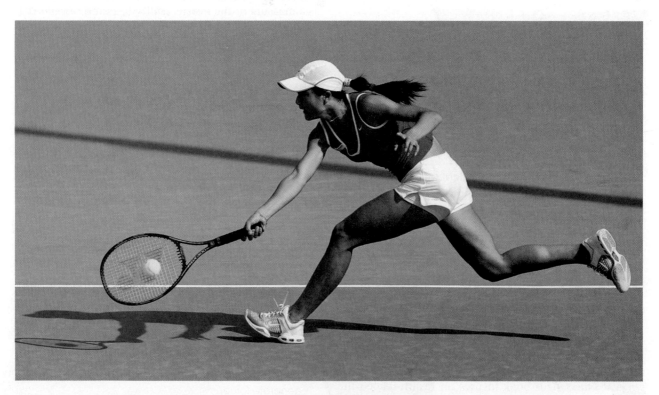

Swinging a tennis racquet repeatedly during a tennis match requires a high level of muscular endurance.

Individual needs for flexibility vary. Certain athletes (such as gymnasts and divers) require great flexibility to accomplish complex movements. The average individual requires less flexibility than an athlete, but everyone needs some flexibility for common tasks such as reaching for something on a high shelf. Research suggests that flexibility prevents some types of muscle-tendon injuries and may be useful in reducing low back pain (43, 44).

Body Composition

Body composition refers to the relative amounts of fat and lean tissue in your body. Body composition is included as a component of health-related physical fitness because having a high percentage of body fat is associated with an increased risk of developing CVD, type 2 diabetes, and some cancers. It also increases the risk of developing joint inflammation (arthritis). In general, excess fat elevates the risk of numerous health problems.

Lack of physical activity has been shown to play a major role in gaining body fat. Conversely, regular exercise is an important factor in promoting the loss of body fat and the maintenance of a healthy body weight.

MAKE SURE YOU **KNOW...**

■ Health-related physical fitness consists of five components: cardiorespiratory endurance, muscular strength, muscular endurance, flexibility, and body composition.

—MasteringHealth™

Lifestyle Management Is the Key to Wellness

 Explain how lifestyle plays a role in overall wellness and why it is important to assess your current health habits.

A lifestyle that incorporates healthy behaviors will promote wellness and increase your quality of life. The following behaviors will greatly increase your chances of achieving total wellness:

■ Be physically active and exercise on a regular basis

■ Avoid prolonged periods of sitting

■ Maintain a healthy weight

■ Consume a healthy diet

■ Manage stress

■ Avoid drug and tobacco use

■ Limit alcohol consumption

■ Reduce your risk of injury

■ Get regular medical exams and avoid exposure to infectious diseases

■ Maintain healthy relationships with family and friends

■ Practice spiritual wellness by finding purpose in your life and focusing on the positive aspects of your life

■ Engage in an occupation that provides satisfaction and fulfillment

■ Live within your financial means and manage your money responsibly

MAKE SURE YOU **KNOW...**

■ A lifestyle that incorporates healthy behaviors will promote wellness and enhance your quality of life.

■ Reducing or eliminating unhealthy behaviors and making healthy choices will lead to higher levels of wellness.

—MasteringHealth™

How Does Behavior Change Occur?

 Explain the process of behavior change and name and describe the six phases that are part of the stages of change model.

Numerous theories of behavior change have been proposed. A highly successful model is the **stages of change model** (also called the transtheoretical model); this theory predicts that behavior change occurs in steps or stages. This model is frequently used in programs aimed at modifying health-related behaviors (such as smoking cessation and addiction recovery).

The stages of change model incorporates six stages:

1. **Precontemplation.** Individuals in the *precontemplation* stage have no current plans to change their unhealthy behavior. They might not realize the need to change, or they simply may not want to change. Moving from this stage to the next requires increased knowledge about the benefits of healthy behaviors so that the need for change is recognized.

---

muscular endurance Ability of a muscle to generate a submaximal force over and over again.

flexibility Ability to move joints freely through their full range of motion.

body composition The relative amounts of fat and fat-free tissue (muscle, organs, bone) found in the body.

stages of change model A framework for understanding how the process of behavior change occurs; includes six stages.

Health Hazards of Prolonged Sitting

The term "sedentary" refers to the absence of physical activity. Often, sedentary individuals engage in prolonged periods of sitting, commonly due to occupations that require sitting at a desk or in a car or truck for hours at a time. A recent study reported that U.S. children and adults spend more than 55% of their day in sedentary pursuits (46).

Research reveals that prolonged sitting is associated with higher risks of cardiovascular disease and all-cause mortality (46, 47). Even among people who exercise 30–60 minutes a day, there is a strong association between prolonged sitting and increased risk of mortality (46). This suggests that prolonged sitting is unhealthy and that exercising regularly does not compensate for long periods of sitting. Prolonged sitting increases your risk of developing both obesity and type 2 diabetes (46). It also increases your risk of developing high blood pressure and other cardiovascular diseases (46, 47).

In summary, prolonged sitting is a major health risk that cannot be offset by regular exercise. So what can we do? First, we must reduce the amount of time we spend being sedentary during work and leisure time. Second, we must increase our physical activity as much as possible every day. Even small changes such as

standing while on the phone, taking regular walking breaks, and climbing extra sets of stairs can make a difference.

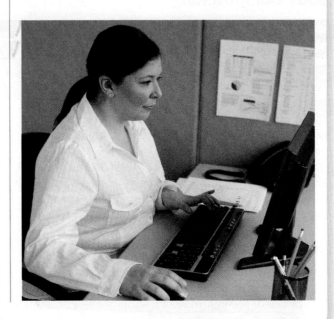

2. **Contemplation.** In the *contemplation* stage, a person is aware of the need to change and intends to make a change within the next several months. However, people in this stage are often unclear about how to accomplish this change. To advance beyond this stage, additional information and details about how to initiate behavior change are needed.

3. **Preparation.** During the *preparation* stage, the person plans to take action within a month. He or she acknowledges the benefits of behavior change and is aware of the process required. In some cases, the person might have created a plan for change.

4. **Action.** In the *action* stage, the person is actively doing things to bring about behavior change. This phase requires motivation and commitment. Relapse is common during this stage, and the individual could regress to the previous stage.

5. **Maintenance.** After sustaining the behavior change for 6 months, the person enters the *maintenance*

stage. At this point, the change has become a habit and requires less conscious effort. As this stage progresses, the temptation to resume old habits steadily decreases. The length of time that a person spends in each of the previous stages is highly individual, and people often move back and forth between the stages several times before they are able to make the behavior change permanent.

6. **Termination.** After a person has maintained a behavior for more than 5 years, they have reached the final stage. Reaching this stage means that the healthy behavior has become normal behavior, and there is no fear of relapse. People in this stage have attained an improved self-image and are capable of maintaining their target behavior.

hear it!

CASE STUDY

How can Anita change her behavior in college? Listen to the online case study at MasteringHealth™.

Assessing Your Current Health Habits

Before you can change a behavior, you must first recognize that the behavior is unhealthy and that you are capable of change. You can use the lifestyle assessment inventory in Laboratory 1.2 to increase your awareness of behaviors that impact your health.

Changing can be difficult, so it is best to start by selecting one *target behavior* you want to change. To improve your chances of success, it is wise to make your first behavior change goal a relatively easy one. For example, you could decide to give up the soda you usually consume between classes and drink water instead. When you succeed in modifying your first unhealthy behavior, move to a second target behavior and continue to build on your successes over time.

MAKE SURE YOU **KNOW**...

- To change a behavior, you must first recognize that the behavior is unhealthy and that you can make changes.
- The stages of change model states that behavior change occurs in six stages: precontemplation, contemplation, preparation, action, maintenance, and termination.
- Assessing your current lifestyle and habits is an important first step in changing unhealthy behaviors.

MasteringHealth™

Staying Motivated and Eliminating Barriers to Change

LO Discuss the strategies and tactics that are effective in maintaining motivation for change and eliminating barriers to change.

Now that you have identified target behaviors that need to be modified, it is time to launch your action plan for change. To do this, you must be motivated to make a change. *Motivation* is the drive that provides direction and gives you the persistence to achieve your goals. Two important elements that can assist in building motivation are examining the benefits of behavior change and increasing self-efficacy.

Evaluating the Benefits of Behavior Change

To achieve change, you must believe that the benefits of change outweigh the costs. Reminding yourself of the short- and long-term benefits provides motivation. Consider the following example of smoking cessation:

- **Short-term benefits.** Since cigarettes are expensive, quitting smoking results in more money in your pocket. There will be no more smoky smell in your home or on your clothes, and food will taste better.

- **Long-term benefits.** Quitting smoking reduces your risk of numerous chronic diseases, including lung disease, cancer, and heart disease. When you stop smoking, your skin improves and your risk of several eye diseases is reduced.

After carefully reviewing the short- and long-term benefits of smoking cessation, focus on those that are most important to you. Although the short-term benefits can be a strong motivating factor, the long-term benefits are extremely important and will impact the remainder of your life.

Increasing Self-Efficacy

The term **self-efficacy** refers to the belief that you can accomplish a specific goal or task. Therefore, increasing self-efficacy improves your chances of achieving behavior change. Strategies to improve self-efficacy include developing an internal locus of control, using visualization and self-talk techniques, and gaining strength from role models and encouragement from supportive people.

Locus of Control This psychological concept refers to how strongly people believe that they have control over events in their lives. People who believe that they can control most of the events that occur in their life possess an **internal locus of control**. In contrast, those with an **external locus of control** believe that factors beyond their control determine the course of their lives. People with an internal locus of control are often happier and have more confidence. When you believe that you have the power to take action, you will have the confidence and motivation to move forward and make changes that will improve your health.

While some people have an exclusively internal or external locus of control, most people fall somewhere in between. Fortunately, it is possible to develop an internal locus of control by learning which aspects of life we can and cannot control and then focusing on changing those factors that can be modified. Simply realizing deep down that you have the power to make decisions that will positively impact your life will help in shifting from an external to internal locus of control.

---

self-efficacy A person's belief in his or her ability to accomplish a specific goal.

internal locus of control Perception that one has control of most of the events of one's life.

external locus of control Perception that the events of one's life are outside of his or her control.

Visualization and Self-Talk Another way to increase and maintain your motivation for change is to visualize yourself engaging in a new healthy behavior. For example, imagine yourself taking a walk after dinner instead of reaching for a cigarette. Visualize breathing in fresh air instead of smoke and how much healthier you feel. Visualization is a powerful tool that can be used to create a new self-image of you as a healthier, happier person.

Self-talk is the internal dialogue we all have with ourselves that can be positive or negative. When positive, it serves as another powerful tool to help you achieve behavior change. You can become your own best cheerleader. Mentally affirming that you are strong and capable of making the desired change supports your commitment to change.

Role Models You probably know people who have reached one or more of the goals you are striving for These individuals can serve as positive role models. You can gain motivation by learning how these people succeeded and telling yourself, "If they can do it, so can I."

In addition to people you know, positive role models can also be found on television shows, in books, and via online blogs and forums. Many people are proud of their improved health status and are willing to share the strategies that worked for them. Just keep in mind that we are all individuals, so you have to consider advice from others in light of what you know will work for you.

Social Support Support and encouragement from others can be a major source of motivation. Surround yourself with friends and family members who encourage your efforts. A friend who wants to make the same behavior changes that you do can make a big difference in helping you achieve a goal. For instance, finding a "fitness buddy" to work out with provides both moral support and companionship. You can encourage each other and hold each other accountable.

Identifying and Eliminating Barriers to Change

As you work toward your goals, you may encounter some potential barriers to change. Awareness of these barriers is the first step in avoiding or overcoming them. Six common barriers are lack of knowledge, lack of motivation, denial, perceived invulnerability, low self-efficacy, and lack of social support.

Lack of Knowledge Not knowing what needs to change is a fundamental barrier to behavior change. If you are unaware that a change is necessary to improve your health, change will not occur. If you have not yet completed Laboratory 1.2, do it now so you can evaluate behaviors that may need to change to improve your overall wellness.

Lack of Motivation Without motivation, change will not occur. Applying the strategies discussed earlier to increase your motivation for change will eliminate this barrier.

Denial Failing to accept that one or more of your behaviors needs modification is another barrier to change. Many people are in denial about negative behaviors such as consuming too much alcohol or eating too many sweets. Being willing to face the fact that some of your current behaviors can endanger your health eliminates this barrier.

Perceived Invulnerability People who do not believe that they are susceptible to a health problem are unlikely to make changes to reduce risk. Some individuals are unrealistically optimistic about their chances of avoiding lifestyle-related health problems. Extensive research reveals that today's chronic health problems are largely due to poor lifestyle choices. No matter our age, we all need to understand that our choices directly affect our current and future health status.

Low Self-Efficacy As discussed earlier, increasing your self-efficacy will remove this barrier and improve your ability to achieve positive behavior change.

Lack of Social Support Social support can play a big role in motivating us toward positive change. In contrast, a lack of social support can be a barrier to success. It is essential to surround yourself with people who are supportive of your goals. Sometimes, friends or family members will feel threatened by your new behavior and will attempt to get you to resume your old ways. If this occurs, you can explain why making the change is important to you. If this doesn't work, then it is often best to limit your contact with "naysayers," at least during the early stages of your change process.

MAKE SURE YOU **KNOW...**

- Motivation is the incentive or drive to perform a task or achieve a goal; successful behavior change requires motivation.
- Examining the benefits of behavior change and increasing self-efficacy can help you stay motivated for behavior change.

■ Visualization, positive self-talk, positive role models, and social support are factors that contribute to increasing self-efficacy.

■ Six common barriers to change are lack of knowledge, lack of motivation, denial, perceived invulnerability, low self-efficacy, and lack of social support. Identifying and eliminating barriers is key to successful change.

— MasteringHealth™

Your Plan for Behavior Change

LO **8** Explain the necessity of SMART goals and create a behavior change action plan that addresses at least one health-related target behavior.

Now it's time to put together a plan of action. Begin with a list of the target behaviors you identified in Laboratory 1.2 that require change and select your first target behavior to modify.

Your key to success is a plan that includes:

■ Setting specific and appropriate goals

■ Documenting these goals in a behavior change contract

■ Creating a specific plan of action

■ Monitoring your progress toward each goal

■ Creating a plan to deal with challenges and relapses

■ Establishing meaningful rewards for achieving your goals

Goal Setting

Setting realistic short-term and long-term goals is essential for effective behavior change. Using the SMART criteria for goal setting ensures that your goals are appropriate and achievable. SMART stands for Specific, Measureable, Attainable, Realistic, and Time frame:

Specific You should establish a concrete goal that targets a specific area for improvement and clearly defines the outcome you want to achieve. Example: *I want to lose 10 pounds of body weight.*

Measureable Your goal should be measureable to provide tangible evidence that progress is being made. Progress can only be tracked when your goals are quantifiable. Example: *I will weigh myself once a week.*

Attainable Set goals that can be achieved. If you set goals that are out of your reach, you will lose your motivation early on and risk not accomplishing your goal. Example: *With appropriate diet and exercise, I will lose weight.*

Realistic Realistic means *doable*. Establish goals that are within reasonable limits and can be reached within the time frame established. Example: *Losing 10 pounds in 10 weeks is realistic for many people.*

Time Frame Establish an appropriate time frame for achieving your goals. Establishing an unrealistic time frame only leads to frustration. Example: *I will lose 10 pounds in 10 weeks.*

Behavior Change Contract

A behavior change contract records your goal(s) and identifies barriers to success and strategies you will use to overcome these barriers (see the blank contract at the front of the book). This written contract will include your goals and your specific plans for changing your behavior. It should be signed by you and a witness (a person close to you who will support your efforts). Completing the behavior change contract helps you think through your plan, and having another person sign the contract provides a partner for support and accountability.

Plan of Action

It is likely that you will identify multiple behaviors that need to change. Remember, you do not need to change all of your unhealthy behaviors at the same time. In fact, trying to make too many changes at once is difficult and reduces your chances for success.

When deciding which changes you want to make first, consider the effort it will take to change each of them. Some behaviors, such as flossing your teeth regularly, are simple and change is relatively easy. Other changes such as quitting smoking or improving your diet require more time and effort. While many people can successfully change more than one behavior at a time, it is usually best to start with one target behavior. Your initial success will increase your confidence and motivate you to tackle more complex challenges.

A well-conceived plan is required to achieve any goal. Before you develop your plan, you need accurate information. You can use this book and its online resources as a starting point. Your instructor may point you to additional resources. You might also need to seek out additional assistance from a counselor, fitness specialist, or support group. Make sure that any outside resources are reputable individuals or groups that are qualified to provide the information and guidance you need (see the Consumer Corner box on the next page).

Putting your plan into action requires commitment and the resolve to see it through. As you move forward, review the strategies you have learned and focus on those that are most effective for you. Remember, you *can* control your destiny and make positive lifestyle changes.

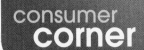

Finding Credible Health Information

Large amounts of health-related information can be found in books, magazines, on television, and online. Some information is supported by scientific research, but a significant amount lacks scientific support. Some can be outright dangerous. How do you know what to believe? To avoid being misled—or even worse, being scammed—you need to develop a healthy skepticism. The next time you encounter health information, ask yourself the following questions:

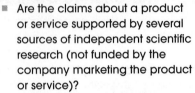

- Are the claims about a product or service supported by several sources of independent scientific research (not funded by the company marketing the product or service)?
- Are the "experts" endorsing a product or service really experts in the field, or do these individuals have a financial interest in the product or service?

- Do the claims made seem too good to be true?
- How do you know that a dietary supplement actually contains the ingredients shown on the label? What potential risks may be associated with the product?
- Are statements about a specific health practice supported by high-quality scientific studies published in peer-reviewed research journals?

If the quality or safety of a product or service can't be verified by reputable sources, this should raise a red flag. You may want to seek out the opinion of a trusted professional or health-care practitioner. Numerous sources of credible information can be found within the Centers for Disease Control and Prevention and National Institutes of Health websites (www.cdc.gov and www.nih.gov). Complete Laboratory 1.6 to learn more.

Monitoring Your Progress

Monitoring your progress provides guidance and ongoing motivation. Self-monitoring helps to identify factors that trigger and reinforce your unhealthy choices; it also provides greater awareness of your positive behaviors.

Dealing with Challenges and Relapses

As you make progress, obstacles are inevitable, so it is important that you anticipate problems. This is known as *relapse prevention* and involves tactics designed to prevent your returning to an unhealthy behavior. You must identify high-risk situations that are likely to trigger an unhealthy choice and develop a plan for avoiding or eliminating those situations.

As you work toward your goals, it is common to accomplish a certain level of change and then experience a few relapses before progress begins again. Evidence indicates that most people make several attempts at change before achieving success. A setback does not mean failure, and you can still get back on track. A relapse provides an opportunity to remember your reasons for wanting to make the change, and this can be very motivating.

Rewards for Achieving Your Goals

Providing yourself with a reward for good behavior will reinforce your efforts. Plan these rewards in advance to coincide with achieving a specific goal. Your rewards should be meaningful and not linked to food or alcohol. For example, you might treat yourself to a movie or a visit to a favorite location.

MAKE SURE YOU **KNOW...**

- A well-designed action plan based on SMART goals is a helpful tool for successful behavior change.
- A behavior change contract documents your goals and is witnessed by another person.
- Keeping a record of your progress can help you stay on track.
- Setbacks and challenges are inevitable; when you plan for them, you can refocus and move forward.
- Your plan should include meaningful and healthy rewards for reaching your goals.

MasteringHealth™

steps ▶ FOR BEHAVIOR CHANGE

Do you have trouble making healthy behavior changes?

Answer the following questions about your typical efforts to change a health behavior.

Y N
☐ ☐ Do you have a specific game plan?
☐ ☐ Do you get help from your friends and family?
☐ ☐ Do you set goals?
☐ ☐ Do you reward yourself for your successes?

If you answered no to most or all of the questions, then you should consider using the behavior change contract in the front of the text.

Tips for Using a Behavior Change Contract and Behavior Change Strategies

Tomorrow, you will:

☑ Talk to a friend about signing a behavior change contract with you.

☑ Write out a short- and a long-term SMART goal that you can work to achieve this semester.

☑ Determine your rewards for reaching your goals.

Within the next 2 weeks, you will:

☑ Assess your progress toward reaching your goals and adjust your goals if you realize they are not realistic.

☑ Determine which behavior change strategies will work best for you and add them to your behavior change contract.

☑ Reward yourself if you reach your short-term goal!

By the end of the semester, you will:

☑ Assess your progress toward your long-term goal and reward yourself if you achieve it.

☑ Set new goals to achieve.

☑ Continue to use behavior change strategies to help maintain your new healthy behaviors.

Sample Program for increasing physical activity

Scan to plan your individualized program for increasing physical activity.

If you have a busy schedule and find it difficult to fit exercise into your day, there are still ways you can increase your physical activity. You might not get the same increase in your fitness level as someone who participates in regular exercise, but you can still improve your health. Getting a pedometer and working to walk 10,000 steps per day, increasing your lifestyle physical activity, and getting small bouts of moderate activity throughout the day are a few things you can do to become more active.

Try using stairs rather than the elevator, walking to classes rather than driving, walking to complete errands, and walking extra aisles when grocery shopping. Consider trying a fitness DVD or online fitness video, and invite a friend or roommate to join you for a fun social experience.

	Activity Time	Monday	Tuesday	Wednesday	Thursday	Friday	Saturday	Sunday

Goals: Increase steps by 250 per day to reach the target goal of 10,000 steps per day, and increase general physical activity. The number of weeks to reach the goal of at least 10,000 steps per day will vary depending on your starting point.

	Activity Time	Monday	Tuesday	Wednesday	Thursday	Friday	Saturday	Sunday
Week 1	**Lunch Break**		10 min walk		10 min walk		10 min walk	10 min walk
	Study Break	1 set of 25 crunches, 1 set of 15 push-ups, 1 set of 15 dips		1 set of 25 crunches, 1 set of 15 push-ups, 1 set of 15 dips		1 set of 25 crunches, 1 set of 15 push-ups, 1 set of 15 dips	10 min walk	10 min walk
Week 2	**Lunch Break**		15 min walk		15 min walk		15 min walk	15 min walk
	Study Break	1 set of 25 crunches, 1 set of 20 push-ups, 2 sets of 10 dips	15 min yoga DVD	1 set of 25 crunches, 1 set of 20 push-ups, 2 sets of 10 dips	15 min yoga DVD	1 set of 25 crunches, 1 set of 20 push-ups, 2 sets of 10 dips	15 min walk	15 min walk (morning) 15 min yoga DVD (afternoon)
Week 3	**Lunch Break**		15 min walk		15 min walk		20 min walk	20 min walk
	Study Break	2 sets of 25 crunches, 2 sets of 15 push-ups, 2 sets of 15 dips	20 min yoga DVD	2 sets of 25 crunches, 2 sets of 15 push-ups, 2 sets of 15 dips	20 min yoga DVD	2 sets of 25 crunches, 2 sets of 15 push-ups, 2 sets of 15 dips	20 min walk	20 min walk (morning) 20 min yoga DVD (afternoon)

study plan

Customize your study plan—and master your health!—in the Study Area of **MasteringHealth.**

summary

hear it! STUDY REVIEW

To hear an MP3 Chapter Summary, scan here or visit the Study Area in MasteringHealth™.

LO **1** ■ U.S. life expectancy is expected to decrease. Cardiovascular disease is the leading cause of death, followed by cancer and respiratory diseases. Lifestyle has the greatest impact on our risk of disease.

■ *Wellness* is defined as optimal health. It is achieved by practicing a healthy lifestyle, which includes regular physical activity, proper nutrition, eliminating unhealthy behaviors, avoiding high-risk activities, and managing stress.

■ Total wellness can be achieved only by a balance of physical, emotional, intellectual, spiritual, social, environmental, occupational, and financial wellness. The components of wellness interact and influence each other.

LO **2** ■ *Healthy People 2020* is a U.S. government initiative that established wellness goals for the nation.

These goals include attaining high-quality, longer lives, reducing the risk of injury and premature death, achieving health equity, eliminating disparities, and improving the health of all groups within the population.

LO **3** ■ Regular exercise offers many health benefits, including reducing the risk of cardiovascular disease, diabetes, and certain types of cancer. It also increases bone mass, maintains physical working capacity as one ages, increases longevity, and improves psychological well-being and quality of life.

LO **4** ■ The five major components of health-related physical fitness are cardiorespiratory endurance, muscular strength, muscular endurance, flexibility, and body composition.

LO **5** ■ Optimal wellness can be achieved by reducing or eliminating unhealthy behaviors and making healthy lifestyle choices.

LO **6** ■ A behavior change can only occur when a person first develops the understanding that a behavior is unhealthy and has the desire to make a change.

■ According to the stages of change model, there are six stages of behavior change:

precontemplation, contemplation, preparation, action, maintenance, and termination.

■ Assessing your current lifestyle is the first step in planning to improve health-related habits.

LO 7 ■ Successful behavior change requires motivation.

■ Strategies shown to be effective in maintaining motivation include thinking about the benefits of change, increasing self-efficacy, visualizing how one's life will be better as a result of the change, using positive self-talk, seeking out positive role models, and obtaining support and encouragement from others.

■ Common barriers to change include lack of knowledge, lack of motivation, denial, perceived

invulnerability, low self-efficacy, and lack of social support. Accomplishing change requires identifying and overcoming barriers.

LO 8 ■ SMART goals are: Specific, Measureable, Attainable, Realistic, and associated with a specific Time frame.

■ A written behavior change contract provides accountability.

■ A well-designed action plan is based on SMART goals and includes strategies for dealing with the setbacks that will inevitably occur.

■ It is advisable to track your progress and use meaningful, healthy rewards to recognize your success in reaching your goals.

study questions

review it! QUIZZES

Find more review questions online at MasteringHealth™.

LO 1 1. _____ **A** _____ is *not* a component of wellness.
   a. Exercise   c. Social health
   b. Spiritual health d. Emotional health

2. List and describe the eight components of wellness.

LO 2 3. Which of the following is not a *Healthy People 2020* objective?
   a. Increase the proportion of adults who get sufficient sleep.
   b. Reduce the proportion of persons engaging in binge drinking of alcoholic beverages.
   c. Increase the proportion of physician office visits that include counseling or education related to nutrition or weight.
   d. All of the choices are *Healthy People 2020* objectives.

LO 3 4. _____ is any body movement produced by skeletal muscles that results in energy expenditure.
   a. Exercise   c. Physical activity
   b. Physical fitness d. Health-related fitness

5. Which of the following is a health benefit of regular physical activity?
   a. reduced risk for osteoporosis
   b. reduced risk for heart disease
   c. improved psychological well-being
   d. all of the above

LO 4 6. Which of the following is *not* a component of health-related fitness?

   a. muscular strength
   b. body composition
   c. agility
   d. flexibility

7. List and describe the five components of health-related fitness.

LO 5 8. Provide at least five examples of lifestyle choices that contribute to wellness.

LO 6 9. A person in the _____ **B** _____ stage of change has been fully participating in the new health behavior for less than 6 months.
   a. maintenance   c. contemplation
   b. action   d. new activity

LO 7 10. Which of the following should be considered when you are planning to make a behavior change?
   a. number of behaviors you want to change and effort involved
   b. motivation for behavior change
   c. current behavior patterns
   d. all of the above

11. Identify four major barriers to behavior change and explain how they could be eliminated.

LO 8 12. What does the acronym SMART stand for?
   a. specific, manageable, accountability, revisable, time-sensitive
   b. sensitive, multiple, action-oriented, reasonable, time-stamped
   c. specific, measurable, attainable, realistic, time frame
   d. short-term, measurable, accountability, realistic, tough

13. Outline the steps involved in launching a plan for behavior change.

suggested reading

Brooks, G. A., N. Butte, W. Rand, J. Flatt, and B. Caballero. Chronicle of the Institute of Medicine physical activity recommendation: How a physical activity recommendation came to be among dietary recommendations. *American Journal of Clinical Nutrition* 79:921S–930S, 2004.

Brown, D., D. Brown, G. Heath, L. Balluz, W. Giles, E. Ward, and A. Mokdad. Association between physical activity dose and health-related quality of life. *Medicine and Science in Sports and Exercise* 36:890–896, 2004.

Bushman, B. (Ed.). *ACSM's Complete Guide to Health and Fitness.* Champaign, IL: Human Kinetics, 2011.

Hamilton, M.T., G. Healy, D. Dunstan, T. Zderic, and N. Owen. Too little exercise and too much sitting: inactivity physiology and the need for new recommendations on sedentary behavior. *Current Cardiovascular Risk Reports.* 2:292-298, 2008.

Haskell, W. L., et al. Physical activity and public health: Updated recommendation for adults from the American College of Sports Medicine and the American Heart Association. *Medicine and Science in Sports and Exercise* 39:1423–1434, 2007.

Howley, E., and D. Thompson. *Fitness Professional's Handbook*, 6th ed. Champaign, IL: Human Kinetics, 2012.

Powers, S., and E. Howley. *Exercise Physiology: Theory and Application to Fitness and Performance*, 9th ed. New York: McGraw-Hill, 2015.

Rahl, R. L. *Physical Activity and Health Guidelines.* Champaign, IL: Human Kinetics, 2010.

helpful weblinks

do it! WEBLINKS

For links to the organizations and websites listed, visit MasteringHealth™.

American College of Sports Medicine

Comprehensive website providing information, articles, equipment recommendations, how-to articles, books, and position statements about all aspects of health and fitness. **www.acsm.org**

American Heart Association

Offers the latest information about ways to reduce your risk of heart and vascular diseases. Site includes -information about exercise, diet, and heart disease. **www.heart.org**

Healthy People

Provides information about the U.S. government's initiative to improve health and wellness for the American people. **www.healthypeople.gov**

WebMD

Contains the latest information on a variety of health-related topics, including diet, exercise, and stress. Links to nutrition, fitness, and wellness topics. **www.webmd.com**

Name _____ Date _____

Wellness Evaluation

The purpose of this quantitative wellness evaluation is to determine your current state of wellness. In the form below, you will be asked specific lifestyle questions about each of the eight components of wellness. After completion of each section, tally and record the total number of points that you scored in the section. When you complete all sections of this inventory, tally the total number of points earned in all sections and use the information provided at the end of the laboratory to determine your level of wellness.

PERSONAL WELLNESS ASSESSMENT:

Circle the number that describes you best.

Physical Wellness

	Rarely, if ever	Sometimes	Most of the time	Always
1. I exercise for ≥30 minutes/day on 3 or more days per week.	1	2	3	4
2. I am physically active most days of the week.	1	2	3	4
3. I maintain a healthy body weight.	1	2	3	4
4. I always use my seatbelt when driving or riding in a car.	1	2	3	4
5. I never drink and drive and I do not ride with anyone who has been drinking.	1	2	3	4
6. I obey traffic rules and speed limits.	1	2	3	4
7. I consistently get 7-9 hours of sleep.	1	2	3	4
8. I am able to sleep peacefully through the night.	1	2	3	4
9. I eat a variety of foods including fruits and vegetables.	1	2	3	4
10. I avoid skipping meals.	1	2	3	4
11. I rarely eat processed foods and/or sweets.	1	2	3	4
12. I consume less than two alcoholic beverages a day.	1	2	3	4
13. I never get intoxicated.	1	2	3	4
14. I do not binge drink.	1	2	3	4
15. I never smoke or use smokeless tobacco.	1	2	3	4
16. I do not use illegal drugs.	1	2	3	4
17. I use prescription medications only for their intended purpose.	1	2	3	4
18. I get annual medical examinations.	1	2	3	4
19. I am not sexually active *or* I always practice safe sex (e.g., using condoms or being involved in a monogamous relationship)	1	2	3	4
Total points:	_____			

Social Wellness

	Rarely, if ever	Sometimes	Most of the time	Always
20. I have a happy and satisfying relationship with my spouse or boyfriend/girlfriend.	1	2	3	4
21. I have good relationships with my close friends.	1	2	3	4
22. I get a great deal of love and support from my family.	1	2	3	4
23. I work to have good communication skills.	1	2	3	4
24. I am able to express my feelings to people close to me.	1	2	3	4
Total points: _____				

Emotional Wellness

	Rarely, if ever	Sometimes	Most of the time	Always
25. I find it easy to relax.	1	2	3	4
26. I regularly participate in activities and hobbies that I enjoy.	1	2	3	4
27. I rarely feel tense or anxious.	1	2	3	4
28. I am able to cope with daily stresses without undue emotional stress.	1	2	3	4
29. I have not experienced a major stressful life event in the last year.	1	2	3	4
30. I do not suffer from depressive or anxiety disorders.	1	2	3	4
31. I do not have an eating disorder.	1	2	3	4
32. I am able to accept responsibility for my own feelings and actions.	1	2	3	4
Total points: _____				

Intellectual Wellness

	Rarely, if ever	Sometimes	Most of the time	Always
33. I attend classes regularly.	1	2	3	4
34. I keep informed about current events.	1	2	3	4
35. I seek opportunities to learn new things.	1	2	3	4
36. I have an open mind regarding ideas that may be different than mine.	1	2	3	4
Total points: _____				

Environmental Wellness

	Rarely, if ever	Sometimes	Most of the time	Always
37. I am not exposed to second-hand smoke.	1	2	3	4
38. I use sunscreen regularly and/or limit my sun exposure.	1	2	3	4
39. I carpool or use physical activity for transportation when possible.	1	2	3	4
40. I recycle regularly.	1	2	3	4
41. I limit my exposure to harmful environmental contaminants.	1	2	3	4
Total points: _____				

Spiritual Wellness

	Rarely, if ever	Sometimes	Most of the time	Always
42. I have a sense of meaning and purpose in my life.	1	2	3	4
43. I am satisfied with my level of spirituality.	1	2	3	4
44. I work to develop my spiritual health.	1	2	3	4
Total points: _____				

Occupational Wellness

	Rarely, if ever	Sometimes	Most of the time	Always
45. My college major/and or occupation is fulfilling and rewarding.	1	2	3	4
46. I enjoy my personal interactions with colleagues at school or my place of work.	1	2	3	4
Total points: _____				

Financial Wellness

	Rarely, if ever	Sometimes	Most of the time	Always
47. I am happy with my current level of savings.	1	2	3	4
48. I live within my budget (i.e., means).	1	2	3	4
49. I feel confident that I will have enough money in retirement.	1	2	3	4
50. I have enough "disposable" income.	1	2	3	4
Total points: _____				

Grand total points (all components of wellness): _____

Evaluating Your Wellness Score in Each of the Eight Components of Wellness

Use your total points score in each of the eight components of wellness to determine where you stand on the wellness scale (see charts below). If you score below excellent on any of the individual components of wellness, this aspect of your lifestyle needs attention. Use the information contained in this book to develop your strategies to achieve an excellent level of total wellness.

INTERPRETATION OF YOUR SCORES IN EACH WELLNESS COMPONENT (WELLNESS RATING)

Excellent: If your total points are within the excellent range, you are practicing a healthy lifestyle in this component of wellness. Keep up the good work!

Good: If your total points are within the good range, your health practices are above average but there is room for improvement.

Needs improvement: If your total points are within the needs improvement range, your health practices are below average and you may be taking unnecessary health risks. Clearly, room for improvement exists.

Needs major improvement: If your total points are within the needs major improvement range, your health practices are poor and you are likely taking unnecessary health risks.

Physical Wellness

Ideal score = 76 points

Your score _____

Your wellness rating _____

Needs major improvement	Needs improvement	Good	Excellent
19–29 points	30–59 points	46–60 points	61–76 points

Social Wellness

Ideal score = 20 points

Your score _____

Your wellness rating _____

Needs major improvement	Needs improvement	Good	Excellent
5–7 points	8–11 points	12–15 points	16–20 points

Emotional Wellness

Ideal score = 32 points

Your score

Your wellness rating _____

Needs major improvement	Needs improvement	Good	Excellent
8–12 points	13–18 points	19–25 points	26–32 points

Intellectual Wellness

Ideal score = 16 points

Your score _____

Your wellness rating _____

Needs major improvement	Needs improvement	Good	Excellent
4–6 points	7–9 points	10–12 points	13–16 points

Environmental Wellness

Ideal score = 20 points

Your score _____

Your wellness rating _____

Needs major improvement	Needs improvement	Good	Excellent
5–7 points	8–11 points	12–15 points	16–20 points

Spiritual Wellness

Ideal score = 12 points

Your score _____

Your wellness rating _____

Needs major improvement	Needs improvement	Good	Excellent
3–4 points	5–6 points	7–9 points	10–12 points

Occupational Wellness

Ideal score = 8 points

Your score _____

Your wellness rating _____

Needs major improvement	Needs improvement	Good	Excellent
2 points	3–4 points	5–6 points	7–8 points

Financial Wellness

Ideal score = 16 points

Your score _____

Your wellness rating _____

Needs major improvement	Needs improvement	Good	Excellent
4–6 points	7–9 points	10–12 points	13–16 points

Record your scores and wellness rating (i.e., excellent, good, etc.) in the table below. Which components of wellness do you need to improve?

Evaluating Your Total Wellness Level on the Wellness Continuum

Component of Wellness	Ideal Score	Your Score	Your Wellness Rating
Physical			
Social			
Emotional			
Intellectual			
Environmental			
Spiritual			
Occupational			
Financial			

Use your grand total score (i.e., sum of each of the eight components of wellness) to determine where you stand on the total wellness scale (see below). If you score below excellent on the continuum of total wellness, one or more aspects of your lifestyle needs behavior modification. Use the information obtained in Laboratory 1.2 to identify specific health behaviors that need to be modified to improve your overall wellness.

WHAT YOUR TOTAL WELLNESS SCORE MEANS

Ideal score = 200 points

Your score = _____

Scores of 160–200: Excellent!

If your total points are within the excellent range, you practice a healthy lifestyle and are enjoying total wellness. Keep up the good work!

Scores of 120–159: Good

If your total points are within the good range, your health practices are above average but there is room for improvement on your overall level of wellness.

Scores of 80–119: Needs improvement

If your total points are within the needs improvement range, many of your health practices are below average and you are taking unnecessary health risks. Clearly, behavior modification is required to improve your overall level of wellness.

Scores of 50–79: Needs major improvement

If your total points are within the needs maj or improvement range, most of your health practices are poor and you are exposed to many unnecessary health risks. Clearly, major behavior modification is required to improve your overall level of wellness.

Wellness continuum

Needs major improvement	Needs improvement	Good	Excellent
50–79 points	80–119 points	120–159 points	160–200 points

Low level of well-being ← — — — — — — — — — — — — — — — — — → High level of well-being

laboratory 1.5

do it! LABS
Complete Lab 1.5 online in the
study area of MasteringHealth.com

Name _____ Date _____

Par-Q and You

The following questionnaire can also be used to determine your readiness to engage in a fitness program.

Physical Activity Readiness
Questionnaire - PAR-Q
(revised 2002)

PAR-Q & YOU

(A Questionnaire for People Aged 15 to 69)

Regular physical activity is fun and healthy, and increasingly more people are starting to become more active every day. Being more active is very safe for most people. However, some people should check with their doctor before they start becoming much more physically active.

If you are planning to become much more physically active than you are now, start by answering the seven questions in the box below. If you are between the ages of 15 and 69, the PAR-Q will tell you if you should check with your doctor before you start. If you are over 69 years of age, and you are not used to being very active, check with your doctor.

Common sense is your best guide when you answer these questions. Please read the questions carefully and answer each one honestly: check YES or NO.

YES	NO		
☐	☐	1.	Has your doctor ever said that you have a heart condition <u>and</u> that you should only do physical activity recommended by a doctor?
☐	☐	2.	Do you feel pain in your chest when you do physical activity?
☐	☐	3.	In the past month, have you had chest pain when you were not doing physical activity?
☐	☐	4.	Do you lose your balance because of dizziness or do you ever lose consciousness?
☐	☐	5.	Do you have a bone or joint problem (for example, back, knee or hip) that could be made worse by a change in your physical activity?
☐	☐	6.	Is your doctor currently prescribing drugs (for example, water pills) for your blood pressure or heart condition?
☐	☐	7.	Do you know of <u>any other reason</u> why you should not do physical activity?

If you answered

YES to one or more questions

Talk with your doctor by phone or in person BEFORE you start becoming much more physically active or BEFORE you have a fitness appraisal. Tell your doctor about the PAR-Q and which questions you answered YES.

- You may be able to do any activity you want — as long as you start slowly and build up gradually. Or, you may need to restrict your activities to those which are safe for you. Talk with your doctor about the kinds of activities you wish to participate in and follow his/her advice.
- Find out which community programs are safe and helpful for you.

NO to all questions

If you answered NO honestly to <u>all</u> PAR-Q questions, you can be reasonably sure that you can:
- start becoming much more physically active — begin slowly and build up gradually. This is the safest and easiest way to go.
- take part in a fitness appraisal – this is an excellent way to determine your basic fitness so that you can plan the best way for you to live actively. It is also highly recommended that you have your blood pressure evaluated. If your reading is over 144/94, talk with your doctor before you start becoming much more active.

DELAY BECOMING MUCH MORE ACTIVE:
- if you are not feeling well because of a temporary illness such as a cold or a fever – wait until you feel better; or
- if you are or may be pregnant – talk to your doctor before you start becoming more active.

PLEASE NOTE: If your health changes so that you then answer YES to any of the above questions, tell your fitness or health professional. Ask whether you should change your physical activity plan.

<u>Informed Use of the PAR-Q</u>: The Canadian Society for Exercise Physiology, Health Canada, and their agents assume no liability for persons who undertake physical activity, and if in doubt after completing this questionnaire, consult your doctor prior to physical activity.

No changes permitted. You are encouraged to photocopy the PAR-Q but only if you use the entire form.

NOTE: If the PAR-Q is being given to a person before he or she participates in a physical activity program or a fitness appraisal, this section may be used for legal or administrative purposes.

"I have read, understood and completed this questionnaire. Any questions I had were answered to my full satisfaction."

SIGNATURE _____ DATE_____

SIGNATURE OF PARENT _____ WITNESS _____
or GUARDIAN (for participants under the age of majority)

Note: This physical activity clearance is valid for a maximum of 12 months from the date it is completed and becomes invalid if your condition changes so that you would answer YES to any of the seven questions.

Physical Activity Readiness Questionnaire (PAR-Q) © 2002. Used with permission from the Canadian Society for Exercise.

Name _____ Date _____

Evaluating Fitness and Health Products

Complete this activity to evaluate fitness advertisements you see or hear regularly. Find three examples (from magazines, TV or radio ads, or online) of claims on fitness or health products. Answer the following questions for each of your products.

1. Are the claims about this product supported by several scientific studies that are independent of the company producing the product?

   _____

   _____

2. If the answer to question 1 is "no," are you confident that the product is both safe and effective? Explain your answer.

   _____

   _____

   _____

3. What are the credentials of the author or person endorsing the product? Is the information provided by an expert in the field of exercise science or health?

   _____

   _____

   _____

4. Are the benefits of the product realistic?

   _____

   _____

   _____

5. Does the ad contain gimmick words, such as "quick," "spot reduce," or "just minutes a day"?

   _____

   _____

   _____

6. Is the main purpose of the ad to provide useful information or only to sell a product?

   _____

   _____

   _____

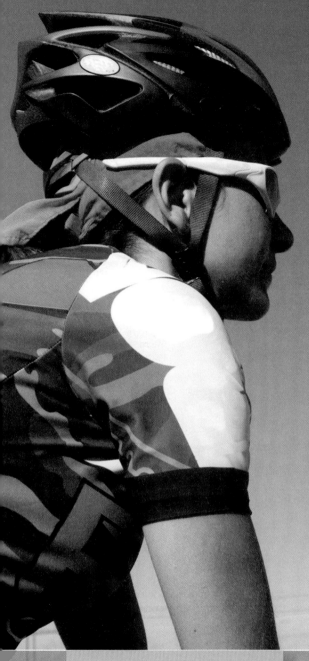

2

General Principles of Exercise for Health and Fitness

AS INTRODUCED IN Chapter 1, the benefits of regular exercise are numerous. People differ widely in regard to their athletic ability and sports-related skills, but everyone can experience health benefits from regular exercise. Many important health benefits can be obtained by simply changing from a sedentary lifestyle to an active lifestyle that includes moderate exercise most days of the week. Additional health benefits can be achieved by exercising more often and at higher intensities.

This chapter will discuss the general principles of exercise training that are required to improve your physical fitness. The basic concepts presented here apply to men and women of all ages and fitness levels. You will learn more about the individual components of health-related physical fitness—cardiorespiratory fitness, muscular strength and endurance, flexibility, and body composition—in the next four chapters and learn how to put these components together into a complete fitness program (Chapter 7).

Principles of Exercise Training to Improve Physical Fitness

 List and describe the guiding principles of exercise training designed to improve physical fitness.

Although everyone's exercise training program will vary according to personal needs, the general principles of physical fitness are universal. The more you exercise, and the greater the variety of activities you do, the more fit you'll be. In the following sections we describe the training concepts of overload, progression, specificity, recuperation, and reversibility, all of which affect the progress you'll make as you design and carry out your exercise training program.

Overload Principle

To improve physical fitness, the major exercise-related organ systems of the body (i.e., the muscular and cardiorespiratory systems) must be stressed. For example, for a skeletal muscle to increase in strength, the muscle must work against a heavier load than normal. This concept illustrates the **overload principle**, and it's a key component of all conditioning programs (1, 2) (**FIGURE 2.1**). We achieve an overload by increasing the intensity of exercise, such as by using heavier weights.

You can also achieve overload by increasing the time (i.e., duration) of exercise. For instance, to increase muscular endurance, a muscle must be worked over a longer duration than normal, such as by performing a greater number of exercise repetitions. To improve flexibility and increase the range of motion at a joint, we must either stretch the muscle to a longer length or hold the stretch for a longer time.

Although overload is important to attaining physical fitness, your workouts should not be exhausting. The

Application of Overload Principle to Increase Fitness Levels

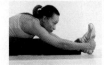
FLEXIBILITY — Stretch farther or longer

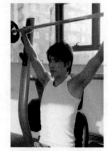
STRENGTH — Increase weight loads

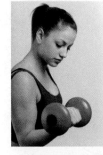
ENDURANCE — Perform more repetitions

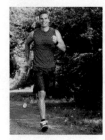
CARDIO-RESPIRATORY — Run farther

FIGURE 2.1 You can use the overload principle to increase your fitness level in each of the key training areas.

often-heard bodybuilding adage "No pain, no gain" is not completely accurate. In fact, you can improve your physical fitness without punishing training sessions.

Principle of Progression

The **principle of progression** is an extension of the overload principle. It states that overload should be increased gradually during the course of a physical fitness program. For example, Becky, a sedentary college-age student who is slightly overweight, might begin her new fitness program with a daily 10-minute walk/jog, then move up to an 11-minute walk/jog in week 2, and by week 5, do a daily 16-minute jog.

The overload in a training program should generally be increased slowly during the first 1–6 weeks of the exercise program. After this initial period, the overload can be increased at a steady and progressive rate during the next 6–20 weeks of training. For best results, the overload should not be increased too slowly or too rapidly. Progressing too slowly will delay improvement in physical fitness, and progressing too quickly can increase your risk of musculoskeletal injuries.

What is a safe rate of progression during an exercise training program? Although people vary in their tolerance for exercise overload, a commonsense guideline to improve physical fitness and avoid overuse injuries is the **ten percent rule** (2). In short, this rule says that the training intensity or duration of exercise should be increased by no more than 10% per week. For example, a runner running 20 minutes per day could increase his or her daily exercise duration to 22 minutes per day (10% of 20 = 2) the following week.

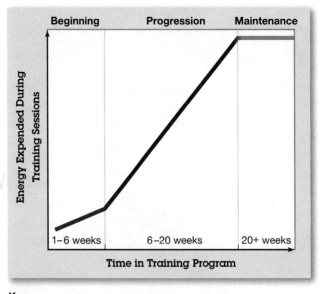

Key

━━━ Beginning of program

━━━ Slow progression during program

━━━ Maintenance

FIGURE 2.2 If you're starting a new exercise program, you'll begin slowly and progress toward doing more exercise at a greater intensity until you reach your desired fitness level. Then you'll develop a maintenance program to sustain your new level of fitness.

consider this! ////////////////

Fewer than 48% of American adults get enough physical activity to meet the guidelines established by the U.S. government.

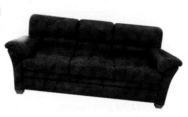

Principle of Specificity

Another key concept in training is the **principle of specificity**, which states that the exercise training effect is specific to those muscles involved in the activity (3). For example, if you perform leg curls, you wouldn't expect your upper arms to benefit, and likewise, your biceps curls aren't going to improve your leg muscles. This is part of the reason why a varied set of exercises is so important to overall physical fitness improvement.

Specificity of training also applies to the types of adaptations that occur in the muscle. For instance, strength training, such as lifting free weights, results in an increase in muscle strength but does not greatly improve the endurance of the muscle. Therefore, strength training is specific to improving muscular strength (4). Similarly, endurance exercise training, such as distance running, results in improved muscular endurance without increasing muscular strength significantly (5). Suppose you want to improve your ability to run a distance of 3 miles. In this case, specific training should include running 3 or more

miles several times a week. This type of training would improve muscular endurance in your legs but would not result in large improvements in leg strength (3).

Once you reach your desired level of physical fitness, you no longer need to increase the training intensity or duration of your physical conditioning. You should instead focus on designing a **maintenance program** to maintain your new fitness level with regular exercise (**FIGURE 2.2**).

---

overload principle Basic principle of physical conditioning that states that in order to improve physical fitness, the body or specific muscles must be stressed.

principle of progression Principle of training that states that overload should be increased gradually.

ten percent rule The training intensity or duration of exercise should not be increased by more than 10% per week.

principle of specificity The effect of exercise training is specific to those muscles involved in the activity.

maintenance program Exercising to sustain a desired level of physical fitness.

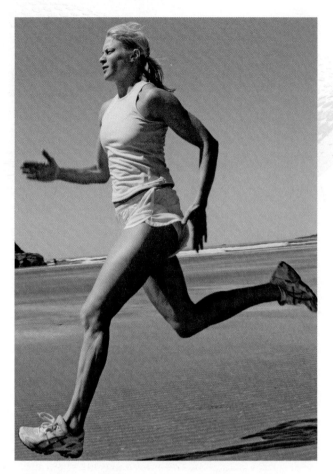

Because running involves the use of the leg muscles, doing it regularly will improve the endurance of those muscles. This is an example of specificity of training.

Principle of Recuperation

Overloading your muscles means stressing them, and they need a period of rest before your next workout. During the recovery period, the body adapts to the exercise stress

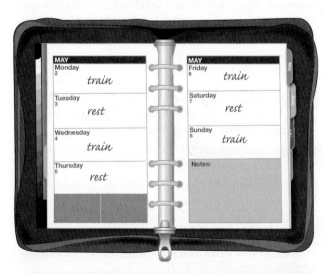

FIGURE 2.3 To maximize benefits and avoid injury, allow adequate rest periods between exercise sessions.

coaching
corner

Don't skip dance Monday!

An important idea associated with a sound exercise program is consistency. If you have always considered fitness optional, it may be helpful to reframe that thought process. Consider adopting the mantra that *daily exercise is nonnegotiable.*

- Schedule your exercise sessions at convenient times of day to ensure consistency.
- Create a schedule of fitness activities that includes several options for cardiorespiratory, strength, and flexibility training.
- Exercise with friends when possible—this enhances both the physical and social dimensions of wellness.
- Develop a backup plan for days when you are less motivated. Some activity is always better than no activity.

by increasing endurance or becoming stronger. In fact, a rest period, usually 24 hours or more, is essential for achieving maximal benefit from exercise. The need for a rest period between exercise training sessions is called the **principle of recuperation** (2) (**FIGURE 2.3**).

consider this! ///////////////////////

Among people who start an exercise program, 50% will drop out within 6 months.

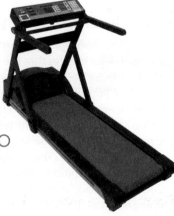

principle of recuperation The body requires recovery periods between exercise training sessions to adapt to the exercise stress. Therefore, a period of rest is essential for achieving maximal benefit from exercise.

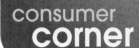
Choosing the Right Exercise Shoe

The right shoe can make it more comfortable for you to exercise and reduce your risk of injury, while the wrong shoe can cause you to avoid your workout or even contribute to injuries. Consider the following factors when buying a pair of workout shoes.

Exercise shoes vary in their design and function. For example, shoes designed for walking are often stiff compared to running shoes, which are more flexible and contain extra cushioning. Shoes for cross-training are designed for activities that involve lateral motion such as volleyball or kickboxing. A good rule of thumb to follow is that if you engage in an activity more than twice a week, buy a shoe designed for that activity.

Feet come in a variety of shapes, and knowing your foot's particular quirks is important in selecting the right shoe. For example, we all differ in the structure of our arch (i.e., the curvature of the bottom of your foot). You can determine your arch type by performing the "wet test." Wet your foot and step on a dry surface to trace your footprint. If you possess flat feet or a low arch, your footprint will reveal the entire sole of your foot, with little or no curve visible. If your footprint shows only a portion of your forefoot and heel with little or no connection between the two, you have high arches. Or

you may have a neutral arch, in which case the wet test shows a distinct curve along the inside of your foot.

Here are some tips for choosing your optimal exercise shoe:

- Exercise shoes are designed with different types of arch supports to accommodate the variance in arch structures. Use the previously discussed "wet test" to determine which type of shoe will best meet your arch-support needs.

- Shop for shoes late in the day. The swelling that occurs in your feet by the end of the day is similar to the swelling they experience during exercise (swelling is due to increased blood flow and fluid collection).

- Make sure that there is a full thumbnail length (approximately 1/2 inch) between the end of your longest toe and the end of the shoe. This ensures that the shoe is long enough for your foot.

- Make sure the front section of the shoe (the toe box) allows the toes to move around.

- The shoe should not feel too tight, but the foot should not slide around in the shoe.

- Do not rely on a break-in period for your shoes to stretch—your shoes should feel good on the day you buy them.

- If in doubt about the correct size, buy the larger size.

Failure to get enough rest between exercise training sessions can result in a fatigue syndrome referred to as **overtraining**. Overtraining can lead to chronic fatigue, increased risk of infection, and injuries. Common symptoms of overtraining include sore and stiff muscles or a feeling of general fatigue the morning after an exercise training session, sometimes called a "workout hangover." The cure is either to increase the duration of rest between workouts or to reduce the intensity of workouts, or both. Although too much exercise is the primary cause of the overtraining syndrome, an inadequate diet, particularly if it's short on carbohydrates and fluids, can also contribute.

Principle of Reversibility

Although rest periods are important to maximizing your benefits from exercise, going too long between exercise sessions (such as days or weeks), or being too inconsistent in your routine, will result in losing the fitness progress you've made (6). To maintain physical fitness, you need to exercise regularly. Indeed, physical fitness cannot be stored. The loss of fitness due to inactivity (i.e., detraining) is an example of the **principle of reversibility**.

How quickly is fitness lost after training has stopped? The answer depends on which component of physical fitness you are considering. For example, if you stop strength training, you will lose muscular strength relatively slowly (4, 7). In contrast, after you stop performing endurance exercise, you will lose muscular endurance relatively rapidly (6) (**FIGURE 2.4**).

For example, 8 weeks after strength training is stopped, only 10% of muscular strength is lost (7). In contrast, 8 weeks after cessation of endurance training, 30–40% of muscular endurance is lost (6). Also, the health benefits of regular exercise are not stored forever and are lost within several months if you stop exercising on a regular basis. Therefore, to achieve a lifetime of health benefits from physical activity, it is important to maintain a regular routine of exercise throughout your lifespan.

---

overtraining Failure to get enough rest between exercise training sessions.

principle of reversibility Loss of fitness due to inactivity.

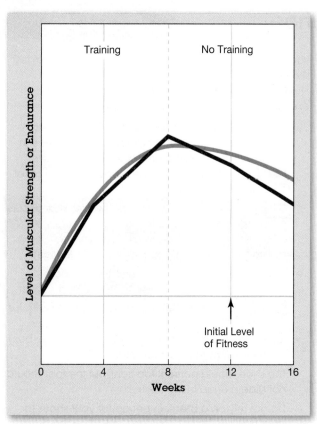

Key

■ Muscular endurance

■ Muscular strength

FIGURE 2.4 Stopping exercise training will reverse gains made in both muscular strength and muscular endurance.

MAKE SURE YOU **KNOW...**

■ Five key principles of exercise training are the overload principle, principle of progression, specificity of exercise, principle of recuperation, and reversibility of training effects.

■ The overload principle states that to improve physical fitness, the body or the specific muscle group used during exercise must be stressed.

■ The principle of progression is an extension of the overload principle and affirms that overload should be increased gradually over the course of a physical fitness training program.

■ The principle of specificity refers to the fact that exercise training is specific to those muscles involved in the activity.

■ The requirement for a rest period between training sessions is called the principle of recuperation.

■ The principle of reversibility refers to loss of physical fitness due to inactivity.

MasteringHealth™

Designing Your Exercise Program

LO **Outline the steps required to design your personal exercise program. Include the key elements of your exercise prescription (goals, warm-up, cool-down, type of exercise, and its frequency, intensity, and duration).**

If you go to a doctor with a bacterial infection and she prescribes an antibiotic as treatment, chances are good that the dose you take is different from the dose that might be prescribed for your 10-year-old brother. Similarly, for each individual there is a correct "dose" of exercise to effectively promote physical fitness, called an **exercise prescription** (6). Exercise prescriptions should be tailored to meet the needs of the individual (3, 6, 8). They should include fitness goals, a mode of exercise (type of activity), a warm-up, a primary conditioning period, and a cool-down. The following sections provide a general introduction to each of these components.

Setting Goals

Establishing fitness goals is the first step in designing your exercise program. If you don't know what you're working toward, you are not likely to achieve it. Thus, setting both short-term and long-term goals is an essential part of an exercise prescription. Visualizing goals such as a leaner, stronger body or an improved competitive performance will provide motivation as you begin your exercise program. Attaining your fitness goals improves self-esteem and provides the incentive needed to make a lifetime commitment to regular exercise.

The importance of fitness goals cannot be overemphasized. Goals provide structure and motivation for a personal fitness program.

The Importance of a Warm-Up

A **warm-up** is a brief (5–15-minute) period of exercise that precedes a workout. In general, a warm-up should include low-intensity, whole-body exercises that are similar to those you will perform during your workout. The purpose of a warm-up is to elevate muscle temperature and increase blood flow to those muscles that will be involved in the workout (1). It is possible that a warm-up may reduce the risk of muscle and tendon injuries. You can find some specific warm up exercises in Laboratory 2.1.

see it!

ABC VIDEOS

Watch the ABC Video "3 Big Mistakes Sabotaging Your Workout" at MasteringHealth™.

---

exercise prescription The individualized amount of exercise that will effectively promote physical fitness for a given person.

warm-up Brief (5–15-minute) period of exercise that precedes a workout.

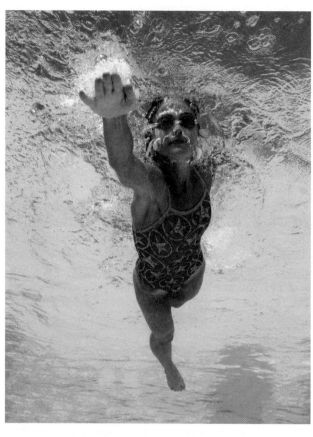

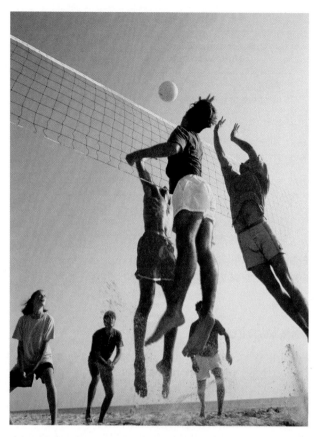

Swimming and volleyball are both excellent for the cardiovascular system. Swimming puts less stress on the joints and is considered a low-impact activity, while volleyball puts more stress on joints and is considered a high-impact activity.

EXAMINING THE EVIDENCE Too Much Exercise Increases Your Risk of Illness

Research indicates that intense exercise training (or overtraining) reduces the body's immunity to disease (13). In contrast, light to moderate exercise training boosts the immune system and reduces the risk of infections (28). The relationship between exercise training and the risk of developing an upper respiratory tract infection (e.g., a cold) is shown in the figure in this box. The J-shaped curve indicates that moderate exercise training reduces the risk of infection, whereas high-intensity and long-duration training increases the risk of infection.

The explanation for this relationship is complex, but it appears that too much exercise increases levels of stress hormones in the body that weaken the immune system. Depressed immune function increases your risk for developing an infection when you are exposed to bacteria or viruses.

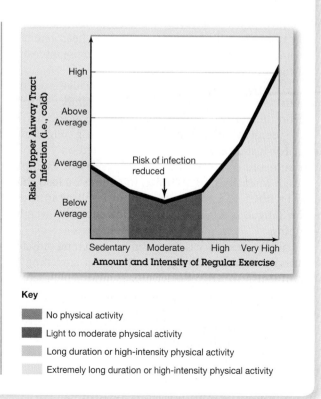

Key

- No physical activity
- Light to moderate physical activity
- Long duration or high-intensity physical activity
- Extremely long duration or high-intensity physical activity

The FITT Principle

Major components of the workout	Examples
Frequency (Number of days per week)	3 days per week
Intensity (Intensity of exercise performed)	Moderate
Time (Duration of exercise)	30 minutes
Type (Mode of exercise)	Running

FIGURE 2.5 The FITT principle encompasses the components of your exercise prescription.

The Workout

Regardless of the activity, the major components of the exercise prescription that define the workout are Frequency, Intensity, Time (duration) and Type (mode) of exercise; these are known as the *FITT principle* (**FIGURE 2.5**).

The **frequency of exercise** is the number of times per week that you intend to exercise. The recommended frequency of exercise to improve most components of health-related physical fitness is 3–7 times per week (1, 2).

The **intensity of exercise** is the amount of physiological stress or overload placed on the body during the exercise. The method for determining the intensity of exercise varies with the type of exercise performed. For example, as you expend more energy during exercise, your heart rate will increase, so measuring heart rate has become a standard means to determine exercise intensity during cardiorespiratory fitness training.

Whereas heart rate can be used to gauge exercise intensity during strength training, the number of repetitions performed before muscular fatigue occurs is more useful for monitoring intensity during weight lifting. For instance, a load that can be lifted only 5 to 8 times before complete muscular fatigue is an example of high-intensity weight lifting. In contrast, a load that can be lifted 40 to 60 times without resulting in muscular fatigue is an illustration of low-intensity weight training.

Finally, flexibility is improved by stretching muscles beyond their normal lengths. Intensity of stretching is monitored by the degree of tension felt during the stretch. Low-intensity stretching results in only minor tension on the muscles and tendons. In contrast, high-intensity stretching places great tension or moderate discomfort on the muscle groups being stretched.

The third aspect of the primary conditioning period is the **time (duration) of exercise**—that is, the amount of time spent performing the primary workout. Note that the duration of exercise does not include the time involved in the warm-up or cool-down. Research reveals that 20–30 minutes per exercise session (performed three or more times per week) is the minimum amount of time required to significantly improve cardiorespiratory endurance. **FIGURE 2.6** (on page 43) shows a physical activity pyramid that can help you identify types of physical activities that increase your fitness level and how frequently you should perform them.

Every exercise prescription includes at least one **type of exercise**. For example, to improve cardiorespiratory fitness you could select activities such as running, swimming, or cycling. To ensure that you will exercise regularly, choose activities that you enjoy doing, that are easily available to you, and that carry a low risk of injury.

The various types of exercise can be classified as *high-impact* or *low-impact*, based upon the amount of stress placed upon joints during the activity. Because of the high correlation between high-impact activities and injuries, many exercise science experts recommend low-impact activities for beginners or people at higher risk for injury (such as older or overweight individuals). Examples of low-impact activities include walking, cycling, swimming, and some forms of dance. High-impact exercise activities include running, basketball, and vigorous dance (such as Zumba®).

The Importance of the Cool-Down

The **cool-down** is a 5- to 15-minute period of low-intensity exercise that immediately follows the primary conditioning period. For instance, a period of slow walking might be used as a cool-down following a running workout. A cool-down period lowers body temperature after exercise and allows blood to return from the muscles toward the heart (3–6). During exercise, large amounts of blood are pumped to the working muscles. Once exercise stops, blood tends to pool in large blood vessels (veins) that return blood from the exercised muscles to the heart. Failure to redistribute pooled blood after exercise could result in your feeling lightheaded or even fainting. You can prevent blood pooling after a workout by doing low-intensity exercise that uses the same muscles you used during the workout.

Personalizing Your Workout

Although the same general principles of exercise training apply to everyone, no two people are the same, so each person's exercise prescription will be slightly different. Your exercise prescription should be based on your general health, age, fitness status, musculoskeletal condition, and body composition.

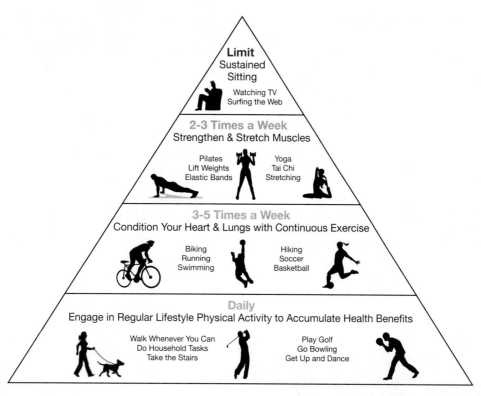

FIGURE 2.6 This physical activity and exercise pyramid shows examples of activities you can incorporate into your fitness program and daily life.

MAKE SURE YOU **KNOW...**

- The "dose" of exercise required to effectively promote physical fitness is called the exercise prescription.

- Components of the exercise prescription include fitness goals, type of exercise, the warm-up, the workout, and the cool-down. You can use the FITT principle (frequency, intensity, time, and type of exercise) in designing your fitness program.

- Exercise training programs should be individualized based on factors that include your age, health status, and fitness.

MasteringHealth™

Health Benefits of Exercise: How Much Is Enough?

 LO **3** Explain how much exercise is required to achieve health benefits.

Exercise training to improve sport performance differs from exercise performed to achieve health benefits. Exercise training for sport performance typically includes long workouts (60–180 minutes/day) involving high-intensity exercise. Components of skill- or sport-related fitness include balance, coordination, agility, speed, power, and reaction time.

In contrast, exercising to obtain health benefits does not require high intensity or long training sessions to produce results. In fact, any type of exercise or physical activity can be beneficial. Research reveals that too many hours spent sitting increases the risk for 34 different chronic diseases and conditions including type 2 diabetes, cardiovascular disease, and obesity (9). In fact, as discussed in Chapter 1, growing evidence suggests

frequency of exercise The number of times per week that one exercises.

intensity of exercise The amount of physiological stress or overload placed on the body during exercise.

time (duration) of exercise The amount of time invested in performing the primary workout.

type of exercise The specific type (mode) of exercise to be performed.

cool-down A 5- to 15-minute period of low-intensity exercise that immediately follows the primary conditioning period.

that prolonged sitting (>10 hours/day) may have more negative health risks than smoking (10, 11)! It follows that simply getting up from your chair and taking brief activity breaks will produce health benefits by reducing your risk of numerous diseases.

While even low levels of physical activity provide some health benefits, evidence indicates that moderate to high levels of physical activity are required to provide major health benefits (12–16). The theoretical relationship between physical activity and health benefits is illustrated in **FIGURE 2.7**. Note that the minimum level of exercise required to achieve some health benefits is the **threshold for health benefits**. Most experts believe that 30–60 minutes of moderate- to high-intensity exercise performed 3–5 days per week will surpass the threshold for health benefits and will reduce the risk of all causes of death (15–21). (See Laboratory 2.3 to determine whether you're engaging in enough physical activity to achieve health benefits.)

The U.S. government has provided physical activity guidelines for Americans. These guidelines recommend that adults ages 18–64 perform at least 150 minutes of moderate-intensity exercise or 75 minutes of vigorous-intensity aerobic physical activity per week (24). Fortunately, the activity doesn't need to be done all at once and can be divided into two to three segments of exercise throughout the day (18–25). If you walk briskly for 15 minutes to get to your class in the morning and then take a 15-minute bike ride in the afternoon, you've attained the goal of incorporating 30 minutes of moderate exercise into your day.

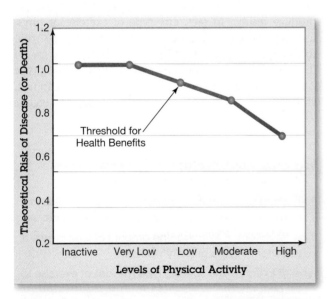

FIGURE 2.7 The relationship between physical activity and improved health benefits. Note that as the level of regular physical activity increases, the theoretical risk of disease (or death) decreases.
Source: Data from References 15, 26, 27.

Note that 30 minutes of moderate-intensity exercise may be insufficient to prevent weight gain in individuals who need additional exercise and calorie restriction to prevent fat gain. Also, although 30 minutes of exercise per day will result in health improvements, people are likely to achieve additional benefits if they exercise for longer periods of time (19, 24).

Are some forms of exercise better than others for obtaining health benefits? There is no short answer to this question. Nonetheless, numerous activities, including running, swimming, cycling, and walking, can improve your health.

MAKE SURE YOU **KNOW...**

- Although low levels of physical activity can provide some health benefits, moderate-to-high levels of physical activity are required to provide major health benefits.

- The threshold for health benefits is the minimum level of exercise required to achieve some health benefits.

MasteringHealth™

steps ▶ FOR BEHAVIOR CHANGE

Are you a couch potato?

Answer the following questions to find out whether you could use more daily physical activity.

Y   N

☐ ☐ Do you usually drive to your destinations, even for short trips to the corner store?

☐ ☐ Do you tend to take the elevator instead of the stairs?

☐ ☐ Does your evening routine involve hours of inactivity (e.g., sitting in front of the computer or television)?

☐ ☐ When you drive to a store for shopping, do you tend to park as close to the store entrance as possible?

☐ ☐ Do you always use a remote control to adjust the volume on your stereo or change the channel on your television?

If you answered "yes" to more than one question, you may be a bit too sedentary.

Tips to Incorporate More Physical Activity Into Your Daily Routine

Tomorrow, you will:

☑ Walk or ride your bike for short trips and errands; walk to class if you live close to or on campus.

☑ Get off the bus a stop early, and walk the rest of the way.

☑ Take the stairs instead of the elevator.

Within the next 2 weeks, you will:

☑ Go for a walk or a bike ride with a friend or family member instead of settling in to watch television after dinner.

By the end of the semester, you will:

☑ Forgo an hour of Internet time every day to walk the dog or play basketball or tennis with a friend.

Removing Barriers to Physical Activity

LO **4** List the four major barriers to physical activity and describe strategies that can be used to overcome each barrier.

Despite the many benefits of an active lifestyle, the level of physical activity remains low for most Americans. For example, the Centers for Disease Control and Prevention (CDC) reports that less than half of all adults engage in enough physical activity to produce health benefits according to the physical activity guidelines. Moreover, rates of physical activity vary across states and regions of the country. For example, residents of Southern states are more likely to be physically inactive compared to people in other regions. In general, men are more likely than women to meet the physical activity threshold for health benefits, and younger adults are more likely to be physically active than older adults.

There are four major barriers that contribute to this low level of exercise activity: lack of time, social and environmental influences, inadequate resources, and a lack of motivation/commitment. Without question, the most significant of these barriers is the lack of motivation and commitment to establish a regular exercise program. Completion of Laboratory 2.4 will assist you in identifying and overcoming your personal barriers to physical activity.

MAKE SURE YOU **KNOW...**

- Fewer than 50% of adults in the United States meet the required physical activity guidelines to achieve the threshold for health benefits.

- Barriers to physical activity include a lack of time, social and environmental influences, inadequate resources, and lack of motivation to participate in regular exercise.

MasteringHealth™

live it!

ASSESS YOURSELF

Assess your physical activity with the *How Much Do I Move?* Take Charge Of Your Health! Worksheet online at MasteringHealth™.

threshold for health benefits The minimum level of physical activity required to achieve some of the health benefits of exercise.

study plan

Customize your study plan—and master your health!—in the Study Area of **MasteringHealth.**

summary

hear it! STUDY REVIEW

To hear an MP3 Chapter Summary, scan here or visit the Study Area in MasteringHealth™.

LO 1
- Five key principles of exercise training are the overload principle, principle of progression, specificity of exercise, principle of recuperation, and reversibility of training effects.

- The overload principle (the most important principle of exercise training) states that to improve physical fitness, the body or muscle group used during exercise must be stressed.

- The principle of progression asserts that overload should be increased gradually during the course of a physical fitness program.

- The principle of specificity holds that exercise training is specific to those muscles involved in a given activity.

- The need for a rest period between exercise training sessions is called the principle of recuperation.

- Physical fitness can be lost due to inactivity; this is called the principle of reversibility.

LO 2
- The components of an exercise prescription include fitness goals, type of activity, a warm up, the workout, and a cool-down.

- The FITT principle defines the major components of the workout as **F**requency of exercise, **I**ntensity of exercise, **T**ime (duration) of exercise, and **T**ype of exercise.

- All exercise training programs should be tailored to meet the objectives of the individual, taking into consideration age, health and fitness status, musculoskeletal condition, and body composition.

LO 3
- The minimum level of physical activity required to achieve some of the health benefits of exercise is the threshold for health benefits.

LO 4
- There are four major barriers to performing physical activity: lack of time, social and environmental influences, inadequate resources, and a lack of motivation and commitment.

study questions

review it! QUIZZES

Find more review questions online at MasteringHealth™.

LO 1
1. Which of the following is NOT a key principle of exercise training?
   a. principle of specificity
   b. principle of progression
   c. principle of recuperation
   d. principle of overcompensation

2. Define overtraining and discuss how the principle of recuperation can prevent overtraining.

3. Define the overload principle and cite one practical example of how to apply this principle in exercise training.

4. What happens to physical fitness if you stop training?

LO 2
5. What are the main purposes of a warm-up and a cool-down?

6. What are the components of the exercise prescription?

7. How does the principle of progression apply to the exercise prescription?

8. Why should the exercise prescription be individualized?

LO 3
9. The current public health recommendation is for adults to achieve a minimum of _____ minutes of moderate-intensity physical activity each day.
   a. 15   c. 30
   b. 20   d. 60

10. Why is the threshold for health benefits an important concept?

LO 4
11. What are the major barriers that prevent people from engaging in physical activity?

12. List at least one strategy that has been shown to be effective in overcoming each of the four barriers to physical activity.

suggested reading

Blair, S. N. Physical inactivity: The biggest public health problem of the 21st century. *British Journal of Sports Medicine* 43:1–2, 2009.

Bushman, B. (Ed). *ACSM's Complete Guide to Fitness and Health*. Champaign, IL: Human Kinetics, 2011.

Howley, E., and D. Thompson. *Fitness Professional's Handbook*. Champaign, IL: Human Kinetics, 2012.

Murphy, M. H., S. N. Blair, and E. M. Murtagh. Accumulated versus continuous exercise for health benefit: A review of empirical studies. *Sports Medicine* 39:29–43, 2009.

Powell, K., A. Paluch, and S. Blair. Physical activity for health: What kind? How much? How intense? On top of what? *Annual Review of Public Health*. 32:349–395, 2011.

Powers, S., and E. Howley. *Exercise Physiology: Theory and Application to Fitness and Performance*, 9th ed. New York: McGraw Hill, 2015.

helpful weblinks

do it! WEBLINKS

For links to the organizations and websites listed, visit MasteringHealth™.

American College of Sports Medicine

Offers information about exercise, health, and fitness. **www.acsm.org**

American Heart Association

Provides the latest news and research about ways to reduce your risk of heart and vascular diseases. Includes information about exercise, diet, and heart disease. **www.heart.org**

Medline Plus

Contains up-to-date information on a variety of -health-related issues, including exercise and physical fitness. **www.nlm.nih.gov/medlineplus**

U.S. Department of Health and Human Services

Provides the *2008 Physical Activity Guidelines for Americans*. **www.health.gov/paguidelines**

WebMD

Gives the latest information on a variety of -health-related topics, including diet, exercise, and stress. Includes links to nutrition, fitness, and wellness topics. **www.webmd.com**

laboratory 2.1

do it! LABS
Complete Lab 2.1 online in the
study area of **MasteringHealth.com**

Name _____ Date _____

Warming Up

Use the following activities to warm up your body for aerobic activities such as jogging, walking, or cycling. Perform the stretching exercises slowly, holding each stretch for 20 to 30 seconds. Do not bounce or jerk the muscle. Do each stretch at least once and up to three times.

CARDIOVASCULAR WARM-UP
Walk briskly or jog slowly for 5 minutes.

STRETCHES

Calf Stretch for Gastrocnemius and Soleus
Stand with your right foot about 1 to 2 feet in front of your left foot, with both feet pointing forward. Keeping your left leg straight, lunge forward by bending your right knee and pushing your left heel backward. Hold this position. Then pull your left foot in slightly and bend your left knee. Shift your weight to your left leg and hold. Repeat this entire sequence with the left leg forward.

Scan to view a demonstration video of the calf stretch.

Sitting Toe Touch for Hamstrings
Sit on the ground with your right leg straight and your left leg tucked close to your body. Reach toward your outstretched right foot as far as possible with both hands. Repeat with the left leg.

Scan to view a demonstration video of the hamstring stretch.

Step Stretch for Quadriceps and Hip
Step forward and bend your front knee about 90 degrees, keeping your knee directly above your ankle. Lift and stretch the opposite leg backward so that it is parallel to the floor. Rotate your hips forward and slightly down to stretch. Your arms can be at your sides or resting on top of your forward thigh. Repeat on the other side.

Scan to view a demonstration video of the hip flexor stretch.

Leg Hug for the Hip and Back Extensors
Lie flat on your back with both legs straight. Bending your knees, bring your legs up to your torso, and grasp both legs behind the thighs. Pull both legs in to your chest and hold.

Scan to view a demonstration video of the knee-to-chest stretch.

Side Stretch for the Torso
Stand with feet shoulder-width apart, knees slightly bent, and pelvis tucked under. Raise one arm over your head, and bend sideways from the waist toward your lowered arm. Support your torso by placing the hand of your resting arm on your hip or thigh for support. Repeat on the other side.

Scan to view a demonstration video of the side stretch.

You can also repeat these same exercises after a workout to cool down.

1. Did you notice an increase in heart rate during the cardiovascular warm-up? _____

2. In which stretch did you feel the most tightness? _____

3. Do you think the sample warm-up is adequate for the activities you plan to do as part of your exercise program? If not, what exercises would you add?

_____

_____

laboratory 2.2

do it! LABS
Complete Lab 2.2 online in the
study area of **MasteringHealth.com**

Name _____ Date _____

Which Physical Activities Work Best for You?

As you design your personal fitness program, think about the activities you currently enjoy most and least and about new activities you would like to try. Which can you incorporate into your program?

Answer the following questions in the spaces provided.

1. List the fitness/wellness activities in which you have participated or are currently participating.

   _____

2. Which of these activities did you enjoy the most? Why?

   _____

3. What are some new activities you might enjoy? (See the list at the end of the lab for additional options.)

   _____

   _____

4. What components of physical fitness do you think these activities affect? For instance, jogging improves cardiovascular fitness, whereas weight lifting increases muscular strength.

   _____

   _____

5. What areas of physical fitness would you like to improve? Develop a list of exercise activities that will improve each area of physical fitness that you want to target.

   _____

   _____

EXAMPLES OF EXERCISE AND PHYSICAL ACTIVITY

- Walking or jogging on a treadmill
- Walking or cycling to work
- Cycling on an upright or recumbent exercise bike
- Walking, jogging, or cycling outdoors
- Zumba®, kickboxing class, or martial arts
- Weight or resistance training
- Yoga
- Pilates
- Hiking
- Rock climbing
- Elliptical trainer
- Sport activities (e.g., soccer, basketball, tennis, racquetball)

laboratory 2.3

do it! LABS
Complete Lab 2.3 online in the
study area of **MasteringHealth.com**

Name _____   Date _____

Using a Pedometer to Count Your Steps

One way to determine your level of daily physical activity is to use a pedometer to measure the number of steps you take in a day. A pedometer is a small portable device that contains a sensor and, often, software applications to estimate the distance walked and the number of calories expended. The accuracy of pedometers can vary from device to device, but many pedometers are reasonably accurate if they are worn in the optimal position (such as on a belt clip). However, carrying a pedometer in a pocket or handbag tends to reduce its accuracy. Moreover, some pedometers record movement other than walking (e.g., bending to tie your shoes), and therefore some "false steps" may show up on your daily step count.

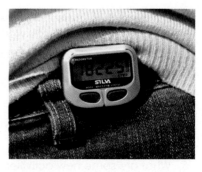

A pedometer worn at the waist.

Experts currently recommend 10,000 steps per day to reach a level of physical activity that is considered to be an active lifestyle with positive health benefits. Do you think you meet this goal?

DIRECTIONS:

Wear a pedometer for a day and note your number of steps. Write in the total number below. Then set a goal for the number of steps you want to take per day, and list some strategies for incorporating more steps into your day. Track the number of steps you take every day for the next 2 weeks, and note your progress toward your goal.

Goal number of steps/day: _____   **Number of steps for day 8:** _____

Number of steps for day 1: _____   **Number of steps for day 9:** _____

Number of steps for day 2: _____   **Number of steps for day 10:** _____

Number of steps for day 3: _____   **Number of steps for day 11:** _____

Number of steps for day 4: _____   **Number of steps for day 12:** _____

Number of steps for day 5: _____   **Number of steps for day 13:** _____

Number of steps for day 6: _____   **Number of steps for day 14:** _____

Number of steps for day 7: _____

ANALYSIS:

1. Did you meet your goal for number of daily steps on most days? Yes/No
2. Are you walking at least the recommended 10,000 steps per day? Yes/No
3. If not, think about how you can incorporate more steps into your daily routine. List below four ways to increase the amount of walking you do daily:

_____

_____

_____

_____

laboratory 2.4

do it! LABS
Complete Lab 2.4 online in the
study area of **MasteringHealth.com**

Name _____ Date _____

Identifying Barriers to Physical Activity

This lab will assist you in identifying the major barriers that prevent you from participating in regular physical activity and exercise. Listed below are the primary reasons why most people do not engage in regular physical activity and exercise. Please read each statement and select the number in the answer box that best applies to you. At the end of this exercise, add up the total number of points in each of the four major categories of barriers to physical activity.

BARRIER CATEGORY 1 ■ Lack of time

How likely are you to say this?	Unlikely	Likely	Very Likely
My day is too busy for exercise. I cannot find the time to include regular physical activity.	0	1	2
Physical activity takes too much time away from work and my family commitments.	0	1	3
My periods of free time during the day are too short to exercise.	0	1	3

BARRIER CATEGORY 2 ■ Social and environmental influences

How likely are you to say this?	Unlikely	Likely	Very Likely
None of my friends or family members are interested or involved in physical activity.	0	1	2
I am embarrassed to exercise in front of other people.	0	1	3
My school or place of work does not provide an environment that permits exercising.	0	1	3

BARRIER CATEGORY 3 ■ Lack of resources

How likely are you to say this?	Unlikely	Likely	Very Likely
I do not have access to walking/jogging trails, swimming pools, or bike paths.	0	1	2
It is too expensive to join a health club or purchase exercise equipment.	0	1	3
My school or place of work does not provide shower facilities or an exercise facility.	0	1	3

BARRIER CATEGORY 4 ■ Lack of motivation

How likely are you to say this?	Unlikely	Likely	Very Likely
I have been considering exercise but I can't seem to get started.	0	1	2
It is easy for me to find an excuse not to exercise.	0	1	3
I would like to exercise but I have difficulty sticking to a commitment.	0	1	3

SCORING AND USING YOUR RESULTS

Add up the total number of points scored in each of the four barrier categories and record your scores in the space provided below. If you scored 2 or more points in any category, this indicates that this category represents one of your major barriers to becoming physically active.

Barrier category 1. Lack of time: Total points = _____

Barrier category 2. Social and environmental influences: Total points = _____

Barrier category 3. Lack of resources: Total points = _____

Barrier category 4. Lack of motivation: Total points = _____

PLANNING YOUR NEXT STEPS

Now that you've identified your major barriers to becoming physically active, your next move is to develop strategies to remove each barrier. The chart below provides suggestions for strategies that can assist you in eliminating barriers.

Barrier	Suggestions for overcoming physical activity barriers
Lack of time	1. Identify available time slots in your day that could be used to exercise. 2. Select a time during your day to replace a sedentary activity with physical activity, such as riding a bike instead of driving. 3. Increase the length of your day to include a time slot for exercise.
Social and environmental influences	1. Encourage your family and friends to exercise. 2. Identify new friends who are already physically active, and make plans to exercise with them. 3. Plan social activities that involve exercise.
Lack of resources	1. Select activities that do not require expensive equipment, such as walking, calisthenics, or jumping rope. 2. Identify inexpensive exercise facilities that are available in your community (park and recreation programs, worksite programs, etc.) 3. Use commonplace areas to incorporate exercise, such as the stairs in your apartment building.
Lack of motivation	1. Write down your exercise goals and put them in a place where you see them every day. 2. Plan your day around a time to exercise. 3. Join an exercise class. 4. Pack a bag with your exercise clothes and place it somewhere you will see it before leaving for work or school.

In the space provided below, list your personal physical activity barriers that were not addressed earlier in this laboratory.

Personal barrier #1. _____

How will you remove this barrier? _____

Personal barrier #2. _____

How will you remove this barrier? _____

Personal barrier #3. _____

How will you remove this barrier? _____

Personal barrier #4. _____

How will you remove this barrier? _____

3

Cardiorespiratory Endurance: Assessment and Prescription

LEARNING OUTCOMES

1 Define *cardiorespiratory endurance* and $\dot{V}O_2$ *max* and explain the importance of $\dot{V}O_2$ max as a measure of cardiorespiratory endurance.

2 Name the major components of the cardiorespiratory system and describe their functions.

3 Explain how ATP is used for energy during exercise and identify the energy systems involved in the production of ATP for muscular contraction.

4 Discuss the roles and adaptations of the cardiovascular and respiratory systems during exercise and training and identify the major changes that occur in skeletal muscles and the cardiorespiratory system in response to aerobic training.

5 Explain the benefits of developing cardiorespiratory fitness.

6 Describe the common field tests used to measure a person's level of cardiorespiratory fitness by estimating $\dot{V}O_2$ max.

7 Outline the general components of an exercise prescription designed to improve cardiorespiratory fitness.

8 Develop an individualized exercise prescription for improving cardiorespiratory endurance.

9 List and describe several types of training used to improve cardiovascular fitness.

10 Present ideas for staying motivated and managing your time to include adequate amounts of aerobic exercise.

DEVELOPING cardiorespiratory endurance (also called cardiorespiratory fitness or aerobic fitness) is beneficial for a number of everyday activities. Walking or biking around your campus to get to class requires cardiorespiratory fitness. Other everyday activities, such as cleaning your dorm room or apartment, or carrying a full backpack, are easier when you have a higher level of cardiorespiratory fitness. Leisure time and social activities, such as a weekend hike, a camping trip with friends, or a night out dancing, are more enjoyable with higher cardiorespiratory fitness.

We discussed the health benefits of exercise and the general principles of exercise training in Chapters 1 and 2. In this and the next two chapters we describe how to assess your level of each health-related fitness component and show you how to design a comprehensive, scientifically based exercise program to meet your health and fitness goals. First, we'll define cardiorespiratory endurance and then discuss some basic cardiovascular physiology.

What Is Cardiorespiratory Endurance?

 LO **1** Define *cardiorespiratory endurance* and $\dot{V}O_2$ *max* and explain the importance of $\dot{V}O_2$ max as a measure of cardiorespiratory endurance.

Cardiorespiratory endurance is the ability to perform **aerobic exercise**, such as walking, swimming, jogging or cycling, for a prolonged period of time. It is effective in promoting increased energy availability, weight loss, and reducing the risk of cardiovascular disease. Because of this, many exercise scientists consider cardiorespiratory endurance the most important component of health-related physical fitness (1, 2).

The most valid measurement of cardiorespiratory fitness is $\dot{V}O_2$ **max**, or maximal aerobic capacity, which is the maximum amount of oxygen the body can take in and use during exercise. In simple terms, $\dot{V}O_2$ max is a measure of the endurance of both the cardiorespiratory system and the exercising skeletal muscles. (To see examples of VO2 max tests, go to www.topendsports.com and search for "$\dot{V}O2$ max tests.")

MAKE SURE YOU **KNOW...**

- Cardiorespiratory endurance is the ability to perform aerobic exercise for a prolonged period of time and is one of the most important health-related fitness components.

- $\dot{V}O_2$ max is a measure of cardiorespiratory endurance.

MasteringHealth™

The Cardiorespiratory System

 LO **2** Name the major components of the cardiorespiratory system and describe their functions.

The cardiorespiratory system is made up of the cardiovascular system (the heart and blood vessels) and the respiratory system (the lungs and muscles involved in respiration). Together these systems deliver oxygen and nutrients throughout the body and remove waste products (such as carbon dioxide) from tissues. Exercise challenges the cardiorespiratory system because it increases the demand for oxygen and nutrients in the working muscles.

The Cardiovascular System

The heart is a pump, about the size of your fist, that contracts and generates pressure to move blood through the blood vessels throughout the body. Actually, the heart is considered two pumps in one. The right side pumps oxygen-depleted (deoxygenated) blood to the lungs in a pathway called the **pulmonary circuit**, and the left side pumps oxygen-rich (oxygenated) blood to tissues throughout the body through a pathway called the **systemic circuit**. **FIGURE 3.1** (page 55) illustrates the path of blood through the heart and lungs.

There are different types of blood vessels in the circulatory system. With the exception of the pulmonary artery (which carries oxygen-depleted blood from the heart to the lungs), **arteries** carry oxygen-rich blood away from the heart to the rest of the body. Except for the pulmonary vein (which carries oxygen-rich blood from the lungs to the heart), **veins** carry oxygen-depleted blood from the body's tissues back to the heart.

consider this! //////////////////////

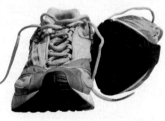

About 75% of college students use on-campus recreation centers, and students who work out the most have higher GPAs than their sedentary counterparts.

(*Sources:* National Intramural-Recreational Sports Association and Purdue University)

FIGURE 3.1 Blood flow though the cardiorespiratory system.

1. Oxygen-depleted blood enters the right side of the heart. Blood is pumped through the right atrium and ventricle and then to the lungs in the pulmonary circuit.
2. Blood gets oxygenated in the lungs and then goes back to the heart.
3. Blood enters the left side of the heart and is pumped through the left atrium and ventricle.
4. Blood leaves the heart through the aorta to be circulated throughout the body. This part of the system is the systemic circuit.

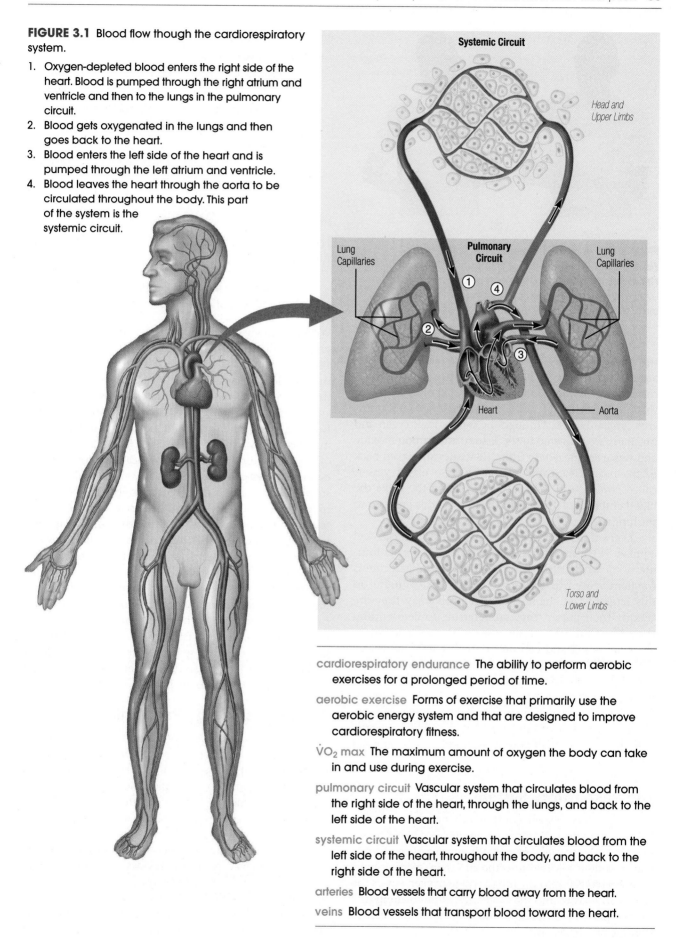

cardiorespiratory endurance The ability to perform aerobic exercises for a prolonged period of time.

aerobic exercise Forms of exercise that primarily use the aerobic energy system and that are designed to improve cardiorespiratory fitness.

$\dot{V}O_2$ max The maximum amount of oxygen the body can take in and use during exercise.

pulmonary circuit Vascular system that circulates blood from the right side of the heart, through the lungs, and back to the left side of the heart.

systemic circuit Vascular system that circulates blood from the left side of the heart, throughout the body, and back to the right side of the heart.

arteries Blood vessels that carry blood away from the heart.

veins Blood vessels that transport blood toward the heart.

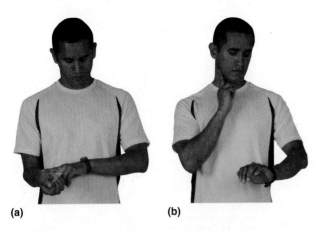

(a)   (b)

FIGURE 3.2 You can measure heart rate at either **(a)** the radial artery in the wrist just under the thumb or **(b)** the carotid artery in the neck below the jawline. See Laboratory 3.3 at the end of the chapter for detailed instructions and links to demonstration videos.

Blood is pumped from the left side of the heart into the aorta, the largest artery in the body. From the aorta, arteries branch into smaller vessels called *arterioles,* which further branch into **capillaries**. The capillaries have walls that are one cell thick, through which oxygen and nutrients can easily pass. Through the capillaries, oxygen and nutrients are delivered to the tissues, and carbon dioxide and waste are picked up from the tissues and taken back to the heart. The capillaries merge into bigger vessels called *venules,* and then into veins. From the veins the blood enters the right side of the heart and is pumped to the lungs.

Every time your heart pumps (beats), you can feel a pulse. The number of times your heart beats per minute is known as the **heart rate**. Measuring heart rate is frequently used to gauge exercise intensity (more on this later in the chapter). When people say they are "taking their pulse," they are referring to determining their heart rate. The easiest places to take your pulse are your radial and carotid arteries. The radial artery is located on the inside of your wrist just below your thumb, and the carotid artery can be found along the neck (see **FIGURE 3.2**). The amount of blood that is pumped with each heartbeat is called **stroke volume**. The product of heart rate and stroke volume is **cardiac output**, which is the amount of blood that is pumped per minute.

The Respiratory System

The respiratory system controls our breathing. In the lungs, carbon dioxide from oxygen-depleted blood passes into tiny air sacs called **alveoli**. When we exhale, the carbon dioxide is released into the air. Then, as we inhale, we bring oxygen into the lungs, where oxygen enters the alveoli and passes into the capillaries. From the lungs the oxygen-rich blood travels to the left side of the heart to start the process again.

How Do We Get Energy for Exercise?

LO Explain how ATP is used for energy during exercise and identify the energy systems involved in the production of ATP for muscular contraction.

We have discussed the importance of getting oxygen to the muscles and having energy for prolonged exercise. But, why is it important to get more oxygen to the muscles, and what do we mean by *energy*? Energy is the fuel needed to make the muscles move for activity, and we get that energy from the breakdown of food. However, food energy cannot be used directly by the muscles. Instead, the energy released from the breakdown of food is used to make a biochemical compound called **adenosine triphosphate (ATP)**. ATP is made and stored in small amounts in muscle and other cells. The breakdown of ATP releases energy that your muscles can use to contract and make you move and it is the only compound in the body that can provide this immediate source of energy. Therefore, for muscles to contract during exercise, a supply of ATP must be available.

The body uses two "systems" in muscle cells to produce ATP. One system does not require oxygen and is called the **anaerobic** (without oxygen) system. The second requires oxygen and is called the **aerobic** (with oxygen) system. The aerobic system is the primary system for developing cardiorespiratory endurance, which is why we need to get oxygen to the muscles.

Anaerobic Energy Production

Most of the anaerobic ATP production in muscle occurs during **glycolysis**, the process that breaks down carbohydrates in cells. In addition to ATP, glycolysis often results in the formation of **lactic acid**, and this pathway for ATP production is often called the *lactic acid system*. This system uses only carbohydrates as an energy source. Carbohydrates are supplied to muscles from blood sugar (glucose) and from muscle stores of glucose called *glycogen*.

The anaerobic pathway provides ATP at the beginning of exercise and for short-term (30–60 seconds) high-intensity exercise. Exercise that is intense and less than 2 minutes in duration, such as a 60- to 80-second 400-meter sprint, relies primarily on this system. During this type of intense exercise, muscles produce large amounts of lactic acid because the lactic acid system is operating at high speed.

Aerobic Energy Production

For exercise that lasts longer than a minute, anaerobic production of ATP begins to decrease, and aerobic production of ATP starts to increase. The aerobic system requires oxygen for the chemical reactions to make ATP. Activities of daily living and many types of exercise depend on ATP production from the aerobic system.

While the anaerobic system uses only carbohydrates as a fuel source, aerobic metabolism can use fats, carbohydrates, and protein to produce ATP, though for a healthy person who eats a balanced diet, proteins have a limited role during exercise—carbohydrates and fats are the primary sources. In general, at the beginning of exercise, carbohydrates are the main fuel broken down during aerobic ATP production. During prolonged exercise (longer than 20 minutes), there is a gradual shift from carbohydrates to fats as an energy source (see **FIGURE 3.3**).

The Energy Continuum

Although we often speak of aerobic versus anaerobic exercise, in reality many types of exercise use both systems. **FIGURE 3.4(a)** (page 58) illustrates the anaerobic-aerobic energy continuum as it relates to exercise duration. Anaerobic energy production is dominant during short-term exercise, and aerobic energy production predominates during long-term exercise. For example, a 100-meter dash uses anaerobic energy sources almost exclusively. At the other end of the energy spectrum, running a marathon uses mostly aerobic production of ATP, because the exercise involves 2 or more hours of continuous activity. Running a maximal-effort 800-meter race (in a period of

2-3 minutes) is an example of an exercise that uses almost an equal amount of aerobic and anaerobic energy sources.

FIGURE 3.4(b) (page 58) applies the anaerobic-aerobic energy continuum to various sports activities. Weight lifting, gymnastics, and wrestling are examples of sports that use anaerobic energy production almost exclusively. Boxing and skating (1,500 meters) require an equal contribution of anaerobic and aerobic energy production. During cross-country skiing and jogging, on the other hand, aerobic energy production dominates. To view a video that shows you how you can train the different energy systems, search www.youtube.com for "3-zone cardiorespiratory training using the ACE IFT model".

MAKE SURE YOU **KNOW...**

- ATP is used for energy during exercise.
- Anaerobic energy production does not require oxygen, uses carbohydrates for fuel, and supplies energy for short-term, high-intensity exercises.
- Aerobic energy production requires oxygen to make ATP; can use carbohydrates, fats, or proteins for fuel; and is used for longer-duration exercises.
- Many activities use both energy systems.

MasteringHealth™

capillaries Thin-walled vessels that permit the exchange of gases (oxygen and carbon dioxide) and nutrients between the blood and tissues.

heart rate The number of heart beats per minute.

stroke volume The amount of blood pumped per heartbeat (generally expressed in milliliters).

cardiac output The amount of blood the heart pumps per minute.

alveoli Tiny air sacs in the lungs that are the site of gas exchange.

adenosine triphosphate (ATP) A high-energy compound that is synthesized and stored in small quantities in muscle and other cells. The breakdown of ATP results in a release of energy that can be used to fuel muscular contraction.

anaerobic Without oxygen; in cells, pertains to biochemical pathways that do not require oxygen to produce energy.

aerobic With oxygen; in cells, pertains to biochemical pathways that use oxygen to produce energy.

glycolysis Process during which carbohydrates are broken down in cells. Much of the anaerobic ATP production in muscle cells occurs during glycolysis.

lactic acid By-product of glucose metabolism, produced primarily during intense exercise (greater than 50%–60% of maximal aerobic capacity).

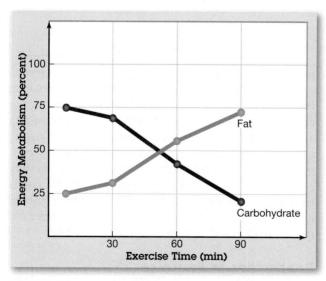

FIGURE 3.3 After about 60 minutes of exercise, the body begins to use more fat and fewer carbohydrates for ATP production.

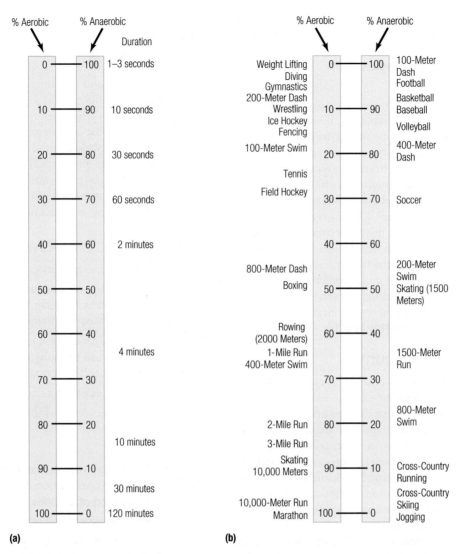

FIGURE 3.4 Contributions of aerobically and anaerobically produced ATP to energy metabolism during exercise. **(a)** Contributions as a function of exercise duration. **(b)** Contributions for various sports activities.

What Happens to the Cardiorespiratory System with Exercise and Training?

 LO **4** Discuss the roles and adaptations of the cardiovascular and respiratory systems during exercise and training and identify the major changes that occur in skeletal muscles and the cardiorespiratory system in response to aerobic training.

You have probably noticed that when you go for a run or spend more than a few minutes on an exercise bike, your heart rate increases and you start to sweat. These reactions are due to specific needs of your body during exercise.

During an exercise session and after a regular exercise program, your cardiorespiratory system undergoes several **responses** and **adaptations**. Responses are the changes that occur during and immediately after exercise. For example, your increased heart rate and heavy breathing after you walk up a hill are responses. Adaptations are the changes you will see if you stick with a regular exercise program. Your ability to walk up that hill without getting winded after a few weeks of regular aerobic exercise is the result of adaptations to the cardiorespiratory system. As the cardiorespiratory system gets stronger, it does not have to work as hard for the same level of exercise.

Responses to Exercise

When you exercise, active muscles need more oxygen and nutrients to maintain their activity, so your cardiac output has to increase. The elevated heart rate you experience during exercise contributes to the increased cardiac output. Increases in stroke volume also increase cardiac output, enabling your working muscles to get enough oxygen to produce energy. The arteries going to the working muscles dilate (expand) to deliver the increased blood and oxygen to the exercising muscles.

The respiratory system also has to respond to the demands of exercise by maintaining constant levels of oxygen and carbon dioxide in the blood. Exercise increases the amount of oxygen the body uses and the amount of carbon dioxide produced. Therefore, breathing rate increases to bring more oxygen into the body and to remove the carbon dioxide. As you exercise at higher intensities, breathing increases rapidly, enhancing the removal of carbon dioxide.

Adaptations to Exercise

Regular endurance exercise training results in adaptations in the cardiovascular, respiratory, skeletal muscle, and energy-producing systems.

Endurance training results in several adaptations in the cardiovascular system (3). One thing you may notice as your cardiorespiratory fitness level increases is that your resting heart rate decreases. This occurs because your heart is able to pump more blood per heartbeat, so it does not have to beat as many times per minute to get the same amount of blood throughout the body. The maximum number of times your heart beats per minute does not increase with aerobic exercise training, but your maximal stroke volume does, and as stroke volume increases, maximal cardiac output increases. Remember that cardiac output is the amount of blood that is pumped through the body per minute. Because the maximal amount of blood your heart can pump per minute increases, the maximal amount of oxygen you can use during exercise (your $\dot{V}O_2$ max) increases.

Aerobic exercise training does not alter the structure or function of the respiratory system, but it does increase the endurance of the muscles involved in the breathing process (3). The diaphragm, located below the lungs, and other key muscles of respiration can work harder and longer without fatigue. This improvement in respiratory muscle endurance may reduce the feeling of being out of breath during exercise and eliminate the pain in the side (often called a stitch) that people sometimes experience when beginning an aerobic exercise program.

Endurance training also increases the muscles' capacity to produce aerobic energy. The practical results of this adaptation are that the body is better able to use fat to produce energy and that muscular endurance increases (3). Note that these changes occur only in those muscles used for exercise or activity. For example, endurance training using a stationary exercise cycle results in improved muscular endurance in leg muscles, but it has little effect on arm muscles. Also, although endurance

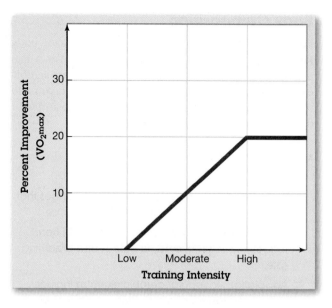

FIGURE 3.5 The relationship between training intensity and improvements in $\dot{V}O_2$ max following a 12-week training period.

training improves muscle tone, you will not see significant increases in muscle size or strength.

Recall that many exercise physiologists consider $\dot{V}O_2$ max the best single measure of cardiorespiratory fitness. Therefore, improved $\dot{V}O_2$ max is an important adaptation resulting from regular aerobic exercise training. In general, 12 to 15 weeks of endurance exercise produces a 10% to 30% improvement in $\dot{V}O_2$ max (3). This is the result of adaptations of the cardiorespiratory system, improved aerobic capacity of the aerobic muscles, and increased maximal cardiac output. The benefits of the increase are that your body can deliver and use more oxygen during exercise, muscular endurance improves, and you experience less fatigue during routine daily activities.

In general, a person who begins an aerobic exercise program with a low $\dot{V}O_2$ max will have greater increases than a person with a high $\dot{V}O_2$ max at the outset. The increase in $\dot{V}O_2$ max is directly related to the intensity of the training program, with high-intensity training programs producing greater increases than low-intensity and short-duration programs (4) (**FIGURE 3.5**). Note that poor nutritional habits will impede improvements in $\dot{V}O_2$ max.

responses Changes that occur during exercise to help you meet the demands of the exercise session. These changes return to normal levels shortly after the exercise session.

adaptations Semi permanent changes that occur over time with regular exercise. Adaptations can be reversed when a regular exercise program is stopped for an extended period of time.

Body Composition

Endurance training generally produces a loss of body fat and healthier body composition (3). However, a loss of body fat is not guaranteed. If you begin an aerobic exercise program with the goal of losing weight, you also need to consider the amount of exercise you do and your dietary habits.

MAKE SURE YOU **KNOW**...

- Responses are short-term changes that occur during exercise, and adaptations are changes that occur over time as a result of regular exercise.
- Responses to exercise include increases in heart rate, stroke volume, cardiac output, and breathing rate.
- Adaptations to regular aerobic exercise include decreased resting heart rate, increased stroke volume, improved ability to use fats for fuel, and improved body composition.

————— MasteringHealth ™

What Are the Health Benefits of Cardiorespiratory Endurance?

LO Explain the benefits of developing cardiorespiratory fitness.

Health and fitness are not the same, and there are differences between physical activity and exercise. Regular physical activity can lead to health improvements such as a reduced risk for heart disease even if you do not have a structured exercise program. However, without a structured program, you probably will not see significant changes in your cardiorespiratory endurance level.

Among the most significant health benefits of cardiorespiratory fitness are a lower risk of cardiovascular disease (CVD) and increased longevity. Also, people who exercise to improve their cardiorespiratory fitness have a reduced risk of type 2 diabetes, lower blood pressure, and increased bone density in weight-bearing bones (5).

In addition to physical health benefits, there are also psychological health benefits associated with regular aerobic exercise training, including a higher level of self-esteem and a more positive body image (6). This relationship is due to multiple factors. First, there is a sense of accomplishment that comes from starting and maintaining a regular exercise program and meeting personal goals. Regular exercise also improves muscle tone and helps with weight management, both of which can have a positive impact on appearance. Improved sleep quality is another psychological benefit of regular exercise (7). Fit individuals tend to sleep longer without interruptions (enjoy more restful sleep) than do less-fit people. A better

night's rest translates into a more complete feeling of being mentally restored.

Benefits of cardiorespiratory endurance also extend to activities of daily living. More energy for work and play is a commonly reported benefit; fit individuals can perform more work with less fatigue. People with high levels of cardiorespiratory fitness often say they exercise because it makes them feel better.

MAKE SURE YOU **KNOW**...

- Regular exercise is needed to improve your cardiorespiratory endurance.
- There are numerous physical and psychological health benefits of regular aerobic exercise, including reduced risk for CVD and type 2 diabetes, increased longevity, and improved self-esteem and body image.

————— MasteringHealth ™

Evaluation of Cardiorespiratory Endurance

LO Describe the common field tests used to measure a person's level of cardiorespiratory fitness by estimating $\dot{V}O_2$ max.

The most accurate means of measuring cardiorespiratory fitness is the laboratory assessment of $\dot{V}O_2$ max (3, 8). However, direct measurement of $\dot{V}O_2$ max requires expensive equipment and is very time-consuming, so it is not practical for general use. Fortunately, there are numerous field tests for estimating $\dot{V}O_2$ max (9–12). Each of these tests has a margin of error, but they are valid measures, and the practical advantages outweigh the disadvantages. This section will explain some of the common ways you can easily estimate your $\dot{V}O_2$ max, and you can use Laboratory 3.1A–D for this purpose.

One of the simplest and most accurate assessments of cardiorespiratory fitness is the **1.5-mile run test**. This test is based on the idea that people with a higher level of cardiorespiratory fitness can run 1.5 miles faster than those with a lower level (11).

The objective of the test is to complete a 1.5-mile run in the shortest possible time. Regular exercisers and people with active lifestyles can probably complete the 1.5-mile distance running or jogging. Because this test requires you to run the 1.5 miles as fast as you can, it is not the best option for sedentary people over age 30. Nor is it a good choice for people who have a very low fitness level due to medical reasons, for individuals with joint problems, or for obese individuals. For these less-active individuals, a walk test or cycle ergometer test is better suited. Laboratory 3.1A provides instructions for performing the 1.5-mile run test and recording the score.

The 1-mile walk test is another common field test to estimate cardiorespiratory fitness. The walk test is based on the same idea as the 1.5-mile run test: that people who have higher cardiorespiratory fitness will be able to complete the test faster than those with low cardiorespiratory fitness. This test is particularly good for sedentary individuals (12, 13). However, people with joint problems should consider a non-weight-bearing test, such as the cycle test described next. See Laboratory 3.1B for instructions on how to perform the 1-mile walk test and how to determine your score.

consider this! ///////////////////////

$\dot{V}O_2$ max begins to decrease around age 25 and decreases at a rate of about 1% per year, but athletes who train into their 80s maintain $\dot{V}O_2$ max levels near those seen in 20- to 30-year-olds (14).

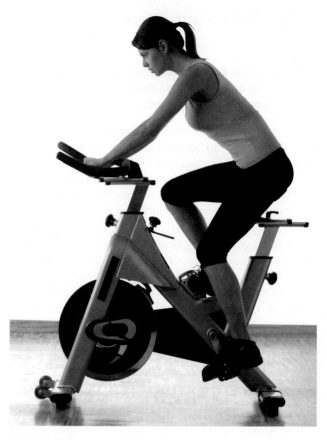

FIGURE 3.6 A cycle ergometer can be used to assess cardiorespiratory endurance.

Two other tests that can be used to assess your cardiorespiratory endurance are the cycle ergometer test and the step test. A **cycle ergometer** test (see **FIGURE 3.6** and to see examples of cycle ergometers, go to www.youtube.com and search for "cycle ergometers.") is ideal for people with joint problems because, unlike walking or jogging, it does not involve a weight-bearing activity. The cycle ergometer test is a submaximal cycle test based on the principle that individuals with high cardiorespiratory fitness levels have a lower exercise heart rate at a standard workload than less-fit individuals (9). You can use Laboratory 3.1C to estimate your $\dot{V}O_2$ max according to your heart rate and the workload used during the cycle ergometer test.

Finally, the step test (to see examples of the step test, go to www.youtube.com and search for "step test.") can be performed by people at all fitness levels. Additionally, this test does not require expensive equipment, and it can be performed in a short amount of time. However, the step test is not recommended for overweight individuals or for people with joint problems. The step test is based on the principle that your heart rate "recovers," or returns to resting levels, faster after exercise when you have a high level of cardiorespiratory fitness. Therefore, individuals with a higher cardiorespiratory fitness will have a lower heart rate during a 3-minute period immediately following the test

compared to less-fit individuals (3). Also, be aware that this test requires stepping at a consistent rate and accurately taking your heart rate multiple times, so there is more chance for error. You can use Laboratory 3.1D to perform the step test and to find the norms for step test results in a college-age population (18–25 years).

MAKE SURE YOU **KNOW...**

- Common tests to assess cardiorespiratory fitness include the 1.5-mile run, the 1-mile walk, the cycle ergometer test, and the step test.
- Obese individuals and people with joint problems should avoid weight-bearing cardiorespiratory assessment tests. Sedentary individuals should avoid the 1.5-mile run test.

—MasteringHealth™

1.5-mile run test One of the simplest and most accurate assessments of cardiorespiratory fitness.

cycle ergometer A stationary exercise cycle that provides pedaling resistance so the amount of work can be measured.

Designing Your Aerobic Exercise Program

 LO **7** Outline the general components of an exercise prescription designed to improve cardiorespiratory fitness.

Once you know your level of cardiorespiratory fitness, you can design an appropriate exercise plan to meet your goals. Setting goals and developing an action plan to meet long- and short-term goals are key to making healthy behavior changes. Starting and maintaining your aerobic exercise program will be much easier if you set goals first and then plan your program specifically to meet those goals. Many fitness experts agree that lack of goals is a major contributor to the high dropout rates seen in many organized fitness programs (15, 16).

Each exercise session will include the warm-up, workout, and cool-down phases (Chapter 2). Within the workout phase you need to consider the frequency, intensity, time, and type (mode) of exercise. Also, it is important to consider the stage of the program—the initial conditioning, progression, or maintenance phase.

The Warm-Up

Every workout should begin with a warm-up of 5 to 10 minutes of low-intensity exercise. Stretching can also be done prior to your workout but is most helpful in increasing flexibility if done after the workout. If you take a class such as step aerobics or spinning, your instructor will lead you through an appropriate warm-up. If you do other aerobic exercises, such as jogging or swimming, then you will need to plan your own warm-up. Typically, the warm-up will include a lower-intensity activity that is similar to or the same as your workout activity. For example, you might walk or jog as warm-up for a run or swim a couple of laps more slowly than you would for the rest of your swim workout. Then, as you start the workout phase, you will gradually increase your intensity to the desired level.

The Workout

The components of an exercise prescription to improve cardiovascular fitness include the components of the FITT principle: frequency, intensity, time (duration), and type (mode) of exercise.

Frequency The general recommendation for exercise frequency is 3 to 5 sessions per week to achieve near-optimal gains in cardiorespiratory fitness with minimal risk of injury. However, cardiorespiratory fitness gains can be achieved with as few as 2 exercise sessions per week (8). You typically will not see significantly greater improvements in your cardiorespiratory fitness if you exercise more than 5 days per week. Additionally, greater exercise

frequency entails a greater risk of injury, which generally is not offset by any added benefit of a greater frequency.

You might have to start with 2 or 3 days per week and increase the frequency as you progress through your program. You should also consider the amount of rest between exercise sessions. A general rule is to exercise no more than 3 days in a row and to rest no more than 3 days in a row, especially if you are doing the same exercise each session.

Intensity Cardiorespiratory fitness improves when the training intensity is at least 50% of $\dot{V}O_2$ max; this level is often called the **training threshold**. While training at exercise intensities close to $\dot{V}O_2$ max does produce an increase in fitness, it also increases risk for injury. Therefore, the recommended optimal range of exercise intensity for improving health-related physical fitness is between 50% and 85% $\dot{V}O_2$ max.

You cannot readily assess your percent $\dot{V}O_2$ max during exercise, but you can use heart rate to monitor exercise intensity. $\dot{V}O_2$ max and heart rate both increase linearly as exercise intensity increases. We also know that maximal heart rate is reached at $\dot{V}O_2$ max. This relationship, coupled with the fact that heart rate is easily monitored, makes monitoring heart rate a practical way to monitor exercise intensity.

How do you know what your heart rate should be during exercise? We can calculate a **target heart rate (THR)** range. **FIGURE 3.7** illustrates the pattern of heart rate during an exercise session. Because the tests we described to assess cardiorespiratory endurance are submaximal tests, we have to estimate maximal heart rate.

Before we explain how to determine your target heart rate range, let's discuss how to measure your heart rate.

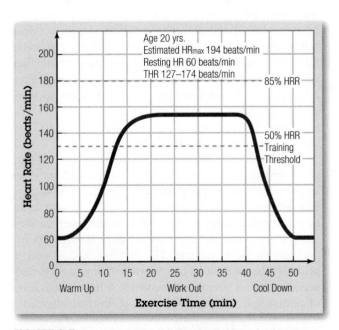

FIGURE 3.7 Sample workout in the target heart rate range.

Figure 3.2 (page 56) shows how to locate the radial (wrist) and carotid (neck) pulse, and Laboratory 3.3 provides the opportunity to practice monitoring your heart rate. When you find your pulse, make sure you use your index and middle finger. Do not use your thumb to take your pulse because it also has a pulse and you will not be able to distinguish between the two pulses for an accurate heart rate. If you are using the carotid pulse, be careful to press lightly on your neck. There is a receptor in the carotid artery that responds to changes in pressure, and too much pressure will make your heart rate slow down.

It is best to check your resting heart rate for 30 or 60 seconds when you are very relaxed (e.g., first thing in the morning). However, your heart rate drops quickly when you stop exercising, especially as your fitness level increases, so you should measure your exercise heart rate for a shorter time frame, 10 or 15 seconds. Laboratory 3.3 provides instructions for determining the number of beats per minute when you take your pulse for less than a full minute. See **TABLE 3.1** for the typical heart rate ranges.

Maximal heart rate (HR$_{max}$) decreases with age and can be estimated by this formula:

$$HR_{max} = 206.9 - (.67 \times \text{age in years})$$

For example, we can estimate a 20-year-old college student's maximal heart rate by the formula

$$HR_{max} = 206.9 - (.67 \times 20) = 194 \text{ bpm}$$

To determine your THR, we next have to determine your **heart rate reserve (HRR)**. Heart rate reserve is the difference between your maximal heart rate and resting heart rate:

$$HRR = HR_{max} - \text{resting HR}$$

Let's assume that our 20-year-old college student's resting heart rate is 60 beats per minute (bpm). Then,

$$HRR = 194 - 60 = 134 \text{ bpm}$$

After determining the HRR, we can calculate 50% and 85% of his HRR. These two heart rates will determine how far above his resting heart rate he needs to raise his heart rate to be exercising at the desired percentage of his $\dot{V}O_2$ max.

$$0.50 \times 134 = 67 \text{ bpm}$$

$$0.85 \times 134 = 114 \text{ bpm}$$

The final step in determining the THR is to add the resting heart rate back to the values just calculated. This step is done because the resting heart rate is the starting point. Our student's THR is calculated as follows:

$$67 + 60 = 127 \text{ bpm}$$
$$114 + 60 = 174 \text{ bpm}$$
$$THR = 127 - 174 \text{ bpm}$$

TABLE 3.1 ■ Heart Rate Classifications	
Heart Rate	Classification
<60 bpm	Bradycardia*
60 – 100 bpm	Normal range
>100 bpm	Tachycardia

*Many people, especially those who participate in regular aerobic exercise, have a resting heart rate below 60 bpm.

coaching corner

Limit Phone Time!

We are all becoming more and more dependent on our phones. In fact, for some people, smart phone use has become addictive. Recent research has shown that phones now occupy so much of our time that it is affecting our fitness levels. A recent study (17) reports that "high-frequency" phone users engaged in only 58% as much physical activity as "low-frequency" users!

Here are some strategies for managing your phone time:

- Limit phone use to certain times such as between classes, at lunch, etc.
- Use an app that tracks your usage such as Moment for iPhones and Joiku Phone Usage for Android devices. This "reality check" may help with time management.
- Choose activities that let you use your phone while exercising. You can easily ride a stationary bike or use a step machine while texting or surfing the web!
- Create a mobile phone "parking area" where you silence the phone (maybe while charging) during specific times such as while studying or driving.
- Don't sleep with your phone in easy reach. Sleep is critically important to your health, and if you constantly wake up to your phone, you are not getting the proper amount and type of sleep. If you place the phone far enough away so that you have to get up to check it, you are less likely to use it.

training threshold The training intensity above which there is an improvement in cardiorespiratory fitness. This intensity is approximately 50% of $\dot{V}O_2$ max.

target heart rate (THR) The range of heart rates that corresponds to an exercise intensity of approximately 50%–85% $\dot{V}O_2$ max. This range results in improvements in aerobic capacity.

heart rate reserve (HRR) The difference between the maximal heart rate and resting heart rate.

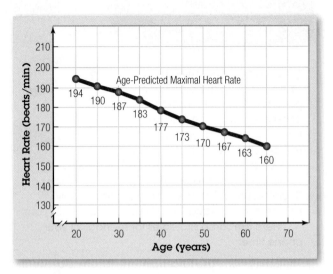

FIGURE 3.8 As you age, your maximal heart rate will decrease.

You can calculate your THR using Laboratory 3.3. Because your maximal heart rate decreases with age, your THR will change as you get older (**FIGURE 3.8**). Also, remember that a lower resting heart rate is an adaptation of aerobic exercise training. As you get older and see changes in your resting heart rate, you should recalculate your THR.

Another way to estimate exercise intensity is the **Borg Rating of Perceived Exertion (RPE)** scale (18). Perceived exertion is how hard you think you are working during exercise. To determine your RPE, take into consideration your efforts in breathing, how much you are sweating, and feelings in your muscles. Do not focus on just one of these aspects of your effort, but consider how they contribute to your overall effort. Because your heart rate increases as your exercise intensity increases, your perception of effort assessed using the RPE scale typically correlates with heart rate during exercise. The RPE scale is a 15-point scale, ranging from 6 to 20. Consider that a resting heart rate might be around 60 beats per minute and a maximal heart rate around 200 beats per minute. So, if you multiply your rating on the RPE scale by 10, it will likely be close to your exercise heart rate. To provide some guidance for using the scale, a value of 6 on the scale means that there is no level of exertion (e.g., standing on the treadmill before your run). Values in the range of 8–11 are common during the warm-up or cool-down phase of the workout. An RPE value between 12 and 16 will correspond with the target heart rate range for most people. Ratings of 12 to 14 are typical for moderate-intensity exercise, while 14 to 16 are common for vigorous-intensity workouts.

Time (Duration) Recall that the duration of exercise does not include the warm-up or cool-down. In general, exercise durations most effective in improving cardiorespiratory fitness are between 20 and 60 minutes (8).

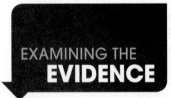

Continuous vs. Interval Training: Benefit vs. Safety?

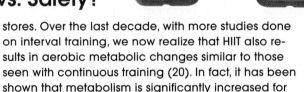

For many years, it was assumed that higher-intensity levels of training meant a higher probability for injuries. Thus, most professionals have guided fitness enthusiasts away from high-intensity workouts. It was also thought that high-intensity work resulted in a shorter total workout time and, therefore, less benefit than long, slow, distance workouts.

However, an accumulation of recent evidence suggests that we need to reexamine that concept. One study (19) concluded that high-intensity interval training (HIIT) results in cardiovascular adaptations that equal or exceed those found with continuous training. It was also shown that skeletal muscle aerobic adaptations to HIIT are equal to those seen with continuous training.

One of the most controversial aspects of the differences in these training methods has been the metabolic adaptations. While it has long been known that continuous training results in an increased ability to metabolize fats during exercise, it was thought that HIIT primarily worked to increase anaerobic energy stores. Over the last decade, with more studies done on interval training, we now realize that HIIT also results in aerobic metabolic changes similar to those seen with continuous training (20). In fact, it has been shown that metabolism is significantly increased for a prolonged period after HIIT!

Although there is the continued concern for increased possibility of injury with more intense exercise, if integrated slowly into your continuous, endurance exercise routine, it appears that it can be done with no increase in injury rate. Kuzy and Zielinski (19) also examined sprinters and long-distance runners and found no difference in injury to Achilles and patellar tendons between the groups. Thus, it appears that HIIT can be safely incorporated into the exercise routine of most individuals.

Interestingly, according to a recent survey of fitness professionals (21), the #1 exercise trend in the United States in 2014 was the use of HIIT as a substitute for or complement to continuous/endurance training.

The time you need to obtain your desired benefits will be specific to your initial level of fitness and your training intensity. For example, a poorly conditioned individual may see improvement in his cardiorespiratory endurance with 20 to 30 minutes of exercise 3 to 5 days per week at his THR. In contrast, a highly trained person may need regular exercise sessions of 40 to 60 minutes duration to improve cardiorespiratory fitness.

When determining your exercise duration, you also have to consider your exercise intensity. If you choose lower-intensity exercise rather than higher-intensity exercise, you will need to factor in a longer duration. For example, training at the lower end of your target heart rate range, around 50% of HRR, might require an exercise duration of 40 to 50 minutes to improve cardiorespiratory fitness. However, if you exercise at a moderate or higher intensity, such as 70% of HRR, you might see similar improvements with only 20 to 30 minutes.

Type Any type of aerobic activities that you enjoy enough to do consistently will help improve and maintain your cardiorespiratory fitness. Also, any activity that uses a large muscle mass (such as the legs) in a slow, rhythmic pattern can improve cardiorespiratory endurance. These activities can be performed for a length of time and at an intensity that will use the aerobic energy system. **TABLE 3.2** lists several activities that have been shown to improve cardiorespiratory fitness.

Because there are many exercises and activities that will improve your cardiorespiratory endurance, it is important to select activities you will enjoy. Another consideration is the risk of injury associated with high-impact activities, such as running. Listen to your body when it comes to choosing a high-impact exercise. If you experience joint pain or discomfort, you should see a health-care provider. You might need to find lower-impact exercises, such as swimming or cycling. Cross training, discussed later in the chapter, is another option to reduce your risk of injury if you enjoy a high-impact exercise. For an example of how to use the FITT principle in designing an exercise program, see **FIGURE 3.9**.

The Cool-Down

Every training session should conclude with a cool-down of light exercises and stretching. Allowing your cardiovascular system to slow down gradually is important: Stopping your workout abruptly can cause blood to pool in the arms and legs, which could result in dizziness, fainting, or both. A cool-down may also decrease the muscle soreness and cardiac irregularities that sometimes occur after a vigorous workout. Although cardiac irregularities are rare in healthy individuals, a cool-down period is still wise to minimize the risk.

A general cool-down of at least 5 minutes involving light exercise such as walking or a lighter intensity of your workout activity can be followed by 5 to 30 minutes

TABLE 3.2 ■ Exercises and Activities That Can Improve Cardiorespiratory Fitness and the Number of Calories Expended per 30-Minute Workout*

Activity	Calories Expended per 30 Minutes
Aerobics classes (moderate intensity step aerobics)	250–400
Bicycling (moderate intensity)	225–375
Bicycling (mountain biking)	250–400
Bicycling (stationary cycle—moderate intensity)	200–325
Circuit training	225–375
Cross-country skiing (moderate intensity)	250–400
Elliptical machine (moderate intensity)	250–400
Hiking	175–300
Rowing machine (moderate intensity)	200–350
Running (8.5-minute mile)	350–500
Skipping rope (moderate pace)	300–450
Soccer	215–350
Spinning classes (moderate intensity)	150–300
Swimming (fast, freestyle)	300–450
Walking (brisk; 3 mph)	150–250
Water aerobics	125–300
Wii Fit game	120–190
Zumba (moderate intensity)	250–400

*These numbers are estimates; the actual numbers will vary depending on body weight.

of flexibility exercises. If you take an exercise class, your instructor will lead you through the cool-down. In general, stretching exercises during the cool-down should focus on the muscles used during training. The type and duration of the stretching session depend on your flexibility goals. If you want to increase the flexibility of particular joints, you may choose to focus your stretching program mainly on those target areas.

Frequency	3–5 times per week
Intensity	50%–85% of HRR
Time	20–60 minutes per session
Type	Jogging

FIGURE 3.9 An example of the FITT principle for improving cardiorespiratory fitness.

Borg Rating of Perceived Exertion (RPE) A subjective way of estimating exercise intensity based on a scale of 6 to 20.

EXAMINING THE **EVIDENCE**

What Is CrossFit and Does It Work?

One of the latest trends in fitness programs is the incorporation of various activities performed at a high intensity into your routine. CrossFit, one such program, has become widely popular in recent years, with more than 10,000 affiliates worldwide. It is a training system that uses constantly varied, functional movements at relatively high intensity. It could be described as "high-intensity power training." CrossFit is also characterized as a community that develops when people perform these workouts together. The communal aspect is credited as being a key part of the program's success.

Is CrossFit effective in improving aerobic endurance and body composition? A recent study addressed this question (22). Researchers tested male and female subjects across a range of initial fitness levels and then trained them for 10 weeks using the CrossFit system. The study found that all subjects, no matter the initial fitness level, increased $\dot{V}O_2$ max by 12% to 14%. In addition, body fat decreased 13% to 19%. Thus, it appears that high-intensity power training can be an effective way to improve fitness and serve as a beneficial addition to your workout program. You can learn more at www.crossfit.com

MAKE SURE YOU **KNOW...**

- Establishing both short-term and long-term fitness goals is essential before beginning a fitness program.

- Each workout should include warm-up, workout, and cool-down phases.

- You need to consider the exercise frequency, intensity, time (duration), and type (mode) for the workout phase.

- Intensity can be monitored using the target heart rate range or Rating of Perceived Exertion.

- Aerobic exercise performed 3 to 5 days per week at 50%–85% of your heart rate reserve for 20–60 minutes is recommended to improve your cardiorespiratory endurance.

MasteringHealth™

Developing an Individualized Exercise Prescription

LO (8) **Develop an individualized exercise prescription for improving cardiorespiratory endurance.**

Anyone beginning a new aerobic exercise program, regardless of initial fitness level or exercise mode, will usually go through three stages: initial conditioning, improvement, and maintenance. In this section we will show you how you can individualize these stages to meet your specific needs and goals. You can use the sample programs for cardiorespiratory endurance on pages 71–73 and Laboratory 3.4 to design your aerobic exercise program.

live it!

ASSESS YOURSELF

Assess your fitness with the At-Home Fitness Test Take Charge of Your Health! Worksheet online in MasteringHealth™.

Initial Conditioning Phase

The initial conditioning stage is to your program what the warm-up is to your workout. Starting slowly will allow the body to adapt gradually to exercise and to avoid soreness, injury, and discouragement. Generally this stage lasts 4 weeks, but it can be as short as 2 weeks or as long as 6 weeks, depending on your initial fitness level (8). For example, if your cardiorespiratory fitness is poor, the initial conditioning stage will likely last closer to 6 weeks, but if you start at a relatively high cardiorespiratory fitness level, 2 weeks might be sufficient.

You should include 10- to 15-minute warm-up and cool-down phases with each workout. In the initial conditioning period of your workout, exercise intensity will be low, typically 40%–60% HRR or RPE of 11–13 (8). For people who have never been involved in a regular exercise program or who have very low fitness, the initial intensity might even be less than the 50% HRR we calculated earlier. It is acceptable to start at an intensity of 40%–50% HRR if that is comfortable for you (8). The duration of the session will likely be short. Initial sessions for a person with very low fitness might be as short as 10 to 15 minutes. At these intensity and duration levels, an exercise frequency of 3 or 4 days is ideal (8).

Here are some key points to remember for your initial conditioning stage:

- Start at an exercise intensity that is comfortable for you.

- Increase your training duration or intensity when you are comfortable, but do not increase intensity and duration at the same time. Gradually increase your duration, and then work on increasing the intensity. Your goal should be 20 to 30 minutes of continuous low to moderate (40%–60% HRR) activity at the end of the initial conditioning phase (8).

- Be aware of new aches or pains. Pain is a symptom of injury and indicates that the body needs rest to repair itself.

steps ▶ STEPS FOR BEHAVIOR CHANGE

How good is your level of cardiorespiratory fitness?

Answer the following questions to assess your level of cardiorespiratory fitness.

Y N

☐ ☐ Do you participate in recreational or competitive sports?

☐ ☐ Can you perform at least 20 minutes of continuous aerobic exercise?

☐ ☐ Can you do your regular household chores without getting out of breath (e.g., cleaning your apartment, walking your dog, mowing the lawn)?

☐ ☐ Can you walk across campus to your classes with little effort?

If you answered yes to three or more questions above, your cardiorespiratory fitness level is probably above average. If you answered yes only to the last two questions, or to none of the questions, you might need to make some improvements.

Tips to Become More Active

Tomorrow, you will:

☑ Take the stairs when possible.

☑ Walk to class instead of driving or taking the bus.

☑ Find a friend to take a walk with you.

Within the next 2 weeks, you will:

☑ Join a club or intramural sports team.

☑ Visit your campus recreation center for options for activity and exercise programs.

☑ Get a pedometer to see how many steps per day you walk. Fewer than 5000 per day indicates a sedentary lifestyle.

By the end of the semester, you will:

☑ Try at least three different types of aerobic activities.

☑ Participate in at least 30 minutes of moderate-intensity aerobic exercise at least 5 days per week.

Improvement Phase

The improvement phase can range from 12 to 40 weeks, and your program will progress more rapidly during this period than in the initial conditioning phase (8). Duration and frequency are increased first, and then the intensity is increased toward the upper end of the THR (60%–85% HRR or RPE of 13–16). The changes should be gradual, with increases in duration of no more than 20% per week until you can do 20 to 30 minutes at a moderate to vigorous intensity (8). Frequency of 3 to 4 days might still be appropriate, but if you want greater changes in your cardiorespiratory endurance, increasing to 5 days might be necessary. A general recommendation is to increase the intensity by no more than 5% of your HRR every sixth exercise session (8). If you are exercising 3 days per week, that means an increase every 2 weeks. As you can see, the changes are gradual, and you should not pressure yourself to make increases faster than you feel comfortable doing.

Maintenance Phase

The average college-age student will generally reach the maintenance phase of the exercise prescription after 16 to 28 weeks of training, but it might take longer for those who started at a low fitness level. In the maintenance stage, you have achieved your fitness goal, and your new goal is to maintain this level of fitness. You still need to exercise regularly, but you do not need to keep increasing all of the components of your exercise prescription.

Several studies have shown that the key factor in maintaining cardiorespiratory fitness is exercise intensity (4). If you keep your intensity at the same level you reached in the final weeks of the improvement phase, you can reduce your frequency. Exercising as few as 2 days

see it!

ABC VIDEOS

How do you keep your heart healthy? Watch the ABC Video "Exercise for Your Heart" at MasteringHealth™.

Don't Let a Disability Stop You!

A temporary or permanent disability can discourage you from exercising, but you can take comfort in knowing that even with most disabilities you can obtain all of the benefits of cardiovascular exercise. If you have an injury that temporarily keeps you from performing your exercise of choice, your physical therapist or physician can help you find suitable alternative exercises to maintain your fitness level. Consulting a physical therapist, physician, or exercise specialist for the best exercise options is also recommended if you have a permanent disability. Additionally, these health professionals will be able to make you aware of any medical complications associated with your disability and how you can address them.

In general, swimming and other water activities are excellent ways to decrease the need to support your body weight and safely exercise capable muscle groups. Other benefits of water exercise include the following:

- They pose little to no risk of falling.

- Flexibility exercises are much easier to do in water.

- Water provides resistance to capable muscle groups. This resistance enables you to progressively overload the intensity and improve the cardiorespiratory system.

- A variety of water aids, including hand paddles, pull-buoys, flotation belts, and kickboards, can be used to help maintain buoyancy and balance as well as help you work in the water.

Basic water safety rules still apply, so be sure to perform water activities with a workout partner or with a lifeguard present.

---

per week can still maintain your fitness level. If you keep to the same frequency and intensity as you achieved during the final weeks of the improvement phase, you can reduce duration to 20 to 25 minutes per session. However, if you hold frequency and duration constant, decreasing intensity by even one-third can significantly decrease your cardiorespiratory endurance. So if you keep up your exercise intensity, you can cut back the duration or frequency and keep your hard-earned benefits.

MAKE SURE YOU **KNOW...**

- Regardless of your initial fitness level, an exercise prescription to improve cardiorespiratory fitness has three phases: initial conditioning, improvement, and maintenance.

- Your exercise program should be tailored to your individual needs and should take into account your current fitness level.

MasteringHealth™

Training Techniques

LO **9** List and describe several types of training used to improve cardiovascular fitness.

Endurance training is a generic term that refers to any type of exercise aimed at improving cardiorespiratory endurance. However, there are numerous endurance training methods that you can use for this purpose. Most common is the use of a continuous activity, such as walking or jogging at a constant intensity. Cross training and interval training are two techniques for people who need some variety or want to make faster gains.

Cross Training

Cross training is the use of multiple training modes. To cross-train, you might take an aerobics class one day, run one day, and swim another day. Some people use cross training to reduce the boredom of performing the same kind of exercise day after day. Cross training also might reduce the risk and frequency of overuse injuries. However, cross training does not provide training specificity. Your cardiorespiratory endurance will improve, but jogging will not improve your swimming, because jogging does not train the arm muscles. Cross training might not be ideal if you are looking to improve your vability in a specific activity, but if you like variety and simply want to increase your cardiorespiratory fitness, it is a great option.

Interval Training

Interval training is typically used by athletes and others who are at a higher fitness level. This type of training includes repeated sessions, or intervals, of relatively intense exercise alternated with lower-intensity periods to rest or recover. Runners, swimmers, and cyclists use interval training to improve their times in competition. People exercising to improve fitness might use interval training to make more rapid increases in their exercise intensity during the improvement stage. Interval workouts are intense training sessions and should not be used on a daily basis; rather, they should be alternated with continuous moderate-intensity exercise sessions.

If you use a gym or other fitness facility, you know the convenience of having equipment such as weights, machines, bikes, treadmills, etc. as part of your fitness program. But some days it's hard to get to the gym, or you get there and then have to wait for access to the equipment. Bodyweight training is an option that can help during such times. Or you can use it to change up your routine. The idea of using the body's weight as resistance during exercise has been around for a long time in the form of calisthenics (think of military and sports team drills). Bodyweight training has had a recent resurgence—a 2014 survey of 3,400 fitness professionals (21) reported it as the #1 fitness trend.

With bodyweight exercises, increasing the number of repetitions will increase endurance, while strength improvements can only be made by increasing the exercise intensity. This is accomplished by changing the mechanics of the movement. For example, not only can you do push-ups with hands outside or inside the shoulder width, you can also do them from an elevated surface, which extends the range of motion for the shoulders and engages more muscle fibers.

The most common bodyweight exercises are push-ups, pull-ups, sit-ups, and squats/lunges. These are very basic exercises, and there are many possible variations and other exercises to try. Visit the Exercise Library at www.acefitness.org for variations of these exercises plus many more.

The duration of the intervals can vary, but a 1- to 5-minute duration is common. Each interval is followed by a rest period, which should be equal to or slightly longer than the interval. For example, if you are running 400-meter intervals on a track and it takes you approximately 90 seconds to complete each run, your rest period between efforts should be at least 90 seconds. An "active rest" period is recommended. If you are running, your rest would be an easy jog or brisk walk to prevent muscle tightness. You do not have to use a track for interval training. You can use a stop watch and do an interval workout anywhere you usually train.

MAKE SURE YOU KNOW...

- Cross training can prevent you from becoming bored with an exercise program and reduce your risk of injury.
- Interval training is used by athletes and more advanced exercisers to produce faster gains in cardiorespiratory endurance.

—MasteringHealth™

How Can You Get Motivated to Be Active?

LO **Present ideas for staying motivated and managing your time to include adequate amounts of aerobic exercise.**

Every year, millions of people make the decision to start an exercise program. Unfortunately, over half of those who begin such a program quit within the first 6 months (16). There are many reasons for this high dropout rate, but lack of time is the most commonly cited reason (16). Although finding time for exercise in a busy schedule is difficult, it is not impossible. The key is to schedule a regular time for exercise and to stick with it. A small investment in time to exercise can reap large improvements in fitness and health.

Think about how much time you have in a week and how much of that time is needed to improve your cardiorespiratory endurance. There are 168 hours in every week, and all you need is three 30-minute workouts to improve cardiorespiratory fitness. Of course, you need to add warm-ups, cool-downs, and showers, which still totals only about 3 hours per week. That leaves you with 165 hours per week to accomplish all of the other things you need to do. The bottom line is that with proper time management, anyone can find time to exercise.

Consider the strategies you learned for behavior change and apply them to your aerobic exercise program. Setting long- and short-term goals is important. Changes happen slowly, and short-term goals will help you monitor your progress to stay on track. Keeping a record of your training program will help you see the small changes that occur on the way to your long-term goal. Keeping your program enjoyable is also important. Exercising with a partner can make your workout more fun and maintain your commitment to a regular exercise routine. Just make sure you choose a partner who is committed and is a good exercise role model.

Finally, some discomfort and soreness is normal after your first several exercise sessions. Do not let these

---

cross training The use of a variety of activities for training the cardiorespiratory system.

interval training Type of training that includes repeated sessions or intervals of relatively intense exercise alternated with lower-intensity periods to rest or recover.

Do you like to exercise with a group? Do you like biking but find it hard to do around campus or in your city? Find a spinning class! Spinning is an aerobic exercise performed on stationary bikes in an indoor group ride led by an instructor. The bike is specially designed so you can quickly change the speed and resistance of pedaling. Being able to make quick changes enables you to mimic cycling

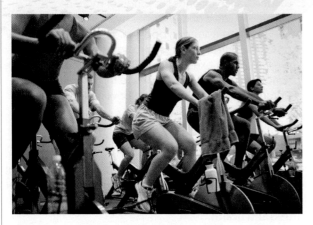

Cycling, whether outside or at the gym, is one popular type of exercise that will improve cardiorespiratory endurance.

Cycle Year-Round Indoors!

in outdoor settings, such as on a long country road or up a mountain. The spinning bikes also are designed to be much more comfortable than typical stationary bikes and feature multiple ways to adjust the seats and handlebars.

Spinning is led by an instructor, so you have the benefit of someone guiding you through your session. The instructor's direction is especially important if you are a beginner, because the instructor can tell you how to make the changes in intensity to fit your experience and fitness level. The classes usually last 30 to 60 minutes, have music for motivation, and use visualization techniques so you can feel as though you were cycling over hills and through valleys.

Spinning is an excellent exercise for improving cardiorespiratory endurance. You can burn up to 600 calories in an hour depending on the speed and resistance, and it is a low-impact activity that is easy on your joints. Additional benefits of spinning include a group setting for support and encouragement and an indoor setting so weather is not a barrier.

feelings discourage you. In a short time the soreness will fade, and the discomfort associated with exercise will disappear. As your fitness level improves, you will feel better and look better. Although reaching and maintaining a healthy level of cardiorespiratory fitness requires time and effort, the rewards are well worth the labor.

MAKE SURE YOU **KNOW...**

- You should apply behavior strategies (Chapter 1) to help maintain your new aerobic exercise program.
- Discomfort and soreness are normal with a new exercise routine but will last for only a brief period.

—— MasteringHealth™

Sample Exercise Prescriptions
for Cardiorespiratory Training

Scan to plan your individualized program for cardiorespiratory training.

Your exercise program should be tailored to your individual needs to meet the goals you set. An important consideration in designing a personal training program is your current fitness level. People with good or excellent cardiorespiratory fitness can start at a higher level and progress more rapidly than people with low cardiorespiratory endurance.

The sample cardiorespiratory training programs below present examples to get help get you started. (You can also use Laboratory 3.4 at the end of this chapter to develop your personal exercise prescription.) These programs are designed for college-age people with varying initial cardiorespiratory fitness levels. Note that in each program, the exercise duration and intensity increase as the program progresses. It is recommended to increase the exercise duration

first and then to increase the exercise intensity once you are comfortable with the new duration. Once you reach the maintenance phase, the exercise duration decreases. Research indicates that the benefits achieved during the improvement phase can be maintained with a shorter duration or with fewer days per week when the exercise intensity is maintained. So, in this example the frequency is increased and the duration is decreased.

The only component missing from this program example is the mode of exercise. That choice is up to you. Just make sure you are participating in aerobic exercise (e.g., waking, jogging, swimming, cycling), and that you select exercises that you will enjoy. To maximize benefits and reduce the risk for injury, you can follow the recommendation of "no more than 3 days on; no more than 3 days off." Also, keep in mind that you can break the workout up into smaller sessions of at least 10–15 minutes within the same day if time is an issue.

Beginner Cardiorespiratory Training Program

	Monday	Tuesday	Wednesday	Thursday	Friday	Saturday	Sunday
			Initial Conditioning				
Week 1	10 min		10 min		10 min		
Week 2	10 min		10 min		10 min		
Week 3	12 min		12 min		12 min		
Week 4	12 min		12 min		12 min		
Week 5	15 min		15 min		15 min		
Week 6	15 min		15 min		15 min		
			Improvement				
Week 7	20 min		20 min		20 min		
Week 8	20 min		20 min		20 min		
Week 9	25 min		25 min		25 min		
Week 10	25 min		25 min		25 min		
Week 11	30 min		30 min		30 min		
Week 12	30 min		30 min		30 min		
Week 13	35 min		35 min		35 min		
Week 14	35 min		35 min		35 min		
Week 15	40 min		40 min		40 min		
Week 16	40 min		40 min		40 min		
Week 17	40 min		40 min		40 min		
Week 18	40 min		40 min		40 min		
			Maintenance				
Week 19	40 min		40 min		40 min		
Week 20	40 min		40 min		40 min		30 min
Week 21	40 min		40 min		40 min		30 min
Week 22	30 min		30 min		30 min		30 min
Week 23	30 min		30 min		30 min		30 min
Week 24	30 min		30 min		30 min		30 min
Week 25	30 min		30 min		30 min		30 min
Week 26	30 min		30 min		30 min		30 min

Intensity Key
60% of HRR
70% of HRR
75% of HRR

Intermediate Cardiorespiratory Training Program

	Monday	Tuesday	Wednesday	Thursday	Friday	Saturday	Sunday
			Initial Conditioning				
Week 1	10 min		10 min		10 min		
Week 2	15 min		15 min		15 min		
Week 3	15 min		15 min		15 min		
Week 4	20 min		20 min		20 min		
			Improvement				
Week 5	25 min		25 min		25 min		
Week 6	25 min		25 min		25 min		
Week 7	25 min		25 min		25 min		
Week 8	30 min		30 min		30 min		
Week 9	30 min		30 min		30 min		
Week 10	35 min		35 min		35 min		
Week 11	35 min		35 min		35 min		
Week 12	40 min		35 min		40 min		
Week 13	40 min		35 min		40 min		
Week 14	40 min		35 min		40 min		
Week 15	40 min		40 min		40 min		
Week 16	40 min		40 min		40 min		30 min
Week 17	40 min		40 min		40 min		30 min
Week 18	40 min		40 min		40 min		30 min
			Maintenance				
Week 19	30 min		30 min		30 min		30 min
Week 20	30 min		30 min		30 min		30 min
Week 21	30 min		30 min		30 min		30 min
Week 22	30 min		30 min		30 min		30 min

Intensity Key
70% of HRR
75% of HRR
80% of HRR

Advanced Cardiorespiratory Training Program

	Monday	Tuesday	Wednesday	Thursday	Friday	Saturday	Sunday
Initial Conditioning							
Week 1	15 min		15 min		15 min		
Week 2	20 min		20 min		20 min		
Improvement							
Week 3	25 min		25 min		25 min		
Week 4	30 min		30 min		30 min		
Week 5	35 min		35 min		35 min		
Week 6	40 min		40 min		40 min		40 min
Week 7	40 min		40 min		40 min		40 min
Week 8	40 min		40 min		40 min		40 min
Week 9	40 min		40 min		40 min		40 min
Week 10	40 min		40 min		40 min		40 min
Week 11	40 min		40 min		40 min		40 min
Week 12	40 min		40 min		40 min		40 min
Week 13	40 min		40 min		40 min		40 min
Week 14	40 min		40 min		40 min		40 min
Maintenance							
Week 15	30 min		30 min		30 min		30 min
Week 16	30 min		30 min		30 min		30 min
Week 17	30 min		30 min		30 min		30 min
Week 18	30 min		30 min		30 min		30 min

Intensity Key
75% of HRR
80% of HRR
80%–85% of HRR

study plan
Customize your study plan—and master your health!—in the Study Area of **MasteringHealth.**

summary

 hear it! STUDY REVIEW
To hear an MP3 Chapter Summary, scan here or visit the Study Area in MasteringHealth™.

LO ①
- Cardiorespiratory endurance is the ability to perform aerobic exercise for a prolonged period of time.

- Many exercise physiologists consider $\dot{V}O_2$ max (the maximum capacity of the cardiorespiratory system to transport and use oxygen during exercise) to be the most valid measurement of cardiorespiratory endurance.

LO ②
- The term *cardiorespiratory system* refers to the cooperative work of the cardiovascular and respiratory systems. The primary function of the cardiovascular system is to transport blood carrying oxygen and nutrients to body tissues. The principal function of the respiratory system is to load oxygen into and remove carbon dioxide from the blood.

LO ③ ■ Adenosine triphosphate (ATP) provides the energy muscles need to move. It is produced by two systems: anaerobic (without oxygen) and aerobic (with oxygen).

■ Anaerobic energy production is the primary source of energy for short-term exercise, and aerobic energy production dominates during prolonged exercise.

LO ④ ■ Responses to exercise are the short-term changes that occur during exercise to meet the immediate demands of exercise. Adaptations are developed over the long term through regular exercise training and will persist if you continue your exercise program.

■ Cardiac output, stroke volume, and heart rate increase as a function of exercise intensity. Breathing rate also increases in proportion to exercise intensity.

LO ⑤ ■ Benefits of cardiorespiratory fitness include a lower risk of disease, feeling better, increased capacity to perform everyday tasks, and improved self-esteem and body image.

LO ⑥ ■ There are many field tests that can be used to estimate $\dot{V}O_2$ max using little or no equipment. These include the 1.5-mile run, the 1-mile walk, the cycle ergometer test, and the step test.

LO ⑦ ■ Setting short-term and long-term fitness goals is an essential first step in beginning a fitness program.

■ The exercise prescription incorporates the warm-up, workout (primary conditioning period), and cool-down. The components of the workout are the frequency, intensity, time (duration), and type (mode) of exercise (FITT).

■ The FITT principle for improving cardiorespiratory endurance calls for a type of exercise that uses large-muscle groups in a slow, rhythmic pattern for 20 to 60 minutes, 3 to 5 times per week.

■ Target heart rate is the range of exercise heart rates between 50% and 85% of heart rate reserve.

LO ⑧ ■ Regardless of your initial fitness level, an exercise prescription for improving cardiorespiratory fitness has three phases: initial conditioning, improvement, and maintenance.

LO ⑨ ■ Cross training and interval training provide alternatives to a continuous workout of the same mode. Cross training can be done by individuals of all fitness levels, but interval training is for those who are more experienced with exercise.

LO ⑩ ■ Maintaining a regular exercise routine requires good time management and choosing physical activities that you enjoy.

study questions

review it! QUIZZES

Find more review questions online in MasteringHealth™.

LO ① 1. Which of the following is *not* an example of aerobic exercise?

    a. running
    b. swimming
    c. abdominal toning class
    d. spinning class

LO ② 2. _____ are the blood vessels that take blood away from the heart.

    a. Arteries   c. Capillaries
    b. Veins   d. Venules

3. What is meant by the term *cardiorespiratory system*?

4. List the major functions of the circulatory and respiratory systems.

5. Why is the heart considered "two pumps in one"?

LO ③ 6. Define *adenosine triphosphate (ATP)*.

7. The anaerobic energy pathway is predominantly responsible for production of ATP during which of the following activities?

    a. wrestling   c. 400-meter swim
    b. 800-meter run   d. 30-minute brisk walk

LO ④ 8. _____ is an adaptation resulting from a regular aerobic exercise program.

    a. Lower maximal heart rate
    b. Lower resting heart rate
    c. Faster breathing rate
    d. All of the above

9. _____ is a response during exercise.

    a. Faster heart rate
    b. Increased cardiac output
    c. Faster breathing
    d. All of the above

LO ⑤ 10. List four benefits of an increase in cardiorespiratory endurance.

LO ⑥ 11. Cardiorespiratory fitness is measured in field tests that determine a person's

    a. HR_{max} c. HRR
    b. $\dot{V}O_2$ max   d. THR

LO 12. Exercise intensity should be at least _____% of heart rate reserve to improve cardiorespiratory endurance.

a. 85   c. 50
b. 70   d. 25

LO 8 13. What are the three phases of the exercise prescription for improving cardiorespiratory fitness?

LO 14. Explain the difference between cross training and interval training.

LO 10 15. Why is time management so important in staying motivated to maintain a regular exercise routine?

suggested reading

Blair, S. N., M. J. LaMonte, and M. Z. Nichaman. The evolution of physical activity recommendations: How much is enough? *American Journal of Clinical Nutrition* 79(5):913S–920S, 2004.

Brisswalter J., M. Collardeau, and A. Rene. Effects of acute physical exercise characteristics on cognitive performance. *Sports Medicine* 32(9):555–566, 2002.

Chobanian, A. V., G. L. Bakris, H. R. Black, W. C. Cushman, L. A. Green, J. L. Izzo Jr., D. W. Jones, B. J. Materson, S. Oparil, J. T. Wright Jr., and E. J. Roccella. National Heart, Lung, and Blood Institute Joint National Committee on Prevention, Detection, Evaluation, and Treatment of High Blood Pressure; National High Blood Pressure Education Program Coordinating Committee. The seventh report of the Joint National Committee on Prevention, Detection, Evaluation, and Treatment of High Blood Pressure: The JNC 7 report. *Journal of the American Medical Association* 289(19):2560–2572, 2003.

Haskell, W. L., et al. Physical activity and public health: Updated recommendation for adults from the American College of Sports Medicine and the American Heart Association. *Medicine and Science in Sports and Exercise* 39:1423–1434, 2007.

Pollock, M. L., and J. H. Wilmore. *Exercise in Health and Disease*, 3rd ed. Philadelphia: W. B. Saunders, 1998.

Powers, S., and E. Howley. *Exercise Physiology: Theory and Application to Fitness and Performance,* 9th ed. New York: McGraw-Hill, 2015.

Rahl, R. L. *Physical Activity and Health Guidelines.* Champaign, IL: Human Kinetics, 2010.

Robertson, R. *Perceived Exertion for Practitioners: Rating Effort with the OMNI Picture System.* Champaign, IL: Human Kinetics, 2004.

Spriet, L. L., and M. J. Gibala. Nutritional strategies to influence adaptations to training. *Journal of Sports Science* 22(1):127–141, 2004.

Warburton, D. E., N. Gledhill, and A. Quinney. Musculoskeletal fitness and health. Canadian Journal of Applied Physiology 26(2):217–237, 2001.

helpful weblinks

do it! WEBLINKS

For links to the organizations and websites listed, go online to MasteringHealth™.

American College of Sports Medicine

Comprehensive website providing information, equipment recommendations, how-to articles, books, and position statements about all aspects of health and fitness. **www.acsm.org**

Everyday Health Fitness

Offers information on injury prevention and treatment, weight training, flexibility, exercise prescriptions, and more. **www.everydayhealth.com** and **www.everydayhealth.com/fitness/articles.aspx**

The Running Page

Contains information about racing, running clubs, places to run, running-related products, magazines, and treating running injuries. **www.runningpage.com**

WebMD

General information about exercise, fitness, and wellness. Great articles, instructional information, and updates. **www.webmd.com**

laboratory 3.1A

do it! LABS
Complete Lab 3.1A online in the
study area of **MasteringHealth.com**

Name _____   Date _____

Measuring Cardiorespiratory Fitness: The 1.5-Mile Run Test

The objective of this test is to complete the 1.5-mile distance as quickly as possible. You can complete the run on an oval track or on any properly measured course. If the run will take place outside, the test is best conducted in moderate weather conditions; avoid running it on very hot or very cold days. A good strategy is to try to keep a steady pace over the entire distance. Performing a practice test is a good way to get familiar with the distance and determine the ideal pace you can maintain. You should use a stopwatch to get an accurate time. You should attempt this test only if you have met the medical clearance criteria (discussed in Chapter 1).

Before the test, perform a 5- to 10-minute warm-up. If you become extremely fatigued during the test, slow your pace or walk—do not overstress yourself! If you feel faint or nauseated or experience any unusual pains in your upper body, stop and notify your instructor.

After you complete the test, cool down and record your time and fitness category from **TABLE 3.3** included in this lab. Locate your time range according to your sex and age group. The fitness classifications are along the top of the table.

Test date: _____   **Finish time:** _____   **Fitness category:** _____

1. Is your fitness classification what you expected based on your current level of activity? If not, why do you think it was higher or lower than expected?

    _____

    _____

2. Write fitness goals for maintaining or improving your cardiorespiratory endurance.

    _____

    _____

TABLE 3.3 ■ Fitness Categories for Cooper's 1.5-Mile Run Test

Estimated Run Time Ratings				
Men	**Excellent**	**Good**	**Fair**	**Poor**
20–29 yrs	<10:10	10:10–11:29	11:30–12:38	>12:38
30–39 yrs	<10:47	10:47–11:54	11:55–12:58	>12:58
40–49 yrs	<11:16	11:16–12:24	12:25–13:50	>13:50
50–59 yrs	<12:09	12:09–13:35	13:36–15:06	>15:06
60–69 yrs	<13:24	13:24–15:04	15:05–16:46	>16.46
Women	**Excellent**	**Good**	**Fair**	**Poor**
20–29 yrs	<11:59	11:59–13:24	13:25–14:50	>14:50
30–39 yrs	<12:25	12:25–14:08	14:09–15:43	>15:43
40–49 yrs	<13:34	13:24–14:53	14:54–16:31	>16:31
50–59 yrs	<14:35	14:35–16:35	16:36–18:18	>18:18
60–69 yrs	<16:34	16:34–18:27	18:28–20:16	>20:16

Source: Reprinted with permission from The Cooper Institute®, Dallas, Texas, from a book called *Physical Fitness Assessments and Norms for Adults and Law Enforcement.* Available online at www.CooperInstitute.org.

laboratory 3.1B

do it! LABS
Complete Lab 3.1B online in the
study area of **MasteringHealth.com**

Name _____ Date _____

Measuring Cardiorespiratory Fitness: The 1-Mile Walk Test

The objective of this test is to walk the 1-mile distance as quickly as possible. You can complete the walk on an oval track or on any properly measured course. You should attempt this test only if you have met the medical clearance criteria (discussed in Chapter 1).

Before the test, perform a 5- to 10-minute warm-up. If you become extremely fatigued during the test, slow your pace—do not overstress yourself! If you feel faint or nauseated or experience any unusual pains in your upper body, stop and notify your instructor.

After you complete the test, cool down and record your time and fitness category from **TABLE 3.4** included in this lab. Locate your time range according to your sex and age group. The fitness classifications are along the top of the table.

Test date: _____

Finish time: _____

Fitness category: _____

1. Is your fitness classification what you expected based on your current level of activity? If not, why do you think it was higher or lower than expected?

   _____

   _____

2. Write fitness goals for maintaining or improving your cardiorespiratory endurance.

   _____

   _____

TABLE 3.4 ■ Fitness Classification for 1-Mile Walk Test

Men	Excellent	Good	Average	Poor	Very Poor
13–19 yrs	<12:30	12:30–14:00	14:01–16:00	16:01–17:30	>17:30
20–29 yrs	<13:00	13:00–14:30	14:31–16:30	16:31–18:00	>18:00
30–39 yrs	<13:30	13:30–15:30	15:31–17:30	17:31–19:00	>19:00
40+ yrs	<14:00	14:00–16:00	16:01–18:30	18:31–21:30	>21:30
Women	**Excellent**	**Good**	**Average**	**Poor**	**Very Poor**
13–19 yrs	<13:30	13:30–14:30	14:31–16:30	16:31–18:00	>18:00
20–29 yrs	<13:30	13:30–15:00	15:01–17:00	17:01–18:30	>18:30
30–39 yrs	<14:00	14:00–16:00	16:01–18:00	18:01–19:30	>19:30
40+ yrs	<14:30	14:30–18:00	18:01–19:30	19:31–20:00	>20:00

Because the 1-mile walk test is designed primarily for older or less-conditioned individuals, the fitness categories listed here do not include a "superior" category.

Source: From Rockport Fitness Walking Test. Copyright © 1993 The Rockport Company, Inc.

laboratory 3.1C

do it! LABS
Complete Lab 3.1C online in the
study area of **MasteringHealth.com**

Name _____   Date _____

Measuring Cardiorespiratory Fitness: Submaximal Cycle Test

This test is performed with a partner. While you are exercising, your partner will help by setting the workload for the test, checking your pedal rate, and taking your heart rate. The work performed on a cycle ergometer is commonly expressed either in *kilopond meters per minute (KPM)* or in watts. Your instructor will explain how to use the KPM and watts settings to adjust the workload.

Warm up for 3 minutes without using any resistance (unloaded pedaling). Your instructor will tell you how to adjust the workload. Set the appropriate load for your age, sex, and level of conditioning (**TABLE 3.5**), and begin pedaling at the rate of 50 revolutions per minute (RPM). Your instructor will set a metronome so you know how fast to pedal. Exercise for a 5-minute period. Your partner will take your heart rate during a 15-second period between minutes 4.5 and 5 of the test.

Cool down for 3 to 5 minutes without resistance. Record your heart rate (15-second count) below, and calculate your relative $\dot{V}O_2$ max using **TABLE 3.6** (page 79). After calculating your relative $\dot{V}O_2$ max locate your fitness category in **TABLE 3.7** (page 79).

Test date: _____

Heart rate (15-second count) during minute 5 of test: _____

Fitness category: _____

1. Is your fitness classification what you expected based on your current level of activity? If not, why do you think it was higher or lower than expected?

   _____

   _____

2. Write fitness goals for maintaining or improving your cardiorespiratory endurance.

   _____

   _____

To calculate your relative $\dot{V}O_2$ max using Table 3.6, locate your 15-second heart rate in the left-hand column; then find your estimated $\dot{V}O_2$ max in the appropriate column on the right. For example, the second column from the left contains the absolute $\dot{V}O_2$ max (expressed in mL/min) for male subjects using the 900-KPM work rate. The third column from the left contains the absolute $\dot{V}O_2$ max (expressed in mL/min) for women using the 600-KPM work rate, and so on. After determining your absolute $\dot{V}O_2$ max, calculate your relative $\dot{V}O_2$ max (mL/kg/min) by dividing your $\dot{V}O_2$ max expressed in mL/min by your body weight in kilograms (1 kilogram = 2.2 pounds). For example, if your body weight is 70 kilograms and your absolute $\dot{V}O_2$ max is 2631 mL/min, your relative $\dot{V}O_2$ max is approximately 38 mL/kg/min ($2631 \div 70 = 37.6$). After computing your relative $\dot{V}O_2$ max, use Table 3.7 to identify your fitness category.

TABLE 3.5 ■ Work Rates for Submaximal Cycle Ergometer Fitness Test

Men	Pedal Speed (RPM)	Load (watts)	Load (kilopond meters)
Up to 29 yrs	50	150	900
30 yrs or above	50	50	300
Women	**Pedal Speed (RPM)**	**Load (watts)**	**Load (kilopond meters)**
Up to 29 yrs (or well conditioned)	50	100	600
30 yrs or above (or poorly conditioned)	50	50	300

TABLE 3.6 ■ Cycle Ergometer Fitness Index for Men and Women

15-Second Heart Rate	Estimated Absolute $\dot{V}O_2$ max (mL/min)		
	Men@900-KPM Work Rate (mL/min)	Women@600-KPM Work Rate (mL/min)	Men or Women@300-KPM Work Rate (mL/min)
28	3560	2541	1525
29	3442	2459	1475
30	3333	2376	1425
31	3216	2293	1375
32	3099	2210	1325
33	2982	2127	1275
34	2865	2044	1225
35	2748	1961	1175
36	2631	1878	1125
37	2514	1795	1075
38	2397	1712	1025
39	2280	1629	—
40	2163	1546	—
41	2046	1463	—
42	1929	1380	—
43	1812	1297	—
44	1695	1214	—
45	1578	1131	—

After determining your relative $\dot{V}O_2$ max (mL/kg/min) using Table 3.6, find your appropriate fitness category.

TABLE 3.7 ■ Cardiorespiratory Fitness Norms for Men and Women Based on

Estimated $\dot{V}O_2$max Fitness Ratings (mL/kg/min)						
Men	Superior	Excellent	Good	Fair	Poor	Very Poor
18–29 yrs	>56.1	51.1–56.1	45.7–51.0	42.2–45.6	38.1–42.1	<38.1
30–39 yrs	>54.2	48.9–54.2	44.4–48.8	41.0–44.3	36.7–40.9	<36.7
40–49 yrs	>52.8	46.8–52.8	42.4–46.7	38.4–42.3	34.6–38.3	<34.6
50–59 yrs	>49.6	43.3–49.6	38.3–43.2	35.2–38.2	31.1–35.1	<31.1
60–69 yrs	>46.0	39.5–46.0	35.0–39.4	31.4–34.9	27.4–31.3	<27.4
Women	Superior	Excellent	Good	Fair	Poor	Very Poor
18–29 yrs	>50.1	44.0–50.1	39.5–43.9	35.5–39.4	31.6–35.4	<31.6
30–39 yrs	>46.8	41.0–46.8	36.8–40.9	33.8–36.7	29.9–33.7	<29.9
40–49 yrs	>45.1	38.9–45.1	35.1–38.8	31.6–35.0	28.0–31.5	<28.0
50–59 yrs	>39.8	35.2–39.8	31.4–35.1	28.7–31.3	25.5–28.6	<25.5
60–69 yrs	>36.8	32.3–36.8	29.1–32.2	26.6–29.0	23.7–26.5	<23.7

Source: Reprinted with permission from The Cooper Institute®, Dallas, Texas, from a book called *Physical Fitness Assessments and Norms for Adults and Law Enforcement.* Available online at www.CooperInstitute.org.

laboratory 3.1D

do it! LABS
Complete Lab 3.1D online in the
study area of **MasteringHealth.com**

Name _____   Date _____

Measuring Cardiorespiratory Fitness: Step Test

To complete this test, you need a step or bench that is approximately 18 inches high, such as a locker room bench or a sturdy chair. The step test lasts for 3 minutes, and then heart rate is assessed in the 3.5 minutes following the test. You will need a metronome to help you maintain the step rate.

To perform this test, you will step up and down at a rate of 30 complete steps per minute. If you set the metronome to 60 tones per minute, you will step with each tone, making a complete step (up, up, down, down) every 2 seconds. Note that it is important that you straighten your knees during the "up" phase of the test. After you complete the test, sit quietly in a chair or on the step bench, and take your heart rate for 30 seconds at the following times:

- 1 to 1.5 minutes post exercise
- 2 to 2.5 minutes post exercise
- 3 to 3.5 minutes post exercise

Maintaining the 30-step-per-minute cadence and accurately taking your heart rate are very important for getting a good estimate from the step test. To determine your fitness category, add the three 30-second heart rates obtained during the period after exercise.

Record your heart rates below, and use Table 3.8 on this page to determine your fitness category.

Scan to view a demonstration video of the step test.

Test date: _____

Recovery heart rate post exercise (bpm)

1–1.5 min: _____   **Total (recovery index):** _____

2–2.5 min: _____   **Fitness category:** _____

3–3.5 min: _____

Throughout the test, make sure to maintain correct form with your back straight.

1. Is your fitness classification what you expected based on your current level of activity? If not, why do you think it was higher or lower than expected?

   _____

   _____

2. Write fitness goals for maintaining or improving your cardiorespiratory endurance.

   _____

   _____

TABLE 3.8 ■ Norms for Cardiorespiratory Fitness Using the Sum of Three Recovery Heart Rates Obtained Following the Step Test

	3-Minute Step Test Recovery Index					
	Superior	Excellent	Good	Average	Poor	Very Poor
Men	95–117	118–132	133–147	148–165	166–192	193–217
Women	95–120	121–135	136–153	154–174	175–204	205–233

Fitness categories are for college-age men and women (age 18–25 years) at the University of Florida who performed the test on an 18-inch bench.

laboratory 3.2

do it! LABS
Complete Lab 3.2 online in the
study area of **MasteringHealth.com**

Name _____   Date _____

Assessing Cardiorespiratory Fitness for Individuals with Disabilities

This test uses arm exercise and is for people who cannot perform exercise that requires use of the legs (people in wheelchairs or with leg or foot injuries). To perform this assessment, you will need an arm crank ergometer. Your instructor will adjust the ergometer to the correct height and position for the test.

First, do a warm-up with no resistance. Then your instructor will increase the resistance, and you will perform a 2-minute stage. Rest 5 to 10 minutes. Then, after your instructor increases the workload, perform another 2-minute period of arm exercise. Repeat this cycle until you cannot complete 2 minutes of exercise at a given workload. Your instructor will tell you the workload for the last stage in which you completed the full 2 minutes of exercise. You can use that number and the calculation below to determine your $\dot{V}O_2$ max.

$$\dot{V}O_2 \text{ max} = 3 \times (\text{work rate*})/\text{body weight in kg}^\dagger + 3.5$$

* Your instructor will give you this value.

† Weight in kg = weight in lb ÷ 2.2

Table 3.7 (page 79) in Laboratory 3.1C has the fitness classifications that correspond to your $\dot{V}O_2$ max. Because this test uses arm exercise, which involves a smaller muscle mass than leg or whole-body exercise, your $\dot{V}O_2$ max estimate will be a slight underestimate.

Fitness category: _____

1. Is your fitness classification what you expected based on your current level of activity? If not, why do you think it was higher or lower than expected?

    _____

    _____

2. Write fitness goals for maintaining or improving your cardiorespiratory endurance.

    _____

    _____

Name _____ Date _____

Determining Target Heart Rate

Scan to view
demonstration
videos of locating
the radial and
carotid pulses.

radial pulse   carotid pulse

Practice taking your pulse at both the carotid and radial locations. You can feel the carotid pulse next to the larynx, beneath the lower jaw. The radial pulse is located on the inside of the wrist, directly in line with the base of the thumb. Use a timer to count for 15, 30, and 60 seconds. To determine your heart rate in beats per minute (bpm), multiply your 15-second count by 4, and your 30-second count by 2.

Try locating and taking the pulse of a classmate at both the radial and carotid locations. Record your resting pulse counts in the spaces provided.

Carotid Pulse Count (self)	Heart Rate (bpm)	Radial Pulse Count (self)	Heart Rate (bpm)
15 seconds × 4		× 4	
30 seconds × 2		× 2	
60 seconds × 1		× 1	

Carotid Pulse Count (partner)	Heart Rate (bpm)	Radial Pulse Count (partner)	Heart Rate (bpm)
15 seconds × 4		× 4	
30 seconds × 2		× 2	
60 seconds × 1		× 1	

The target heart rate (THR) range is calculated in the following steps:

STEP 1: Calculate your estimated maximal heart rate (HR_{max}).

$HR_{max} = 206.9 - (0.67 \times age)$

STEP 2: Calculate your heart rate reserve (HRR) by subtracting your resting heart rate from your HR_{max} (use the 60-second count from above).

$HRR = HR_{max} -$ resting heart rate

HRR = _____ − _____

HRR = _____

STEP 3: Calculate 50% and 85% HRR (use decimal values).

Lower end of THR = 0.50 × (HRR) = _____

Upper end of THR = 0.85 × (HRR) = _____

STEP 4: Add your resting heart rate back to these values.

50% HRR + resting heart rate = _____

85% HRR + resting heart rate = _____

THR _____ bpm to _____ bpm

1. Which of the resting pulses did you find easiest to locate on yourself?

    _____ Carotid _____ Radial

2. Which resting pulse was easiest to locate on your partner?

    _____ Carotid _____ Radial

3. Which of the two locations would you prefer to use when taking your pulse to determine exercise heart rate?

    _____ Carotid _____ Radial

    Why? _____

do it! LABS
Complete Lab 3.4 online in the
study area of **MasteringHealth.com**

Name _____ Date _____

Developing Your Personal Exercise Prescription

Develop your personal exercise program based on your current fitness level and goals. Record the appropriate information in the spaces provided below.

Week	Phase	Intensity (% of HRR or RPE)	Exercise Mode	Duration (min/day)	Monday	Tuesday	Wednesday	Thursday	Friday	Saturday	Sunday
1											
2											
3											
4											
5											
6											
7											
8											
9											
10											
11											
12											
13											
14											
15											
16											

Review the behavior change strategies (discussed in Chapter 1), and write two strategies that can help you begin or maintain your aerobic exercise program (e.g., substituting behaviors—I will take a walk and talk with my friend Mary after class instead of having a text conversation with her).

_____
_____
_____
_____

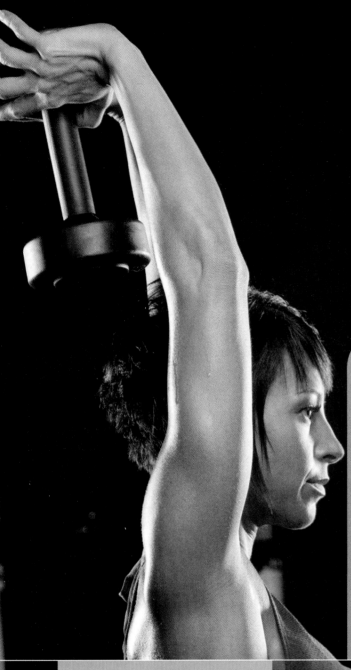

4

Improving Muscular Strength and Endurance

CAN YOU IMAGINE running the 26 continuous miles of a marathon or biking the 2,241 miles in the Tour de France? Or would you consider competing in the Strongman/Strongwoman competitions? These extraordinary feats of human performance are possible because of the human body's great capacity for muscular strength and endurance. While not everyone will compete in a bike race or other athletic event, improved muscular strength and endurance offers numerous everyday benefits for everyone.

The Need for Muscular Strength and Endurance in Daily Living

 LO **1** Describe the need for muscular strength and endurance over the lifespan.

When you climb a flight of stairs or carry a heavy book bag across campus, you're relying on your muscular strength and endurance to perform the task without becoming exhausted. If you've ever worked in a job that required you to shuttle loaded trays of food among tables or move boxes from point A to point B, you've relied on strength and endurance to earn your living. And if you play competitive or recreational sports, your skill level is determined in large part by the strength and endurance of your muscles. Whether we're aware of it or not, the strength and endurance of our muscles affects our physical performance numerous times every day.

Muscular strength and endurance are related, but they are not the same thing (Chapter 1). Muscular strength is the ability of a muscle to generate maximal force. In simple terms, muscular strength is the amount of weight that an individual can lift during one maximal effort. In contrast, muscular endurance is the ability to generate force over and over again. In general, increasing muscular strength by exercise training will also increase muscular endurance. However, training to improve muscular endurance does not significantly improve muscular strength.

Muscular strength and endurance can be increased and maintained with strength-training and endurance-training programs. In addition, regular strength training promotes numerous health benefits. For example, incidence of low back pain, a common problem in both men and women, can be reduced with appropriate strengthening exercises for the lower back and abdominal muscles (1). Further, studies demonstrate that muscle-strengthening exercises may reduce the occurrence of joint and/or muscle abnormalities and injuries that occur during physical activity (2). Strength training can also delay the decrease in muscle strength experienced by sedentary older individuals (3) and may help prevent osteoporosis.

Another important benefit of strength training is that it increases **resting metabolic rate** in larger muscles (4). Resting metabolic rate (also called *resting energy expenditure*) includes the energy required to drive the heart and respiratory muscles and to build and maintain body tissues. An elevated metabolic rate allows the body to burn more calories throughout the day. Conversely, a lower metabolic rate burns fewer calories, thereby leading to weight gain.

How does strength training influence resting metabolic rate? One of the primary results of strength training is an increase in muscle mass in relation to body fat. An increase of 1 pound of muscle elevates resting metabolism by approximately 2%–3%. This increase can be magnified with larger gains in muscle. For instance, a 5-pound increase in muscle mass results in a 10%–15% increase in resting metabolic rate. Changes of this magnitude can play an important role in helping you lose weight or maintaining desirable body composition throughout life. Although overall body weight may increase slightly as muscle mass increases, fat mass should decrease. Clothing may fit better, and self-image is likely to improve.

see it!
ABC VIDEOS

How do you increase your core strength? Watch the ABC Video "Improve Your Abs" at MasteringHealth™.

MAKE SURE YOU **KNOW...**

- Muscular strength and endurance are important for numerous daily tasks. Strength training can reduce low back pain, reduce the incidence of exercise-related injuries, decrease the incidence of osteoporosis, and help maintain functional capacity that normally decreases with age.

- Muscular strength is the ability to generate maximal force, whereas muscular endurance is the ability to generate force over and over again.

- Strength training can improve a muscle's resting metabolic rate.

——————————— MasteringHealth™

How Muscles Work: Structure and Function

LO **2** Describe the basic anatomy and physiology of muscle; differentiate between muscle exercise and muscle action; name the muscle fiber types and explain their functional differences; and list the factors that determine muscular strength.

There are about 600 skeletal muscles in the human body, and their primary function is to provide force for physical movement. When the muscles shorten or lengthen during a **muscle action**, they apply force to the bones, causing the body to move.

The skeletal muscles also are responsible for maintaining posture and regulating body temperature through the mechanism of shivering (which results in heat production). Because all fitness activities require the use of skeletal muscles, anyone beginning a physical fitness program should understand basic muscle structure and function.

Muscle Structure

Skeletal muscle is a collection of long, thin cells called *fibers*. These fibers are surrounded by a dense layer of connective tissue called **fascia** that holds the individual fibers together and separates muscle from surrounding tissues (**FIGURE 4.1**).

Muscles are attached to bones by connective tissues known as **tendons**. Muscular action causes the tendons to pull on the bones, thereby causing movement. Muscles cannot push the bones; they can only pull them. Many of the muscles involved in movement are illustrated in **FIGURE 4.2** on page 88.

Muscle Function

Muscle actions are regulated by electrical signals from motor nerves, which originate in the spinal cord and send messages to individual muscles throughout the body. A motor nerve and an individual muscle fiber make contact at a neuromuscular junction (see **FIGURE 4.3** on page 89). Note from the figure that each motor nerve branches and then connects with numerous individual muscle fibers.

The motor nerve and all of the muscle fibers it controls comprise a **motor unit**. Motor units come in various sizes, depending on how many muscle fibers they contain. A motor nerve can innervate a few muscle fibers for fine motor control, such as blinking the eye, or it can innervate many muscle fibers for gross motor movement, such as kicking a ball.

A muscle action begins when a message to develop tension (called a nerve impulse) reaches the neuromuscular junction. The arrival of the nerve impulse triggers the action process by permitting the interaction of contractile proteins in muscle. Just as the nerve impulse initiates the contractile process, the removal of the nerve signal from the muscle "turns it off." That is, when a motor nerve ceases to send signals to a muscle, the muscle action stops. Occasionally, however, an uncontrolled muscular action occurs, which results in a muscle cramp or a muscle twitch.

Muscle Exercise and Muscle Action

Skeletal muscle exercise is classified into three major categories: **isotonic**, **isometric**, and **isokinetic**. Isotonic (also called *dynamic*) exercise results in movement of a body part at a joint. Most exercise or sports activities are isotonic. For example, lifting a dumbbell involves movement of the forearm and is therefore classified as an isotonic exercise.

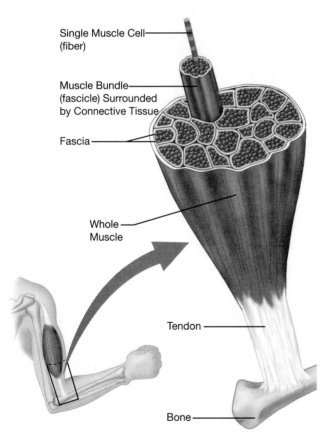

FIGURE 4.1 The structure of skeletal muscle.

Single Muscle Cell (fiber)

Muscle Bundle (fascicle) Surrounded by Connective Tissue

Fascia

Whole Muscle

Tendon

Bone

Source: Johnson, Michael D., *Human Biology: Concepts and Current Issues,* 4th Ed., © 2008. Reprinted and Electronically reproduced by permission of Pearson Education, Inc., Upper Saddle River, New Jersey.

resting metabolic rate The amount of energy expended during all sedentary activities. Also called *resting energy expenditure.*

muscle action The shortening of a skeletal muscle (causing movement) or the lengthening of a skeletal muscle (resisting movement).

fascia Dense but thin layer of connective tissue that surrounds the muscle.

tendons Fibrous connective tissue that attaches muscle to bone.

motor unit A motor nerve and all of the muscle fibers it controls.

isotonic Type of exercise in which there is movement of a body part. Most exercise or sports skills are isotonic exercise. Also called *dynamic* exercise.

isometric Type of exercise in which muscular tension is developed but the body part does not move. Also called *static* exercise.

isokinetic Type of exercise that can include concentric or eccentric muscle actions performed at a constant speed using a specialized machine.

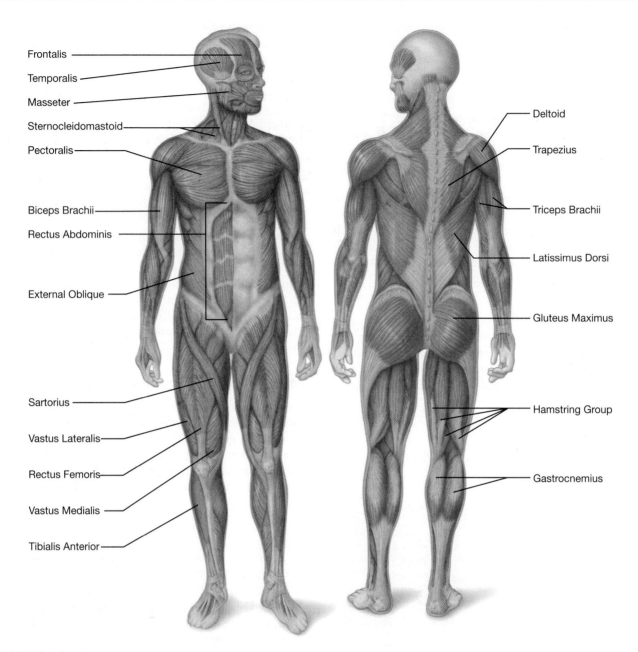

FIGURE 4.2 Major muscles of the human body.

Source: Johnson, Michael D., *Human Biology: Concepts and Current Issues,* 4th Ed., © 2008. Reprinted and Electronically reproduced by permission of Pearson Education, Inc., Upper Saddle River, New Jersey.

An isometric (also called *static*) exercise requires the development of muscular tension but results in no movement of body parts. A classic example of isometric exercise is pressing the palms of the hands together. Although there is tension within the muscles of the arms and chest, the arms do not move. Isometric exercises are an excellent way to develop strength during the early stages of an injury rehabilitation program.

Isokinetic exercise is performed at a constant velocity; that is, the speed of muscle shortening or lengthening is regulated at a fixed, controlled rate. This is generally accomplished by using a machine that provides an accommodating resistance throughout the full **range of motion**.

Muscle action can similarly be classified as isometric, concentric, or eccentric, depending on the activity the muscle needs to perform. Like isometric exercise, isometric muscle action is static and does not involve any joint movement. An isometric muscle action occurs during isometric exercise.

A **concentric muscle action** causes movement of the body part against resistance or gravity; it occurs when the muscle shortens. Concentric muscle actions (also called *positive work*) can be performed during isotonic or isokinetic exercise. For example, the upward movement of the arm during a bicep curl (see **FIGURE 4.4** on the following page) is an example of a concentric muscle action.

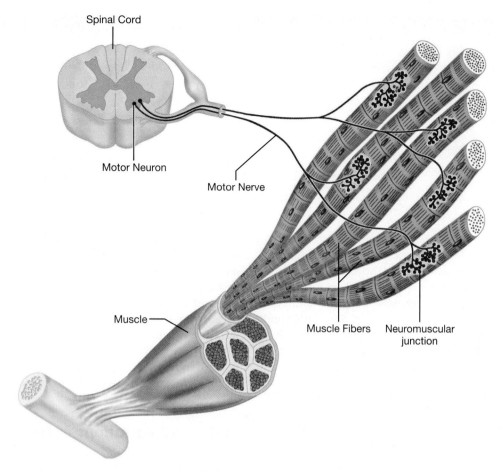

FIGURE 4.3 A motor unit. Two motor nerves from the central nervous system are shown innervating several muscle fibers. With one impulse from the motor nerve, all fibers respond.

Concentric Action

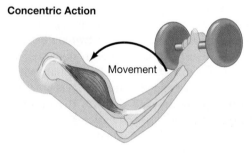

Movement

Eccentric Action

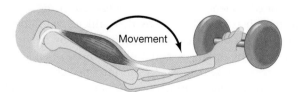

Movement

FIGURE 4.4 Concentric and eccentric muscle actions in an isotonic exercise. The muscle shortens during a concentric action and lengthens during an eccentric action.

In contrast, **eccentric muscle action** (also called *negative work*) controls movement with resistance or gravity; it occurs when the muscle lengthens. The downward or lowering phase of the bicep curl is controlled as the biceps muscle lengthens (Figure 4.4); the muscle develops tension, but the force developed is not great enough to prevent the weight from being lowered.

Types of Muscle Fibers

Although all skeletal muscles do the same thing—contract for skeletal movement—the fibers within them have

range of motion The amount of movement possible at a joint.

concentric muscle action Action in which the muscle develops tension as it shortens against resistance and/or gravity. Also called *positive work*.

eccentric muscle action Action in which the muscle develops tension as it lengthens while controlling the movement with gravity. Also called *negative work*.

TABLE 4.1 ■ Properties of Human Skeletal Muscle Fiber Types

Properties	FIBER TYPE		
	Slow-Twitch (Type I)	Fast-Twitch (Type IIa)	Fast-Twitch (Type IIx)
Contraction speed	Slow	Faster	Fastest
Resistance to fatigue	Highest	Higher	Low
Predominant energy system	Aerobic	Aerobic and anaerobic	Anaerobic
Force generation	Low	Higher	Highest
Color	Red	White (pink)	White
Best suited for	Endurance events (10 K race - Marathon)	Middle-distance events (1500-m to 3000-m races)	Short-distance or fast events (100-m sprint)

different characteristics that determine how efficiently they function (5). There are two major classifications of skeletal muscle fibers: *slow-twitch* (also called type I), and *fast-twitch* (also called type II) Type II fibers can be further categorized into two subclasses: type IIa and type IIx. **TABLE 4.1** compares the properties of slow-twitch and fast-twitch fibers. Because most human muscles contain a mixture of all three fiber types, it is helpful to understand each type before beginning the strength-training process.

Slow-Twitch Fibers As the name implies, **slow-twitch fibers** (also called type I fibers) contract slowly and produce low force. However, these fibers are highly resistant to fatigue. Slow-twitch fibers appear red or darker in color because of the numerous capillaries that supply blood to the fibers. They have the capacity to produce large quantities of adenosine triphosphate (ATP) aerobically, which makes them ideally suited for low-force, prolonged exercise such as walking or slow jogging. Because of their resistance to fatigue, most postural muscles are composed primarily of slow-twitch fibers.

Fast-Twitch Fibers The subclass of **fast-twitch fibers** known as *type IIx* fibers function in a manner opposite to that of slow-twitch fibers. They contract rapidly and generate great amounts of force but fatigue quickly. These fibers have a low aerobic capacity and appear white because they are supplied by only a few capillaries. Type IIx fibers are well equipped to produce ATP anaerobically, but only for a short time. Due to their ability to contract rapidly and produce large amounts of force, fast-twitch fibers are used during activities that require very rapid or forceful movement such as jumping, sprinting, and heavy weight lifting. These fibers are the most easily damaged during strenuous exercise, causing soreness.

The subclass of fast-twitch fibers known as *type IIa* exhibit a combination of characteristics found in both fast- and slow-twitch fibers. They contract rapidly and produce high force (almost to the level of type IIx fibers), but they are fatigue-resistant because they have a well-developed aerobic capacity, similar to slow-twitch fibers. They have a light red (pink) appearance that is darker than type IIx fibers but not as red as slow-twitch fibers.

Visualizing Muscle Fiber Types An example of the different muscle fiber types can be seen in chicken meat. Some chicken meat is white and other parts are darker (reddish) in color. The dark meat of a chicken (the legs and thighs) contains primarily slow-twitch fibers. Because these fibers are slow to fatigue, the bird is able to walk around most of the day. White meat (the breast and wings) is composed mostly of type IIx fibers. This class of fast-twitch fibers allows the bird to fly but only for short distances because they are quick to fatigue.

Individual Variations in Fiber Type

While there are individual variations, the average non-athlete generally has equal numbers of all three fiber types. Research has shown a relationship between muscle fiber type and athletic success. For example, champion endurance athletes, such as marathon runners, have a predominance of slow-twitch fibers. This finding makes sense because endurance sports require muscles with high fatigue resistance. In contrast, elite sprinters, such as 100-meter runners, have more fast-twitch fibers.

Muscle fiber type has also been suggested as a link to obesity and diabetes (6, 7). Individuals with a predominance of fast-twitch muscle fibers may be more susceptible to obesity and diabetes than those with a predominance of slow-twitch muscle fibers.

Some evidence has shown that fibers can be converted from one type to another. For example, endurance training has been shown to cause some fiber conversion between the fast-twitch type IIa and type IIx fibers. However, there is limited evidence of fast-twitch fibers converting to slow-twitch fibers (8). This means that athletes who do well in short distances can stretch their careers by moving to intermediate distances, and athletes who do well at long distances can also move to the intermediate distances. But a long-distance athlete would not be very successful switching to a short-distance event.

Although endurance exercise training has been shown to cause some fiber conversion, the number and percentage of skeletal muscle fiber types are strongly influenced by genetics (5).

Recruitment of Muscle Fibers during Exercise

Many types of exercise use only a small fraction of the muscle fibers available in a muscle group. For example, walking at a slow speed may use fewer than 30% of the muscle fibers in the legs. More intense types of exercise, however, require more force. To generate this force, a greater number of muscle fibers must be made to contract.

The process of involving more muscle fibers to produce increased muscular force is called **fiber recruitment**. **FIGURE 4.5** illustrates the order in which muscle fibers are recruited as the intensity of exercise increases. Note that during low-intensity exercise, only slow-twitch fibers are used. As the exercise intensity increases, fibers are progressively recruited, from slow-twitch to intermediate fibers and finally to fast-twitch fibers. High-intensity activities, such as weight training, recruit large numbers of fast-twitch fibers. Why does this matter? By understanding which types of fibers are used for various exercises, you will better understand why you are working a particular muscle or muscle group in a particular way.

Muscular Strength

Two physiological factors determine the amount of force that a muscle can generate: the size of the muscle and the number of fibers recruited during the contraction. Muscle size is the primary factor. The larger the muscle, the greater the force it can produce.

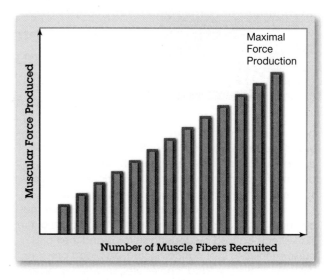

FIGURE 4.6 The relationship between recruitment of motor units and production of muscular force.

Although there is no difference in the chemical makeup of muscle in men and women, men tend to have more muscle mass and are therefore generally stronger. The larger muscle mass is due to higher levels of the hormone testosterone in men, which helps build muscle. The fact that testosterone promotes an increase in muscle size has led some athletes to use drugs in an attempt to improve muscular strength (see Examining the Evidence on the following page).

The other significant factor that determines how much force is generated is the number of fibers recruited for a given movement. The more muscle fibers that are stimulated, the greater the total muscle force generated; this is because the force generated by individual fibers is cumulative (**FIGURE 4.6**).

Muscle fiber recruitment is regulated voluntarily through the nervous system. That is, we decide how much effort to put into a particular movement. For instance, when we choose to make a minimal effort to lift an object, we recruit only a few motor units, and the

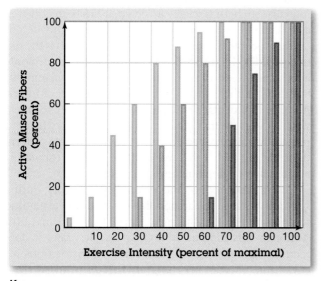

Key

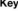 Slow-Twitch (Type I) Fibers

▨ Fast-Twitch (Type IIa) Fibers

▨ Fast-Twitch (Type IIx) Fibers

FIGURE 4.5 The relationship between exercise intensity and recruitment of muscle fiber type.

slow-twitch fibers Red muscle fibers that contract slowly and are highly resistant to fatigue. These fibers have the capacity to produce large quantities of ATP aerobically. Also known as *type I fibers*.

fast-twitch fibers Muscle fibers that contract rapidly but fatigue more quickly than slow-twitch fibers. There are two types: *type IIa* and *type IIx*.

fiber recruitment Process of involving more muscle fibers to increase muscular force.

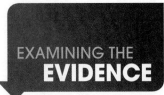

Anabolic Steroid Use Increases Muscle Size But Has Serious Side Effects

The abuse of *anabolic steroids* (synthetic forms of the hormone testosterone) and their precursors has mushroomed over the past several decades. The fierce competition in body building and other sports that require strength and power has driven both men and women to risk serious health consequences in the quest to develop large muscles.

The large doses of steroids needed to increase muscle mass produce several health risks. A partial list of the side effects caused by abusing steroids and their precursors includes liver cancer, increased blood pressure, increased levels of "bad" cholesterol, severe depression, and prostate cancer. Prolonged use and high doses of steroids can be lethal.

One of the most popular chemical precursors to testosterone, androstenedione, is used to increase blood testosterone with the intent to increase strength, lean body mass, and sexual performance. However, research indicates that androstenedione does not significantly increase strength and/or lean body mass.

Another precursor to testosterone production in the body, dehydroepiandrosterone (DHEA), has also been used to increase testosterone in the body. DHEA is also advertised as a weight-loss and anti-aging supplement capable of improving libido, vitality, and immunity levels. However, the best evidence demonstrates that DHEA supplementation does not increase testosterone concentrations or increase strength in men, and it may have masculinizing effects in women.

---

muscle develops limited force. However, if we decide to exert maximal effort to lift a heavy object, many muscle fibers are recruited, and a larger force is generated.

MAKE SURE YOU **KNOW...**

- Skeletal muscle is composed of various types of fibers that are attached to bone by tendons.

- Skeletal muscle actions are regulated by signals coming from motor nerves. A motor unit consists of a motor nerve and all the muscle fibers it controls.

- Exercise can be isometric, isotonic, or isokinetic. Isometric actions do not result in movement, while isotonic actions move a body part.

- Isometric exercise involves isometric muscle action. Isotonic and isokinetic exercises use concentric actions (muscle shortens) and eccentric actions (muscle lengthens).

- Slow-twitch muscle fibers shorten slowly but are fatigueresistant. Fast-twitch fibers are classified into two types: Type IIx shorten rapidly but fatigue rapidly, and type IIa fibers shorten quickly but fatigue slowly.

- The process of involving more muscle fibers to produce increased muscular force is called fiber recruitment.

- Two factors determine muscularforce: the size of the muscle and the number of fibers recruited.

 MasteringHealth™

Evaluation of Muscular Strength and Endurance

LO **3** Describe the methods used to evaluate a person's muscular strength and endurance.

Muscular strength can be assessed by the **one-repetition maximum (1 RM) test**, which measures the maximum amount of weight that can be lifted one time. Although the 1 RM test for muscular strength is widely accepted, it has been criticized as unsuitable for use by older individuals or highly deconditioned people (9), for whom the major concern is the risk of injury. The 1 RM test should therefore be attempted only after several weeks of strength training, which will improve both skill and strength and thus reduce the risk of injury. An older or sedentary individual would probably require 6 weeks of exercise training prior to the 1 RM test, whereas a physically active college-age person could probably perform the 1 RM test after 1 to 2 weeks of training. See Laboratory 4.1 for a step-by-step walk-through of the 1 RM test.

To further reduce the possibility of injury during strength testing, researchers have developed a method to estimate the 1 RM using a series of submaximal lifts. Although this method is slightly less accurate, it does reduce the risk of injury. You can read instructions for performing this test in Laboratory 4.2.

Muscular endurance is usually evaluated with two simple tests: the **push-up test** and either the **sit-up test** or the **curl-up test**. Push-ups require endurance in the shoulder, arm, and chest muscles, whereas sits-ups and curl-ups primarily require endurance in the abdominal muscles. To learn how to perform these tests and assess your own muscular endurance, turn to Laboratory 4.4 at the end of the chapter.

MAKE SURE YOU **KNOW...**

- The 1 RM test can be used to evaluate muscular strength.

- To reduce the possibility of injury, the estimated 1 RM test can be performed instead of the 1 RM test.

- The push-up and sit-up (or curl-up) tests are used to evaluate muscular endurance.

MasteringHealth™

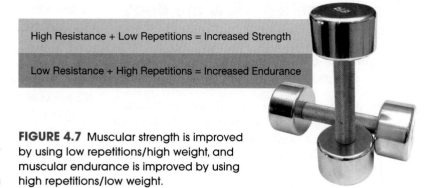

High Resistance + Low Repetitions = Increased Strength

Low Resistance + High Repetitions = Increased Endurance

FIGURE 4.7 Muscular strength is improved by using low repetitions/high weight, and muscular endurance is improved by using high repetitions/low weight.

Principles for Designing a Strength and Endurance Program

 Discuss the general principles for developing a strength and endurance training program.

We discussed the general principles for developing training programs to improve physical fitness in Chapter 2. Before moving on to the specifics of how to develop a strength-training program, let's discuss how two training principles, overload and specificity, factor into the design of a muscular strength- and endurance-training program.

Progressive Overload

The concept of **progressive overload** applies to both strength training and endurance exercise. If your goal is to develop strong biceps muscles, you must progressively increase the resistance (load) that you lift. For example, you may begin your program using 10-pound dumbbells and perform one set of 8 repetitions 3 times a week. As this exercise becomes easier, you can progressively increase the workload by increasing the weight, increasing the number of sets to 2 and then 3, and/or increasing the number of repetitions up to 12.

Specificity of Training

The principle of **specificity of training** states that development of muscular strength and endurance is specific to both the muscle group that is exercised and the training intensity. Only those muscles that are trained will improve in strength and endurance. For example, to improve the strength of the back muscles, you need to train the specific muscles involved with movement of the back.

The intensity of training will determine whether the muscular adaptation is primarily an increase in strength or in endurance (**FIGURE 4.7**). High-intensity training (such as lifting heavy weights 6 to 8 times) increases muscular strength but yields only limited improvements in muscular endurance. Conversely, high-repetition, low-intensity training (such as lifting light weights 20 times or more) increases muscular endurance but yields only limited improvements in muscular strength.

MAKE SURE YOU **KNOW...**

- In the context of strength and endurance training, the progressive overload principle means that you need to progressively increase the amount of resistance with which you train.

- The intensity of training determines whether you primarily increase muscular strength or endurance. High-intensity training will increase muscle strength and size; low-intensity training will increase muscular endurance.

MasteringHealth™

---

one-repetition maximum (1 RM) test Measurement of the maximum amount of weight that can be lifted one time.

push-up test Fitness test designed to evaluate endurance of shoulder and arm muscles.

sit-up test Test used to evaluate abdominal and hip muscle endurance.

curl-up test Test used to evaluate abdominal muscle endurance.

progressive overload Application of the overload principle to strength and endurance exercise programs.

specificity of training The concept that the development of muscular strength and endurance, as well as cardiorespiratory endurance, is specific to both the muscle group exercised and the training intensity.

Strength Training: How the Body Adapts

 LO **5** List and explain the physiological adaptations to strength training.

What physiological changes result from strength training? How quickly can you gain muscular strength? Do men and women differ in their responses to weight-training programs? Let's address these questions next.

Physiological Changes Due to Weight Training

You now know that programs designed to improve muscular strength can do so only by increasing muscle size and/or by increasing the number of muscle fibers recruited. Strength training alters both these factors (10). Research has shown that strength-training programs increase muscular strength first by altering fiber recruitment patterns, and then by increasing muscle size.

Increase in muscle size is due primarily to an increase in fiber size, called **hypertrophy** (10). Most research has shown that strength training has little effect on the formation of new muscle fibers, a process called **hyperplasia**. The role of hyperplasia in the increase in muscle size due to strength training remains controversial (11). Regardless, the increase in muscle size depends on diet, the muscle fiber type (fast-twitch fibers may hypertrophy more than slow-twitch fibers), blood levels of testosterone, and the type of training program.

Although strength training does not result in significant improvements in cardiorespiratory fitness (12), a regular weight-training program can provide positive changes in both body composition and flexibility. For most men and women, rigorous weight training results in an increase in muscle mass and a loss of body fat, both of which decrease the percentage of body fat.

Performing weight-training exercises over the full range of motion at a joint can improve flexibility (9). In fact, many diligent weight lifters have excellent flexibility. Thus, the notion that weight lifting causes inflexibility is generally incorrect.

Rate of Strength Improvement with Weight Training

How rapidly does strength improvement occur? The answer depends on your initial strength level. Strength gains occur rapidly in untrained people, and more gradually in individuals with relatively higher strength levels. In fact, for a novice lifter, strength gains can occur very quickly (13). These rapid gains tend to motivate the lifter to stick with a regular weight-training program.

Gender Differences in Response to Weight Training

Men and women do not differ in their initial responses to weight-training programs (14). On a percentage basis, women gain strength as rapidly as men during the first 12 weeks of a strength-training program. However, with long-term weight training, men generally exhibit a greater increase in muscle size than do women. The reason is that men have 20 to 30 times more testosterone than women have.

MAKE SURE YOU **KNOW...**

- Muscle size increases primarily because of hypertrophy (increase in size) of muscle fibers.
- Strength training promotes positive changes in both body composition and flexibility.
- The rate of improvement in weight training depends on initial strength level.
- Early in a weight-training program, women gain strength as quickly as men do.

———————— MasteringHealth™

Designing a Training Program for Increasing Muscular Strength

 LO **6** Name at least three safety concerns for any weight-training program and describe the three basic types of weight-training programs.

There are numerous approaches to designing weight-training programs. Any program that adheres to the basic principles described earlier will improve strength and endurance. However, the type of weight-training program that you develop for yourself depends on your goals and the types of equipment available to you. There are several other factors to consider in developing a weight-training program; we discuss those next.

Safety Concerns

Before beginning any weight-training program, you need to think about safety. Follow these safety guidelines when weight training:

- When using free weights (such as barbells), have spotters (helpers) help you perform the exercises. The purpose of a spotter is to help you complete a lift if you are unable to do it on your own. Using weight machines reduces the need for spotters.

- Be sure that the collars on the ends of the bars of free weights are tightly secured to prevent the weights from falling off. Dropping weight plates on toes and feet can result in serious injuries. Again, many weight machines have safety features that reduce the risk of dropping weights.

- Warm up properly before doing any weight-lifting exercise. You can warm up for lifting by performing a few repetitions with very light weights.

- Do not hold your breath during weight lifting. Instead, follow this breathing pattern: Exhale while lifting the weight, and inhale while lowering it. Also, breathe through both your nose and mouth.

- Although debate continues as to whether high-speed weight lifting yields greater strength gains than slow-speed lifting, slow movements may reduce the risk of injury. Make sure that you move slowly enough to maintain total control of the weights at all times.

- Use light weights in the beginning so that you can maintain the proper form through the full range of motion in each exercise. This is particularly important when you are lifting free weights.

Types of Weight-Training Programs

Weight-training programs specifically designed to improve strength and those designed to improve muscular endurance differ mainly in the number of repetitions and the amount of resistance (10). A combination of low repetition and high resistance appears to be the optimal training method to increase strength; moreover, this type of training improves muscular endurance as well. In contrast, a program of high repetition and low resistance improves endurance but results in only small strength increases, particularly in less-fit individuals.

As with types of muscle exercise, weight-training programs can be divided into three general categories: isotonic, isometric, and isokinetic.

Isotonic Programs Isotonic programs involve contracting a muscle against a movable load (usually a free weight or weights on a weight machine). The load is lifted on the up phase using concentric muscle action and then lowered on the down phase using eccentric muscle action. Isotonic programs are the most common type of weight-training program in use today.

Weight-training machines are ideal for the beginning exerciser because the weight is mounted to a cable or chain. If you were unable to complete a lift using a heavy weight and accidentally let go of the bar, the weights would slam down on the weight stack without injuring you or anyone else. In addition, machines allow a single joint to be isolated and exercised.

Free weights are preferred by many serious weight lifters because they can be used to exercise multiple joints. For example, the squat exercise involves muscles of the hip, knee, and ankle, thus allowing three joints to be exercised during one movement.

Isometric Programs An isometric strength-training program is based on the concept of contracting a muscle at a fixed angle against an immovable object, using an isometric muscle action. Interest in strength training increased dramatically during the 1950s with the finding that maximal strength could be increased by contracting a muscle for 6 seconds at two-thirds of maximal tension once per day for 5 days per week. Although subsequent studies suggested that these claims were exaggerated, it is generally agreed that isometric training can increase muscular strength and endurance (15).

Two important aspects of isometric training make it different from isotonic training. First, in isometric training, the development of strength and endurance is specific to the joint angle at which the muscle group is trained (15). Therefore, if you use isometric techniques, you will need to perform isometric contractions at several different joint angles if you want to gain strength and endurance throughout a full range of motion. In contrast, because isotonic contractions generally involve the full range of joint motion, strength is developed over the full movement pattern.

Second, the static nature of isometric muscle action can lead to breath holding (called a **Valsalva maneuver**), which can reduce blood flow to the brain and cause dizziness and fainting. In an individual at high risk for coronary disease, the maneuver could be extremely dangerous and should always be avoided. Remember: Continue to breathe during any type of isometric or isotonic exercise.

Isokinetic Programs Recall that isokinetic exercise involves concentric or eccentric muscle action performed at a constant speed (*isokinetic* refers to constant speed of movement). Isokinetic training is a relatively underused strength-training method, so limited research exists to describe its strength benefits compared with those of isometric and isotonic programs.

Isokinetic exercises require the use of machines that govern the speed of movement during muscle actions. The first isokinetic machines available were very expensive and were used primarily in clinical settings for injury rehabilitation. Recently, less expensive machines use a piston device (much like a shock absorber on a car) to limit the speed of movement throughout the range of the exercise.

live it!
ASSESS YOURSELF

Assess your exercise I.Q. with the *Test Your Exercise I.Q.* Take Charge of Your Health! Worksheet online at MasteringHealth™.

---

hypertrophy Increase in muscle fiber size.

hyperplasia Increase in the number of muscle fibers.

Valsalva maneuver Holding the breath during an intense muscle contraction; can reduce blood flow to the brain and cause dizziness and fainting.

steps FOR BEHAVIOR CHANGE

Are you reluctant to strength train?

Answer the following questions to assess the barriers that prevent you from starting a strength-training program.

Y   N

☐ ☐ I feel intimidated by other people in the strength-training facility.

☐ ☐ I cannot find time in my schedule to exercise.

☐ ☐ I do not know how to use the various machines or free weights.

☐ ☐ I do not know how to begin a strength-training program.

If you answered yes to more than one question, check out the following tips to help you break through the barriers.

Tips to Ease Yourself into a Strength-Training Routine

Tomorrow, you will:

☑ Research the fitness facilities in your area. Fitness facilities cater to a wide range of clients, from beginners to professional body builders. Try to find one that is convenient, affordable, and contains enough of the basic equipment to meet your strength-training goals.

Within the next 2 weeks, you will:

☑ Join a fitness facility. After doing your research for a facility, join the one that meets the criteria above and also makes you feel welcome and comfortable.

☑ Take an orientation tour through the fitness facility to familiarize yourself with the machines and equipment.

☑ Consider hiring a personal trainer at the facility if you feel you need more individualized instruction. Most facilities have fitness professionals who will assess your overall strength and suggest a starting program.

By the end of the semester, you will:

☑ Make a commitment to set aside 30–60 minutes a day for training, and do not allow others to interfere with your personal time. Personal fitness does require a time commitment, but you are worth the investment.

MAKE SURE YOU **KNOW...**

- The greatest strength gains are made with a training program using low repetitions and high resistance, while the greatest improvements in endurance are made using high repetitions and low resistance.

- Isotonic programs include exercises with movable loads. Isometric training includes exercises in which a muscle contracts at a fixed angle against an immovable object. Isokinetic exercises involve machines that govern the speed of movement during muscle contraction.

 MasteringHealth™

Exercise Prescription for Weight Training

LO 7 **Explain how the concepts of frequency, intensity, and duration are applied to weight training.**

An understanding of the general concepts of frequency, intensity, and duration (or time) of exercise is required to improve physical fitness (Chapter 2). Although these same concepts apply to improving muscular strength and endurance through weight training, the terminology used to monitor the intensity and duration of weight training is unique. For example, the intensity of weight training is measured not by heart rate but by the number of *repetition*

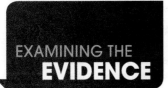

Does Creatine Supplementation Increase Muscle Size and Strength?

Creatine (Cr) is marketed as a muscle-building dietary supplement that can help you achieve significant increases in muscle size and strength. Does it work? Is it safe? Let's investigate how it is used by the body and learn what current research suggests about its effectiveness.

Your diet provides energy sources for all types of exercise. For activities requiring powerful bursts (sprints) or high forces (resistance training), one of the most important energy sources is Cr, particularly in fast-twitch muscle fibers. During these activities, phosphorylated creatine (PCr) is an immediate source to replenish ATP. In fact, the best evidence suggests that Cr contributes most of the energy needed for activities that involve less than a minute of intense work.

You need about 2 grams of Cr in your diet per day to maintain normal levels. Meat and fish are the primary sources. However, Cr can be reduced significantly in active individuals who engage in repeated bouts of high speed/high force exercises. Research shows that supplementation can prevent depletion and may, in some people, increase the amount stored by the body.

A number of studies have examined the effect of Cr supplementation on exercise performance. The consensus seems to be that while not increasing peak force output by the muscle, PCr might increase the amount of work done (~8%) in repeated, short duration, maximal work bouts. The mechanism of this enhancement is not yet clearly documented but is most likely due to increasing the available PCr and prolonging the total work time and, thus, the stimulus for muscle adaptation.

While the beneficial effects of Cr continue to be debated, the potential for unwanted side-effects exists. High doses of Cr taken for extended periods of time may damage the kidneys, liver, and/or heart, although a direct link has not been firmly established. In the short term, Cr can cause stomach pain, nausea, diarrhea, and muscle cramping. As Cr is taken up by the muscle, water is also taken in, causing muscle swelling and increased weight gain. This swelling has been purported to be muscle hypertrophy accompanied by increases in strength but obviously, swelling doesn't increase strength. For more information, go to http://www.nlm.nih.gov/ and search for creatine supplementation.

---

maximums. Similarly, the duration of weight training is measured not by actual time but by the number of sets performed. Let's discuss these two concepts briefly.

The intensity of exercise in both isotonic and isokinetic weight-training programs is measured by the repetition maximum (RM). Recall from earlier in the chapter that 1 RM is the maximal load that a muscle group can lift one time. Similarly, 6 RM is the maximal load that can be lifted six times. Therefore, the amount of weight lifted is greater when you perform a low number of RM than a high number of RM; that is, the weight lifted while you perform 4 RM is greater than the weight lifted while you perform 15 RM.

The number of repetitions (reps) performed consecutively without resting is called a **set**. For example, if you lift 6 RM, 1 set = 6 reps. Because the amount of rest required between sets will vary among individuals depending on how fit they are, the duration of weight training is measured by the number of sets performed, not by actual time.

Although experts disagree as to the optimum number of reps and sets required to improve strength and endurance, they do agree on some general guidelines. To improve strength, 3 sets of 6 reps for each exercise are generally recommended. Applying the concept of progressive

resistance to a strength-training program involves increasing the amount of weight to be lifted a specific number of reps. For example, suppose that 3 sets of 6 reps were selected as your exercise prescription for increasing strength. As the training progresses and you become stronger, the amount of weight you lift must be increased. A good rule of thumb is that once you can perform 10 reps easily, you should increase the load to a level at which 6 reps are again maximal. **FIGURE 4.8** on page 98 illustrates the relationship between strength improvement and various combinations of reps and sets.

A key point in Figure 4.8 is that programs involving 3 sets result in the greatest strength gains. The reason is that the third set requires the greatest effort and thus is the greatest overload for the muscle. Although it may seem that adding a fourth set would elicit even greater gains, most studies suggest that performing 4 or more sets results in overtraining and decreased benefits.

To improve muscular endurance, 4 to 6 sets of 15 to 18 reps for each exercise are recommended. Note that you

---

set Number of repetitions performed consecutively without resting.

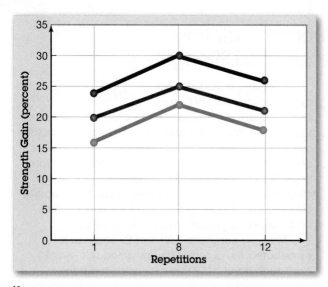

Key

⬤━⬤ 1 Set

⬤━⬤ 2 Sets

⬤━⬤ 3 Sets

FIGURE 4.8 Strength gains from a resistance-training program consisting of various sets and repetitions. All programs were performed 3 days a week for 12 weeks. Note that in this program, the greatest strength gains (+30% improvement) were obtained using 3 sets of 8 reps per set.

can improve endurance either by increasing the number of reps progressively while maintaining the same load, or by increasing the amount of weight while maintaining the same number of reps. The advantage of the latter program is that it would also improve muscular strength.

Most research suggests that 2 to 3 days of exercise per week is optimal for strength gains (5). However, studies have also shown that once the desired level of strength has been achieved, one high-intensity training session per week is sufficient to maintain the new level of strength. Finally, although limited research exists regarding the optimal frequency of training to improve muscular endurance, 3 to 5 days per week appear to be adequate (13).

MAKE SURE YOU **KNOW...**

■ Progressively overloading a muscle can be accomplished by changing the frequency, intensity, and/or duration of the activity. Increasing the weight lifted increases the intensity of the exercise. Increasing repetitions increases the duration of the exercise.

■ Exercising 2 to 3 days per week is optimal for strength gains, and one high-intensity session per week is sufficient to maintain new strength levels. Exercising 3 to 5 days per week is adequate to improve muscular endurance.

——MasteringHealth™

Starting and Maintaining a Weight-Training Program

LO Differentiate between the starter, slow progression, and maintenance phases of weight-training programs.

As with any plan for behavior change, you should begin your weight-training program with both short- and long-term goals. Be sure to establish realistic short-term goals that you can reach in the first several weeks of training. Reaching these goals will help motivate you to continue training.

Developing an Individualized Exercise Prescription

An exercise prescription for strength training has three stages: the starter phase, the slow progression phase, and the maintenance phase.

The primary objective of the **starter phase** is to build strength gradually without developing undue muscular soreness or injury. You can accomplish this by starting your weight-training program slowly—beginning with light weights, a high number of repetitions, and only 1 set per exercise, gradually working up to 2 sets per exercise. The recommended frequency of training during this phase is twice per week. The duration of this phase varies from 1 to 3 weeks, depending on your initial strength fitness level. A sedentary person might spend 3 weeks in the starter phase, whereas a moderately trained person may spend only 1 to 2 weeks.

The **slow progression phase** may last 4 to 20 weeks, depending on your initial strength level and your long-term strength goal. The transition from the starter phase to the slow progression phase involves three changes in the exercise prescription: increasing the frequency of training from 2 to 3 days per week; increasing the amount of weight lifted (and decreasing the number of repetitions); and increasing the number of sets performed from 2 to 3. The objective of the slow progression phase is to gradually increase muscular strength until you reach your desired level.

After reaching your strength goal, your long-term objective is to maintain this level of strength; this is the **maintenance phase** of the strength-training exercise prescription. Maintaining strength will require a lifelong weight-training effort. You will lose strength if you do not continue to exercise. The good news is that the effort required to maintain muscular strength is less than the initial effort needed to gain strength: Research has shown that as little as one workout per week is required to maintain strength (16).

See the sample programs on pages 101–103 to develop your exercise prescription for weight training.

Supine Exercises

The 5-point contact principle (explained in the "Coaching Corner" box on this page) applies most easily to supine exercises such as bench presses, flys, incline or decline presses, and triceps extensions. For example, when doing a bench press, check the points from head to toe. The back of your head, your upper back and your lower back/buttocks should be in contact with the bench. The bottom of each foot should be in contact with the floor. If your feet do not reach the floor, place a step at the end of the bench. The step should be a height that allows you to place your feet flat with your knees in line with your hips. If your knees are above your hips, the step is too high.

Seated or Standing Exercises

If you are in a seated or standing position, you can still use the 5-point contact principle as a safety measure. Imagine you have a wall behind you. Your head should be touching the imaginary wall with your chin level to the floor. Stand with your shoulders and lower back/buttocks to the imaginary wall. Maintain a slight pinch in your shoulder blades and *do not* arch your back more than normal. Both feet should be flat on the floor.

Motivation to Maintain Strength Fitness

 LO 9 List at least three things you can do to motivate yourself to begin and continue a weight-training program.

The problems associated with starting and maintaining weight-training programs are similar to those associated with cardiorespiratory training. You must find time to train regularly, so good time management is critical.

Another key feature of any successful exercise program is that training must be fun. You can make weight training fun in a variety of ways. First, find an enjoyable place to work out. Locate a facility that contains the type of weights you want to use and in which you feel comfortable and motivated. Second, develop a realistic weight-training routine. Designing a training routine

Any weight-training program must place a major emphasis on safety and injury prevention. Improper posture and body alignment can result in significant injury. One of the ways you can check your form is to use the *5-point contact principle*. While this principle applies primarily to exercises performed in the supine position (lying on the back), it can also be applied to seated and standing exercises. If each of the five areas of the body is in contact with the bench or the floor, it increases stability and reduces the risk of injury. The five points of contact are:

■ Back of the head
■ Upper back
■ Lower back/buttocks
■ Bottom of right foot
■ Bottom of left foot

These five points of contact ensure that you have proper alignment and support for your spine and lower back, which is especially important if you are lifting heavy weights. Check yourself for the five points of contact before each exercise set. If a spotter is available, have him or her check these during the set.

that is too hard may be good for improving strength but will not increase your desire to train. Therefore, design a program that is challenging but fun. Weight training is often more enjoyable with a partner. When looking for a workout buddy, ask a friend who is highly motivated to exercise and has strength abilities similar to yours.

starter phase The beginning phase of an exercise program. The goal of this phase is to build a base for further physical conditioning.

slow progression phase The second phase of an exercise program. The goal of this phase is to increase muscular strength beyond the starter phase.

maintenance phase The third phase of an exercise program. The goal of this phase is to maintain the increase in strength obtained during the first two phases.

Strength Training for Older Adults

According to the Centers for Disease Control and Prevention (CDC), in 2012, 2.4 million people age 65 and older were treated in emergency rooms for injuries due to falls. Nearly 23,000 people over age 65 died as a result of injuries sustained in falls. In an effort to combat the number and minimize the severity of the falls, the American Academy of Orthopedic Surgeons (AAOS) and the National Athletic Trainers Association (NATA) are teaming up to help older Americans avoid falls and reduce the severity of injuries when falls do occur. The two organizations have established guidelines that call for older adults to keep muscles and bones strong by strength training with weight-bearing and resistance exercise.

Weight-bearing exercises increase bone density and help prevent osteoporosis. Research has shown that resistance training can enhance muscle mass and function even in 90-year-old subjects. Seniors can increase their lean muscle mass, improve dynamic balance, and increase their strength by participating in a well-designed strength-training program 2 or 3 days a week.

Sources: Centers for Disease Control and Prevention and The Merck Company Foundation. *The State of Aging and Health in America 2013.* Whitehouse Station, NJ: The Merck Company Foundation, 2007; Kim, S., and T. Lockhart. Effects of 8 weeks of balance or weight training for the independently living

Although the benefits of weight training are numerous, recent studies have shown that improved appearance, elevated self-esteem, and the overall feeling of well-being that result from regular weight training are the most important factors in motivating people to continue to train regularly. Looking your best and feeling good about yourself are excellent reasons to maintain a regular weight-training program. In addition, your elevated resting metabolic rate can help you burn calories more efficiently throughout the day, so even if you put on a few extra pounds of muscle mass, your clothes will fit better and you will look better.

Sample Exercise Prescriptions for Weight Training

Scan to plan your individualized program for weight training.

As with training to improve cardiorespiratory fitness, the exercise prescription for improving muscular strength must be tailored to the individual. Before starting a program, review the guidelines and precautions listed in **FIGURE 4.9** on the following page.

The sample programs below illustrate the stages of a suggested strength-training exercise prescription. When you reach the strength goals of the program, the maintenance phase begins. You will use the same routine as you used during the progression phase, but you'll need to perform the routine only once per week.

The isotonic strength-training program contains exercises that are designed to provide a whole-body workout.

Although you can perform some exercises using either machines or free weights, keep in mind that safety and proper lifting techniques are especially important when using free weights.

Follow the exercise routines described and illustrated on pages 104–110, and develop your program using the guidelines provided. This selection of exercises is designed to provide a comprehensive strength-training program that focuses on the major muscle groups. You can also use Table 4.2 to help you plan a program that works the total body. To avoid overtraining any one muscle group, be aware of which muscle groups are involved in an exercise. Note that it is not necessary to perform all exercises in one workout session; you can perform half of the exercises on one day and the remaining exercises on another day.

1. Warm up before beginning a workout. This involves 5 to 10 minutes of movement (calisthenics) using all major muscle groups.

2. Start slowly. The first several training sessions should involve limited exercises and light weight!

3. Use the proper lifting technique, as shown in the isotonic strength-training exercises in this chapter. Improper technique can lead to injury.

4. Follow all safety rules.

5. Always lift through the full range of motion. This not only develops strength throughout the full range of motion but also helps you maintain flexibility.

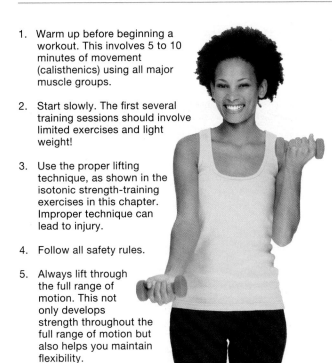

FIGURE 4.9 Follow these guidelines and precautions prior to beginning a strength-training program.

TABLE 4.2 ▪ Total-Body Resistance-Training Program

Target Area	Muscles	Without Weights	With Weights
Arms	Biceps	Pull-up	Biceps curl
	Triceps	Push-up	Triceps extension
Chest	Pectoralis major	Push-up, dip	Fly, chest press, bench press
Upper back	Trapezius, rhomboids	Pull-up	Upright row
Abdomen	Rectus abdominis, obliques	Curl-up, plank	Abdominal curl
Back	Erector spinae, Latissimus dorsi	Back extension	Lateral pulldown, back extension
Legs	Gluteus maximus	Lunge	Leg press
	Quadriceps	Lunge	Leg extension, leg press
	Hamstrings	Lunge	Hamstring curl
	Gastrocnemius, soleus	Heel raise	Calf raise

Starter Phase (For Beginner-Level Lifters Using Isotonic Strength-Training Exercises)

Choose exercises from Table 4.2 and on pages 104–110.

Weight = RM for the number of reps (e.g., 15 reps done with a 15 RM weight, etc.)						
	Mon	Tues	Wed	Thur	Fri	Sat
Week 1	1 set/15 reps/ lower body	1 set/15 reps/ upper body		1 set/15 reps/ lower body	1 set/15 reps/ upper body	
Week 2	2 sets/15 reps/ lower body	2 sets/15 reps/ upper body		2 sets/15 reps/ lower body	2 sets/15 reps/ upper body	
Week 3	2 sets/15 reps/ lower body	2 sets/15 reps/ upper body		2 sets/15 reps/ lower body	2 sets/15 reps/ upper body	

Slow Progression Phase (For Intermediate-Level Lifters Using Isotonic Strength-Training Exercises)

Choose exercises from Table 4.2 and on pages 104–110.

Weight = RM for the number of reps (e.g., 12 reps done with a 12 RM weight, etc.)						
	Mon	**Tues**	**Wed**	**Thur**	**Fri**	**Sat**
Week 4	2 sets/12 reps/ upper body	2 sets/12 reps/ lower body		2 sets/12 reps/ upper body	2 sets/12 reps/ lower body	
Week 5	2 sets/12 reps/ upper body	2 sets/12 reps/ lower body		2 sets/12 reps/ upper body	2 sets/12 reps/ lower body	
Week 6	3 sets/12 reps/ upper body	3 sets/12 reps/ lower body		3 sets/12 reps/ upper body	3 sets/12 reps/ lower body	
Week 7	3 sets/12 reps/ upper body	3 sets/12 reps/ lower body		3 sets/12 reps/ upper body	3 sets/12 reps/ lower body	
Week 8	3 sets/12 reps/ upper body	3 sets/12 reps/ lower body		3 sets/12 reps/ upper body	3 sets/12 reps/ lower body	
Week 9	3 sets/12 reps/ upper body	3 sets/12 reps/ lower body		3 sets/12 reps/ upper body	3 sets/12 reps/ lower body	
Week 10	3 sets/12 reps/ upper body	3 sets/12 reps/ lower body		3 sets/12 reps/ upper body	3 sets/12 reps/ lower body	
Week 11	3 sets/12 reps/ upper body	3 sets/12 reps/ lower body		3 sets/12 reps/ upper body	3 sets/12 reps/ lower body	
Week 12	3 sets/12 reps/ upper body	3 sets/12 reps/ lower body		3 sets/12 reps/ upper body	3 sets/12 reps/ lower body	
Week 13	3 sets/12 reps/ upper body	3 sets/12 reps/ lower body		3 sets/12 reps/ upper body	3 sets/12 reps/ lower body	
Week 14	3 sets/12 reps/ upper body	3 sets/12 reps/ lower body		3 sets/12 reps/ upper body	3 sets/12 reps/ lower body	
Week 15	3 sets/10 reps/ upper body	3 sets/10 reps/ lower body		3 sets/10 reps/ upper body	3 sets/10 reps/ lower body	
Week 16	3 sets/10 reps/ upper body	3 sets/10 reps/ lower body		3 sets/10 reps/ upper body	3 sets/10 reps/ lower body	
Week 17	3 sets/10 reps/ upper body	3 sets/10 reps/ lower body		3 sets/10 reps/ upper body	3 sets/10 reps/ lower body	
Week 18	3 sets/10 reps/ upper body	3 sets/10 reps/ lower body		3 sets/10 reps/ upper body	3 sets/10 reps/ lower body	
Week 19	3 sets/10 reps/ upper body	3 sets/10 reps/ lower body		3 sets/10 reps/ upper body	3 sets/10 reps/ lower body	
Week 20	3 sets/10 reps/ upper body	3 sets/10 reps/ lower body		3 sets/10 reps/ upper body	3 sets/10 reps/ lower body	

Maintenance Phase (For Advanced-Level Lifters Using Isotonic Strength-Training Exercises)

Choose exercises from Table 4.2 and on pages 104–110.

Weight = RM for the number of reps (e.g., 8 reps done with an 8 RM weight, etc.)						
	Mon	Tues	Wed	Thur	Fri	sat
Week 21	3 sets/8 reps/ upper body	3 sets/8 reps/ lower body		3 sets/8 reps/ upper body	3 sets/8 reps/ lower body	
Week 22	3 sets/8 reps/ upper body	3 sets/8 reps/ lower body		3 sets/8 reps/ upper body	3 sets/8 reps/ lower body	
Week 23	3 sets/8 reps/ upper body	3 sets/8 reps/ lower body		3 sets/8 reps/ upper body	3 sets/8 reps/ lower body	
Week 24	3 sets/8 reps/ upper body	3 sets/8 reps/ lower body		3 sets/8 reps/ upper body	3 sets/8 reps/ lower body	
Week 25	3 sets/8 reps/ upper body	3 sets/8 reps/ lower body		3 sets/8 reps/ upper body	3 sets/8 reps/ lower body	
Week 26	3 sets/8 reps/ upper body	3 sets/8 reps/ lower body		3 sets/8 reps/ upper body	3 sets/8 reps/ lower body	
Week 27	3 sets/8 reps/ upper body	3 sets/8 reps/ lower body		3 sets/8 reps/ upper body	3 sets/8 reps/ lower body	
Week 28	3 sets/8 reps/ upper body	3 sets/8 reps/ lower body		3 sets/8 reps/ upper body	3 sets/8 reps/ lower body	
Week 29	3 sets/8 reps/ upper body	3 sets/8 reps/ lower body		3 sets/8 reps/ upper body	3 sets/8 reps/ lower body	
Week 30	3 sets/8 reps/ upper body	3 sets/8 reps/ lower body		3 sets/8 reps/ upper body	3 sets/8 reps/ lower body	
Week 31	3 sets/6 reps/ upper body	3 sets/6 reps/ lower body		3 sets/6 reps/ upper body	3 sets/6 reps/ lower body	
Week 32	3 sets/6 reps/ upper body	3 sets/6 reps/ lower body		3 sets/6 reps/ upper body	3 sets/6 reps/ lower body	
Week 33	3 sets/6 reps/ upper body	3 sets/6 reps/ lower body		3 sets/6 reps/ upper body	3 sets/6 reps/ lower body	
Week 34	3 sets/6 reps/ upper body	3 sets/6 reps/ lower body		3 sets/6 reps/ upper body	3 sets/6 reps/ lower body	
Week 35	3 sets/6 reps/ upper body	3 sets/6 reps/ lower body		3 sets/6 reps/ upper body	3 sets/6 reps/ lower body	
Week 36	3 sets/6 reps/ upper body	3 sets/6 reps/ lower body		3 sets/6 reps/ upper body	3 sets/6 reps/ lower body	
Maintain	3 sets/6 reps/ upper body	3 sets/6 reps/ lower body		3 sets/6 reps/ upper body	3 sets/6 reps/ lower body	

EXERCISE 4.1 BICEPS CURL

PURPOSE To strengthen the **elbow flexor muscles** (biceps, brachialis, brachioradialis)

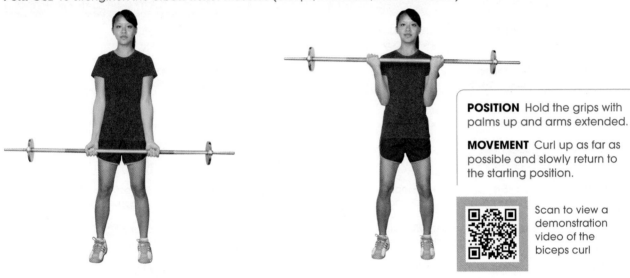

POSITION Hold the grips with palms up and arms extended.

MOVEMENT Curl up as far as possible and slowly return to the starting position.

Scan to view a demonstration video of the biceps curl

EXERCISE 4.2 TRICEPS EXTENSION

PURPOSE To strengthen the muscles on the **back of the upper arm** (triceps)

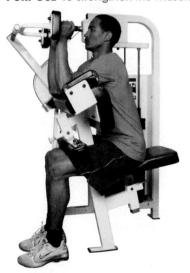 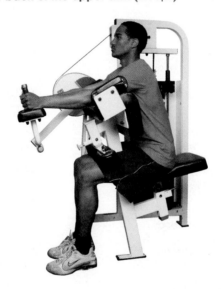

POSITION Sit upright with elbows bent.

MOVEMENT With the little-finger side of the hand against the pad, fully extend the arms and then slowly return to the original position.

Scan to view a demonstration video of the triceps extension

EXERCISE 4.3 DUMBBELL FLY

PURPOSE To strengthen the muscles of the **chest** (pectoralis major) and **shoulder** (anterior deltoid)

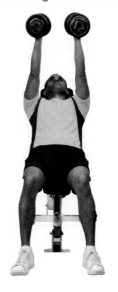
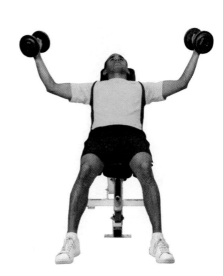

POSITION Lie on an incline bench set at an angle between 45 and 60 degrees. (This can also be done lying flat on the bench.) Hold the dumbbells in front of your body with arms slightly flexed at the elbows.

MOVEMENT Inhale, then lower the dumbbells until your elbows are at shoulder height. Raise the dumbbells while exhaling.

Scan to view a demonstration video of the dumbbell fly.

EXERCISE 4.4 UPRIGHT ROW

PURPOSE To strengthen the muscles of the **neck** (trapezius), **arms** (biceps) and **shoulder** (deltoids)

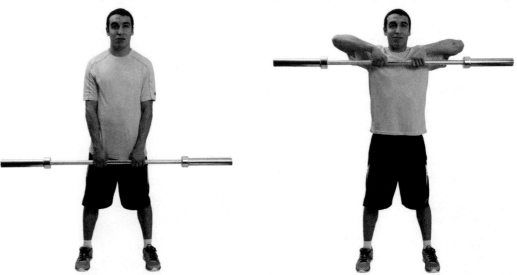

POSITION Stand with your weight equally distributed on both feet and bend legs slightly. Make sure to maintain erect posture with head up, looking straight ahead. Grasp the bar with an overhand grip and keep hands shoulder width apart.

MOVEMENT Raise the bar slowly to chest level and then slowly lower to arms length. Make sure that your elbows are higher than the weights at all times while maintaining total control of the speed of the bar.

CAUTION Beginners and people with lower back problems should use very light weight or a dumbbell at first.

Scan to view a demonstration video of the upright row.

exercises

exercises — Some Exercises for Increasing Muscular Strength

EXERCISE 4.5 LUNGE

PURPOSE To strengthen the muscles of the **hip** (gluteus maximus, hamstrings), **knee** (quadriceps), and **lower back** (erector spinae)

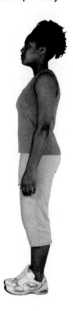
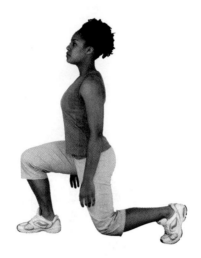

POSITION Stand with your feet hip-width apart.

MOVEMENT Lunge forward, putting all of the weight on your leading leg. Do not let the knee of your leading leg move in front of toes. Keep your knee in line with your ankle. Vary the stride length by taking a simple step forward to involve the quadriceps, or a large step forward to place more stress on the hamstrings and gluteals while stretching the quadriceps and hip flexors.

Scan to view a demonstration video of the lunge.

EXERCISE 4.6 LEG EXTENSION

PURPOSE To strengthen the muscles in the **front of the upper leg** (quadriceps (rectus femoris, vastus lateralis, vastus intermedius, vastus medialis))

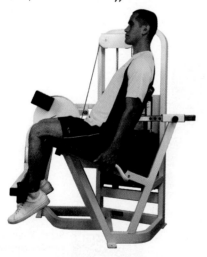
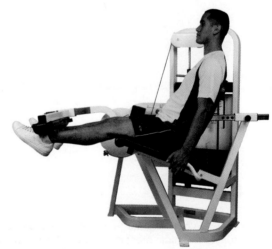

POSITION Sit in a nearly upright position and grasp the handles on the side of the machine. Position your legs so the pads of the machine are against the lower shin.

MOVEMENT Extend the legs until they are completely straight and then slowly return to the starting position.

Scan to view a demonstration video of the leg extension.

106

EXERCISE 4.7 HAMSTRING CURL

PURPOSE To strengthen the muscles on the **back of the upper leg** and **buttocks** (hamstrings (biceps femoris, semi-membranosus, semitendinosis))

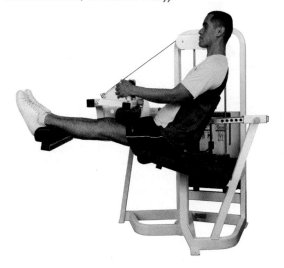

POSITION In a seated position, extend legs so the pads of the machine are just below the calf muscles.

MOVEMENT Curl the legs by pushing down on the pads to at least a 90-degree angle and then slowly return to the original position.

 Scan to view a demonstration video of the hamstring curl.

EXERCISE 4.8 ABDOMINAL CURL

PURPOSE To strengthen the **abdominal muscles** (rectus abdominis, external oblique, internal oblique)

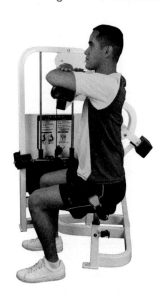
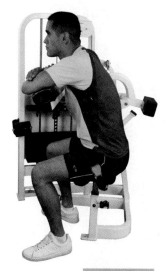

POSITION Sit on the bench and place crossed arms on the padded armrest.

MOVEMENT Bend forward until you feel the abdominals engage. Slowly return to starting position.

 Scan to view a demonstration video of the abdominal curl.

EXERCISE 4.9 BACK EXTENSION

PURPOSE To strengthen the muscles of the **lower back** (erector spinae, quadratus lumborum)

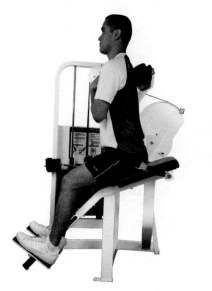
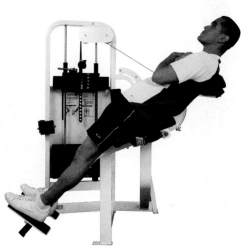

POSITION Sit with your upper back positioned against the back pads, and your feet flat on the platform. Push back against the pads until the spine is straight. Cross your arms over your chest and straighten your spine.

MOVEMENT Press backward against the back pad and slowly extend at the hip, keeping your spine straight. Slowly return to the starting position, keeping the spine straight.

EXERCISE 4.10 BENCH PRESS

PURPOSE To strengthen the muscles in the **chest**, the **front of the shoulders** (pectoralis major, anterior deltoid), and the **back of the upper arm** (triceps)

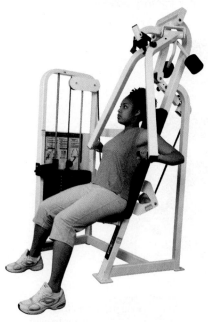
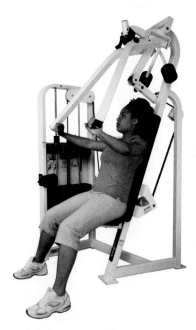

POSITION Sit on the bench with the bench press hand grips level with your chest and your feet flat on the floor.

MOVEMENT Grasp the bar handles and press outward until your arms are completely extended. Return slowly to the original position.

CAUTION Do not arch your back while performing this exercise.

Scan to view a demonstration video of the bench press.

EXERCISE 4.11 PULLOVER

PURPOSE To strengthen the muscles of the **chest** (pectoralis major), **abdomen** (rectus abdominus) and **back** (latissimus dorsi)

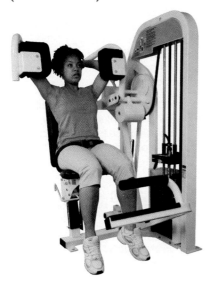 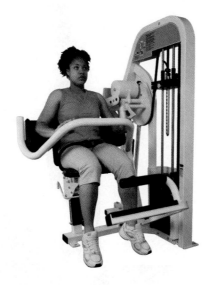

POSITION Sit with your elbows against the padded ends of the movement arm and grasp the bar behind your head.

MOVEMENT Press forward and down with your arms, pulling the bar overhead and down to your abdomen. Slowly return to the original position.

 Scan to view a demonstration video of the pullover.

EXERCISE 4.12 DIP

PURPOSE To strengthen the muscles of the **chest** (pectoralis major), **arms** (triceps) and **shoulders** (deltoids)

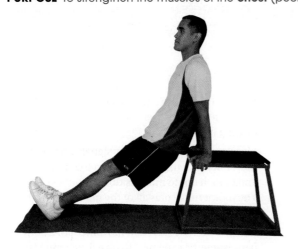 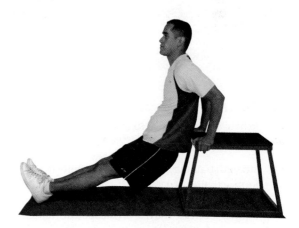

POSITION Stand in front of a platform or a box, facing forward. Place both hands on the platform behind you.

MOVEMENT Dip down until the elbows are at 90-degree angles. Return to starting position.

 Scan to view a demonstration video of the dip.

PURPOSE To strengthen the **calf muscles** (gastrocnemius, soleus)

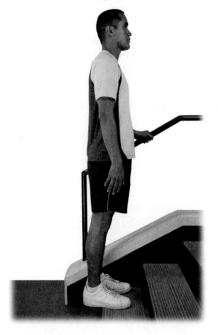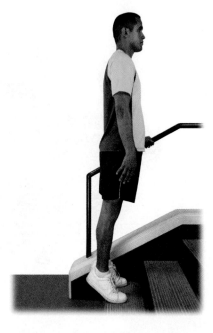

POSITION Stand with your feet flat on the floor, or on the edge of a step.

MOVEMENT Raise yourself up using the ankle joint only, and lower yourself back to starting position.

Scan to view a demonstration video of the toe raise.

study plan

Customize your study plan—and master your health!—in the Study Area of **MasteringHealth.**

summary

hear it! STUDY REVIEW

To hear an MP3 Chapter Summary, scan here or visit the Study Area in MasteringHealth™.

 LO **1** ■ Strength training can improve our ability to perform activities of daily life. It can also reduce low back pain, reduce the incidence of exercise-related injuries, decrease the risk of osteoporosis, and help maintain functional capacity as we age.

■ Muscular strength is the ability of a muscle to generate maximal force. This refers to the amount of weight that an individual can lift during one maximal effort. Muscular endurance is the ability of a muscle to generate force repeatedly. Increasing muscular strength through exercise will also increase muscular endurance. In contrast, training to improve muscular endurance does not always result in improved muscular strength.

LO **2** ■ Skeletal muscle is composed of a collection of long, thin cells (fibers). Muscles are attached to bone by thick connective tissue (tendons). Muscle actions result in the tendons pulling on bone, causing movement.

■ Muscle action is regulated by signals coming from motor nerves, which originate in the spinal cord and branch out to muscles throughout the body. The motor nerve plus all of the muscle fibers it controls make up a motor unit.

■ Isotonic exercises result in movement of a body part. Isometric exercises involve developing tension within the muscle but result in no movement of body parts. Concentric muscle actions (positive work) involve muscle shortening. In contrast, eccentric muscle actions (negative contractions) involve muscle lengthening.

■ Human skeletal muscle can be classified into two major fiber types: slow-twitch (also called type I) and fast-twitch (also called type II, with two subclasses: type IIa and IIx). The percentages of slow-twitch and fast-twitch fibers vary among individuals. Slow-twitch fibers shorten slowly but are highly fatigue resistant. Fast-twitch (IIx) fibers shorten rapidly but fatigue rapidly. Fast-twitch (IIa) fibers combine the characteristics of fast- and slow-twitch fibers—they contract rapidly and are resistant to fatigue.

- The process of involving more muscle fibers to produce increased muscular force is called fiber recruitment. Two physiological factors determine the amount of force that can be generated by a muscle: the size of the muscle and the number of fibers recruited.

LO 3
- A test used to assess muscular strength is the one-repetition maximum (1 RM) test.

- Muscular endurance can be evaluated using the push-up test and either the sit-up test or the curl-up test.

LO 4
- The overload principle states that a muscle will increase in strength and/or endurance only when it works against a workload that is greater than normal. Progressive overload is the application of the overload principle to strength and endurance exercise programs.

LO 5
- Strength training improves muscular strength initially by altering fiber recruitment patterns (increasing the number of fibers recruited) and then by increasing muscle size.

- Muscle size is increased primarily because of an increase in fiber size (hypertrophy).

LO 6
- A weight-training program using low repetitions and high resistance results in the greatest strength gains; a program using high repetitions and low resistance results in the greatest improvement in muscular endurance.

- Isotonic exercise involves contracting a muscle against a movable load (usually a free weight or weights on a weight machine).

- Isometric exercise is based on contracting a muscle at a fixed angle against an immovable object (using isometric muscle action).

- Isokinetic exercise requires the use of machines that govern the speed of movement during muscle contraction throughout the range of motion.

LO 7
- The number of repetitions of an exercise performed without resting is referred to as a set.

- Progressively overloading a muscle can be done by changing the frequency, intensity, and/or duration of the exercise.

- To achieve strength gains, it is necessary to work out 2 to 3 times per week. Once the desired strength level is achieved, one high-intensity workout per week can maintain that level. Exercising 3 to 5 days per week is recommended to improve muscular endurance.

LO 8
- A strength-training program ideally consists of three phases: the starter phase, lasting 1 to 3 weeks, followed by a slow progression phase lasting 4 to 20 weeks, and the maintenance phase that continues for life.

LO 9
- To maintain motivation for strength training, it is important to manage your time to include workouts and to find ways to make the workout fun, such as having a workout partner and finding a gym or other facility that you like.

- Motivation can also stem from improvements in health, physical appearance, and self-esteem that result from training.

study questions

review it! QUIZZES

Find more review questions online at MasteringHealth™.

LO 1
1. Muscular strength is defined as the ability of a muscle to
   a. generate force over and over again.
   b. generate maximal force.
   c. shorten as it moves a resistance.
   d. increase in size.

2. Which of the following is a benefit of a regular strength-training program?
   a. reduces the incidence of back pain
   b. increases $\dot{V}O_2$ max
   c. reduces the incidence of colds
   d. increases endurance exercise capacity

3. List at least three reasons why training for strength and endurance is important.

LO 2
4. What type of muscle action occurs as the muscle lengthens and controls the movement with resistance and/or gravity?
   a. concentric action
   b. eccentric action
   c. isometric action

5. A slow-twitch muscle fiber
   a. contracts slowly and produces small amounts of force.
   b. contracts rapidly and generates great amounts of force.
   c. contracts rapidly, produces great force, and fatigues rapidly.
   d. fatigues rapidly and is ideal for short bursts of activity.

6. Name the three muscle fiber types and describe the characteristics of each type.

7. Explain how muscle fiber type relates to success in various types of athletic events.

8. How does the pattern of muscle fiber recruitment change with increasing intensities of contraction?

9. List the factors that determine muscular strength.

10. Distinguish between isometric, concentric, and eccentric muscle actions.

11. Define the following terms: *motor unit, isotonic exercise, isometric exercise, isokinetic exercise,* and *static contraction.*

LO ③ 12. Define the concept of 1 RM.

LO ④ 13. Define *progressive overload* and explain how this concept is applied in strength training.

14. Explain specificity of training.

15. Compare and contrast training to increase strength versus training to increase endurance.

LO ⑤ 16. Define *hypertrophy* and *hyperplasia.*

17. What types of physiological changes result from strength training and how do these occur?

LO ⑥ 18. Describe the Valsalva maneuver and the effect this has on the body.

19. Which of the following should be the general rule to follow to increase strength in a weight-training program?
   a. high resistance—high repetitions
   b. low resistance—low repetitions
   c. low resistance—high repetitions
   d. high resistance—low repetitions

LO ⑦ 20. What frequency of exercise is needed to produce gains in muscle strength?

LO ⑧ 21. List the phases of strength- and endurance-training programs and explain how the phases differ.

LO ⑨ 22. Why is it important that your strength-training program be challenging enough to produce results but not too difficult?

suggested reading

American College of Sports Medicine. Quantity and quality of exercise for developing and maintaining cardiorespiratory, musculoskeletal, and neuromotor fitness in apparently healthy adults: Guidance for prescribing exercise. *Medicine and Science in Sports and Exercise* 43(7):1334–1359, 2011.

Baechle, T. R., and R. Earle. *Essentials of Strength Training and Conditioning,* 3rd ed. Champaign, IL: Human Kinetics, 2008.

Bishop P. A., E. Jones, and A. K. Woods. Recovery from training: A brief review. *Journal of Strength and Conditioning Research* 22(3):1015–1024, 2008.

Folland, J. P., and A. G. Williams. The adaptations to strength training: Morphological and neurological contributions to increased strength. *Sports Medicine* 37(2):145–168, 2007.

Hoffman, J. (Ed.). *National Strength and Conditioning Association's Guide to Program Design.* Champaign, IL: Human Kinetics, 2012.

Hurley, B., E. D. Hanson, and A. K. Sheaff. Strength training as a countermeasure to aging muscle and chronic disease. *Sports Medicine* 41(4):289–306, 2011.

Knuttgen, H. G. Strength training and aerobic exercise: Comparison and contrast. *Journal of Strength and Conditioning Research* 21(3):973–978, 2007.

Krieger, J. W. Single vs. multiple sets of resistance exercise for muscle hypertrophy: A meta-analysis. *Journal of Strength and Conditioning Research* 24(4):1150–1159, 2010.

Martel, G. F., S. M. Roth, F. M. Ivey, J. T. Lemmer, B. L. Tracy, D. E. Hurlbut, E. J. Metter, B. F. Hurley, and M. A. Rogers. Age and sex affect human muscle fiber adaptations to heavy-resistance strength training. *Experimental Physiology* 91(2):457–464, 2006.

Phillips, S. M. The science of muscle hypertrophy: Making dietary protein count. *Proceedings of the Nutrition Society* 70(1):100–103, 2011.

Phillips, S. M., and R. A. Winett. Uncomplicated resistance training and health-related outcomes: Evidence for a public health mandate. *Current Sports Medicine Report* 9(4):208–213, 2010.

Zatsiorsky, V. M., and W. J. Kraemer. *Science and Practice of Strength Training,* 2nd ed. Champaign, IL: Human Kinetics, 2006.

helpful weblinks

do it! WEBLINKS

For links to the organizations and websites listed, visit MasteringHealth™.

American College of Sports Medicine

Comprehensive website that provides equipment recommendations, how-to articles, book recommendations, and position statements about all aspects of health and fitness. **www.acsm.org**

Muscle Physiology

In-depth presentation of how muscle works. **people.eku. edu/ritchisong/301notes3.htm**

WebMD

General information about exercise, fitness, and wellness. Great articles, instructional information, and updates. **http://www.webmd.com**

WikiBooks

Part of the Human Physiology series highlighting Muscular Physiology. **http://en.wikibooks.org**

laboratory 4.1

do it! LABS
Complete Lab 4.1 online in the
study area of **MasteringHealth.com**

Name _____ Date _____

Evaluating Muscular Strength: The 1 RM Test

The 1 RM test is used to measure muscular strength. You can use the following procedure to determine your 1 RM:

1. Begin with a 5- to 10-minute warm-up using the muscles to be tested.
2. For each muscle group, select an initial weight that you can lift without undue stress.
3. Gradually add weight until you reach the maximum weight that you can lift at one time. If you can lift the weight more than once, add additional weight until you reach a level of resistance such that you can perform only one repetition. Remember that a true 1 RM is the maximum amount of weight that you can lift one time.

The seated chest press and the leg press are two common exercises used to perform the 1 RM test. The seated chest press measures upper-body muscular strength, and the leg press measures muscular strength in the lower body.

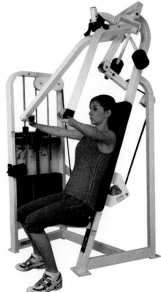
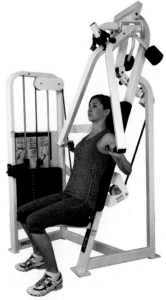

Scan to view a demonstration video of the chest press.

The seated chest press can be used to evaluate upper-body muscular strength.

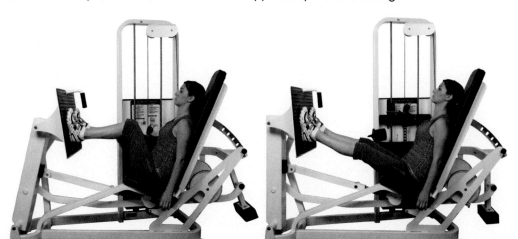

Scan to view a demonstration video of the leg press.

A leg press can be used to evaluate lower-body muscular strength.

Your muscular strength score is the percentage of your body weight lifted in each exercise. To compute your strength score, divide your 1 RM weight in pounds by your body weight in pounds, and then multiply by 100. For example, suppose a 150-pound man has a seated chest press 1 RM of 180 pounds. This individual's muscular strength score for the seated chest press is computed as

$$\frac{1 \text{ RM weight}}{\text{body weight}} \times 100 = \text{muscle strength score}$$

Therefore,

$$\text{muscle strength score} = \frac{180 \text{ pounds}}{150 \text{ pounds}} \times 100 = 120$$

TABLE 4.3 and **TABLE 4.4** on page 116 list strength score norms for college-age men and women for the seated chest press and leg press, respectively. According to **TABLE 4.3**, a muscular strength score of 120 on the seated chess press places a college-age man in the "good" category.

In the spaces below, record your muscular strength score and fitness category for the 1 RM tests for the leg press and seated chess press.

Age: _____   **Body weight:** _____ **lb**

Date: _____

Exercise	1 RM (lb)	Muscular Strength	Fitness Category
Seated chest press			
Leg press			

GOAL SETTING

1. Based on your results, write a goal to maintain or improve your current fitness level. For example, if you scored "fair" on this test, your goal might be to improve your fitness level to a "good" rating. If your fitness level indicated a score of "excellent," your goal might be to maintain your current fitness status.

   Goal: _____

2. Write three strategies for how you intend to achieve the goal you wrote. For example, one strategy for improving your current fitness status might be to perform 1 set of 10 repetitions at 50% of your 1 RM, 3 times a week. To progressively overload the muscles, increase the number of sets, and increase the weight load by 5–10 lb.

   1. _____

      _____

   2. _____

      _____

   3. _____

      _____

Muscular strength score calculation is based on: Roitman, J. (Ed.). *ACSM's Resource Manual for Guidelines for Exercise Testing and Prescription*. Philadelphia: Lippincott, Williams, & Wilkins, 2001.

TABLE 4.3 ■ Strength Score Norms for the Seated Chest Press

Locate your fitness level for upper-body muscular strength using your seated chest press score.

Men	Superior	Excellent	Good	Average	Poor	Very Poor
20–29 yrs	>147	130–147	114–129	99–113	89–98	<89
30–39 yrs	>123	110–123	98–109	88–97	79–87	<79
40–49 yrs	>109	98–109	88–97	80–87	73–79	<73
50–59 yrs	>96	88–96	79–87	71–78	64–70	<64
60+ yrs	>87	80–87	72–79	66–71	58–65	<58
Women	Superior	Excellent	Good	Average	Poor	Very Poor
20–29 yrs	>90	80–90	70–79	59–69	52–58	<52
30–39 yrs	>76	70–76	60–69	53–59	48–52	<48
40–49 yrs	>71	62–71	54–61	50–53	44–49	<44
50–59 yrs	>61	55–61	48–54	44–47	40–43	<40
60+ yrs	>64	54–64	47–53	43–46	39–42	<39

1 RM seated bench press with bench press weight ratio = weight pushed/body weight X 100.

TABLE 4.4 ■ Strength Score Norms for the Leg Press

Locate your fitness level for lower-body muscular strength using your seated leg press score.

Men	Superior	Excellent	Good	Average	Poor	Very Poor
20–29 yrs	>227	213–227	197–212	183–196	164–182	<164
30–39 yrs	>207	193–207	177–192	165–176	153–164	<153
40–49 yrs	>191	182–191	168–181	157–167	145–156	<145
50–59 yrs	>179	171–179	158–170	146–157	133–145	<133
60+ yrs	>172	162–172	149–161	138–148	126–137	<126
Women	Superior	Excellent	Good	Average	Poor	Very Poor
20–29 yrs	>181	168–181	150–167	137–149	123–136	<123
30–39 yrs	>160	147–160	133–146	121–132	110–120	<110
40–49 yrs	>147	137–147	123–136	113–122	103–112	<103
50–59 yrs	>136	125–136	110–124	99–109	89–98	<89
60+ yrs	>131	118–131	104–117	93–103	86–92	<86

1 RM seated leg press with leg press weight ratio = weight pushed/body weight X 100.

laboratory 4.2

do it! LABS
Complete Lab 4.2 online in the
study area of **MasteringHealth.com**

Name _____ Date _____

Evaluating Muscular Strength: The Estimated 1 RM Test

You can use the following procedure to determine your estimated 1 RM for any particular lift (e.g., chest press and leg press for this lab):

1. First, perform a set of 10 repetitions using a light weight.

2. Next, add 5 lb and perform up to 10 repetitions.

3. Repeat this process until you reach a weight that you can lift only 5 times. This is called your repetitions maximum (RM) for that weight. Therefore, when you find the weight that you can press only 5 times, that is your 5 RM weight

Be sure to have an experienced instructor supervise the process so that your 5 RM weight can be discovered in fewer than five trials. Rest a few minutes after each trial to recover.

After determining your 5 RM, you can use **TABLE 4.5** on page 118 to estimate your 1 RM. For example, if your 5 RM for the chest press is 100 lb., then the estimate for the 1 RM would be about 115 lb.

Remember, strength is largely determined by your body size. Thus, to determine your "standardized" muscle strength from the estimated 1 RM, use the same formula that you used in Laboratory 4.1:

$$\text{muscle strength score} = \frac{\text{1 RM weight}}{\text{body weight}} \times 100$$

Record your muscular strength scores below, and use Table 4.3 or Table 4.4 in Laboratory 4.1 to determine your fitness category.

Age: _____   **Body weight:** _____ **lb**

Date: _____

Exercise	1 RM (lb)	Muscular Strength	Fitness Category
Seated chest press			
Leg press			

GOAL SETTING

1. Based on your results, write a goal to maintain or improve your current fitness level. For example, if your score was "fair" on this test, your goal might be to improve your fitness level to a "good" rating. If your fitness level indicated a score of "excellent," your goal might be to maintain your current fitness status.

   Goal: _____

2. Write three strategies for how you intend to achieve the goal you wrote. For example, one strategy for improving your current fitness status could be to perform 1 set of 10 repetitions at 50% of your 1 RM, 3 times a week. To progressively overload the muscles, increase the number of sets, and increase the weight load by 5–10 lb.

   1. _____
   _____
   2. _____
   _____
   3. _____
   _____

Muscular strength score calculation is based on: Roitman, J. (Ed.). *ACSM's Resource Manual for Guidelines for Exercise Testing and Prescription.* Philadelphia: Lippincott, Williams, & Wilkins, 2001.

Table 4.5 ■ 1 RM Prediction Table

In the left column, find your 5 RM weight for either the chest press or the leg press exercise. Then go to the specific column for each exercise to find your estimated 1 RM.

	Chest Press	Leg Press
5RM Wt (lb)	1 RM Predicted	1 RM Predicted
10	13	42
15	19	48
20	24	53
25	30	59
30	35	64
35	41	70
40	47	75
45	52	81
50	58	86
55	64	92
60	69	97
65	75	103
70	81	108
75	86	114
80	92	119
85	98	125
90	103	130
95	109	136
100	115	141
105	120	147
110	126	152
115	132	158
120	137	163
125	143	169
130	149	174
135	154	180
140	160	185
145	165	190
150	171	196
155	177	201
160	182	207
165	188	212
170	194	218
175	199	223
180	205	229
185	211	234
190	216	240
195	222	245
200	228	251
205	233	256

5RM Wt (lb)	Chest Press 1 RM Predicted	Leg Press 1 RM Predicted
210	239	262
215	245	267
220	250	273
225	256	278
230	262	284
235	267	289
240	273	295
245	279	300
250	284	306

Source: Adapted from Reynolds et al., Prediction of one repetition maximum strength from multiple repletion maximum testing and anthropometry. *Journal of Strength and Conditioning Research.* 20(3):584-592, 2006.

laboratory 4.3

do it! LABS
Complete Lab 4.3 online in the
study area of **MasteringHealth.com**

Name _____   Date_____

Tracking Your Progress

Use the log below to chart your strength-training progress. Record the date, number of sets, reps, and the weight for each of the exercises listed in the left column.

Date				
Exercise	St/Rp/Wt	St/Rp/Wt	St/Rp/Wt	St/Rp/Wt
Biceps curl (see Exercise 4.1)				
Triceps extension (see Exercise 4.2)				
Dumbbell fly (see Exercise 4.3)				
Upright rows (see Exercise 4.4)				
Lunges (with or without weights) (see Exercise 4.5)				
Abdominal curl (see Exercise 4.8)				
Quadriceps extension (see Exercise 4.6)				
Hamstring curl (see Exercise 4.7)				
Bench press or chest press (see Exercise 4.10)				

St / Rp / Wt = Sets / Reps / Weight *Example:* 2 / 6 / 80=2 sets of 6 reps each with 80 lb.

laboratory 4.4

do it! LABS
Complete Lab 4.4 online in the
study area of **MasteringHealth.com**

Name _____ Date _____

Measuring Muscular Endurance: The Push-Up and Curl-Up Tests

THE STANDARD PUSH-UP TEST

Perform the standard push-up test as follows:

Scan to view a demonstration video of the push-up test.

1. Position yourself on the ground in push-up position (Figure a). (Note that you can instead use the modified push-up position shown in Figures c and d.) Place your hands about shoulder-width apart, and extend your legs in a straight line with your weight on your toes.

2. Lower your body until your chest is within 1 to 2 inches off the ground (Figure b), and raise yourself back to the up position. Be sure to keep your back straight and to lower your entire body as a unit.

3. Select a partner to count your push-ups and time your test (test duration is 60 seconds). Warm up with a few push-ups, and rest for 2 to 3 minutes after the warm-up to prepare for the test.

4. When your partner says "Go," start performing push-ups. Have your partner count your push-ups aloud, and ask him or her to let you know periodically how much time remains.

5. Record your score and fitness classification (from **TABLE 4.6** on page 122) in the chart on page 123.

THE STANDARD PUSH-UP

Scan to view a demonstration video of the standard push-up.

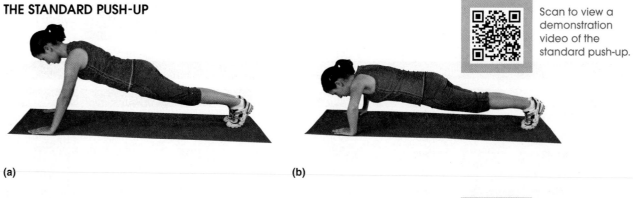

(a)   (b)

THE MODIFIED PUSH-UP

Scan to view a demonstration video of the modified push-up.

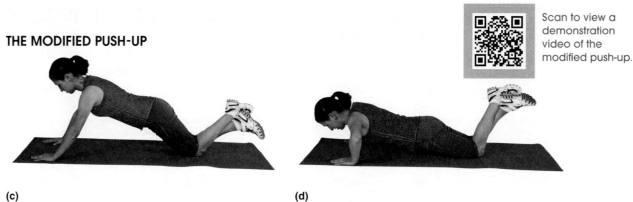

(c)   (d)

THE CURL-UP TEST

You can perform the curl-up test as follows:

1. Lie on your back with your legs shoulder-width apart, your knees bent 90 degrees, your arms straight at your sides, and your palms flat on the mat (Figure a).
2. Extend your arms so that your fingertips touch a strip of tape perpendicular to your body. A second strip of tape is located toward the feet and parallel to the first (10 centimeters apart).
3. Use the cadence provided on a metronome set to 50 beats per minute. Slowly curl up your upper spine until your fingers touch the second strip of tape. Then slowly return to the lying position with your head and shoulder blades touching the mat and your fingertips touching the first strip of tape. Breathe normally throughout, exhaling during the curling up stage.
4. Have your partner count the number of consecutive curl-ups you do in 1 minute, maintaining the metronome cadence and without pausing, to a maximum of 25. Record your score and fitness classification (from **TABLE 4.7**) in the chart on page 123.

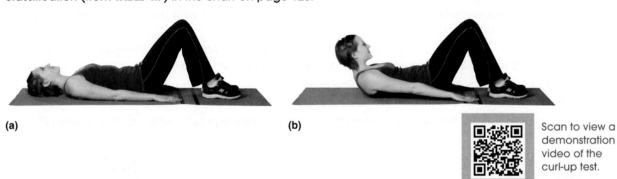

(a)   (b)

Scan to view a demonstration video of the curl-up test.

TABLE 4.6 ■ Norms for Muscular Endurance Using the Push-Up and Modified Push-Up Tests

Men	Superior	Excellent	Good	Fair	Poor	Very Poor
20–29 yrs	≥62	47–61	37–46	29–36	22–28	≤21
30–39 yrs	≥52	39–51	30–38	24–29	17–23	≤16
40–49 yrs	≥40	30–39	24–29	18–23	11–17	≤10
50–59 yrs	≥39	25–38	19–24	13–18	9–12	≤8
60+ yrs	≥28	23–27	18–22	10–17	6–9	≤5
Women (modified push-up)	**Superior**	**Excellent**	**Good**	**Fair**	**Poor**	**Very Poor**
20–29 yrs	≥45	36–44	30–35	23–29	17–22	≤16
30–39 yrs	≥39	31–38	24–30	19–23	11–18	≤10
40–49 yrs	≥33	24–32	18–23	13–17	6–12	≤5
50–59 yrs	≥28	21–27	17–20	12–16	6–11	≤5
60+ yrs	≥20	15–19	12–14	5–11	2–4	≤1
Women (full push-up)	**Superior**	**Excellent**	**Good**	**Fair**	**Poor**	**Very Poor**
20–29 yrs	≥42	28–41	21–27	15–20	10–14	≤9
30–39 yrs	≥39	23–38	15–22	11–14	8–10	≤7
40–49 yrs	≥20	15–19	13–14	9–12	6–8	≤5
50–59 yrs	—	—	—	—	—	—
60+ yrs	—	—	—	—	—	—

— indicates data not available.

Source: Reprinted with permission from The Cooper Institute®, Dallas, Texas from a book called *Physical Fitness Assessments and Norms for Adults and Law Enforcement.* Available online at www.CooperInstitute.org.

TABLE 4.7 ■ Norms for Muscular Endurance Using the Curl-Up Test

Men	Excellent	Very Good	Good	Fair	Needs Improvement
15–19 yrs	25	23–24	21–22	16–20	≤15
20–29 yrs	25	21–24	16–20	11–15	≤10
30–39 yrs	25	18–24	15–17	11–14	≤10
40–49 yrs	25	18–24	13–17	6–12	≤5
50–59 yrs	25	17–24	11–16	8–10	≤7
60–69 yrs	25	16–24	11–15	6–10	≤5
Women	Excellent	Very Good	Good	Fair	Needs Improvement
15–19 yrs	25	22–24	17–21	12–16	≤11
20–29 yrs	25	18–24	14–17	5–13	≤4
30–39 yrs	25	19–24	10–18	6–9	≤5
40–49 yrs	25	19–24	11–18	4–10	≤3
50–59 yrs	25	19–24	10–18	6–9	≤5
60–69 yrs	25	17–24	8–16	3–7	≤2

Source: Canadian Physical Activity, Fitness & Lifestyle Approach: CSEP-Health & Fitness Program's Appraisal and Counselling Strategy, 3rd edition, © 2003. Reprinted with permission from the Canadian Society for Exercise Physiology.

Age: _____

Date: _____

Number	Fitness Category
Push-ups (1 min):	
Curl-ups (1 min):	

GOAL SETTING

1. Based on your results, write a goal to maintain or improve your current fitness level. For example, if your score was "fair" on this test, your goal might be to improve your fitness level to a "good" rating. If your fitness level indicated a score of "excellent," your goal might be to maintain your current fitness status.

   Goal: _____

2. Write three strategies for how you intend to achieve your goal. For example, a strategy for improving your current fitness status might be to perform 1 set of 10 push-ups (or curl-ups), 3 times a week. To progressively overload the muscles, increase the number of sets to 2 and then 3.

   1. _____
      _____

   2. _____
      _____

   3. _____
      _____

Source: Curl-up test from *Canadian Physical Activity, Fitness & Lifestyle Approach: CSEP-Health & Fitness Program's Appraisal and Counselling Strategy,* 3rd edition, © 2003. Reprinted with permission from the Canadian Society for Exercise Physiology.

laboratory 4.5

do it! LABS
Complete Lab 4.5 online in the
study area of **MasteringHealth.com**

Name _____   Date _____

Measuring Core Strength and Stability

Position a watch on the ground where you can easily see it.

1. Assume the basic press-up position, with your elbows on the ground (see the figure below). Hold this position for 60 seconds.
2. Lift your right arm off the ground. Hold this position for 15 seconds.
3. Return your right arm to the ground, and lift your left arm off the ground. Hold this position for 15 seconds.
4. Return your left arm to the ground, and lift your right leg off the ground. Hold this position for 15 seconds.
5. Return your right leg to the ground, and lift your left leg off the ground. Hold this position for 15 seconds.
6. Lift your left leg and right arm off the ground. Hold this position for 15 seconds.
7. Return your left leg and right arm to the ground, and lift your right leg and left arm off the ground. Hold this position for 15 seconds.
8. Return to the basic press-up position (elbows on the ground). Hold this position for 30 seconds.

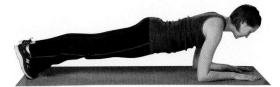

Basic press-up position

Scan to view a demonstration video of the basic press-up.

ANALYSIS

Analysis of the result involves comparing it with the results of previous tests. It is expected that, with appropriate training between each test, the analysis would indicate an improvement.

If you were able to complete this test, you have good core strength. If you were unable to complete the test, then repeat the routine 3 or 4 times a week until you can.

Source: Modified from the Core Muscle Strength Test by Brian Mackenzie, www.brianmac.co.uk/coretest.htm.

GOAL SETTING

1. Based on your results, write a goal to maintain or improve your current core strength and stability. For example, if you were able to hold the position for 60 seconds in step 1 but were unable to lift your right arm off the ground (step 2), your goal might be to work on completing step 2 and step 3. If you completed all steps, your goal could be to maintain your current core strength and stability.

   Goal: _____

2. Write three strategies for how you intend to achieve your goal. For example, an objective for improving your current fitness status might be to perform steps 3 and 4 three times a week. To progressively overload the muscles, increase to steps 5 and 6.

   1. _____
      _____
   2. _____
      _____
   3. _____
      _____

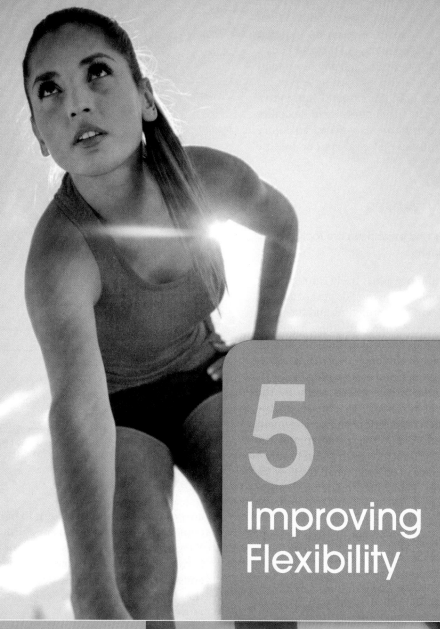

5
Improving Flexibility

1. Define *flexibility* and explain the five factors that limit movement.

2. Describe how the stretch reflex works and how it can be avoided during flexibility exercises.

3. List the benefits of improved flexibility and explain why flexibility is important for a healthy back.

4. Define *posture* and explain how good and bad posture differ.

5. Name and describe two common tests used to evaluate flexibility and the factors measured by each test.

6. Define four stretching techniques and explain the purposes of each; also, list the essential components and time frame of an exercise program designed to increase flexibility.

GYMNASTS AND ICE SKATERS are not the only people who need to maintain adequate flexibility. When you bend down to tie your shoes or reach up to pull a sweatshirt over your head, you're relying on your body's flexibility to perform these tasks. In fact, any movement that requires stretching, reaching, or twisting is possible because you enjoy a range of motion around your joints. Most of us do not appreciate the importance of flexibility as a fitness component until we experience an injury resulting in pain or stiffness that restricts our routine movements.

How Flexibility Works

 Define *flexibility* **and explain the five factors that limit movement.**

Flexibility is the ability to move joints freely through their full range of motion. People vary in their degrees of flexibility because of differences in body structure, and the range of motion of most joints can decline with disuse. Tightness of the muscles, tendons, and connective tissue surrounding a joint can limit your range of motion; however, this restriction can be eliminated through proper stretching.

Joint range of motion is determined partly by the shapes and positions of the bones that make up the joint and partly by the composition and arrangement of muscles, tendons, and connective tissue around the joint (1, 2). Although the structure of the bones cannot be altered, the soft tissues can be lengthened to allow for greater range of motion. Remember, moderate tension to the muscles being stretched can make a significant improvement in your flexibility over time.

Of course, there are some movements that you will not be able to do, no matter how much you stretch, without causing yourself harm. You can't bend your fingers backward, for example, or rotate your arm 360 degrees at the elbow. The reason is that you are limited in the range of motion at your joints by your body's anatomy.

Structural Limitations to Movement

There are five primary anatomical factors that limit movement (see **FIGURE 5.1**):

1. *The shape of the bones* determines the amount of movement possible at each joint. For example, because of the way they are structured, ball and socket joints, such as the shoulder and hip, have greater range of motion than hinge joints, such as the elbow and knee.

2. *A stiff muscle* will limit the range of motion at a joint; likewise, a warmed-up muscle will be more flexible and allow a greater range of motion.

3. *The connective tissue* within the joint capsule provides stability at the joint. **Ligaments**, for example,

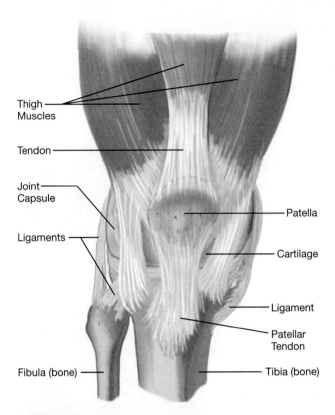

FIGURE 5.1 A view of the knee joint and the anatomical structures that influence movement.

Source: Based on Johnson, Michael D., *Human Biology: Concepts and Current Issues, 7th Ed.,* © 2014. Reprinted and Electronically reproduced by permission of Pearson Education, Inc., Upper Saddle River, New Jersey.

are positioned around the joint to prevent the bone ends from coming apart, as in a dislocation injury. They prevent movements that a normal, healthy joint is not supposed to make. **Cartilage** covers the ends of the bones and creates a better fit between the bones, which helps eliminate unnecessary movements.

4. *Tendons*, which connect muscles to bones and to connective tissue surrounding joints, are extensions of the muscle tissue. If the muscle is tight, the tendon will also be tight.

5. *Tight skin* can limit the range of motion at a joint.

Exercise aimed at improving flexibility does not change the structure of bone, but it alters the soft tissues (muscles, joint connective tissue, and tendons) that contribute to flexibility. The resistance of various soft tissues to total joint flexibility breaks down as follows: joint capsule (47%), muscle (41%), tendon (10%), and skin (2%). Note that the structures associated with the joint capsule, muscles, and tendons provide most of the body's resistance to movement. Therefore, flexibility exercises must alter the resistance of one of these three to increase the range of motion around a joint.

MAKE SURE YOU **KNOW...**

- Flexibility is the range of motion of a joint; it allows you to bend, twist, and reach without experiencing pain or stiffness.

- Stretching can alleviate tightness at a joint.

- The structural and physiological limits to flexibility are due to the characteristics of bone; muscles; connective tissue within the joint capsule, such as ligaments and cartilage; the tendons, which connect muscles to bones and to connective tissue surrounding joints; and skin.

—MasteringHealth™

Stretching and the Stretch Reflex

 Describe how the stretch reflex works and how it can be avoided during flexibility exercises.

Stretching muscles and tendons is desirable because these soft tissues can lengthen over time and thus improve flexibility. In contrast, stretching the ligaments in the joint capsule is undesirable because it can lead to a loose joint that would be highly susceptible to injury.

When a doctor taps you below the knee with a rubber hammer, your knee extends. This is a **stretch reflex** caused by the rapid stretching of the **muscle spindles** within the quadriceps muscles that move the knee joint. Activating the stretch reflex is counterproductive to flexibility, because during the stretch the muscle shortens rather than lengthens. (Remember that the goal of stretching is to lengthen the muscle.) Fortunately, you can avoid the stretch reflex if you stretch the muscles and tendons very slowly. In fact, if you hold a muscle stretch for several seconds, the muscle spindles allow the muscle being stretched to further relax and permit an even greater stretch (2, 3). Therefore, stretching exercises are most effective when they avoid promoting a stretch reflex.

Muscle spindles are one type of **proprioceptor**, specialized receptors in muscles and tendons that provide feedback to the brain about the position of the body parts. When you were learning to catch a ball, you had to look at the position of your arms and hands to make sure they were in line with the path of the ball. As your catching skills improved, you no longer had to look at your arm position to know that it was lined up with the ball. The proprioceptors in your muscles and tendons provided feedback to your brain about where your arm was positioned. The proprioceptors within the muscles are muscle spindles, and the proprioceptors within the tendons are **Golgi tendon organs**.

MAKE SURE YOU **KNOW...**

- If muscle spindles are stretched suddenly, they initiate a stretch reflex that causes the muscle to contract and shorten. However, if muscles are stretched slowly, the stretch reflex can be avoided.

- The proprioceptors (muscle spindles and Golgi tendon organs) monitor the muscles and tendons and report their positions to the brain.

—MasteringHealth™

Benefits of Flexibility

 List the benefits of improved flexibility and explain why flexibility is important for a healthy back.

Although increased flexibility provides numerous benefits, including increased joint mobility, efficient body movement, and good posture (1, 3, 4), there is no research evidence to support the idea that it reduces the incidence of muscle injury during exercise. In fact, one critical review article suggests that stretching may contribute to injury (5). However, most studies suggest that stretching offers protection from muscle injury when combined with a general warm-up, and improved flexibility does help keep your joints healthy and can prevent lower back pain. Let's look at these benefits more closely.

---

flexibility The ability to move joints freely through their full range of motion.

ligaments Connective tissues within the joint capsule that hold bones together.

cartilage Tough connective tissue that forms a pad on the end of long bones such as the femur, tibia, and humerus. Cartilage acts as a shock absorber to cushion the weight of one bone on another and to provide protection from the friction due to joint movement.

stretch reflex Involuntary contraction of a muscle due to rapid stretching of that muscle.

muscle spindles Type of proprioceptor found within muscle.

proprioceptor Specialized receptor in muscle or tendon that provides feedback to the brain about the position of body parts.

Golgi tendon organs Type of proprioceptor found within tendons.

Keeping Joints Healthy

Joints will suffer from lack of movement if you do not regularly engage them. If a joint is not moved enough, or has a limited range of motion, scar tissue can form that further restricts the joint motion and can be painful to the point that you may not be able to move the joint. The shoulder joint is particularly susceptible to such scar tissue formation. Mild stretching on a daily basis can prevent a joint from becoming immobile.

Joint mobility is also important for keeping the joint lubricated. Joints contain synovial fluid, which is needed to reduce friction and decrease wear and tear. Moving the joint helps circulate the synovial fluid, which in turn reduces the friction on the cartilage between the bones. Too much friction can damage cartilage, setting the stage for arthritis. Mild stretching can improve the mobility of the joint and promote normal wear on the cartilage covering the ends of the bones.

Stretching also directly affects the joints by reducing tension within the fibers of a muscle. When a muscle is stretched, these fibers are free to slide past one another, and the tension is literally worked out of the muscle. Reduced muscle tension reduces the tension exerted by the tendon as it crosses the joint. The force of the muscle exerted through the tendon on the bone can cause the bone ends in the joint to be pulled closer together, thus limiting the joint's range of motion. In essence, stretching can have the same effects on muscle tension as a manual muscle massage, at a much lower cost.

Preventing Lower Back Pain

Another benefit of improved flexibility is that it can help prevent lower back problems. Lower back pain (LBP) is sometimes called a **hypokinetic disease**, that is, a disease associated with a lack of exercise. The weak abdominal muscles commonly seen in sedentary individuals and the lack of flexibility in the hip flexor muscles are two common causes of LBP.

The abdominal muscles play a significant role in keeping the pelvic girdle in a neutral alignment with the spine **(FIGURE 5.2)**. When the abdominal muscles are weak, the pelvis tilts forward and creates an increased hyperextension (forward curve), called *lordosis*, in the lower back. The muscles that flex the hip can affect the pelvis in the same way; however, they pull the pelvis forward when they are tight. Stretching these muscles and strengthening the abdominal muscles are important to keep the pelvis in a neutral alignment.

In addition to the abdominal muscles and the hip flexor muscles, the hamstrings and the lower back muscles also attach to the posterior side of the pelvis and can affect its alignment. The hamstring muscles exert a downward pull on the pelvis, whereas the lower back muscles exert an upward pull. Keeping all four muscle groups in balance helps keep the pelvis in a neutral alignment with

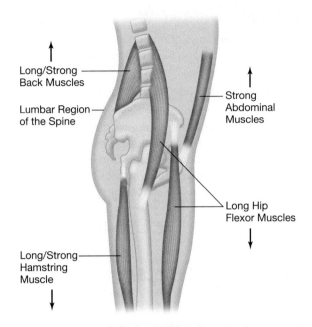

Long/Strong Back Muscles

Lumbar Region of the Spine

Strong Abdominal Muscles

Long Hip Flexor Muscles

Long/Strong Hamstring Muscle

FIGURE 5.2 Strong abdominal and hip flexor muscles, balanced with strong back and hamstring muscles, help keep the spine and pelvis in neutral alignment, thereby lowering the risk of LBP.

the lumbar region of the spine and thus diminishes the likelihood for LBP.

Up to 80% of people will experience LBP, and approximately 15% of Americans will be disabled by LBP in their lifetime (6). Men and women are affected equally by back pain, usually between the ages of 25 and 60. Most pain in the lower back goes away in a few days or weeks. Lower back pain that lasts for longer than 6 months is considered chronic.

People who regularly carry heavy backpacks are at increased risk of lower back problems. In one study (7), curvature of the spine significantly increased as subjects carried weight high on the back rather than on the lower back. Although this study did not examine resulting back problems from the chronic wearing of a backpack, the findings certainly suggest that long-term backpack use can result in misalignment in the lower back.

The psychological, social, and physical costs of lower back pain are high, as are the economic costs. The medical, insurance, and business/industry costs are generally considered to be in the billions of dollars per year. Developing and maintaining healthy lower back function requires a balance of flexibility, strength, and endurance. **TABLE 5.1** outlines the top contributors to lower back pain, and the stretching you can do to help maintain a healthy back.

see it!

ABC VIDEOS

Watch an ABC Video about the "Do's and Don'ts of Stretching" at MasteringHealth™.

TABLE 5.1 ■ Top Potential Contributors to Lower Back Pain and Sample Exercises to Maintain a Healthy Back	
Contributor to LBP	**Exercise**
Poor lower back lumbar flexibility	Modified hurdler's stretch (Exercise 5.5) Lower back stretch (Exercise 5.8)
Poor hamstring flexibility	Leg stretch (Exercise 5.4) Modified hurdler's stretch (Exercise 5.5)
Poor gluteal flexibility	Hip and gluteal stretch (Exercise 5.7)
Poor strength of the anterior and lateral abdominals	Curl-ups (page 144)
Poor flexibility of the back extensor muscles	Lower back stretch (Exercise 5.8)

MAKE SURE YOU **KNOW...**

- Improved flexibility increases joint mobility and joint health, increases resistance to muscle injury, helps prevent lower back problems, allows for efficient body movement, and improves posture and personal appearance.

- Flexibility of the hamstrings and lower back and strong abdominal muscles are important for a healthy back.

— MasteringHealth ™

Preventing Poor Posture

LO Define *posture* and explain how good and bad posture differ.

Posture is the position of your joints that you hold while standing or sitting. Good posture is the result of holding positions that place the least amount of strain on the supporting muscles and ligaments around your joints. By routinely holding your body in good posture, you are maintaining the proper balance between the length and tension of all of the muscles around the joints.

Bad posture occurs when you hold positions that stretch muscles on one side of a joint, while shortening them on the other side. This can place undue strain on muscles, ligaments, and joints that will, over time, cause misalignment, pain, and possible damage to joints. Thus, bad posture leads to worse posture!

By incorporating strength and flexibility exercises into your daily routine, you can help correct any imbalances that you may have in your posture and prevent problems from occurring in the future. Here are some benefits of good posture:

- Minimizes any abnormal wear on joint surfaces that could result in arthritis.

- Reduces the stress on the ligaments holding the joints of the spine together.

- Prevents the spine from becoming fixed in abnormal positions, which may help prevent nerve stress and associated pains.

- Prevents fatigue because muscles are being used more efficiently.

- Prevents strain or overuse problems.

- Prevents backache and muscular pain.

- Contributes to a good appearance.

Use Laboratory 5.1 to evaluate your posture and then determine how your flexibility (determined in the next section) might be affecting your posture. Then make sure to include in your exercise routine those flexibility exercises that can help with correcting imbalances around joints.

MAKE SURE YOU **KNOW...**

- Posture refers to the position of your joints that you hold while standing or sitting.

- Strength and flexibility exercises can help you correct imbalances in your posture.

— MasteringHealth ™

Evaluating Flexibility

LO Name and describe two common tests used to evaluate flexibility and the factors measured by each test.

Flexibility is joint specific. That is, you might be flexible in one joint but lack flexibility in another. You may also notice that you are more flexible on one side of your body than the other. This disparity is often due to more frequent use of the dominant side of the body.

Although no single test is representative of total body flexibility, measurements of trunk and shoulder flexibility are commonly evaluated. The **sit-and-reach test** measures the ability to flex the trunk, which means stretching the lower back muscles and the muscles in the back of the thigh (hamstrings). In Laboratory 5.2, the first figure illustrates the sit-and-reach test using a sit-and-reach box.

The **shoulder flexibility test** evaluates the range of motion at the shoulder. See Laboratory 5.2 at the end of the chapter for a walk-through of the sit-and-reach and shoulder flexibility tests.

---

hypokinetic disease Disease associated with a lack of exercise.

sit-and-reach test Fitness test that measures the ability to flex the trunk.

shoulder flexibility test Fitness test that measures the ability of the shoulder muscles to move through their full range of motion.

Once you complete the sit-and-reach test and the shoulder flexibility test, you will better understand how flexible or inflexible you are. Both active and inactive individuals are often classified as average or below average for trunk and shoulder flexibility. In fact, only individuals who regularly perform stretching exercises are likely to possess flexibility levels that exceed the average. Regardless of your current flexibility classification, your flexibility goal should be to reach a classification of above average (i.e., good, excellent, or superior).

MAKE SURE YOU **KNOW**...

- Flexibility measurements are joint specific.
- Two popular tests to evaluate flexibility are the sit-and-reach test and the shoulder flexibility test.

MasteringHealth™

consider this! //////////////////////

Contrary to popular belief, weight lifting does not decrease flexibility. In fact, the use of proper form during weight lifting can actually increase flexibility.

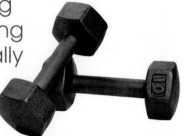

EXAMINING THE **EVIDENCE**
Can Yoga Improve Your Fitness Levels?

Yoga is an ancient discipline that originated thousands of years ago in India. It involves physical, mental, and spiritual aspects, and there are various forms (schools) of practice. Some forms place more emphasis on meditation and spiritual practice, and others focus primarily on enhancing the health of the body.

Hatha yoga refers to any form that incorporates *asanas* (physical postures). Various types of hatha yoga are practiced in the Western world (see chart below for common types). A 2012 Harris poll (see www.yogajournal.com) found that 20 million people in the United States practice yoga and another 40 million plan to try it.

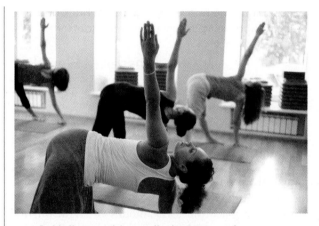

Type of Yoga	Description
Ashtanga	Involves a rigorous series of postures.
Bikram (also known as hot yoga)	Postures are performed in a heated room to promote sweating.
Hatha	General term that describes any form of yoga based on a series of physical postures.
Iyengar	Emphasizes proper alignment in poses and involves the use of props for assistance.
Restorative	Uses props and passive poses to encourage relaxation.
Vinyasa	Rigorous practice that involves a flow of poses with smooth transitions and may include music.

One major purpose of a yoga practice is to reduce stress. The practice is designed to connect body, mind, and spirit through specific breathing patterns and physical movements. Yoga participants report better sleep, increased energy levels, less stiffness, reduced blood pressure, and improved circulation.

But is there evidence that yoga can improve physical fitness? As you have learned, overload stress is required to produce physiological adaptation in our body. Thus, an exercise must cause a large volume of blood flow to induce cardiorespiratory adaptations (increased $\dot{V}O_2$ max). Muscles must be overloaded with heavier weights to increase strength and endurance. While the benefits of yoga have been debated by researchers, recent studies have shown how the body adapts to a regular yoga practice. It is clear that yoga improves flexibility, since the postures stretch muscles around joints (8). It was also shown that strength, cardiovascular measures, and maximal aerobic fitness were not altered after yoga training (8).

The takeaway is that yoga offers some of the same benefits that exercise can have on certain aspects of mental health, and there is solid evidence that a regular practice can significantly increase joint flexibility. To date, most evidence suggests that yoga doesn't increase aerobic capacity or strength in healthy young adults.

Designing a Flexibility Training Program

 Define four stretching techniques and explain the purposes of each; also, list the essential components and time frame of an exercise program designed to increase flexibility.

Because flexibility training is a key part of any fitness program, you'll want to include stretching exercises in your fitness routine. As with designing programs for the other fitness components, your first step will be to set short- and long-term goals. Do you want to become more flexible in the shoulders, or is your aim more to improve your hamstring and lower back flexibility? No matter what your goal, you will want to think about how you will get there before you begin your new flexibility training routine. Also consider keeping a record of your workouts and improvements to follow your progress and plan your future training schedule.

Once you've set your goals, you can consider the types of stretches to include in your program. Three kinds of stretching techniques are commonly used to increase

---

steps ▶ FOR BEHAVIOR CHANGE

Are you too stiff?

Answer the following questions to help determine whether you would benefit from increased flexibility.

Y N
☐ ☐ Do you often feel as though you have a stiff neck?
☐ ☐ Is your mobility impaired when you turn your head to the left or right?
☐ ☐ Do you have difficulty washing your own back?
☐ ☐ Does your lower back feel stiff when you sit at your desk for prolonged periods of time?
☐ ☐ Do your ankles and feet feel stiff when you get out of bed in the morning?

If you answered yes to more than one question, check out the following tips.

Tips to Improve Flexibility

Tomorrow, you will:

☑ Sit on the edge of your bed when you wake up and make 10 small and 10 large circles to the right and then to the left with your right foot. Repeat with your left foot.

☑ Use the shower as an opportunity to incorporate stretching. Let the warm water hit the back of your neck, shoulders, and upper back. Perform 10 shoulder rolls forward, 10 backward, and 10 neck tilts to the left and right while the shower spray is aimed at your neck and shoulders.

☑ Stretch if your neck feels stiff when you are working at your desk. Perform 5 minutes of gentle neck stretches and shoulder rolls at the top of every hour.

Within the next 2 weeks, you will:

☑ Try to increase the flexibility in your shoulders by holding a washcloth in your right hand as you reach behind your head. Try to grasp the washcloth with your left hand as you reach behind your back. By the end of the first 2 weeks, you should be able to reach it. Try pulling the washcloth up and down as you grasp it in both hands, increasing your range of motion with each up-and-down movement.

By the end of the semester, you will:

☑ Find a physioball for prolonged sitting. If your lower back is stiff after sitting for prolonged periods of time, try sitting on a physioball instead of a desk chair. The smaller muscles of the spine will be exercised as you balance on the physioball.

EXAMINING THE EVIDENCE

When Muscles Cramp

A muscle cramp is one of the most common problems encountered in sports and exercise. For many years, the primary causes of muscle cramps were thought to be dehydration and/or electrolyte imbalances. Accordingly, drinking enough fluids and ensuring that the diet contains sufficient amounts of sodium (from table salt, for example) and potassium (e.g., from bananas) have long been encouraged as preventive measures. When muscles cramp, stretching and/or massage have been used to relieve the cramping until electrolyte balance can be restored.

More recent research, however, suggests that cramping may be due to abnormal spinal control of motor neuron activity, especially when a muscle contracts while shortened (9). For example, the cramping that often occurs in the calf muscles of recreational swimmers when their toes are pointed may occur because those calf muscles are contracting while they are shortened.

The most prevalent risk factors for cramps during exercise are muscle fatigue and poor stretching habits (failure to stretch regularly and long enough during each session). Other risk factors include older age, higher body mass index, and a family history of muscle cramps.

If cramping occurs, you should do the following:

- Passively stretch the muscle. Such stretching induces receptors that sense the stretch to initiate nerve impulses that inhibit muscle stimulation.

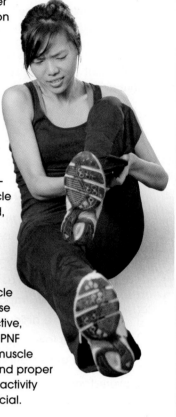

- Drink plenty of water to avoid dehydration or electrolyte imbalances. Sports drinks can help replenish glucose and electrolytes, but do not use salt tablets or drink fluids containing caffeine.

- Seek medical attention if multiple muscle groups are involved, because this could be a sign of more serious problems.

Although no strategies for preventing muscle cramping during exercise have been proven effective, regular stretching using PNF techniques, correcting muscle balance and posture, and proper training for the exercise activity involved may be beneficial.

---

flexibility: **dynamic stretching**, **ballistic stretching**, and **static stretching**. A fourth type of stretching called **proprioceptive neuromuscular facilitation (PNF)** is often used in rehabilitation settings (2, 9).

Dynamic stretching is equally effective for exercise programs and sports training. The fluid, exaggerated movements in dynamic stretches mimic the movements of many exercises. Ballistic stretching, in contrast, involves rapid and forceful bouncing movements to stretch the muscles. The movements of ballistic stretching are more likely to cause injury, so exercises to warm up the muscles prior to stretching are helpful. Ballistic stretches may be most beneficial to athletes involved in quick, explosive movements. With ballistic stretching, the athlete trains the nervous system and the muscles to adapt to the movements that she routinely performs. However, for the average fitness enthusiast seeking to increase flexibility, ballistic movements may activate the stretch reflex, injuring muscles and tendons. For this reason, ballistic stretching techniques are not usually incorporated into a non-athlete's fitness program.

Most people will benefit from incorporating dynamic, static, and PNF techniques into their fitness program. We'll discuss static and PNF stretching techniques next.

Static Stretching

Static stretching is extremely effective for improving flexibility (2, 4). Static stretching involves slowly lengthening a muscle to a point at which further movement is limited (slight discomfort is felt) and holding this position for a fixed period of time, normally 20–30 seconds, and repeating it 3–4 times, to improve flexibility (4). Compared with ballistic stretching, the risk of injury to the muscles or tendons is minimal with static stretching. When performed during the cool-down period, static stretching may reduce the muscle stiffness associated with some exercise routines (2, 4).

You can perform static stretches at home, and you don't need any special equipment to do them. You can even do them while watching television or sitting at your computer. See Exercises 5.1 through 5.12 for examples of static stretches.

Proprioceptive Neuromuscular Facilitation

Proprioceptive neuromuscular facilitation (PNF) combines stretching with alternately contracting and relaxing muscles. There are two common types of PNF stretching:

Skipping stretches may seem like a time saver, but the return on your time invested in stretching is significant. The following tips can help you make the most of your stretch time.

- Stretching is essential and more productive at the end of a workout than at the beginning. Stretch when it matters most!

- Perform stretches that involve more than one joint at a time.

- Stretch only to a point of mild discomfort and then gradually ease out of the stretch. Try achieving a mind-body connection through stretching and rhythmical breathing. Inhale deeply as you feel your muscles lengthen and exhale deeply as you relax out of the stretch. Repeat 2-3 times and move on to the next stretch.

- Notice if you have different ranges of motion in the major joints. Are there imbalances? Measure your range of motion at each joint and work to improve it over a realistic time period.

- Enhance your experience by listening to your favorite music while you stretch.

---

contract–relax (CR) stretching and *contract–relax/antagonist contract (CRAC) stretching.* The CR stretch technique calls for first contracting the muscle to be stretched. Then, after the muscle is relaxed, it is slowly stretched. The CRAC method calls for the same contract–relax routine but adds the contraction of the **antagonist** muscle, the muscle on the opposite side of the joint. The purpose of contracting the antagonist muscle is to promote a reflex relaxation of the muscle to be stretched.

How do PNF techniques compare with ballistic and static stretching? First, PNF has been shown to be safer and more effective in promoting flexibility than ballistic stretching (9). Second, studies have shown PNF programs to be equal to, or in some cases superior to, static stretching for improving flexibility (10).

Passive and Active Stretching

Some PNF stretches cannot be done alone—that is, they require a partner. The partner supplies resistance to the body part during the contraction of the antagonist muscles, thus preventing the body part from moving. This sequence of movements allows the muscle to relax more than in a static stretch, and greater range of motion can be achieved. The only drawback to this type of stretch is that the partner must provide resistance, which can be very tiring over a short period of time.

The following steps illustrate how a CRAC procedure can be done with a partner (**FIGURE 5.3**):

1. After the assistant moves the limb in the direction necessary to stretch the desired muscles to the point of tightness (where mild discomfort is felt), the exerciser isometrically contracts the muscle being stretched for 3–5 seconds and then relaxes it.

2. The exerciser then moves the limb in the opposite direction of the stretch by isometrically contracting the antagonist muscles. The exerciser holds this isometric contraction for approximately 5 seconds, during which time the muscles to be stretched relax. While the desired muscles are relaxed, the assistant may increase the stretch of the desired muscles.

3. The exerciser then isometrically contracts the antagonist muscles for another 5 seconds, which relaxes the desired muscles, and the assistant again stretches the desired muscles to the point of mild discomfort.

This cycle of three steps is repeated 3 to 5 times.

Some PNF stretches can also be done without a partner (**FIGURE 5.4**). Using a towel or other object to provide resistance can achieve the same benefits without fatiguing an assistant.

---

dynamic stretching Stretching that involves moving the joints through the full range of motion to mimic a movement used in a sport or exercise.

ballistic stretching Type of stretch that involves sudden and forceful bouncing to stretch the muscles.

static stretching Stretching that slowly lengthens a muscle to a point where further movement is limited.

proprioceptive neuromuscular facilitation (PNF) Series of movements combining stretching with alternating contraction and relaxation of muscles.

antagonist The muscle on the opposite side of a joint.

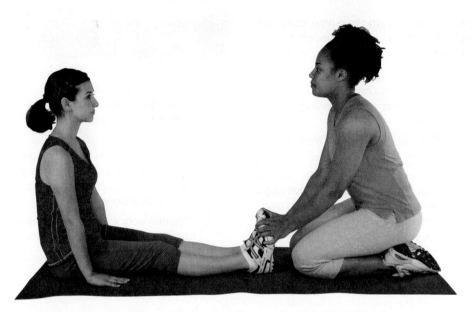

FIGURE 5.3 An example of a partner-assisted CRAC procedure for stretching the calf muscles. The exerciser contracts the calf muscles against resistance provided by the assistant. Then, unassisted, the exerciser contracts the shin (antagonist) muscles, thereby relaxing the calf muscles. Finally, while the exerciser continues contracting the shin muscles, the assistant stretches the calf muscles.

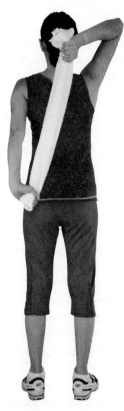

FIGURE 5.4 You can use a towel to do some PNF stretches without a partner.

MAKE SURE YOU **KNOW...**

- Ballistic stretching involves sudden, forceful bouncing.

- Dynamic stretching involves moving the joints through a range of motion that is specific to a sport or activity.

- Static stretches involve stretching a muscle to the limit of movement and holding the stretch for an extended period of time.

- Proprioceptive neuromuscular facilitation (PNF) combines stretching with alternating contraction and relaxation of muscles to improve flexibility.

- Stretching exercises should be performed 2–5 days per week for 10–30 minutes each day.

- The intensity of a stretch is considered to be maximal when "mild discomfort" is felt.

- You can minimize your risk of injury during stretches by avoiding hazardous exercises and making sure to perform stretches correctly.

MasteringHealth™

Sample Exercise Prescriptions for flexibility

Scan to plan your individualized program for flexibility.

So what are the best frequency, intensity, time (duration), and type for your stretching routine (the FITT principle)? The answers vary according to your present level of flexibility, among other factors, but a good rule of thumb is that the first 3 weeks, or starter phase, of a stretching regimen should begin with two stretching sessions per week (see example programs below). Then, in the slow progression phase of the program, add another session during week 6 and another during week 9. Another session, or more, can be added in the maintenance phase beginning in week 12.

Initially, the duration of each training session should be approximately 5 minutes and should increase gradually to approximately 20 minutes (depending on the number of stretches you perform) after 6–12 weeks of stretching during the slow progression phase. The physiological rationale for increasing the duration of stretching is that each stretch position is held for progressively longer durations as the program continues. For example, begin by holding each stretched position for 15 seconds, then add 5 seconds over at least a week, until you reach about 30 seconds. Start by performing each of the exercises once (1 rep), and progress to 4 reps. Thus, the frequency and duration of a stretching exercise prescription should be 2–5 days per week for 10–30 minutes each day. Keep in mind that the total "overload" is what is important! To get 2 minutes of a stretch, you can do 4 reps for 30 seconds, or you can do 8 reps for 15 seconds.

What about the intensity of stretching? In general, a limb should not be stretched beyond a position of mild discomfort. The intensity of stretching is increased by extending the stretch to the limits of your range of motion. Your range of motion will gradually increase as your flexibility improves during the training program.

To improve overall flexibility, all major muscle groups should be stretched. Just because you have good flexibility in the shoulders does not mean your flexibility will be good in the hamstrings. Exercises 5.1 through 5.12 illustrate the proper methods of performing 12 different stretching exercises. Integrate these exercises into the programs outlined on page 152.

In considering the type of exercises to be performed, these exercises are designed to be used in a regular program of stretching to increase flexibility. For safety reasons, all flexibility programs should consist of either PNF or static stretching exercises. The exercises presented involve the joints and major muscle groups for which range of motion tends to decrease with age and disuse. The exercises include both static and PNF movements and may require a partner.

Some stretches that were once thought to improve flexibility are now known to be potentially damaging to the musculoskeletal system. The photos starting on page 143 show some common exercises that may cause injury along with substitute exercises that accomplish the same goals.

To avoid injury, be sure to follow these guidelines:

1. Don't hold your breath. Try to breathe as normally as possible during the exercise.
2. Do not fully extend the knee, neck, or back.
3. Do not stretch muscles that are already stretched.
4. Do not stretch to the point that joint pain occurs.
5. Avoid overstretching when having someone assist you with passive stretches. Make sure you communicate about the end of the range of motion.
6. Avoid forceful extension and flexion of the spine.

Starter Phase (Beginner Flexibility Training Program)

	Mon	Tues	Wed	Thurs	Fri
Week 1	1 rep/12 stretches/10 sec			1 rep/12 stretches/10 sec	
Week 2	1 rep/12 stretches/10 sec			1 rep/12 stretches/10 sec	
Week 3	2 rep/12 stretches/10 sec			2 rep/12 stretches/10 sec	

Slow Progression Phase (Intermediate Flexibility Training Program)

	Mon	Tues	Wed	Thurs	Fri
Week 4	2 rep/12 stretches/ 15 sec			2 rep/12 stretches/ 15 sec	
Week 5	2 rep/12 stretches/ 15 sec			2 rep/12 stretches/ 15 sec	
Week 6	2 rep/12 stretches/ 15 sec	2 rep/12 stretches/ 15 sec		2 rep/12 stretches/ 15 sec	
Week 7	2 rep/12 stretches/ 15 sec	2 rep/12 stretches/ 15 sec		2 rep/12 stretches/ 15 sec	
Week 8	3 rep/12 stretches/ 20 sec	3 rep/12 stretches/ 20 sec		3 rep/12 stretches/ 20 sec	
Week 9	3 rep/12 stretches/ 20 sec	3 rep/12 stretches/ 20 sec		3 rep/12 stretches/ 20 sec	3 rep/12 stretches/ 20 sec
Week 10	3 rep/12 stretches/ 20 sec	3 rep/12 stretches/ 20 sec		3 rep/12 stretches/ 20 sec	3 rep/12 stretches/ 20 sec
Week 11	4 rep/12 stretches/ 30 sec	4 rep/12 stretches/ 30 sec		4 rep/12 stretches/ 30 sec	4 rep/12 stretches/ 30 sec

Maintenance Phase (Advanced Flexibility Training Program)

	Mon	Tues	Wed	Thurs	Fri
Week 12	4 rep/12 stretches/ 30 sec	4 rep/12 stretches/ 30 sec	4 rep/12 stretches/ 30 sec	4 rep/12 stretches/ 30 sec	4 rep/12 stretches/ 30 sec
Week 13	4 rep/12 stretches/ 30 sec	4 rep/12 stretches/ 30 sec	4 rep/12 stretches/ 30 sec	4 rep/12 stretches/ 30 sec	4 rep/12 stretches/ 30 sec
Week 14	4 rep/12 stretches/ 30 sec	4 rep/12 stretches/ 30 sec	4 rep/12 stretches/ 30 sec	4 rep/12 stretches/ 30 sec	4 rep/12 stretches/ 30 sec
Week 15	4 rep/12 stretches/ 30 sec	4 rep/12 stretches/ 30 sec	4 rep/12 stretches/ 30 sec	4 rep/12 stretches/ 30 sec	4 rep/12 stretches/ 30 sec
Week 16	4 rep/12 stretches/ 30 sec	4 rep/12 stretches/ 30 sec	4 rep/12 stretches/ 30 sec	4 rep/12 stretches/ 30 sec	4 rep/12 stretches/ 30 sec
Maintain	4 rep/12 stretches/ 30 sec	4 rep/12 stretches/ 30 sec	4 rep/12 stretches/ 30 sec	4 rep/12 stretches/ 30 sec	4 rep/12 stretches/ 30 sec

EXERCISE 5.1 LOWER LEG STRETCH

PURPOSE To stretch the **calf** muscles (gastrocnemius, soleus) and the **Achilles' tendon**.

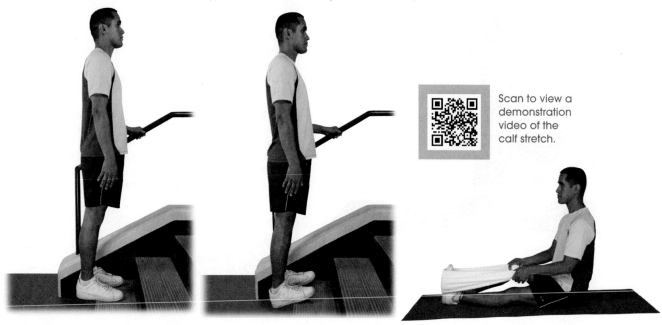

Scan to view a demonstration video of the calf stretch.

POSITION Stand on the edge of a surface that is high enough to allow your heel to drop lower than your toes. Have a support nearby to hold for balance.

MOVEMENT Rise up on your toes as far as possible for several seconds, then lower your heels as far as possible. Shift your body weight from one leg to the other for added stretch of the muscles.

VARIATION Sit on the floor with leg outstretched, loop a towel under the ball of your foot, and gently pull your foot upward so that the top of the foot moves closer to your shin. Another variation (not pictured) is to sit on the floor with one leg outstretched and the other leg flexed, with the sole of your foot along the knee of your other leg. Reach down, grasp the toes of the outstretched leg, and gently pull the foot upward so that the top of the foot moves closer to the shin.

EXERCISE 5.2 SHIN STRETCH

PURPOSE To stretch the muscles of the **shin** (tibialis anterior, extensor digitorum longus, extensor hallucis longus).

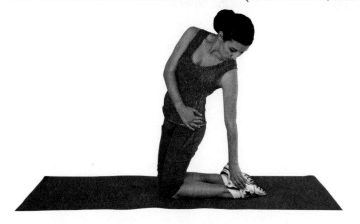

POSITION Kneel on both knees, with your trunk rotated to one side and the hand on that side pressing down on your ankle.

MOVEMENT While pressing down on your ankle, move your pelvis forward; hold for several seconds. Repeat on the other side.

Scan to view a demonstration video of the shin stretch.

EXERCISE 5.3 THIGH STRETCH

PURPOSE To stretch the muscles in the front of the **thigh** (quadriceps) of the extended (rear) leg.

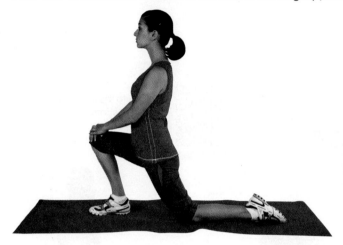

POSITION Kneel on one knee, resting your rear shin and foot flat on the floor. Place both hands on the forward knee. *Note*: If you need more stability, you can place your hands on the floor on either side of the forward foot.

MOVEMENT Slide your rear leg backward so that the knee is slightly behind your hips; then press your hips forward and down, and hold for several seconds. While stretching, maintain approximately a 90-degree angle at the knee of the front leg. Switch the positions of the legs to stretch the other thigh.

Scan to view a demonstration video of the thigh stretch.

EXERCISE 5.4 LEG STRETCH

PURPOSE To stretch the muscles on the **back of the hip** (gluteus maximus), the **back of the thigh** (hamstrings), and the **calf** (gastrocnemius and soleus).

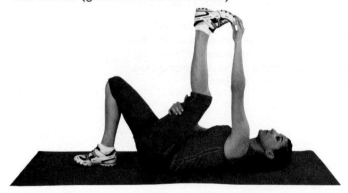

POSITION Lying on your back, bring one knee toward your chest, and grasp your toes with the hand on the same side. Place the opposite hand on the back of the leg just below the knee.

MOVEMENT Pull your knee toward your chest while pushing your heel toward the ceiling and pulling your toes toward your shin. Straighten your knee until you feel sufficient stretch in the muscles of the back of the leg, and hold for several seconds. Repeat for the other leg.

EXERCISE 5.5 MODIFIED HURDLER'S STRETCH

PURPOSE To stretch the **lower back muscles** (erector spinae) and muscles in the **back of the thigh** (hamstrings).

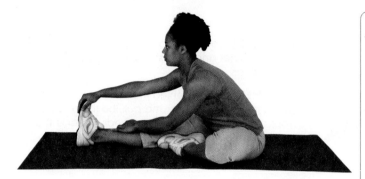

POSITION Sit on a level surface with one leg out in front, bend the other knee, and place the sole of the foot alongside the knee of the outstretched leg.

MOVEMENT Reach down and grab the ankle or toes of the outstretched leg. Keeping your head and trunk straight, lean your trunk forward, and attempt to touch your chest to your knee. Hold for several seconds. Return to the upright position, and alternate legs.

VARIATION Grasp the toes of the extended leg, and pull your toes toward your shin while stretching. This will also stretch the calf muscles (gastrocnemius and soleus).

 Scan to view a demonstration video of the modified hurdler's stretch.

EXERCISE 5.6 INNER THIGH STRETCH

PURPOSE To stretch the muscles on the **inside of the thighs** (adductors and internal rotators).

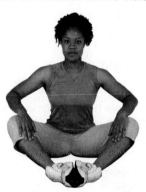

POSITION Sit with the bottoms of your feet together and place your hands just below your knees.

MOVEMENT Try to raise your knees while pushing down with your hands and forearms. Then relax, and, using your hands, press your knees toward the floor; hold for several seconds.

 Scan to view a demonstration video of the inner thigh stretch.

EXERCISE 5.7 HIP AND GLUTEAL STRETCH

PURPOSE To stretch the muscles at the **hip** (gluteals, tensor fasciae latae).

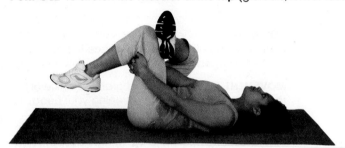

POSITION Lie on your back, with one leg crossed over the other and both shoulders and both arms on the floor.

MOVEMENT Grasp behind the knee of the leg that is not crossed over, and pull the thigh toward your chest. Hold for several seconds. Reverse the positions of the legs, and repeat the stretch.

Scan to view a demonstration video of the hip and gluteal stretch.

EXERCISE 5.8 LOWER BACK STRETCH

PURPOSE To stretch the muscles of the **lower back** (erector spinae) and **buttocks** (gluteals).

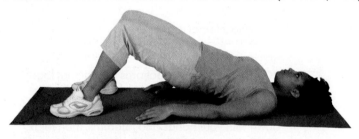

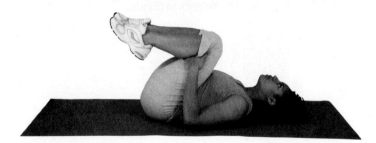

POSITION Lie on your back with your hips and knees bent, your feet flat on the floor, and your arms positioned along your sides.

MOVEMENT First, arch your back and lift your hips off the floor; hold for several seconds. Then relax and return to starting position. Place your hands behind your knees, and pull the knees to your chest. Hold for several seconds.

Scan to view a demonstration video of the lower back stretch.

EXERCISE 5.9 SIDE STRETCH

PURPOSE To stretch the muscles of the **upper arm** (triceps) and **side of the trunk** (latissimus dorsi).

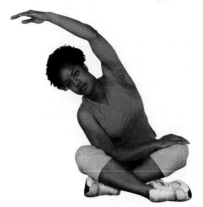

POSITION Sit on the floor with your legs crossed.

MOVEMENT Stretch one arm over your head while bending at your waist toward the side of the opposite arm. With the opposite arm, reach across your chest as far as possible; hold for several seconds. Do not rotate your trunk; try to stretch the muscles on the same side of the trunk as the overhead arm. Alternate arms to stretch the other side of the trunk.

 Scan to view a demonstration video of the side stretch.

EXERCISE 5.10 TRUNK TWISTER

PURPOSE To stretch the muscles of the **trunk** (obliques and latissimus dorsi) and **hip** (gluteus maximus).

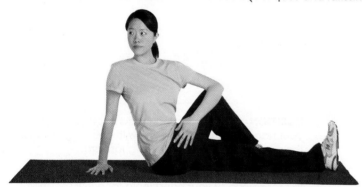

POSITION Sit with your left leg extended, your right leg bent and crossed over your left knee, and your right foot on the floor. Place your right hand on the floor behind your buttocks.

MOVEMENT Placing your left arm on the right side of your right thigh and your right hand on the floor, use your left arm to push against your right leg while twisting your trunk to the right; hold for several seconds. Then assume the starting position with your right leg extended, and stretch the opposite side of the body.

 Scan to view a demonstration video of the trunk twister.

EXERCISE 5.11   CHEST STRETCH

PURPOSE To stretch the muscles across the **chest** (pectoralis major) and **shoulder** (anterior deltoid and biceps).

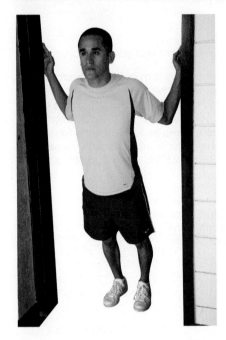

POSITION Stand in a doorway, and grasp the frame of the doorway at shoulder height.

MOVEMENT Press forward on the frame for 5 seconds. Then relax and shift your weight forward until you feel the stretch of muscles across your chest; hold for several seconds.

Scan to view a demonstration video of the chest stretch.

EXERCISE 5.12   NECK STRETCH

PURPOSE To stretch the muscles that rotate the **head** (sternocleidomastoid).

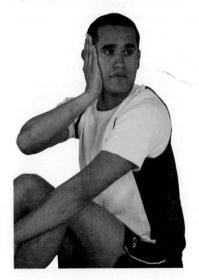

POSITION After turning your head to one side, place your hand against your cheek with your fingers toward the ear and your elbow pointing forward.

MOVEMENT Try to turn your head and neck against the resistance of your hand; hold for a few seconds. Remove your hand and relax, then turn your head as far as possible in the same direction. Repeat the stretch, turning in the other direction.

Scan to view a demonstration video of the neck stretch.

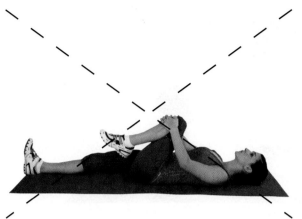

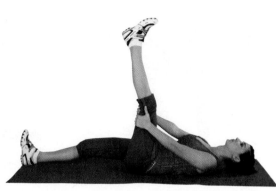

MAY CAUSE INJURY:

KNEE PULL This position places undue stress on the knee joint.

TRY THIS INSTEAD:

LEG PULL Lie on your back and pull your knee toward your chest by pulling on the back of your leg just below the knee. Then extend the knee joint and point the sole of your foot straight up. Continue to pull your leg toward your chest. Repeat several times with each leg.

PURPOSE: To stretch the buttocks and lower back muscles.

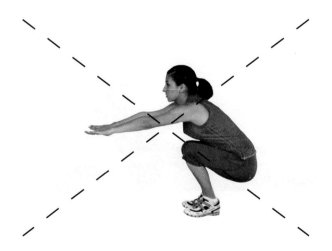

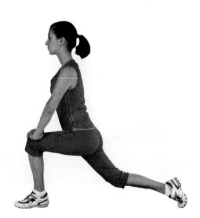

MAY CAUSE INJURY:

DEEP KNEE BEND This movement hyperflexes the knee and "opens" the joint while stretching the ligaments.

TRY THIS INSTEAD:

LUNGE From a standing position, step forward with either foot and touch the opposite knee to the ground. Repeat with the opposite leg.

PURPOSE: To stretch the buttocks and hamstring muscles.

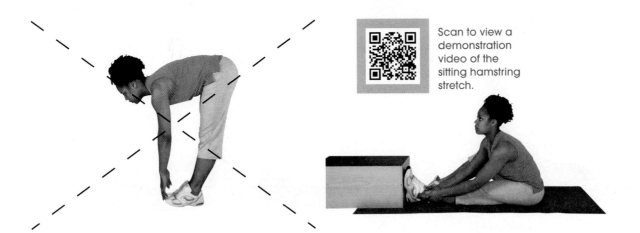

Scan to view a demonstration video of the sitting hamstring stretch.

MAY CAUSE INJURY:

STANDING TOE TOUCH This movement could damage the lower back.

TRY THIS INSTEAD:

SITTING HAMSTRING STRETCH Sit at leg-length from a wall. With your foot on the wall and the other knee bent with the foot between the wall and your buttocks, bend forward, keeping your lower back straight. The bent knee can fall to the side.

PURPOSE: To stretch the buttocks and hamstring muscles.

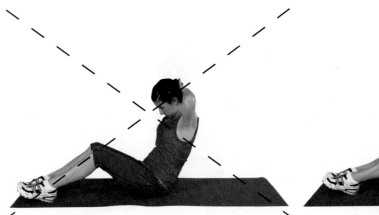

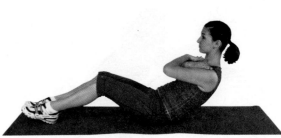

MAY CAUSE INJURY:

SIT-UP (HANDS BEHIND HEAD) This movement could cause hyperflexion of the neck and strain the neck muscles.

TRY THIS INSTEAD

CURL-UP Lie on your back with your knees bent, and cross your arms over your chest. Using your abdominal muscles, curl up until the upper half of your back is off the floor, and then return to the starting position.

PURPOSE: To strengthen the abdominal muscles.

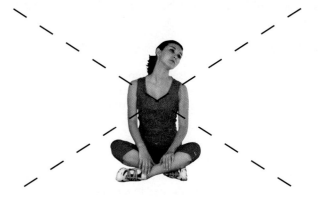

MAY CAUSE INJURY:

NECK CIRCLES This movement hyperextends the neck, which can pinch arteries and nerves as well as damage disks in the spine.

TRY THIS INSTEAD:

NECK STRETCHES Sit with your head and neck straight. Move your head down to flex your neck, and return your head upright. Then slowly turn your head from side to side as far as possible; attempt to point your chin at each shoulder.

PURPOSE: To stretch the muscles of the neck.

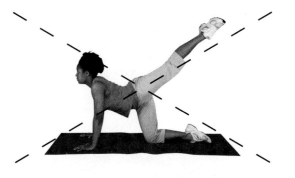

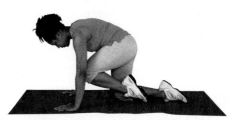

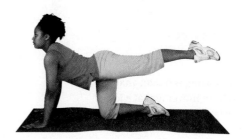

MAY CAUSE INJURY:

DONKEY KICK When kicking the leg back, most people hyperextend the neck and/or back.

TRY THIS INSTEAD:

KNEE-TO-NOSE TOUCH While on your hands and knees, lift one knee toward your nose and then extend that leg to the horizontal position. Alternate legs. Do not lift your leg higher than your hips, and keep your neck in line with your back.

PURPOSE: To stretch the buttocks and lower back muscles.

study plan
Customize your study plan—and master your health!—in the Study Area of **MasteringHealth.com**

summary

hear it! STUDY REVIEW

To hear an MP3 Chapter Summary, scan here or visit the Study Area in MasteringHealth™.

LO **1** ■ Flexibility is the range of motion of a joint.

■ The five structural and physiological limits to flexibility relate to characteristics of bone, muscles, tendons, skin, and connective tissue within the joint capsule.

LO **2** ■ Proprioceptors are constantly monitoring the tension of the muscles and tendons and providing feedback to the brain.

■ If muscle spindles are suddenly stretched, they respond by initiating a stretch reflex that causes the muscle to contract. However, if the muscles and tendons are stretched slowly, the stretch reflex can be avoided.

LO **3** ■ Improved flexibility results in the following benefits: increased joint mobility, prevention of lower back problems, efficient body movement, and improved posture and personal appearance.

LO **4** ■ Posture is the position of the body, specifically of the joints, while standing or sitting.

■ Flexibility exercises are important in maintaining good posture and preventing misalignment and debilitating changes in the musculoskeletal system.

LO **5** ■ Flexibility is evaluated by measuring the range of motion at a particular joint.

■ The sit-and-reach test and the shoulder flexibility test are commonly used to measure flexibility.

LO **6** ■ Designing your flexibility program involves setting short-term and long-term goals and selecting appropriate stretches to meet your goals. It is ideal to incorporate stretching sessions 2–5 days per week.

■ Static stretches involve stretching a muscle to the limit of movement and holding the stretch for an extended period of time. Dynamic stretches involve fluid, exaggerated movements designed to mimic the movements of a given sport or activity.

■ Proprioceptive neuromuscular facilitation (PNF) combines stretching with alternating contraction and relaxation of muscles to improve flexibility. Ballistic stretches may be appropriate for some athletes but are not safe for the general public.

study questions

review it! QUIZZES

Find more review questions online in MasteringHealth™.

LO **1** 1. Which of the following is not an anatomical factor that can limit movement at a joint?
   a. shape of the bones
   b. tight skin
   c. tight tendons
   d. length of the bone

2. Define the following terms: flexibility, range of motion, ligament, tendon, and cartilage.

3. Describe the difference in function between ligaments and tendons.

4. List the factors that limit flexibility. Which factors place the greatest limitations on flexibility?

LO **2** 5. Proprioceptors include which of the following?
   a. motor units
   b. Golgi organs
   c. muscle spindles
   d. both b and c

LO **3** 6. Describe why the stretch reflex should be avoided.

7. Lower back pain is the result of
   a. weak abdominal muscles.
   b. weak hamstring muscles.
   c. hyperextension of the lower back.
   d. all of the above.

8. List three primary reasons why maintaining flexibility is important.

LO **4** 9. List four benefits of having good posture.

LO **5** 10. Describe two common tests used to evaluate flexibility.

LO 11. Static stretching is not advisable for nonathletes.
   a. true
   b. false

12. To avoid injury, most stretching should be done
   a. only at night.
   b. after the muscles have been warmed up.
   c. while watching television.
   d. to the point of pain.

13. Define "antagonist" and explain proprioceptive neuromuscular facilitation.

14. Compare static and ballistic stretching.

15. Briefly outline the exercise prescription to improve flexibility.

suggested reading

American College of Sports Medicine. American College of Sports Medicine position stand: Quantity and quality of exercise for developing and maintaining cardiorespiratory, musculoskeletal, and neuromotor fitness in apparently healthy adults: Guidance for prescribing exercise. *Medicine and Science in Sports and Exercise* 43(7):1334–1359, 2011.

Behm, D. G., and A. Chaouachi. A review of the acute effects of static and dynamic stretching on performance. *European Journal of Applied Physiology* 111(11): 2633–2635, 2011.

Cruz-Ferreira, A., J. Fernandes, L. Laranjo, L. M. Bernardo, and A. Silva. A systematic review of the effects of Pilates method of exercise in healthy people. *Archives of Physical Medicine and Rehabilitation* 92(12):2071–2081, 2011.

da Costa, B. R., and E. R. Vieira. Stretching to reduce work-related musculoskeletal disorders: A systematic review. *Journal of Rehabilitation Medicine* 40(5):321–328, 2008.

Herbert, R. D., M. de Noronha, and S. J. Kamper. Stretching to prevent or reduce muscle soreness after exercise. *Cochrane Database of Systematic Reviews* 6(7):CD004577, 2011.

Herman, S. L., and D. T. Smith. Four-week dynamic stretching warm-up intervention elicits longer-term performance benefits. *Journal of Strength and Conditioning Research* 22(4):1286–1297, 2008.

Jenkins, J., and J. Beazell. Flexibility for runners. *Clinics in Sports Medicine* 29(3):365–377, 2010.

Rubini, E. C., A. L. L. Costa, and P. S. C. Gomes. The effects of stretching on strength performance. *Sports Medicine* 37(3):213–224, 2007.

Small, K., L. McNaughton, and M. Matthews. A systematic review into the efficacy of static stretching as part of a warm-up for the prevention of exercise-related injury. *Research in Sports Medicine* 16(3):213–231, 2008.

helpful weblinks

do it! WEBLINKS

For links to the organizations and websites listed, visit MasteringHealth™.

American College of Sports Medicine

Provides information, articles, and position statements about health and fitness. www.acsm.org

Mayo Clinic

General information about fitness and wellness. Includes flexibility exercises for particular muscle groups, sports, and conditions. http://www.mayoclinic.org/healthy-lifestyle

Yoga

Information and videos on yoga practice, meditation methods, and a healthy lifestyle. www.yogajournal.com.

WebMD

General information about exercise, fitness, and wellness. Great articles, instructional information, and updates. www.webmd.com

TeachPE

Descriptions and demonstrations of stretching exercises. http://www.teachpe.com/stretching/stretches.php

Name _____   Date _____

Assessing Your Posture

Poor posture is all too common and can lead to severe muscle and joint misalignment, possibly resulting in debilitating musculoskeletal problems. In fact, poor posture often progresses so slowly that you may notice its symptoms (back and neck pain, stiffness, increased injury, and reduced range of motion) well before you notice a change in your posture.

The first step to improving posture is finding out what your posture looks like. Then you can compare it to "good" posture and determine the kind of exercise that will help you to correct the misalignments.

STEP 1: Take a Photograph to Determine Your Posture

You can determine what your posture looks like by taking a photograph of yourself standing against a wall. Have a friend or relative photograph you standing against a plain, flat surface, from the back and side.

You can compare your body position to a straight plane by placing a string behind you. Attach the string to an object overhead and then tie a light weight to the other end of the string so that the weight is suspended just above the floor. Stand so the string is centered between your feet in the back view photograph. Center the string on the medial malleolus (bone protrusion on the side of the ankle) in the side view photograph.

STEP 2: Score Your Posture

Once you have the photographs of your posture from the back and side, compare them to the scoring chart on the following page. With each aspect of the posture shown, determine your score from the values shown at the top of the chart.

STEP 3: Review Your Scores

Review each of the posture aspects that you evaluated.

A score of 2 in all the categories indicates that your posture is good. A strength and flexibility exercise program should help you maintain your excellent posture.

If you scored a 1, you might want to find some flexibility exercise that will help you to realign that aspect.

If you scored a 0, begin flexibility exercises now to correct that aspect of your posture. This is important since the misalignment will almost certainly lead to pain and/or permanent alterations to your posture in the future.

Note the date of your assessment in the space provided on the right side of the chart. In 6 weeks, reassess you posture and your scores. Remember: Be conscious of your posture throughout the day. Continue to use both strength and flexibility exercises to help correct any misalignment you detect.

	Good—2	Fair—1	Poor—0	Scores	
Back View				Date 1	Date 2
Head	Head erect, gravity passes directly through center	Head twisted or turned to one side slightly	Head twisted or turned to one side markedly		
Shoulders	Shoulders level horizontally	One shoulder slightly higher	One shoulder markedly higher		
Spine	Spine straight	Spine slightly curved	Spine markedly curved laterally		
Hips	Hips level horizontally	One hip slightly higher	One hip markedly higher		
Knees and Ankles	Feet pointed straight ahead, legs vertical	Feet pointed out, legs deviating outward at the knee	Feet pointed out markedly, legs deviated markedly		
Side View				Date 1	Date 2
Neck and Upper back	Neck erect, head in line with shoulders, rounded upper back	Neck slightly foward, chin out, slightly more rounded upper back	Neck markedly forward, chin markedly out, markedly rounded upper back		
Trunk	Trunk erect	Trunk inclined to rear slightly	Trunk inclined to rear markedly		
Abdomen	Abdomen flat	Abdomen protruding	Abdomen protruding and sagging		
Lower back	Lower back normally curved	Lower back slightly hollow	Lower back markedly hollow		
Legs	Legs straight	Knees slightly hyperextended	Knees markedly hyperextended		

149

laboratory 5.2

do it! LABS
Complete Lab 5.2 online in the
study area of **MasteringHealth.com**

Name _____ Date _____

Assessing Flexibility: Trunk Flexion (Sit-and-Reach) Test and Shoulder Flexibility Test

THE SIT-AND-REACH TEST

To perform the sit-and-reach test, start by sitting upright with your feet flat against a sit-and-reach box. Keeping your feet flat on the box and your legs straight, extend your hands as far forward as possible, and hold this position for 3 seconds. Repeat this procedure 3 times. Your score on the sit-and-reach test is the distance, measured in centimeters, between the edge of the sit-and-reach box closest to you and the tips of your fingers during the best of your three stretching efforts. The edge of the box is set to 26 centimeters.

Note that you should warm up by stretching for a few minutes before you perform the test. To reduce the possibility of injury, avoid rapid or jerky movements during the test. It is often useful to have a partner help by holding your legs straight during the test and by measuring the distance. After completing the test, consult **TABLE 5.2** to locate your flexibility fitness category, and record your scores on the same page.

Scan to view a demonstration video of the sit-and-reach test.

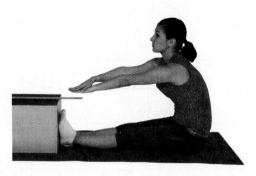

The sit-and-reach test.

THE SHOULDER FLEXIBILITY TEST

To perform the shoulder flexibility test, follow these steps: While standing, raise your right arm and reach down your back as far as possible. At the same time, extend your left arm behind your back and reach upward toward your right hand. The objective is to try to overlap your fingers as much as possible. Your score on the shoulder flexibility test is the distance, measured in inches, of finger overlap.

Measure the distance of finger overlap to the nearest inch. For example, an overlap of 3/4 inch would be recorded as 1 inch. If your fingers fail to overlap, record this score as −1. Finally, if your fingertips barely touch, record this score as 0. After completing the test with the right hand up, repeat the test in the opposite direction (left hand up).

As with the sit-and-reach test, you should warm up with a few minutes of stretching prior to performing the shoulder flexibility test. Again, to prevent injury, avoid rapid or jerky movements during the test. After completing the test, consult **TABLE 5.3** to locate your shoulder flexibility category, and record your scores on the same page.

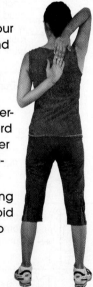

The shoulder flexibility test.

Scan to view a demonstration video of the shoulder flexibility test.

TABLE 5.2 ■ Physical Fitness Norms for Trunk Flexion

Sit-and-Reach Test (centimeters)					
Men	Excellent	Very Good	Good	Fair	Needs Improvement
15–19 yrs	≥ 40	34–39	30–33	25–29	≤ 24
20–29 yrs	≥ 39	34–38	29–33	24–28	≤ 23
30–39 yrs	≥ 38	33–37	28–32	23–27	≤ 22
40–49 yrs	≥ 35	29–34	24–28	18–23	≤ 17
50–59 yrs	≥ 35	28–34	24–27	16–23	≤ 15
60–69 yrs	≥ 33	25–32	20–24	15–19	≤ 14
Women	Excellent	Very Good	Good	Fair	Needs Improvement
15–19 yrs	≥ 43	38–42	34–37	29–33	≤ 28
20–29 yrs	≥ 41	37–40	33–36	28–32	≤ 27
30–39 yrs	≥ 41	36–40	32–35	27–31	≤ 26
40–49 yrs	≥ 38	34–37	30–33	25–29	≤ 24
50–59 yrs	≥ 39	33–38	30–32	25–29	≤ 24
60–69 yrs	≥ 35	31–34	27–30	23–26	≤ 22

Source: Canadian Physical Activity, Fitness & Lifestyle Approach: CSEP-Health & Fitness Program's Appraisal and Counseling Strategy, 3rd Ed., © 2003. Reprinted with permission from the Canadian Society for Exercise Physiology.

TABLE 5.3 ■ Physical Fitness Norms for Shoulder Flexibility

Right Hand Up Score	Left Hand Up Score	Fitness Classification
< 0	< 0	Very poor
0	0	Poor
+1	+1	Average
+2	+2	Good
+3	+3	Excellent
+4	+4	Superior

Note that these norms are for both men and women of all ages. Units for the shoulder flexibility test score are inches and indicate the distance between the fingers of your right and left hands.

Source: Fox, Edward L., Kirby, Timothy, and Fox, Ann Roberts, *Bases of Fitness, 1st Ed.,* © 1987. Reprinted and Electronically reproduced by permission of Pearson Education, Inc., Upper Saddle River, New Jersey.

Date: _____

Sit-and-reach score (centimeters): _____   Fitness category: _____

Shoulder flexibility score (inches)

Left side: _____   Fitness category: _____

Right side: _____   Fitness category: _____

GOAL SETTING

1. Based on your results for the flexibility testing, write a goal to either improve or maintain your fitness category.

2. Write three objectives to help you achieve your goal.

   1. _____

   2. _____

   3. _____

laboratory 5.3

do it! LABS
Complete Lab 5.3 online in the
study area of **MasteringHealth.com**

Name _____   Date _____

Flexibility Progression Log

Use this log to record your progress in increasing flexibility in selected joints. Record the date, hold time, and sets for each of the exercises listed in the left column.

Date							
Exercise	St/Hold	St/Hold	St/Hold	St/Hold	St/Hold	St/Hold	St/Hold
Lower leg stretch (see Exercise 5.1)							
Shin stretch (see Exercise 5.2)							
Thigh stretch (see Exercise 5.3)							
Leg stretch (see Exercise 5.4)							
Modified hurdler's stretch (see Exercise 5.5)							
Inside leg stretch (see Exercise 5.6)							
Hip and gluteal stretch (see Exercise 5.7)							
Lower back stretch (see Exercise 5.8)							
Side stretch (see Exercise 5.9)							
Trunk twister (see Exercise 5.10)							
Chest stretch (see Exercise 5.11)							
Neck stretch (see Exercise 5.12)							

St/Hold = sets and hold time *Example:* 2/30 = 2 sets held for 30 seconds each.

laboratory 5.4

do it! LABS
Complete Lab 5.4 online in the
study area of **MasteringHealth.com**

Name _____ Date _____

Stretching to Prevent or Reduce Lower Back Pain

Stretching exercises are important in maintaining a flexible and healthy back. Our daily activities often result in overuse and -tightening of back muscles. Chronic overuse and straining can cause significant back pain and increase your risk of back injury.

In this lab, you will learn exercises to stretch the muscles of your lower back to help in maintaining flexibility. Performing these stretches will help prevent back pain and may help reduce back aches.

BACK EXTENSION—PRONE

1. Lie on your stomach.
2. Prop yourself up on your elbows, extending your back.
3. Start straightening your elbows, further extending your back.
4. Continue straightening your elbows until you feel a gentle stretch.
5. Hold for 15 seconds.
6. Return to the starting position.
7. Repeat 10 more times.

Scan to view a demonstration video of the back extension stretch.

CAT STRETCH

1. Get down on the floor on your hands and knees.
2. Push your back up toward the ceiling (like a cat arching its back).
3. Continue arching until you feel a gentle stretch in your back.
4. Hold for 15 seconds.
5. Return to the starting position.
6. Repeat 10 more times.

Scan to view a demonstration video of the cat stretch.

THE PELVIC TILT

1. Lie on your back, with your knees bent and feet flat on the floor.
2. Exhale, and press the small of your back against the floor.
3. Hold for 15 seconds.
4. Return to the starting position.
5. Repeat 10 more times.

Scan to view a demonstration video of the pelvic tilt.

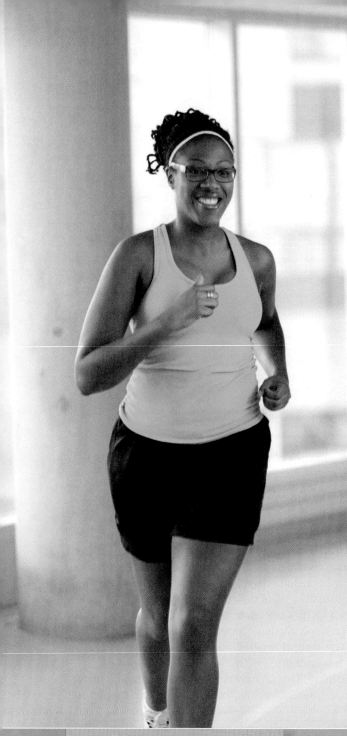
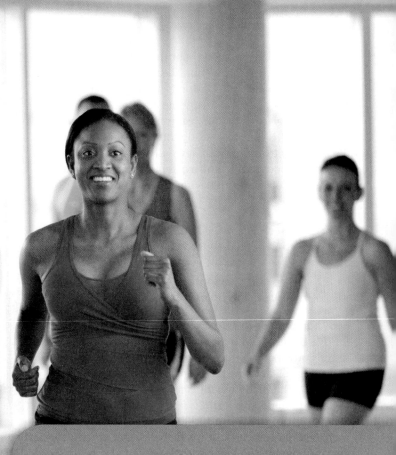

6

Body Composition

LEARNING OUTCOMES

1. Define *body composition* and explain how this measurement relates to body weight.

2. Explain why excess body fat increases health risks, list five chronic conditions associated with obesity, and explain why too little body fat is also a health risk.

3. Describe the methods used to assess body composition and provide the advantages and disadvantages of each.

4. Calculate your ideal body weight.

5. List your goals for achieving your ideal body weight and body composition.

MANY PEOPLE WORRY about their body weight, but how much you weigh is not always a good index of whether your body composition is healthy. In fact, based on height and weight charts, some athletes appear to be 25 pounds overweight but really have very little body fat. How is this possible? Read more to find out! We will discuss how to assess your level of body fat, consider how much body fat is healthy, and examine the health problems associated with having too much body fat.

What Is Body Composition and What Does It Tell Us?

LO **1** Define *body composition* and explain how this measurement relates to body weight.

Body composition refers to the relative amounts of fat and fat-free tissues (e.g., bone, muscle, and internal organs) in the body. Body composition is typically expressed as a percentage of fat in the body. So if a person has 20% body fat, 20% of her body weight is fat mass, and the remaining 80% of her body weight is fat-free or lean body mass. Having a high percentage of body fat is associated with an increased risk of heart disease, diabetes, and other disorders, but having too low a percentage can also be linked to health problems, such as osteoporosis.

Measuring percentage of body fat can help determine whether a person is at a healthy weight, **overweight**, or **obese**. Someone who is "overweight" has a body fat percentage above the level that is considered to be "healthy," based on research examining the relationship between body fatness and rates of disease. A person classified as obese has a very high percentage of body fat, generally over 25% for men and over 35% for women (1–5).

MAKE SURE YOU **KNOW...**

- Body composition refers to the relative amounts of fat and fat-free mass in the body and is generally reported in terms of the percentage of fat in the body.
- Measuring body fat percentage can help determine whether someone is overweight or obese.

MasteringHealth™

How Is Body Composition Related to Health?

LO **2** Explain why excess body fat increases health risks, list five chronic conditions associated with obesity, and explain why too little body fat is also a health risk.

Maintaining a healthy body composition is an important goal to achieve a lifetime of wellness. To determine a

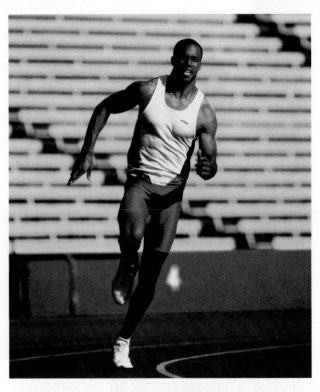

Some muscular athletes can be "overweight" without being over-fat.

healthy body weight, you need to consider the percentage of body fat.

The human body contains two major types of fat: essential fat and storage fat. **Essential fat** is necessary for body functions such as facilitating nerve impulses. Locations of this fat include nerves and cell membranes. Men have approximately 3% of their body weight as essential fat, and women—who carry more fat in their breasts, uterus, and other sex-specific sites—have approximately 12%.

The second type of body fat is called **storage fat**, which is contained within **adipose tissue** (i.e., fat cells) in the body. This fat may be **visceral fat**, which is located around internal organs, or **subcutaneous fat**, located

body composition The relative amounts of fat and fat-free mass in the body.

overweight A weight above the recommended level for health.

obese An excessive amount of fat in the body, typically above 25% for men and 35% for women.

essential fat Body fat that is necessary for physiological functioning.

storage fat Excess fat reserves stored in the body's adipose tissue.

adipose tissue Tissue where fat is stored in the body.

visceral fat Fat stored around the internal organs.

subcutaneous fat Fat stored just beneath the skin.

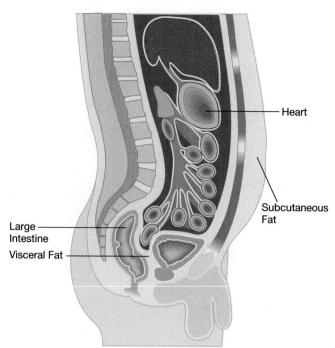

FIGURE 6.1 Storage fat can be visceral or subcutaneous. Visceral fat is stored around the organs; subcutaneous fat is stored between the skin and muscle layers.

just below the skin (**FIGURE 6.1**). Storage fat provides energy for activity, insulates the body to retain heat, and protects against trauma to the body. However, high levels of storage fat, particularly in the visceral region of

the body, increase the risk of numerous diseases including cardiovascular disease, diabetes, and cancer. This is why maintaining a healthy body composition is such an important goal.

In general, a healthy percentage of body fat for young men (20–39 years) can range from 8% to 19%, and for young women (20–39 years), from 21% to 32% (1). However, many public health experts recommend levels at the lower end of these ranges for young adults, 12%–15% and 21%–25% for men and women, respectively (1). For most people, a body fat percentage outside these ranges indicates an unhealthy body weight. However, athletes or very active individuals might have lower values. Some athletic men have as little as 5%–13% fat, and athletic women can have as little as 12%–22% (1). Keep in mind that these values are not recommended for the general population and that you can be healthy if your body fat percentage falls within the ranges mentioned. See **FIGURE 6.2** for recommended ranges of percent body fat according to sex and age.

It is not just *how much* body fat a person carries that can greatly affect his risk for several chronic diseases; *where* he carries it also matters. Fat cells are unequally distributed throughout the body, and the distribution of body fat is determined largely by genetics. We inherit specific fat storage traits that determine the regional distribution of fat. For example, many men have a high number of fat cells in the upper body and as a result store more fat within the abdominal area (around the

Gender	20–39 years		40–59 years		60+ years		Weight Status	Health Risk
	Body Fat	BMI	Body Fat	BMI	Body Fat	BMI		
Men	<8%	<18.5	<11%	<18.5	<13%	<18.5	Under weight	Increased
Women	<21%	<18.5	<23%	<18.5	<24%	<18.5		
Men	8–19%	18.6–24.9	11–21%	18.6–24.9	13–24%	18.6–24.9	Average	Normal
Women	21–32%	18.6–24.9	23–33%	18.6–24.9	24–35%	18.6–24.9		
Men	20–24%	25.0–29.9	22–27%	25.0–29.9	25–39%	25.0–29.9	Over-weight	Increased
Women	33–38%	25.0–29.9	34–39%	25.0–29.9	36–41%	25.0–29.9		
Men	>25%	>30	>28%	>30	>30%	>30	Obese	High
Women	>39%	>30	>40%	>30	>42%	>30		

FIGURE 6.2 Health risks associated with varying levels of body fat for men and women according to age. Note that health risks are increased for both underweight individuals and overweight individuals.

Sources: Data from National Institutes of Health. Assessing Your Weight and Health Risk, 2012. http://www.nhlbi.nih.gov/health/public/heart/obesity/lose_wt/risk.htm and Shah, N. R., and E. R. Braverman. Measuring Adiposity in Patients: The Utility of Body Mass Index (BMI), Percent Body Fat, and Leptin. PLoS ONE 7(4): e33308, 2012.

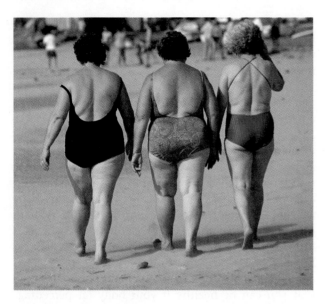

Women tend to store fat in the lower body, around the hips and thighs.

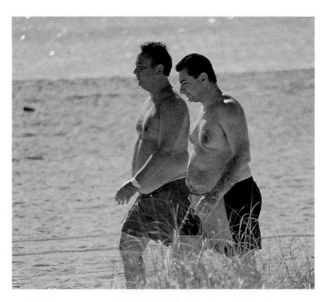

Men tend to store fat in the upper body, around the abdomen.

waist). This is referred to as the **android pattern** of obesity. In contrast, women tend to carry more fat cells in the waist, hips, and thighs of the lower body. This is called the **gynoid pattern** of obesity. People who carry body fat primarily in the abdominal or waist area are at greater risk of developing heart disease and diabetes than are those who store body fat in the hips or lower part of the body (6, 7).

Overweight and Obesity in the United States

Obesity is often defined as a percentage of body fat greater than 25% for men and greater than 35% for women. Current estimates for the United States suggest that nearly 34% of adults and approximately 17% of children and adolescents (ages 2–19) meet the criteria for obesity (8). Obesity is a major health problem in the United States, and numerous diseases have been linked to being too fat. Because of a strong link between obesity and disease, it is estimated that obesity directly contributes to 15%–20% of the deaths in the United States (5).

The burden of obesity has also had a significant effect on health-care costs. Currently, an estimated 10% of all medical costs in the United States are attributed to overweight- and obesity-related health problems. This adds up to the hefty price tag of over $200 billion per year in direct medical costs and this number is predicted to rise sharply in the future (8, 9). The World Health Organization reports that the obesity rates in the United States are the highest in the world and are continuing to climb. The reports are based on studies indicating that the number of obese or overweight people in the United States has increased rapidly during the past 20 years (12). In 2013, no state had a prevalence of obesity less than 20%, 43 states had a prevalence of 25% or more, and 20 states had a prevalence of 30% or more **(FIGURE 6.3)**. The good news is that the increase in adult obesity in the United States is leveling off. The bad news is that 67% of all Americans are either obese or overweight, and there is no evidence of a decrease in the rate of obesity among children (8, 10). Thus, obesity continues to be a major threat to wellness in the United States.

Why are so many Americans obese? There is no single answer. Obesity is related to both genetic traits and lifestyle (3, 11, 12).

consider this! ////////////////////////////

On average, female college students gain about 2 pounds during their first year of college (21). This is down more than 50% from 5 to 10 years ago!

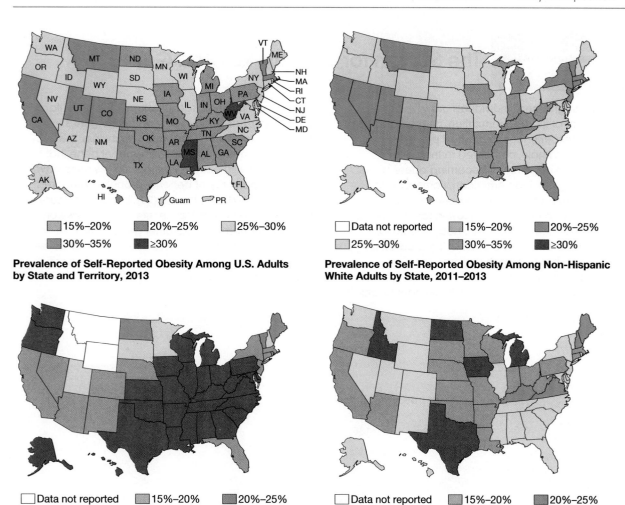

Prevalence of Self-Reported Obesity Among U.S. Adults by State and Territory, 2013

Prevalence of Self-Reported Obesity Among Non-Hispanic White Adults by State, 2011–2013

Prevalence of Self-Reported Obesity Among Non-Hispanic Black Adults by State, BRFSS, 2011–2013

Prevalence of Self-Reported Obesity Among Hispanic Adults by State, 2011–2013

FIGURE 6.3 Obesity prevalence in the United States based on 2013 data. You can see that the rate of obesity varies from region to region. Where does your home state rank?

Source: Centers for Disease Control and Prevention. Overweight and Obesity: Obesity Prevalence Trends. http://www.cdc.gov/obesity/data/prevalence-maps.html

Creeping Obesity Many individuals can experience **creeping obesity**, gradually adding fat over a period of time. This type of slow weight gain is usually attributed to poor diet (including increased food intake) and a gradual decline in physical activity (12). The woman shown in **FIGURE 6.4** is gaining a small amount (one-quarter pound of fat per month or, 3 pounds per year). After four years, she will have gained 12 pounds! The weight gain is so gradual that it typically does not become a concern until years later, when the total weight is more noticeable.

Other factors can also play a role in increased fat accumulation. Even if diet and level of physical activity remain fairly consistent, our metabolism slows as we age. This decrease in metabolic rate often coincides with less time for physical activity due to life changes such as a more demanding job or increased family responsibilities. The end result is less time spent exercising and gradual weight gain.

android pattern Pattern of fat distribution characterized by fat stored in the abdominal region; more common in men.

gynoid pattern Pattern of fat distribution characterized by fat stored in the hips and thighs; more common in women.

creeping obesity A slow increase in body weight and percentage of body fat over several years.

APPRECIATING DIVERSITY The Search for Obesity-Related Genes

Even though obese individuals are found in every segment of the U.S. population, certain subsets of Americans experience the greatest prevalence of obesity. For example, compared to the U.S. population as a whole, the risk of becoming obese is greatest among Mexican American women, African American women, some Native Americans (such as Pima Indians), and children from low-income families. The high prevalence of obesity in these populations places individuals in those groups at the greatest risk of developing obesity-related diseases.

Research efforts to understand the role of genetics in the high prevalence of obesity in these populations are expanding. One large investigation, the Heritage Family Study, has been searching for the genes responsible for both obesity and weight loss. This investigation has identified an important gene that is associated with obesity. People with this gene have 1.7 times greater risk of becoming obese compared to people who do not have it (20). In addition, these individuals are resistant to the effects of exercise on fat mass. Results from this and other genetics studies are expected to provide important information for developing programs that can prevent and treat obesity in high-risk populations.

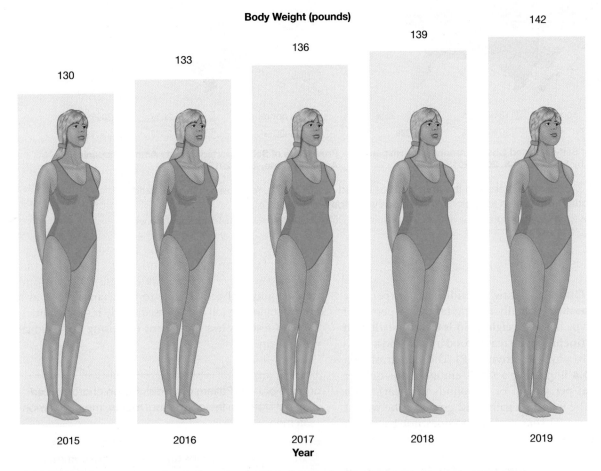

Body Weight (pounds)

130	133	136	139	142
2015	2016	2017	2018	2019

Year

FIGURE 6.4 The concept of creeping obesity. Note the gradual weight gain over a 4-year period.

Source: Byrne, N. M., and A. P. Hills. Biology or behavior: Which is the strongest contributor to weight gain? *Current Obesity Reports* 2(1):65–76, 2013.

Chronic Conditions Associated with Overweight and Obesity

Obesity increases the risk of developing at least 26 diseases. Cardiovascular disease, colon cancer, hypertension (high blood pressure), kidney disease, arthritis, and diabetes are among the most serious (7, 8, 12). While genetic factors play a role in these conditions, lifestyle is the primary determinant of a person's risk.

Cardiovascular Disease Cardiovascular disease (CVD) is the leading cause of death in the United States for both men and women. Obesity is considered a major independent risk factor for coronary heart disease, the leading cause of heart attacks. Obesity has been shown to increase the risk of heart attack by 60%–80% (3, 8, 12).

consider this! ///////////////////

Sedentary adults are over 2.5 times more likely to experience significant weight gain over 10 years compared to adults who exercise vigorously two or more times per week.

Hypertension is more common among overweight and obese individuals. However, on a positive note, blood pressure is usually reduced with weight loss. Obesity is linked to elevated cholesterol levels and unhealthy blood lipid profiles. As with hypertension, the cholesterol profile typically improves with weight loss. High blood pressure and cholesterol levels are also independent risk factors for coronary heart disease, so the combination of obesity with these risk factors poses a significantly greater risk for a heart attack.

Diabetes **Diabetes** is a metabolic disorder characterized by high blood glucose levels; it affects over 18 million people. Chronic elevation of blood glucose is associated with increased incidence of heart disease, kidney disease,

nerve dysfunction, and eye damage. In fact, diabetes is one of the leading causes of death and disability in the United States, and its incidence is increasing.

There is a strong relationship between the onset of type 2 diabetes and body fat: More than 80% of people with this type of diabetes are obese. Type 2 diabetes has traditionally been referred to as *adult-onset diabetes* because its risk increases after age 45. This type of diabetes is largely associated with behavioral factors, such as poor dietary habits, physical inactivity, and obesity. As obesity among young people has increased, so has the incidence of type 2 diabetes among adolescents and young adults.

Type 2 diabetes is also known as non–insulin-dependent diabetes, because insulin is not always required as treatment. In type 2 diabetes, the body can produce insulin, but there is a reduced ability of insulin to transport glucose from the blood to the cells. This problem, called *decreased insulin sensitivity,* results in elevated blood glucose levels. People can have decreased insulin sensitivity but not have blood glucose levels high enough to be diagnosed with diabetes. In this case, a person has *prediabetes,* which is also more common among obese individuals. As with cardiovascular disease, weight loss can significantly reduce the risk of diabetes and help manage the disease. In fact, research has indicated that modest weight loss of 5%–10% can reduce the risk of CVD and type 2 diabetes (13).

hear it!

CASE STUDY

How can Harold manage his body weight and prevent diabetes? Listen to the online case study at MasteringHealth™.

Other Conditions Obesity is a risk factor for some of the most prevalent types of cancers, including breast, prostate, and colon cancer. Overweight and obese individuals are at higher risk for joint problems and osteoarthritis. Sleep apnea (a condition in which a person stops breathing for brief periods while sleeping) and gallbladder disease are more common among obese individuals. Additionally, obese women are more likely to experience menstrual abnormalities, difficulty conceiving, and complications during pregnancy than are women of normal weight.

Mental and Physical Benefits of a Healthy Weight

Maintaining a healthy weight is important for physical health, and it is also associated with certain aspects of mental health. People who are overweight

diabetes Metabolic disorder characterized by high blood glucose levels that is associated with increased risk for cardiovascular disease, kidney disease, nerve dysfunction, and eye damage.

steps ▸ FOR BEHAVIOR CHANGE

Are you at risk for developing diabetes?

Does your body composition, or other factors, put you at increased risk for developing diabetes? To find out whether you are at increased risk, respond true or false to the following statements.

Y N
☐ ☐ I have a BMI that puts me in the overweight or obese category.
☐ ☐ I am under 65 years of age and I get little or no exercise.
☐ ☐ I have a sister or brother with diabetes.
☐ ☐ I have a parent with diabetes.
☐ ☐ I am a woman who has had a baby weighing more than 9 pounds at birth.

In general, the more "true" answers you have, the higher your risk.

Tips to Reduce Your Risk of Diabetes

Tomorrow, you will:

☑ Determine whether you are overweight, and if so, make a plan to lose weight. If you have a BMI above the healthy range, schedule a body composition assessment to determine your level of fat. If your percentage of body fat is above the healthy range, talk to your instructor or a health educator at your campus health center about setting goals and preparing a plan for weight loss.

Within the next 2 weeks, you will:

☑ Get more exercise. Be more active most days of the week. (See Chapter 1 for tips to change your health behavior.)

☑ Incorporate more fresh fruits and vegetables and whole grains into your diet, and cut back on the salt and high-fat foods.

By the end of the semester, you will:

☑ See your health-care provider. A lot of people have diabetes and prediabetes without knowing it.

Source: Based on the American Diabetes Association. Diabetes Risk Test. www.diabetes.org.

---

see it!

ABC VIDEO

Watch the ABC Video "Overweight and Healthy?" at MasteringHealth™.

or obese are more likely to have poor body image and low -self-esteem compared to people of normal weight. An unhealthy body image and poor self-esteem are associated with poor health behavior choices and increased risk for physical and mental health problems, such as depression and increased anxiety (14). Maintaining a healthy body weight will make physical activity and everyday activities easier. Individuals who maintain a healthy body weight have a lower risk of developing major chronic conditions such as cardiovascular disease, type 2 diabetes, and certain types of cancers. Cardiovascular disease and all-cause death rates are also lower in people at their recommended body weights compared to overweight and obese individuals (15).

Health Effects of Too Little Body Fat

Although the current rates of overweight and obesity among U.S. adults indicate there is an obesity epidemic, a small percentage of people suffer from health problems associated with being underweight. As with overweight, underweight can be determined by measuring height, weight, and body fat percentage. However, as with determining overweight and obesity, it is best to use a measure of body composition to determine whether one is underweight. Having close to or below the level of essential body fat is an indicator that an individual might be too thin.

Health problems associated with being underweight are typically related to malnutrition, because the person is likely not eating enough to get all the necessary nutrients. Severe and prolonged malnutrition can result in

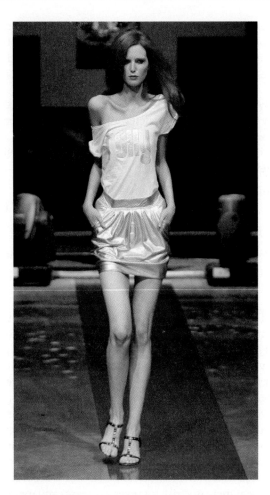

Being underweight can lead to significant health problems.

a loss of muscle mass and strength. Further, underweight individuals are at increased risk for osteoporosis, and underweight women are at increased risk for menstrual abnormalities that can lead to infertility. People with eating disorders, such as anorexia nervosa and bulimia, can experience many other health problems, including heart problems, digestive disorders, kidney damage, anemia, lethargy, muscle weakness, dry skin, and poor immune function.

MAKE SURE YOU **KNOW...**

- Overweight refers to a weight above the recommended level, and obesity refers to an excessive amount of body fat.
- A certain amount of fat is needed for normal physiological functioning, but excess storage fat is associated with increased risk for numerous conditions.
- Rates of obesity in the United States are high and contribute significantly to health-care costs.
- The amount and distribution of excess storage fat can lead to increased risk of illness and death associated with heart disease and diabetes.
- Physical and mental health are affected by unhealthy levels of body fat.
- Having too little body fat can lead to significant health problems.

MasteringHealth™

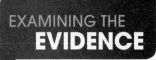
EXAMINING THE EVIDENCE ## Can You Be Fit and Fat?

Although overweight and obesity are associated with numerous unhealthy conditions, and people should always strive for a healthy body weight, it is possible to be fit and overweight. Think about watching your favorite football team. Do all the players look thin and healthy? Probably not. However, because of their intense workouts, even those players with seemingly unhealthy-looking physiques can still be healthy.

Multiple studies have found that overweight individuals can be healthy if they are physically active or fit. The strongest evidence comes from several longitudinal studies. Researchers examined cardiovascular disease and death risk and overall death rates in men and women. Death risk was 1.5 times greater for low-fit participants compared to highly fit participants across both normal and overweight BMI classifications. Those with the highest fitness levels and the lowest BMIs had the lowest risk for disease and death. However,

overweight but highly fit men and women had lower risk for death than their overweight low-fit counterparts and than low-fit men and women of normal weight. Others have found reduced risk for heart disease and death in active and fit overweight and obese individuals.

These findings support the fact that efforts to incorporate regular physical activity into your life are not in vain, no matter your weight. Active, overweight individuals do enjoy the benefits of lower risk of heart disease. Sedentary people who are at a recommended weight should still consider a regular exercise program to minimize their risk of chronic disease.

Sources: Stevens, J., K. Evenson, O. Thomas, J. Cai, and R. Thomas. Associations of fitness and fatness with mortality in Russian and American men in the lipids research clinics study. *Int J Obes,* 28:1463–1470, 2004; Church, T., M. LaMonte, C. Barlow, and S. Blair. Cardiorespiratory fitness and body mass index as predictors of cardiovascular disease mortality among men with diabetes. *Arch Intern Med,* 165:2114–2120, 2005.

Assessing Body Composition

LO **Describe the methods used to assess body composition and provide the advantages and disadvantages of each.**

Several field and laboratory methods are available for assessing body composition. Field methods require little equipment and can be easily administered at a fitness center or gym to determine weight status or body composition. The laboratory measures are used more frequently in research or medical settings. Each measure has strengths and limitations.

Field Methods

Several quick and inexpensive field techniques are used to evaluate body composition and the risk for disease (16). The procedures discussed in this section have been validated and can provide good estimates of your level of body fat or level of disease risk.

Height/Weight Tables The application of height/weight tables to determine whether a person is overweight has a long history of use by many organizations (such as life insurance companies). These tables are designed to determine if an individual is considered to have a body weight greater than normal for a specific height. Although the idea that a simple table can be used to determine if a person is too fat is attractive, there are limits to the usefulness of this approach. The major drawback is that the tables do not reveal how much of the body weight is fat. We now know that an individual can exceed the ideal body weight on a height/weight chart by being heavily muscled or by being over-fat. Because of the poor predictive ability of tables in estimating body fat, most experts do not recommend their use to determine an ideal weight.

Body Mass Index One of the easiest and most common techniques used to determine whether someone is overweight or obese is the **body mass index (BMI)**. The BMI is computed as the ratio of the body weight divided by height (in meters squared; m²):

(Metric Units) $\quad$ BMI = weight(kg) ÷ height(m)²
(*Note:* 1 kg = 2.2 lb and 1 m = 39.37 in.)

(U.S. Units) $\quad$ BMI = weight(lb) ÷ height(in.)² × 703

For example, for an individual who weighs 64.5 kg and is 1.72 m tall, the BMI would be computed as follows:

$$64.5 ÷ 1.72^2 = 64.5 ÷ 2.96 = 21.8$$

The BMI correlates with body fat, but it does not represent the percentage of body fat. Typically, individuals with a low percentage of body fat will have a low BMI, and vice versa. Using the chart in **FIGURE 6.5**, you can estimate your BMI. Next, using the chart in Figure 6.2, determine if your BMI indicates that you are underweight, normal, or overweight. For example, if your BMI is less than 25, you are considered to be at a normal and healthy weight. In contrast, if you have a BMI greater than 30, you are considered obese. This is important because research has indicated that individuals classified as obese according to BMI are at increased risk for several diseases and for death.

BMI is a simple and inexpensive method for determining your weight status, but it has limitations. BMI is not a perfect predictor of obesity: In some cases the

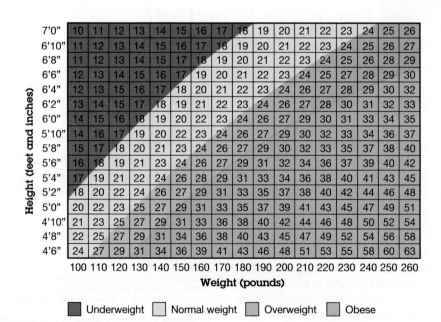

FIGURE 6.5 Estimate your BMI by finding the intersection of your weight and height. For example, if you weigh 150 pounds and your height is 5'8", your BMI would be estimated to be 23.

method can over- or underestimate body fatness. For example, an individual with a low percentage of body fat but a high level of muscularity would typically have a relatively high BMI, which would incorrectly suggest a high percentage of body fat.

Additionally, BMI is not a perfect predictor of body fat percentage. **FIGURE 6.6** illustrates the relationship between BMI and body fat percentage. For example, if you are a male with a BMI of 25, your body fat percentage is estimated to be ~19%. However, your true percentage could be as low as 14% or as high as 24% because several factors (such as muscularity) affect the relationship between BMI and body fat percentage.

Regardless of its flaws, BMI has become a widely used method to estimate body composition because BMI is a both a simple and practical predictor of body fat percentage. BMI is best used to obtain an initial estimate of whether one's percentage is at a healthy level. If your BMI suggests that you have too much body fat, you should follow up a calculation with a measure of body fat percentage, especially if you feel you are at a healthy weight and your BMI indicates otherwise.

Skinfold Assessment Because more than 50% of body fat is subcutaneous fat that lies just beneath the skin, a **skinfold test** can be used to estimate a person's overall body fatness (17). In a skinfold test, subcutaneous fat is measured using an instrument called a skinfold caliper. To be accurate, skinfold tests to estimate body fat for both men and women require at least three skinfold measurement sites (12). The anatomical sites to be measured in men (abdominal, chest, thigh skinfolds) and in women (suprailium, triceps, and thigh skinfolds) are illustrated in Laboratory 6.1. Note that for standardization, all measurements should be made on the right side of the body.

Skinfold measurements to determine body fat can be accurate but generally have a ±3%−4% margin of error (17). Using calibrated metal calipers (instead of plastic) and having a skilled technician do the test are two ways to increase accuracy. Skinfold assessment is an easy measure to obtain and can provide good estimates of body fat when done properly. However, it is not a good measure to assess body composition for obese individuals, because it is often difficult to obtain accurate measures of skinfold thickness. Inaccurate measures of skinfold thickness can be both misleading and discouraging to individuals trying to lose weight and can interfere with setting an appropriate weight goal. Bioelectrical impedance may be a preferred method of estimating body fat for some individuals.

Waist Measurement and Waist-to-Hip Ratio Waist measurements and the **waist-to-hip ratio** can be used to estimate the risk of disease associated with high body fat. Note, however, that these techniques do not provide an estimate of body fat percentage. Nonetheless, they are often good indicators of whether body fat distribution is unhealthy.

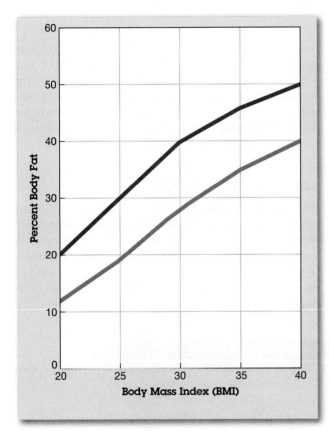

Key

▬▬▬ Women

▬▬▬ Men

FIGURE 6.6 Illustration of the relationship between body mass index (BMI) and percentage of body fat for men and women. Using this figure, you can estimate your % body fat by determining where your BMI intersects with the line representing your gender. For example, if you are female with a BMI of 25, your estimated body fat is ~30%.

Source: Modified from Pasco, J., G. Nicholson, and S. Brennan, M. Kotowicz. Prevalence of Obesity and the Relationship between the Body Mass Index and Body Fat: Cross-Sectional, Population-Based Data. PLoS ONE 7(1): e29580. doi: 10.1371/journal.pone.002958, 2012.

body mass index (BMI) Ratio of body weight (kg) divided by height squared (m^2) used to determine whether a person is at a healthy body weight; BMI is related to the percentage of body fat.

skinfold test A field test used to estimate body composition; representative samples of subcutaneous fat are measured using calipers to estimate the overall level of body fat.

waist-to-hip ratio Ratio of the waist and hip circumferences used to determine the risk for disease associated with the android pattern of obesity.

Waist measurements greater than or equal to 40 inches (102 cm) for men and 35 inches (88 cm) for women are considered health risks and indicate the android pattern of obesity. You can better evaluate your risk according to waist measurement by also considering your BMI (see **TABLE 6.1**). A high waist measurement alone might not indicate increased risk. For example, a high waist measurement for someone who is tall might be proportional to his or her height, and the level of BMI and body fat might be well within the healthy range.

Another way to estimate disease risk according to body fat distribution is the waist-to-hip ratio. An individual with a large fat deposit in the abdominal region would have a high waist-to-hip ratio and would have a higher risk of disease than someone with a lower ratio.

Both waist and hip circumference measurements should be made while the person is standing, using a nonelastic tape. It is important that the person not wear bulky clothing during the measurement, because that could alter the measurements. During measurements, the tape should be placed snugly around the body but should not press into the skin. Record your measurements to the nearest millimeter or sixteenth of an inch. The specific procedure is detailed in Laboratory 6.1.

Laboratory Measures

Body fat measurements performed in a laboratory are considered the gold standard for assessing body composition. However, these techniques require expensive specialized equipment and are often not readily available to the general public. The methods are typically used by researchers or clinicians to determine body fat percentage in research participants or patients.

TABLE 6.1 ■ Ranges and Classification for BMI and Waist Circumference

	BMI	Disease Risk* Relative to Normal Weight and Waist Circumference	
		Men, ≤102 cm Women, ≤88 cm	Men, >102 cm Women, >88 cm
Underweight	<18.5	—	—
Normal	18.5–24.9	—	—
Overweight	25.0–29.9	Increased	High
Obesity			
Class I	30.0–34.9	High	Very high
Class II	35.0–39.9	Very high	Very high
Class III	≥ 40	Extremely high	Extremely high

*Disease risk for type 2 diabetes, hypertension, and cardiovascular disease. Dashes (—) indicate that no additional risk at these levels of BMI was assigned. Increased waist circumference can also be a marker for increased risk even in persons of normal weight.

Source: Data from Gallagher, D., S. B. Heymsfield, M. Heo, S. A. Jebb, P. Murgatroyd, and Y. Sakamoto. Healthy percentage body fat ranges: An approach for developing guidelines based on body mass index. *American Journal of Clinical Nutrition* 72(3):694–701, 2000.

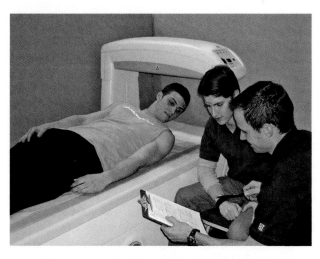

The DXA scan is considered the gold standard for measuring body composition.

Dual Energy X-Ray Absorptiometry **Dual energy X-ray absorptiometry (DXA)** involves taking a low-radiation X-ray scan (involving considerably less radiation than a typical X-ray scan) of the entire body to obtain estimates of body fat percentage. In this procedure, the person lies still on a table while an X-ray arm passes over the body. The scan typically takes about 15 minutes.

The advantage of using DXA is that it provides a measure of total body fat as well as of regional fat distribution. It can also be used to assess bone density as it relates to osteoporosis and osteoporosis risk. However, the technique is generally not used outside research or clinical settings. The equipment is expensive, and because it uses an X-ray, only trained professionals can perform the scan. Therefore, this technique of determining body composition is not commonly available in fitness and wellness centers.

Hydrostatic Weighing **Hydrostatic weighing,** also called underwater weighing, is a technique that involves weighing the individual both on land and in a tank of water to determine body volume and body density. Lean mass has a higher density than water, whereas fat mass is less dense than water. The more muscular person will weigh more under water. Because fat tends to float, the person with more fat will weigh less under water. After the two weights are obtained, they are used to calculate percentage of body fat.

Underwater weighing is very time consuming and requires special equipment. Additionally, this measure does not appeal to most individuals because it involves being completely submerged under water. Thus, this procedure is rarely employed to assess body composition in fitness centers or in college fitness and wellness courses.

Air Displacement **Air displacement** is another method used to assess body composition; it is similar in principle to hydrostatic weighing, but instead of being submerged

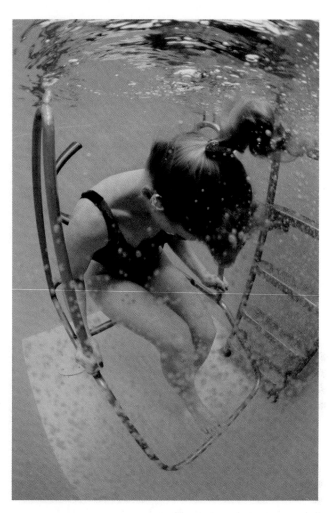

Hydrostatic weighing involves being weighed while submerged in a tank of water.

in water, the individual is seated in a chamber (the Bod Pod®). Computerized sensors are used to estimate the amount of air that is displaced when the participant is in the chamber. From knowing the amount of air displaced, body volume and then body fat can be calculated. Estimates of body fat percentage from air displacement are similar to measures from hydrostatic weighing.

Air displacement is less time consuming than underwater weighing; however, the equipment is expensive, so

---

dual energy X-ray absorptiometry (DXA) Technique for assessing body composition using a low-radiation X-ray; typically used in research or clinical settings and considered a gold-standard measure.

hydrostatic weighing Method of determining body composition that involves weighing an individual on land and in a tank of water.

air displacement Technique used to assess body composition by estimating body volume based on air displaced when a person sits in a chamber.

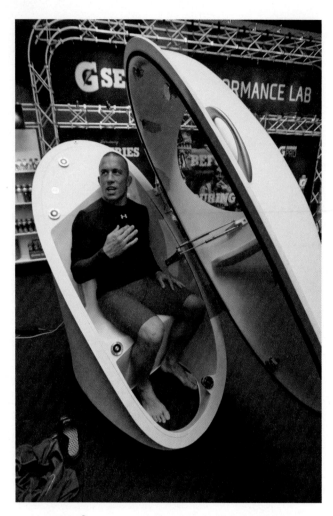

The Bod Pod® uses air displacement to measure body composition.

this technique is not available in most fitness centers. Air displacement is more commonly used in research settings and has gained wide acceptance as a means of estimating the percentage of body fat in adults.

Bioelectrical Impedance Analysis **Bioelectrical impedance analysis (BIA)** is a procedure used in fitness centers as well as in research laboratories. With commercially available BIA monitors, the person either stands on sensors of a scale-like piece of equipment or holds sensors between both hands. In the laboratory, the participant lies on a table with surface electrodes placed at the hand and foot. Then a very low-level electrical current (too low to be felt) is passed through the body between the electrodes or sensors. Because lean tissue contains more water, it is a good conductor of the current. Fat tissue, in contrast, contains less water and impedes the flow of the current. Body fat is estimated according to the resistance to the flow of the current.

BIA can be an accurate technique to estimate body fat in many individuals. However, commercially available BIA instruments can vary in quality and the devices do not provide an accurate estimate of percentage of body fat in all populations (18). For example, the validity of BIA can be influenced by gender, age, body temperature, hydration status, and overall level of fatness. Therefore, prior to using this technique, you should determine if the BIA approach has been validated for individuals in your gender and age category (19). For those populations for which BIA has been shown to be valid, the advantages are numerous, including wide availability of BIA instruments, limited time requirement, and low cost.

A major source of error in the BIA assessment of body fat is a failure to follow precisely the guidelines in regard to exercise, voiding, eating, and drinking prior to the assessment. Failure to comply with the instructions from the manufacturer can significantly impair the accuracy of the measurement.

MAKE SURE YOU **KNOW...**

- There are several laboratory and field methods used to assess body composition and weight status.

- BMI, skinfold, and waist-to-hip ratio are the most common assessments for general use in fitness courses and fitness centers.

- In monitoring the progress of your fitness program, the same method should be used for initial and later measurements of body composition, with the same person doing the measuring.

- Laboratory assessments such as DXA, hydrostatic weighing, air displacement, and BIA provide very good estimates of body composition, but most are not practical for commercial use because of their cost.

MasteringHealth™

Using Body Composition to Determine Your Ideal Weight

LO **Calculate your ideal body weight.**

The fitness categories presented for body composition differ from those for the other components of health-related physical fitness. Whereas "superior" was the highest fitness level for cardiorespiratory, strength, and muscular endurance fitness, the classification of "optimal" is the highest standard for body composition. Any category other than "optimal" is considered

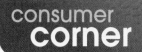

Choose your best method for determining body composition.

Method	Estimates % Body Fat	Advantages	Disadvantages
BMI	No	No cost, no special equipment required, fast, easy, anyone can do	Limited estimate of body composition
Skinfold	Yes	Accurate measurement, low cost, portable device	Trained technician required
Waist-Hip Ratio	No	No cost, no special equipment required, fast, easy, anyone can do	Limited estimate of body composition
DXA	Yes	Very accurate	Certified technician required, high cost, limited availability, time consuming, not portable
Hydrostatic Weighing	Yes	Very accurate, reasonable cost	Trained technician required, limited availability, time consuming, not portable, subjects limited to those who don't fear being submerged in water
Air Displacement (Bod Pod ®)	Yes	Fairly accurate, fast	Trained technician required, moderately high cost, limited availability, not portable
BIA	Yes	Fairly accurate, fast, portable, reasonable cost	Results vary with age, gender, body temperature, diet, and hydration level

unsatisfactory for health-related fitness. Therefore, your goal should be to reach and maintain an optimal body composition.

Research suggests that a range of 8%–19% body fat is an optimal health and fitness goal for men ages 20–39 years, and a range of 21%–32% is optimal for women ages 20–39 years (1, 16). These ranges afford little risk of disease associated with body fatness and permit individual differences in physical activity patterns and diet.

Once you have calculated your body fat percentage and know the optimal range of body fat, how can you determine the desired range of body weight? A typical 20-year-old man who has 30% body fat and weighs 185 pounds can calculate his optimal range of body weight in two simple steps:

Step 1. Compute fat-free weight—that is, the amount of total body weight contained in bones, organs, and muscles:

$$\text{Total body weight-fat weight} = \text{fat-free weight}$$
$$100\% - 30\% = 70\%$$

This means that 70% of total body weight is fat-free weight. Therefore, the fat-free weight for this student is

$$70\% \times 185\,\text{lb} = 129.5\,\text{lb}$$

Step 2. Calculate the optimal weight (which for men is 8%–19% of total body weight): The formula to compute optimal body weight is

Optimal weight
$$= \text{fat-free weight} \div (1 - \text{optimal \% fat})$$

Note that fat percentage should be expressed as a decimal. Thus, for 8% body fat,

$$\text{Optimal weight} = 129.5 \div (1 - 0.08)$$
$$= 140.8 \text{ pounds}$$

For 19% body fat,

$$\text{Optimal weight} = 129.5 \div (1 - 0.19)$$
$$= 159.9 \text{ pounds}$$

In making these calculations, we assume that this individual will maintain his lean body mass and lose fat. So his 129.5 pounds of lean mass will be 81%–92% of his new optimal body weight to achieve a healthy body composition. Hence, the optimal body weight for this individual is between 140.8 and 159.9 pounds.

---

bioelectrical impedance analysis (BIA) Method of assessing body composition by running a low-level electrical current through the body.

Laboratory 6.2 provides an opportunity to compute your optimal body weight using both body fat percentage and body mass index.

MAKE SURE YOU **KNOW...**

- Healthy body weight should be determined based on the optimal level of body fat for your age, height, and gender.
- Ideal weight can be easily calculated if you know your percentage of body fat.

—— MasteringHealth™

Behavior Change: Set Goals and Get Regular Assessments

LO **5** List your goals for achieving your ideal body weight and body composition.

As you attempt to lose or gain weight, it is important to get regular body composition assessments. When we calculated the goal weight based on the optimal level of body fat, we assumed that only fat weight was lost. However, a person experiencing weight loss may also lose water weight and possibly lose lean mass. Incorporating regular aerobic and resistance exercise along with a healthy diet will maximize the amount of fat that is lost and maintain more lean mass.

As the body changes with weight loss or gain, the weights that were originally calculated might not correspond exactly with the desired body fat percentage. In the previous example, the individual might lose 7 pounds and be in the optimal range if he also increased lean mass. Additionally, regular assessments will help you determine whether the weight you are losing is fat and not lean mass. Therefore, it is important to have regular body composition assessments as you try to reach a new goal weight. Note that it is vital to get the same type of body composition measurement when you get follow-up assessments. If possible, it is also recommended that the same person perform the assessment. These factors will reduce measurement errors. The frequency of the assessments will depend on your goal.

MAKE SURE YOU **KNOW...**

- You should have regular body composition assessments when trying to lose or gain weight to ensure the healthiest changes.
- Follow-up assessments should be made using the same method/procedure as the original assessment.

—— MasteringHealth™

study plan

Customize your study plan—and master your health!—in the Study Area of **MasteringHealth.**

summary

hear it! STUDY REVIEW

To hear an MP3 Chapter Summary, scan here or visit the Study Area in MasteringHealth™.

LO **1** ■ Body composition is a measurement of the relative amounts of fat and lean body tissue reported as percentage of body fat.

LO **2** ■ Fat can be essential fat or storage fat. A healthy body weight is based on the recommended amount of body fat.

■ Body composition is an important component of health-related physical fitness because a high percentage of body fat is associated with an increased risk for numerous diseases, including cardiovascular disease, diabetes, and cancer.

■ The distribution of fat affects disease risk associated with overweight and obesity. A very low percentage of body fat also increases risk for disease.

LO **3** ■ Common field techniques used to determine body composition are BMI, skinfold measurement, and the waist-to-hip ratio.

■ Laboratory techniques for estimating body fat are most commonly used in research and clinical settings. DXA is considered the gold-standard measure for estimating body fat.

LO **4** ■ You can calculate your healthy weight range if you know your desired percentage of body fat or BMI.

LO **5** ■ You should have regular body composition assessments when trying to lose or gain weight to monitor your progress in achieving your goals.

study questions

review it! QUIZZES

Find more review questions online in MasteringHealth™.

LO ① 1. Body composition assessments are used to determine the
   a. percentage of water in the body.
   b. percentage of fat in the body.
   c. ratio of height to weight.
   d. ratio of waist to hip size.

LO ② 2. How much essential fat do the average man and woman carry?
   a. 25% and 30%
   b. 3% and 12%
   c. 10% and 20%
   d. 5% and 18%

3. Storing excess fat in the hips and thighs puts an individual at greater risk for cardiovascular disease and diabetes than storing excess fat in the abdomen.
   a. true
   b. false

4. Which of the following is *not* a potential health consequence of being overweight or obese?
   a. low self-esteem
   b. gallbladder disease
   c. osteoarthritis
   d. anemia

5. Which of the following is *not* a potential health consequence of being underweight or having an eating disorder?
   a. malnutrition
   b. menstrual abnormalities
   c. digestive disorders
   d. type 1 diabetes

6. Describe at least several potential health consequences of not maintaining a healthy body composition.

7. Define *overweight* and *obese*. What is the public health impact of overweight and obesity in the United States?

LO ③ 8. Which technique is used to assess disease risk status associated with regional fat distribution?
   a. waist-to-hip ratio
   b. air displacement
   c. underwater weighing
   d. bioelectrical impedance analysis

9. For disease risk and health standards, a BMI of _____ is considered obese.
   a. 27   c. 30
   b. 25   d. 45

10. Which of the following is a common field test used to assess body composition?
   a. waist-to-hip measurement
   b. skinfold test
   c. hydrostatic weighing
   d. DXA

11. A person classified as normal weight based on a BMI in the healthy range can be overweight.
   a. true
   b. false

12. Name and describe the various types of field measurement techniques for assessing body composition and explain the strengths and limitations of each.

LO ④ 13. In the calculation of ideal body weight, the ideal range of body fat for men is
   a. 5-12%.   c. 8-19%.
   b. 6-12%.   d. 12-18%.

LO ⑤ 14. To achieve your ideal body weight, one of your goals should be to
   a. lose weight as fast as possible.
   b. lose both fat and lean tissue.
   c. lose only fat.
   d. gain fat and lean tissue in different proportions.

suggested reading

Bouchard, C., S. Blair, and W. Haskell (Eds.). *Physical Activity and Health.* Champaign, IL: Human Kinetics, 2012.

Bouchard, C., and P. Katzmarzyk (Eds.). *Physical Activity and Obesity.* Champaign, IL: Human Kinetics, 2010.

Church, T., and S. N. Blair. Does physical activity ameliorate the health hazards of obesity? *British Journal of Sports Medicine* 43:80–81, 2009.

Donnelly, J., S. Blair, J. Jakicic, M. Manore, J. Rankin, and B. Smith. American College of Sports Medicine position stand: Appropriate physical activity intervention strategies for weight loss and prevention of weight gain for adults. *Medicine and Science in Sports and Exercise* 41:459–471, 2009.

Heshmat, S. *Eating Behavior and Obesity.* New York: Springer, 2011.

Howley, E., and D. Thompson. *Fitness Professional's Handbook.* Champaign, IL: Human Kinetics, 2012.

Kumanvika, S., R. Brownson, and D. Satcher. *Handbook of Obesity Prevention.* New York: Springer, 2010.

Lee, R., K. McAlexander, and J. Banda. *Reversing the Obesogenic Environment.* Champaign, IL: Human Kinetics, 2011.

Powers, S., and E. Howley. *Exercise Physiology: Theory and Application to Fitness and Performance*, 8th ed. New York: McGraw-Hill, 2012.

Waisted: Abdominal obesity and your health. *Harvard Men's Health Watch* 13:1–6, 2009.

helpful weblinks

do it! WEBLINKS

For links to the organizations and websites listed, visit MasteringHealth™.

American College of Sports Medicine

Comprehensive website providing information, articles, and position statements about all aspects of health and fitness. **www.acsm.org**

American Diabetes Association

Provides diabetes information, including exercise and diet guidelines to reduce your risk. **www.diabetes.org**

American Heart Association

Contains the latest information about ways to reduce your risk of heart and vascular diseases; includes information about exercise, diet, and heart disease. **www.heart.org**

Centers for Disease Control and Prevention Healthy Weight

Offers information about maintaining a healthy weight and a BMI calculator to assess your weight. **www.cdc.gov/**

laboratory 6.1

do it! LABS
Complete Lab 6.1 online in the
study area of **MasteringHealth.com**

Name _____ Date _____

Assessing Body Composition

EQUIPMENT
Tape measure, skinfold caliper, scale

DIRECTIONS
Complete the assessments described below as directed by your instructor. Then record your body composition data and weight classifications for skinfold, waist circumference, waist-to-hip ratio, BMI, and/or other measures in the spaces below.

SKINFOLD TEST

Skinfold Test Sites

 Scan to view a demonstration video of the skinfold measurement of percent body fat.

Men

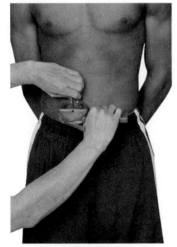
Abdomen

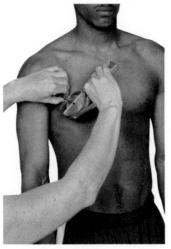
Chest

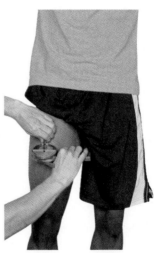
Thigh

Women

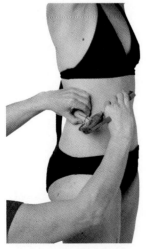
Suprailium

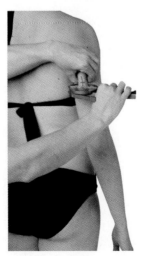
Triceps

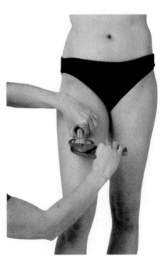
Thigh

To perform skinfold measurements:

- Hold the skinfold between your thumb and index finger.
- Slowly release the tension on the skinfold calipers to pinch the skinfold within ½ inch of your fingers.
- Hold the skinfold, and fully release the tension on the calipers.
- Read the number (the skinfold thickness in millimeters) from the gauge.
- Release the skinfold, and allow the tissue to relax.
- Measure the skinfold thickness at each site.
- Repeat three times, and average the measurements.
- Total the measurements, and use **TABLES 6.2** and **6.3** on pages 175 and 176 to determine the percent body fat.
- Enter your data in the spaces below.

  Sum of 3 skinfolds (mm) _____

  Percent body fat _____

  Classification:

  _____ Underweight

  _____ Normal

  _____ Overweight

  _____ Obese

TABLE 6.2 ■ Percent Body Fat Estimates for Women (from triceps, suprailiac, and thigh skinfolds)								
Sum of Skinfolds (mm)	Age (years)							
	Under 22	23–27	28–32	33–37	38–42	43–47	48–52	53–57	Over 57
23–25	9.7	9.9	10.2	10.4	10.7	10.9	11.2	11.4	11.7
26–28	11.0	11.2	11.5	11.7	12.0	12.3	12.5	12.7	13.0
29–31	12.3	12.5	12.8	13.0	13.3	13.5	13.8	14.0	14.3
32–34	13.6	13.8	14.0	14.3	14.5	14.8	15.0	15.3	15.5
35–37	14.8	15.0	15.3	15.5	15.8	16.0	16.3	16.5	16.8
38–40	16.0	16.3	16.5	16.7	17.0	17.2	17.5	17.7	18.0
41–43	17.2	17.4	17.7	17.9	18.2	18.4	18.7	18.9	19.2
44–46	18.3	18.6	18.8	19.1	19.3	19.6	19.8	20.1	20.3
47–49	19.5	19.7	20.0	20.2	20.5	20.7	21.0	21.2	21.5
50–52	20.6	20.8	21.1	21.3	21.6	21.8	22.1	22.3	22.6
53–55	21.7	21.9	22.1	22.4	22.6	22.9	23.1	23.4	23.6
56–58	22.7	23.0	23.2	23.4	23.7	23.9	24.2	24.4	24.7
59–61	23.7	24.0	24.2	24.5	24.7	25.0	25.2	25.5	25.7
62–64	24.7	25.0	25.2	25.5	25.7	26.0	26.2	26.4	26.7
65–67	25.7	25.9	26.2	26.4	26.7	26.9	27.2	27.4	27.7
68–70	26.6	26.9	27.1	27.4	27.6	27.9	28.1	28.4	28.6
71–73	27.5	27.8	28.0	28.3	28.5	28.8	29.0	29.3	29.5
74–76	28.4	28.7	28.9	29.2	29.4	29.7	29.9	30.2	30.4
77–79	29.3	29.5	29.8	30.0	30.3	30.5	30.8	31.0	31.3
80–82	30.1	30.4	30.6	30.9	31.1	31.4	31.6	31.9	32.1
83–85	30.9	31.2	31.4	31.7	31.9	32.2	32.4	32.7	32.9
86–88	31.7	32.0	32.2	32.5	32.7	32.9	33.2	33.4	33.7
89–91	32.5	32.7	33.0	33.2	33.5	33.7	33.9	34.2	34.4
92–94	33.2	33.4	33.7	33.9	34.2	34.4	34.7	34.9	35.2
95–97	33.9	34.1	34.4	34.6	34.9	35.1	35.4	35.6	35.9
98–100	34.6	34.8	35.1	35.3	35.5	35.8	36.0	36.3	36.5
101–103	35.3	35.4	35.7	35.9	36.2	36.4	36.7	36.9	37.2
104–106	35.8	36.1	36.3	36.6	36.8	37.1	37.3	37.5	37.8
107–109	36.4	36.7	36.9	37.1	37.4	37.6	37.9	38.1	38.4
110–112	37.0	37.2	37.5	37.7	38.0	38.2	38.5	38.7	38.9
113–115	37.5	37.8	38.0	38.2	38.5	38.7	39	39.2	39.5
116–118	38.0	38.3	38.5	38.8	39.0	39.3	39.5	39.7	40.0
119–121	38.5	38.7	39.0	39.2	39.5	39.7	40.0	40.2	40.5
122–124	39.0	39.2	39.4	39.7	39.9	40.2	40.4	40.7	40.9
125–127	39.4	39.6	39.9	40.1	40.4	40.6	40.9	41.1	41.4
128–130	39.8	40.0	40.3	40.5	40.8	41.0	41.3	41.5	41.8

Source: A. S. Jackson and M. L. Pollock, "Practical Assessment of Body Composition," *The Physician and Sportsmedicine*, Vol. 13, No. 5 (1985):76–90. Copyright © 1985 JTE Multimedia, LLC. Reprinted by permission.

Sum of Skinfolds (mm)	Age (years)								
	Under 22	23–27	28–32	33–37	38–42	43–47	48–52	53–57	Over 57
8–10	1. 3	1.8	2.3	2.9	3.4	3.9	4.5	5.0	5.5
11–13	2.2	2.8	3.3	3.9	4.4	4.9	5.5	6.0	6.5
14–16	3.2	3.8	4.3	4.8	5.4	5.9	6.4	7.0	7.5
17–19	4.2	4.7	5.3	5.8	6.3	6.9	7.4	8.0	8.5
20–22	5.1	5.7	6.2	6.8	7.3	7.9	8.4	8.9	9.5
23–25	6.1	6.6	7.2	7.7	8.3	8.8	9.4	9.9	10.5
26–28	7.0	7.6	8.1	8.7	9.2	9.8	10.3	10.9	11.4
29–31	8.0	8.5	9.1	9.6	10.2	10.7	11.3	11.8	12.4
32–34	8.9	9.4	10.0	10.5	11.1	11.6	12.2	12.8	13.3
35–37	9.8	10.4	10.9	11.5	12.0	12.6	13.1	13.7	14.3
38–40	10.7	11.3	11.8	12.4	12.9	13.5	14.1	14.6	15.2
41–43	11.6	12.2	12.7	13.3	13.8	14.4	15.0	15.5	16.1
44–46	12.5	13.1	13.6	14.2	14.7	15.3	15.9	16.4	17.0
47–49	13.4	13.9	14.5	15.1	15.6	16.2	16.8	17.3	17.9
50–52	14.3	14.8	15.4	15.9	16.5	17.1	17.6	18.2	18.8
53–55	15.1	15.7	16.2	16.8	17.4	17.9	18.5	19.1	19.7
56–58	16.0	16.5	17.1	17.7	18.2	18.8	19.4	20.0	20.5
59–61	16.9	17.4	17.9	18.5	19.1	19.7	20.2	20.8	21.4
62–64	17.6	18.2	18.8	19.4	19.9	20.5	21.1	21.7	22.2
65–67	18.5	19.0	19.6	20.2	20.8	21.3	21.9	22.5	23.1
68–70	19.3	19.9	20.4	21.0	21.6	22.2	22.7	23.3	23.9
71–73	20.1	20.7	21.2	21.8	22.4	23.0	23.6	24.1	24.7
74–76	20.9	21.5	22.0	22.6	23.2	23.8	24.4	25.0	25.5
77–79	21.7	22.2	22.8	23.4	24.0	24.6	25.2	25.8	26.3
80–82	22.4	23.0	23.6	24.2	24.8	25.4	25.9	26.5	27.1
83–85	23.2	23.8	24.4	25.0	25.5	26.1	26.7	27.3	27.9
86–88	24.0	24.5	25.1	25.7	26.3	26.9	27.5	28.1	28.7
89–91	24.7	25.3	25.9	26.5	27.1	27.6	28.2	28.8	29.4
92–94	25.4	26.0	26.6	27.2	27.8	28.4	29.0	29.6	30.2
95–97	26.1	26.7	27.3	27.9	28.5	29.1	29.7	30.3	30.9
98–100	26.9	27.4	28.0	28.6	29.2	29.8	30.4	31.0	31.6
101–103	27.5	28.1	28.7	29.3	29.9	30.5	31.1	31.7	32.3
104–106	28.2	28.8	29.4	30.0	30.6	31.2	31.8	32.4	33.0
107–109	28.9	29.5	30.1	30.7	31.3	31.9	32.5	33.1	33.7
110–112	29.6	30.2	30.8	31.4	32.0	32.6	33.2	33.8	34.4
113–115	30.2	30.8	31.4	32.0	32.6	33.2	33.8	34.5	35.1
116–118	30.9	31.5	32.1	32.7	33.3	33.9	34.5	35.1	35.7
119–121	31.5	32.1	32.7	33.3	33.9	34.5	35.1	35.7	36.4
122–124	32.1	32.7	33.3	33.9	34.5	35.1	35.8	36.4	37.0
125–127	32.7	33.3	33.9	34.5	35.1	35.8	36.4	37.0	37.6

TABLE 6.3 ■ Percent Body Fat Estimates for Men (from chest, abdomen, and thigh skinfolds)

Source: A. S. Jackson and M. L. Pollock, "Practical Assessment of Body Composition," *The Physician and Sportsmedicine,* Vol. 13, No. 5 (1985):76–90. Copyright © 1985 JTE Multimedia, LLC. Reprinted by permission.

WAIST CIRCUMFERENCE AND WAIST-TO-HIP RATIO

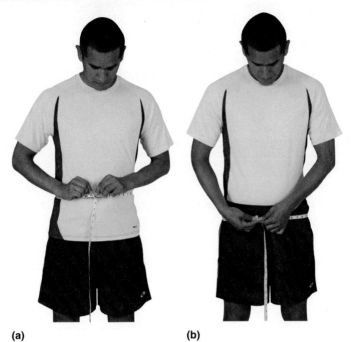

(a)   (b)

Scan to view a demonstration video of the waist and hip circumference measurements.

To perform waist-to-hip circumference measurements:

- Perform the waist measurement first.
- Place the tape at the narrowest point of the waist (a). If the subject's waist does not have a narrow point, place it at the level of the navel. Take the measurement at the end of an exhaled breath.
- For the hip measurement, place the tape around the maximum circumference of the buttocks (b).
- Divide the waist circumference by the hip circumference to determine the waist-to-hip ratio.
- Use **TABLE 6.4** on page 178 to determine the waist-to-hip ratio rating.
- Use Table 6.1 on page 166 to determine your waist measurement rating.
- Enter your data in the spaces below.

Waist measurement _____

Hip measurement   _____

Waist-to-hip ratio   _____

Classification:

_____ Low risk

_____ Moderate risk

_____ High risk

_____ Very high risk

TABLE 6.4 ■ Waist-to-Hip Circumference Ratio Standards for Men and Women

Men	Risk			
	Low	Moderate	High	Very High
20–29 yrs	<0.83	0.83–0.88	0.89–0.94	>0.94
30–39 yrs	<0.84	0.84–0.91	0.92–0.96	>0.96
40–49 yrs	<0.88	0.88–0.95	0.96–1.00	>1.00
50–59 yrs	<0.90	0.90–0.96	0.97–1.02	>1.02
60–69 yrs	<0.91	0.91–0.98	0.99–1.03	>1.03
Women	Risk			
	Low	Moderate	High	Very High
20–29 yrs	<0.71	0.71–0.77	0.78–0.82	>0.82
30–39 yrs	<0.72	0.72–0.78	0.79–0.84	>0.84
40–49 yrs	<0.73	0.73–0.79	0.80–0.87	>0.87
50–59 yrs	<0.74	0.74–0.81	0.82–0.88	>0.88
60–69 yrs	<0.76	0.76–0.83	0.84–0.90	>0.90

Source: Data from Bray, G. A., and D. S. Gray. Obesity. Part I–Pathogenesis. *West J Med* 149(4):429–441, 1988.

BMI

Weight (kg) _____

Height (m^2) _____

BMI   _____

Classification (see Table 6.1 on page 166):

_____ Underweight

_____ Normal

_____ Overweight

_____ Obese

Other Measure: _____

Percent body fat _____

Classification:

_____ Underweight

_____ Normal

_____ Overweight

_____ Obese

QUESTIONS

1. Are your classifications for each assessment similar? If not, why do you think there are discrepancies?

   _____

   _____

2. Which assessment did you feel was most accurate for you, and why?

   _____

   _____

laboratory 6.2

do it! LABS
Complete Lab 6.2 online in the
study area of **MasteringHealth.com**

Name _____   Date _____

Determining a Healthy Body Weight

EQUIPMENT

Results from Laboratory 6.1 and a calculator

DIRECTIONS

If your results from Laboratory 6.1 indicate that you need to lose or gain weight, you should calculate a goal body weight needed to achieve an optimal level of body fat or optimal BMI. Keep in mind that not everyone will need to lose or gain weight. If your weight is within the recommended levels and you are happy with your current body composition, weight maintenance should be your goal.

PART 1

Current weight	_____	*Example:*
Current percent fat	_____	*Current weight* 176
Current BMI	_____	*Current percent fat* 38
Goal percent fat	_____	*Current BMI* 29.3*
Goal BMI	_____	*Goal percent fat* 25–30†
		Goal BMI 20–25

STEP 1: Calculate % of fat-free mass.

1 − _____ (current percent fat‡) = _____ (% fat-free mass)

Example: 1 − (0.38) = 0.62

STEP 2: Calculate fat-free weight.

_____ (% fat-free mass†) × _____ (current body weight) = _____ (fat-free weight)

Example: 0.62 × 176 = 109.12

STEP 3: Calculate optimal weight, lower and upper ends of the range.

_____ (optimal weight) = _____ (fat free weight)/(1 − _____ (optimal percent fat‡)

Calculate for each end of the range.

Example, lower end: 109.12 ÷ (1 − 0.25) = 145.5

Example, upper end: 109.12 ÷ (1 − 0.30) = 155.9

Example optimal range = 146 to 156 pounds

Your optimal range: _____ to _____

---

* We used a height of 65 inches.

† We selected values within the recommended healthy range. You can use the whole range, or you can use part of the range, as we did. The important thing to remember is that your goal should be within the recommended levels for your age and activity level.

‡ Expressed as a decimal.

STEP 4: Calculate BMI based on your optimal weight range.

_____ to _____

Example:

Conversion factor: 1 m = 39.25 in.; 1 lb = 2.2 kg

Convert inches to meters: 65 in. ÷ 39.25 = 1.65 m

Convert pounds to kilograms, lower end: 145.5 lb ÷ 2.2 = 66.1 kg

Calculate BMI, lower end: 66.1 ÷ 1.65^2 = 24.3

Convert pounds to kilograms, upper end: 155.5 lb ÷ 2.2 = 70.9 kg

Calculate BMI, upper end: 70.9 ÷ 1.65^2 = 26.1

BMI: 24.3 to 26.1

PART 2

Repeat the calculations for determining a healthy goal weight, using BMI.

goal weight (kg) = desired BMI × height (m^2)

Calculate for each end of the range.

_____ to _____

QUESTIONS

1. Do the BMI values in part 1 of the lab place you in the recommended range? If not, why not?

   _____

   _____

2. Are there any differences between the BMI values from parts 1 and 2? If so, why?

   _____

   _____

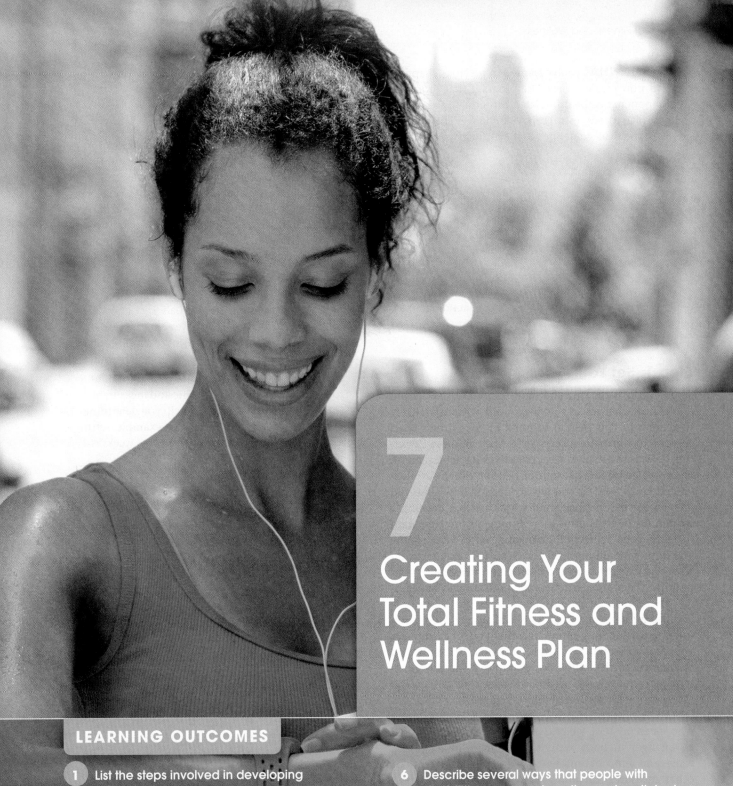

7

Creating Your Total Fitness and Wellness Plan

LEARNING OUTCOMES

1 List the steps involved in developing a fitness plan.

2 Select the training components that will be part of your fitness plan.

3 Describe the strategies that will help you be successful in implementing your exercise program.

4 Explain the importance of fitness during all stages of life.

5 Outline the guidelines for exercise during pregnancy.

6 Describe several ways that people with disabilities can remain active and participate in sports.

7 Describe common physical and mental changes associated with aging, and outline the guidelines for exercise for older adults.

8 List the steps involved in developing and implementing a wellness plan.

BASED ON WHAT you've learned in previous chapters, you can now create an exercise program that promotes all components of health-related physical fitness and a wellness plan for successful behavior change. This chapter presents practical guidelines that will help you achieve these goals.

Steps to Develop a Personal Fitness Plan

LO **1** **List the steps involved in developing a fitness plan.**

Now that you understand the benefits and components of physical fitness, it is time to develop an action plan for personal fitness. This section presents a four-step process for setting up your own fitness program.

Step 1. Set Your Goals

Setting goals is the first and most important step. If you don't know what you're working toward, you are not likely to achieve it. It is helpful to think of your fitness goals as your roadmap to success. The main purpose of setting goals is to establish clear objectives for achievement. Fitness objectives are like mile markers on a highway; they let you know how far you have come and how close you are to your destination. Studies indicate that creating a written list of goals prior to beginning a fitness program increases your chances of maintaining an exercise regime and improving physical fitness. Goals help you focus on what you expect to achieve and define and establish your priorities. They also reinforce your motivation to succeed.

There are three major types of fitness goals. One type is called a *performance goal*. This is a specific short-term, intermediate, or long-term target that you set to improve your cardiorespiratory fitness, muscular strength and endurance, or flexibility. For example, a specific short-term performance goal might be to raise your cardiorespiratory fitness rating from poor to average.

You can also set *body composition goals*. For those who need to lose weight, progress can be measured by changes in body weight, body mass index (BMI), waist and hip circumference, skinfold assessment, or other measures, including how well your clothes fit! Individuals with health issues may set body composition goals such as lowering blood pressure, triglyceride, or cholesterol levels. Respiratory capacity and cardiovascular endurance are affected by one's BMI. Therefore, anyone who wants to increase respiratory capacity and improve cardiovascular endurance will benefit from establishing body composition goals (1, 2). You should also establish *adherence goals*, which are goals to exercise a specific number of days per week. Adherence goals are important because regular exercise is essential to achieve your overall fitness goals.

The following guidelines can help you establish your personal fitness goals:

- **Set realistic short-term goals first.** Short-term goals are typically fitness objectives to be achieved within the first 2 to 6 months of an exercise program. Establishing realistic short-term goals (Laboratory 7.2) is important for two reasons: First, if your goals are too hard to achieve, you may get frustrated and give up. In addition, injuries and illness associated with unrealistic goals are frustrating and can derail your progress. Second, reaching short-term goals will help motivate you to achieve future goals.

- **Set intermediate and long-term goals.** In addition to short-term goals, it is important to set intermediate and long-term fitness goals (Laboratory 7.3). Intermediate goals typically have a time frame of 6 to 12 months, and the time frame for accomplishing long-term goals can range from 1 to 2 years and beyond.

- **Establish measurable goals.** It is important to make your goals both specific and measurable (1) (Laboratory 7.1). This will help you determine when you have reached them. For example, setting a weight-loss goal of 5 pounds within 3 weeks is a measurable (and realistic) goal.

- **Put goals in writing.** Recording your goals in a journal or fitness app is important. You can also post them in a place where you will see them every day to remind you of your fitness objectives. Keeping your goals in mind is essential to achieving them (2).

- **Establish a reward system.** After you reach each of your specific fitness goals, give yourself a reward! Rewards can be intrinsic or extrinsic. Intrinsic rewards originate inside a person and may include feeling good about body composition changes or taking pride in reaching a specific performance goal. Extrinsic rewards can be some type of tangible object such as a pair of trendy sunglasses, new water bottle, or a new blender for making healthy smoothies. You might decide to reward yourself with a subscription to a fitness magazine, hiking or kayaking with friends, reading a book (not required for class!), or simply enjoying a quiet day by yourself. Rewarding achievement is a good way to maintain your motivation while moving on to your next goal (2).

Both short- and long-term goals are flexible. If you begin your program and find that your initial goals were unrealistic they can be modified to better meet your needs and circumstances. You can use fitness testing to determine when you have reached your short-term and long-term objectives. A variety of apps are available that track your fitness goals and your progress toward achieving those goals. See **TABLE 7.1** for an overview of selected apps.

Once you begin your fitness program, be prepared for setbacks such as skipping workouts or falling behind in your

TABLE 7.1 ■ Overview of Selected Fitness Apps

App	Cost	Features	Compatible Devices
FitStar Personal Trainer www.fitstar.com	Free basic program Premium membership $39.99/year	Assesses your needs and fitness level by asking a simple set of questions at the end of every workout, allows workouts to be challenging but not crushing.	Requires iOS 7.1 or later. Compatible with iPhone, iPad, and iPod touch. Optimized for iPhone 5, iPhone 6, and iPhone 6 Plus.
Fitnet www.fit.net	Free	Offers workout videos from personal trainers. Uses the camera on your smartphone or tablet to assess how well you're keeping up with the workout and provides real-time feedback to help improve your performance.	Requires iOS 7.0 or later. Compatible with iPhone, iPad, and iPod touch. Optimized for iPhone 5, iPhone 6, and iPhone 6 Plus. Requires Android 4.1 and up.
WOD (workout of the day) Deck of Cards www.letswod.com	Free	Selected types of CrossFit exercises are dealt from a deck of cards. You can keep drawing new cards until you finish the deck or drop from exhaustion! Can track and log custom workout records, create and save workouts, post results to social media, and manage your workout history.	Requires iOS 4.3 or later. Compatible with iPhone, iPad, and iPod touch. Optimized for iPhone 5. Requires Android 2.2 and up.
Sworkit www.sworkit.com	Sworkit Lite: Free Sworkit Pro: (custom workouts) $2.99	High-intensity body weight workouts ranging from 5 minutes to an hour; includes a countdown clock showing the number of remaining reps. You can choose strength, cardio, yoga, Pilates, or stretching.	Requires iOS 7.0 or later. Compatible with iPhone, iPad, and iPod touch. Optimized for iPhone 5, iPhone 6, and iPhone 6 Plus. Requires Android 4.0 and up.
Spring www.springmoves.com	5-hour trial: Free $3.99/month or $19.99/year	Rhythm-based music for exercise. Select your favorite artists or genres and customize your playlist or use playlists created by professional DJs. Playlists contain songs with a similar range of beats per minute.	Requires iOS 7.0 or later. Compatible with iPhone, iPad, and iPod touch. Optimized for iPhone 5, iPhone 6, and iPhone 6 Plus.
Charity Miles www.charitymiles.org	Free	You can support selected charitable organizations based on your miles run, cycled, and walked, courtesy of corporate sponsors.	Requires iOS 8.0 or later. Compatible with iPhone, iPad, and iPod touch. Optimized for iPhone 5, iPhone 6, and iPhone 6 Plus. Requires Android 4.0 and up.
Endomondo www.endomondo.com	Free	Uses the GPS on your smartphone to track fitness activities. Users begin with an assessment of fitness level, and the app suggests a plan based on your exercise preferences. A virtual trainer tracks your progress.	Requires iOS 7.0 or later. Compatible with iPhone, iPad, and iPod touch. Optimized for iPhone 5, iPhone 6, and iPhone 6 Plus. Android requirements vary by device.
Coach.me www.coach.me	$14.99/week	Virtual coaching service includes support for fitness and diet goals. Helps create a plan for behavior change and monitors your progress via text messaging.	Requires iOS 7.0 or later. Compatible with iPhone, iPad, and iPod touch. Optimized for iPhone 5, iPhone 6, and iPhone 6 Plus. Requires Android 3.0 and up.

progress. An occasional setback is normal (3). However, once you realize that you have stopped making progress, you should work to get back on track as soon as possible. Setbacks can be a signal to review and possibly modify your goals. It is important to assess whether the goals are realistic for your lifestyle. Sometimes just changing the time or day of a workout can help you get back on track.

Step 2. Select Exercises for Your Fitness Program

After establishing your personal fitness goals, the next step is to choose exercises that develop the various components of health-related physical fitness. Remember to target each of the following components.

Cardiorespiratory Endurance Exercises that develop this component involve repetitive movement of large-muscle groups, such as the legs (see Chapter 3). Combining aerobic training techniques to vary your fitness routine will prevent boredom and make it more likely you will accomplish your fitness goals. Just remember that any cardiorespiratory endurance program should be designed to achieve your specific fitness goals (3).

Muscular Strength and Endurance Progressive resistance exercise training is the key to increasing muscular strength and endurance (see Chapter 4). Again, keep

in mind that the use of variations in training such as high-intensity interval training (HIIT) and CrossFit (see Chapter 3) can help keep you motivated in your workouts.

Flexibility Because flexibility is an important part of any fitness program, you should include stretching exercises in your training routine (see Chapter 5). How you incorporate flexibility training into your exercise routine should be guided by your personal fitness goals.

Body Composition Remember, too, that body composition is an important component of health-related physical fitness (see Chapter 6). Achieving a desirable body composition (for health or performance reasons) should be an intermediate and a long-term goal of your total fitness program. Activities in each of the above categories will improve body composition.

Step 3. Plan Your Weekly Fitness Routine

The next step is to plan your weekly fitness routine by determining how much time and energy you will devote to each element of your program. This calculation should be based on the FITT principle—frequency, intensity, time, and type (see Chapter 3). **FIGURE 7.1** illustrates how to apply the FITT principle to each component of a health-related physical fitness program.

	Flexibility Training	Cardiorespiratory Training	Strength Training	High Intensity Interval Training (HIIT)
FREQUENCY	2–7 times/week	3–7 times/week	2–3 times/week	3–6 times/week
INTENSITY	Stretch to position of mild discomfort	50%–85% target heart rate	Completion of one set of reps should result in muscle fatigue	**Cardio** (near maximal intensity*) **Weights** (10–15 rep max weight)
TIME	1–4 repetitions (hold stretch 15-30 seconds)	20–60 minutes per training session	6–15 repetitions each (2–3 sets)	**Cardio** (3–10 sets) (20–60 seconds per set**) **Weights** (3 sets to failure - 60 second rest intervals)
TYPE	Stretching exercises including all major muscle groups	Continuous rhythmic exercise using large muscle groups	Resistance exercises training all muscle groups	**Cardio** (Continuous rhythmic exercise using large muscle groups) **Weights** (all muscle groups)

**Flexibility Training + Cardiorespiratory Training + Strength Training
or Flexibility Training + HIIT
= A well-rounded exercise program**

* Varies with the length of the sets. For example, 20 second sets are more intense than 60 second sets. Rest intervals between sets varies with intensity.

** Sets should be interspersed with low intensity bouts for recovery. For example, sprinting for 20 second sets with 60 second slow jog in between; or sprinting for 60 seconds sets with 30 second slow jog in between.

FIGURE 7.1 This chart can help you apply the FITT principle to each component of health-related physical fitness.

Training to Improve Cardiorespiratory Fitness
Most cardiorespiratory health benefits occur with 120–150 minutes per week of moderate-intensity aerobic exercise. However, training more than 150 minutes per week can provide even more fitness benefits and help to achieve weight-loss goals. HIIT training can provide benefits while reducing total workout time. However, if you use interval training, slow down your rate of progress, since higher-intensity work can result in more soreness and a higher risk of injury. Examples of aerobic activities and their intensity are listed in **TABLE 7.2**.

Training to Improve Muscular Strength and Endurance A training frequency of 2 to 3 days per week—on nonconsecutive days—is recommended to improve muscular strength and endurance (4, 5). You can increase the number of days per week that you train with weights by focusing on different muscle groups on different days. For example, you could do upper body exercises Monday, Wednesday, and Friday, and lower body exercises Tuesday, Thursday, and Saturday. You should progress until you can perform 2 to 3 sets of each exercise, with 6 to 15 repetitions in each set (Figure 7.1).

Training to Improve Flexibility Flexibility exercises should be performed 2 to 7 days per week, with stretches performed on all major muscle groups. One to four repetitions of each exercise for 15 to 30 seconds is recommended (Figure 7.1).

Step 4. Monitor Your Progress

The final step in designing your fitness plan is to create a training log (or begin using a fitness app) to record your progress. A log that tracks your weekly training activities will give you a sense of accomplishment and help motivate you to continue your program (6). **FIGURE 7.2** provides two examples. You should create a log format or choose an app that is easy to use.

Remember that you should monitor your fitness progress in cardiorespiratory endurance and muscular strength by retesting your fitness levels at regularly established intervals—for example, every 3 months—and keeping a record of your improvements. Always use the same test or measure to accurately detect changes in fitness levels over time. For example, if you initially measure your cardiorespiratory endurance using a test like the Rockport Walk Test (7), it is important to use this same test when evaluating future $\dot{V}O_2$ max levels. Using different measures over time will produce inaccurate (and possibly disappointing) results.

MAKE SURE YOU **KNOW...**

- There are four main steps to follow in developing a personal fitness plan: set goals, select activities, plan your weekly routine, and monitor your progress.

- It is important to choose fitness activities that target cardiorespiratory fitness, muscular strength and endurance, and flexibility. Monitor your progress using a training log or fitness app.

- The FITT principle will help you plan your weekly fitness routine.

—— MasteringHealth™

Combining Fitness Training Components

LO **2** **Select the training components that will be part of your fitness plan.**

Once you have selected activities and created exercise programs that target the main components of physical fitness, you are ready to combine these elements into an integrated weekly exercise routine. Sample programs are provided at the end of this chapter. To plan and record your own weekly program, you can use the chart in Laboratory 7.4. Consider the following factors when developing your exercise plan:

- **Fun and variety.** You are more likely to be successful with your fitness program if you choose activities you enjoy. It is also a good idea to add variety by including different types of activities—such as swimming, hiking, rowing, inline skating, and cycling. You may also enjoy classes such as dance, yoga, Pilates, or spinning.

TABLE 7.2 ▪ Aerobic Activities and Intensities	
Type of Activity	Intensity
Bicycling (level and <10 mph)	Moderate
Bicycling (>12 mph)	Vigorous
Golf, pulling clubs	Moderate
Hiking, rigorous	Vigorous
Race-walking	Moderate to vigorous
Rowing	Moderate to vigorous
Running, 12-min. mile	Vigorous
Shoveling snow	Vigorous
Skiing, cross country	Vigorous
Skipping rope	Vigorous
Spinning classes	Moderate to vigorous
Swimming	Moderate to vigorous
Tennis (doubles)	Moderate
Tennis (singles)	Vigorous
Walking 3.0 mph	Moderate
Water aerobics	Moderate

Weekly Exercise Training Log
Name: Dylan Brown
Week: September 9–15

Activity	Mon	Tue	Wed	Thur	Fri	Sat	Sun
Aerobics Class	20 min		20 min	20 min	20 min		30 min
Soccer Practice		30 min		20 min		30 min	
Weight Training	2 sets (8 reps) × 8 exercises		2 sets (8 reps) × 8 exercises		2 sets (8 reps) × 8 exercises		
Stretching		15 min		15 min			15 min
Daily Duration	20 min	30 min	20 min	40 min	20 min	30 min	30 min
Total Weekly Duration	**190 min**						

(a) Conventional Training Plan

Weekly Exercise Training Log
Name: Dylan Brown
Week: September 9–15

Activity	Mon	Tue	Wed	Thur	Fri	Sat	Sun
Cardio Intervals	5 @ 60 sec (20 sec between at slow jog)		9 @ 60 sec (20 sec between at slow jog)		5 @ 60 sec (20 sec between at slow jog)		9 @ 60 sec (20 sec between at slow jog)
Soccer Practice		30 min		20 min		30 min	
Weight Training Intervals	2 sets (10–15 rep max wt. to failure) × 6 exercises		2 sets (10–15 rep max wt. to failure) × 6 exercises		2 sets (10–15 rep max wt. to failure) × 6 exercises		
Stretching		15 min		15 min			15 min
Daily Duration	5 min	30 min	3 min	20 min	5 min	30 min	3 min
Total Weekly Duration	**96 min**						

(b) HIIT Plan

FIGURE 7.2 A weekly exercise training log (or app) is useful in recording your activities and charting your progress. Here are two examples: (a) Conventional workout that incorporates cardio, weights, and flexibility training, plus time allotted for a sport or recreational activity. (b) Alternative workout using HIIT principles.

- **Current fitness level.** Make sure to construct a fitness program that matches your current fitness level. It is counterproductive to design a training plan that is overly ambitious and impossible to complete. You should create a program that is realistic and achievable.

- **Special health issues.** If you have special health concerns—such as type 1 diabetes or asthma—consult your physician before designing your fitness program. Your doctor can provide information that will help you devise a program to safely meet your needs. If you need additional help, consult a certified personal trainer.

- **Muscle strain.** Keep in mind that muscles need time to rest and recover after weight training. For this reason, you should not schedule weight-training sessions for the same muscle groups on consecutive days. Note in the sample exercise programs on pages 199–200 that weight training and running are scheduled on alternating days (also see **TABLE 7.3**). Some people prefer the routine provided by daily gym workouts. You can do this safely by alternating the muscle groups you focus on each day. For example, train your lower body on Mondays and Wednesdays and your upper body on Tuesdays and Thursdays.

- **Flexibility training.** You should perform stretching exercises at least 2 days per week. Table 7.3 shows a stretching program of 3 days per week, but 5 to 7 days per week is considered ideal. As you progress toward your fitness goals, you should add additional stretching days.

TABLE 7.3 ■ Example of a Weekly Exercise Plan							
Activity	Monday	Tuesday	Wednesday	Thursday	Friday	Saturday	Sunday
Running	X		X		X		
Cycling		X		X			X
Weight training		X		X		X	
Stretching	X		X		X		

MAKE SURE YOU **KNOW...**

- Your fitness program will be more successful if you include a variety of physical activities you enjoy.
- Your program should be realistic and correspond to your current fitness level.
- If you have special health concerns, consult your health-care provider and a certified personal trainer when planning your exercise program.
- Strength training should be scheduled to allow muscles to recover (alternate days or muscle groups).
- Stretching exercises should be performed at least 2 days a week, after a warm-up or exercise session when muscles are warm.

MasteringHealth™

Putting Your Plan into Action

LO **3** Describe the strategies that will help you be successful in implementing your exercise program.

After setting your goals, planning your fitness routine, and creating a monitoring system to chart your progress, it is time to launch your plan into action. Remember that planning a fitness program is easier than carrying it out. The following guidelines will help you stick with your plan and succeed in achieving your goals.

- **Take a gradual approach.** Begin your exercise program in a careful, measured way. You may incur injuries such as muscle strain if you push yourself too hard at the start. After adjusting to your routine, you can gradually increase the amount of exercise overload to increase your fitness level. Even small increases in exercise duration and intensity will result in noticeable improvements.

- **Be consistent and methodical.** One key to reaching your fitness goals is to maintain a pattern of regular exercise. If you pick a convenient time and place for your training sessions, you are more likely to stick to your routine.

- **Exercise with friends.** Research shows that exercising with friends can make exercise more fun and increase your motivation (8). Choose a friend with a similar fitness level who shares your exercise goals and is willing to commit to a regular routine. Keep in mind, too, that a canine friend can be a good exercise partner. It has been shown that having a dog will increase your physical activity (9). Dog walking can be a great way to get daily exercise, so your favorite pet may help you reach your goals (10).

- **Vary your training.** Engaging in a variety of fitness activities will make your exercise program more enjoyable and productive. Cross training, for example, has many health and fitness benefits (11). Even simple variations such as changing the time of day or route you walk, run, or cycle can help maintain your interest and enthusiasm.

- **Get enough rest.** Getting adequate sleep plays an important role in any fitness program. Good sleep patterns are critical to overall health and well-being (12, 13). Research indicates that irritability,

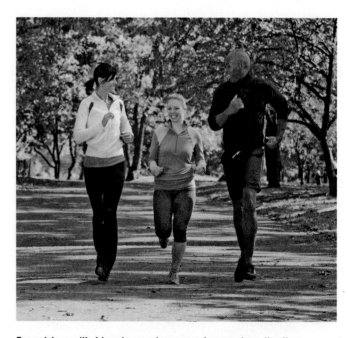

Exercising with friends can increase fun and motivation.

moodiness, and general fatigue are among the first signs of a lack of sleep (14). Most adults need an average of 8 hours of sleep a day, though sleep needs can vary (15). Some people are able to get by on as little as 6 hours of sleep, while others can't perform well unless they've slept for 10 hours. Determine how much sleep you need, and schedule that time into your daily routine (16).

- **Adapt to changing circumstances.** Don't allow changes in your work or class schedule to disrupt your exercise program. If necessary, adjust your exercise routine, but don't give it up. If you are used to exercising outdoors, don't let bad weather or less daylight during winter interfere with your training. Continue your exercise indoors, at home or at a gym or fitness center.

- **Expect backsliding.** At times you may miss a few exercise sessions and lose motivation. This may occur because you feel tired or ill, or because other things get in the way. This type of "backsliding" is common and should not discourage you or keep you from getting your fitness program back on track. See Examining the Evidence for strategies to avoid backsliding.

- **Combine regular exercise with other healthy behaviors.** Although exercise provides major health benefits, it is not a cure-all to achieving good health (17, 18). Other factors, such as a nutrient-dense diet and avoiding smoking and drug abuse, will improve your chances of remaining healthy. Later in this chapter you will learn more about putting together wellness plans for improved healthy behaviors.

MAKE SURE YOU **KNOW**...

- It is important to take a gradual approach and not overdo it when starting your fitness program.
- It is best to exercise in a regular and consistent pattern but also adjust your routine as needed to accommodate changing schedules and circumstances.
- Exercising with friends or pets can be beneficial for some people.
- Varying your training activities can increase motivation.
- Getting enough sleep is critical to the success of your fitness program.
- Backsliding is common and should not be a cause for discouragement.
- Exercise should be combined with other healthy behaviors to ensure good health.

— MasteringHealth™

Fitness Is a Lifelong Process

LO **4** **Explain the importance of fitness during all stages of life.**

Maintaining fitness and wellness is a lifelong process, and your actions today will have a significant impact on your health 10, 20, 40, even 60 or more years from now. Think about the health and fitness levels of your parents, grandparents, or other older adults you know. Whatever age we are, we all need to make wise choices to ensure good health now and in the years to come.

EXAMINING THE EVIDENCE ## How to Avoid Backsliding

Reverting to old habits (backsliding) is common in any behavior change program. Most people who start a new exercise routine have trouble maintaining a regular workout schedule. One key to success is to recognize that backsliding is typical. The following tips may help you stay on track:

- If you slip out of your exercise routine, remember that you can resume it just as easily. Focus on your fitness goals and the health benefits you hope to gain.
- Don't become discouraged. Progress takes time, and a positive attitude is very helpful! Sticking with your program (and varying it as needed) will lead to success.

- If you have a hard time staying motivated, remember that exercise has a positive impact on physical and mental energy. Even if you perform only part of your regular workout, exercise will lift your mood and make you feel better.
- Stay active by walking or running up steps, parking in distant parking spaces, or fitting in just the first 10 or 15 minutes of your usual workout.
- Using a fitness app or keeping a training log will also help you stay on track. A log of your accomplishments can help you take pride in your progress and keep you moving forward toward your goals.

Remember, fitness cannot be stored! The principle of reversibility (discussed in Chapter 2) states that if you stop being active, you lose fitness and the health benefits you worked so hard to achieve.

Changes in Physical Activity Levels

For most adults, rates of physical activity decline with age (19, 20). You have already experienced one of the periods during which a decline in activity is common—starting college. Rates of physical activity tend to drop during periods of major life changes, such as beginning college life, graduating from college, moving to a new town, getting married, or starting a family (21). In situations in which people experience a lot of changes at once, they can become overwhelmed. They may feel that they do not have time to fit in an exercise program with all their other commitments. When you are dealing with a planned event, you can prepare for both the event and any accompanying lifestyle changes, including finding ways to stay active.

Other life-changing events, such as an unexpected death in the family or a sudden job loss, may occur without your having time to prepare. Keep in mind that a lapse in physical activity does not have to lead to the failure of your fitness plan. Scheduling a break and allowing a few days off during times when you feel overwhelmed is fine, as long as you also plan to get back on track. Planning for shortened or modified workouts is another option. Some adults must care for a sick spouse or parent, leaving them less time for exercise.

As you get older, your interests and your body will change, leading to changes in your workout choices. For instance, a long-time runner might have to shift to a lower-impact activity as age weakens his or her joints. The important thing is to be open to new activities (or trying a new sport) and selecting those you enjoy so you can maintain your motivation to keep up a regular exercise routine (see **TABLE 7.4** for a comparison of various activities).

TABLE 7.4 ■ Fitness Evaluation of Various Activities and Sports

Sport/Activity	Cardiorespiratory Endurance	Upper Body Muscular Strength and Endurance	Lower Body Muscular Strength and Endurance	Flexibility	Caloric Expenditure (calories/min)
Aerobic dance	Good	Good	Good	Fair	5–10
Badminton	Fair	Fair	Good	Fair	5–10
Baseball	Poor	Fair	Fair	Fair	4–6
Basketball	Good	Fair	Good	Fair	10–12
Bowling	Poor	Fair	Poor	Fair	3–4
Canoeing	Fair	Good	Poor	Fair	4–10
Cross-country skiing	Excellent/good	Good	Good	Fair	7–15
Downhill skiing	Fair	Fair	Good	Fair	5–10
Golf (walking)	Poor	Fair	Good/fair	Fair	2–4
Gymnastics	Poor	Excellent	Excellent	Excellent	3–4
Handball	Good	Good/fair	Good	Fair	7–12
Ice skating	Good/fair	Poor	Good/fair	Good/fair	5–10
Karate	Fair	Good	Good	Excellent	7–10
Racquetball	Good/fair	Good/fair	Good	Fair	6–12
Roller skating	Good/fair	Poor	Good/fair	Fair	5–10
Running	Excellent	Fair	Good	Fair	8–15
Soccer	Good	Fair	Good	Good/fair	7–17
Tai chi	Good/fair	Good/fair	Good/fair	Fair	5–9
Tennis	Good/fair	Good/fair	Good	Fair	5–12
Volleyball	Fair	Fair	Good/fair	Fair	4–8
Waterskiing	Poor	Good	Good	Fair	4–7
Weight training	Poor	Excellent	Excellent	Fair	4–6
Yoga	Poor	Poor	Poor	Excellent	2–4

Sources: From *Physical Fitness: A Way of Life,* 5/e by Bud Getchell, Alan E. Mikesky and Kay Mikesky. Reprinted by permission of Cooper Publishing Group; Lan, C., S. Chen, and J. Lai. Tai chi. *American Journal of Chinese Medicine* 32:151–160, 2004; Taylor-Pillae, R., and E. Foelicher. Effectiveness of tai chi in improving aerobic capacity: A meta analysis. *Journal of Cardiovascular Nursing* 19:48–57, 2004.

MAKE SURE YOU **KNOW**...

- Fitness is a lifelong process, and exercise needs to be engaged in consistently to maintain health benefits.

- Rates of physical activity decrease with age. Finding activities that you can enjoy as you age is important for staying active.

- Exercising regularly may be difficult during periods of change or transition. Planning ahead (when possible) and adjusting your routine can help you stay active during these times.

MasteringHealth™

Fitness During Pregnancy

LO **5** Outline the guidelines for exercise during pregnancy.

In most cases, women can exercise safely during a normal pregnancy. However, every pregnant woman should consult with her health-care provider before starting a new program or continuing an existing program. This recommendation is especially important for women who were sedentary prior to pregnancy or who have medical conditions that might require special attention (e.g., obesity, hypertension, gestational diabetes). Women who exercise regularly may need to modify their workouts to adjust to changes associated with pregnancy. Exercise has been shown to have numerous benefits for pregnant women, including less weight gain, fewer discomforts, and shorter labor (22). There is also some evidence that exercise might help prevent and treat gestational diabetes (22, 23). Women who maintain regular aerobic exercise during pregnancy can maintain cardiorespiratory fitness, have better posture, retain less weight, and have less back pain than women who remain sedentary. There are risks to the fetus associated with exercise during pregnancy, so knowing one's own body and following the recommended exercise prescription and guidelines is very important.

The exercise prescription for pregnancy endorsed by the American College of Sports Medicine (ACSM) is at least 15 minutes per session for a minimum of 3 days per week. The duration can be gradually increased to 30 minutes of moderate-intensity aerobic exercise most days of the week. Women should avoid exercise or activities with a high risk for falling or that could cause trauma to the fetus (22). Some activities that were engaged in prior to pregnancy might have higher risk due to pregnancy-related changes. For example, joint laxity increases during pregnancy, and joints may feel less stable. Pregnant women who are regular joggers might need to consider walking or jogging on a treadmill for increased safety. Prolonged or high-intensity exercise may impair fetal development, and women should

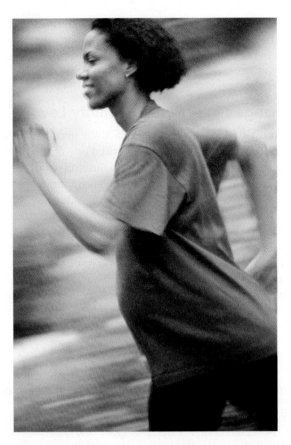

Short-duration, low- to moderate-intensity exercise can be beneficial for a pregnant woman while posing little risk for the fetus.

consult with their health-care providers before continuing any type of intense exercise program (22, 24).

Women who exercise during pregnancy should follow these guidelines (22, 24):

- Do not increase the amount of exercise you typically performed before your pregnancy.

- Do not participate in sports with a high risk of injury.

- Do not use exercises that require lying on the back after the first trimester. The weight of the fetus may reduce blood flow through vessels supplying blood to the lower extremities.

- During the last trimester, avoid exercises that use quick jerking movements, because they may cause joint strains.

- Wear good supportive footwear and adequate breast support.

- Avoid exercising in high-temperature conditions (especially with high humidity too), and wear clothing that will allow your body to dissipate heat. The primary dangers of exercise during pregnancy are elevated body temperature and lack of blood flow to the baby. Aquatic exercise prevents large gains of body heat because water removes heat from the body better than air does.

- Drink plenty of water to maintain hydration. The recommendation is to drink 2 additional glasses of water (8 oz.) for each hour of exercise.

- Monitor exercise intensity using a rating of perceived exertion (RPE). An RPE value of 12–14 is recommended. The talk test can also be used to monitor exercise intensity. Exercise during which you are able to maintain a conversation is considered moderate intensity.

- Stop exercising immediately and call your health-care provider if you experience shortness of breath, dizziness, numbness, tingling, abdominal pain, or vaginal bleeding.

- Light- to moderate-intensity resistance training can be performed. Avoid isometric exercise and the Valsalva maneuver.

- Increase caloric intake by about 300 kcal per day to meet the increased needs due to exercise and pregnancy.

- In most cases, after consulting with their health-care provider women can gradually resume exercise 4 to 6 weeks after delivery.

MAKE SURE YOU **KNOW**...

- Exercise is safe for healthy pregnant women; a workout can consist of aerobic exercise up to 30 minutes at moderate intensity (RPE 12–14) and light- to moderate-intensity resistance training.

- Pregnant women should avoid exercises performed while lying on the back and activities with high risk for falling or fetal trauma.

— MasteringHealth™

Fitness for People with Disabilities

LO **6** Describe several ways that people with disabilities can remain active and participate in sports.

People with a physical disability or mental health/developmental challenge can benefit from the exercise programs described in previous chapters. Depending on their abilities and limitations, some may find it difficult to engage in regular exercise or find an activity that is of interest. It has been shown that regular exercise is especially important to the health of people with physical disabilities (25) and mental/emotional challenges (such as post-traumatic stress disorder) (26). In some cases, it is advisable for individuals with disabilities to exercise under the supervision of a physical therapist or certified personal trainer.

In the past decade, there have been innovative adaptations to individual and group exercise classes and

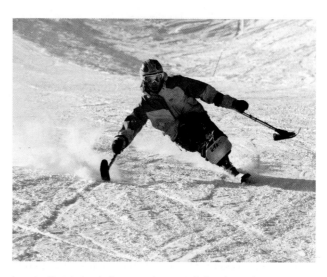

Innovative adaptations make a variety of sports more accessible.

sports and a change in the philosophy of certain games and competitions that have created new opportunities for people of all ability levels. Today, regardless of ability level, there is probably a sport out there for you! Even activities such as water skiing and mountain climbing are accessible to those who want to learn them. Sports for people with a disability are typically divided into two main types: adapted sports and inclusive sports.

Adapted sports (also known as *adaptive sports*) are played solely by people with a disability. The rules of play (and sometimes equipment) have been adapted to make the sport more accessible. Adapted sports programs can usually be found at recreational centers and sports clubs that work specifically with disabled individuals. Some adapted sports organizations are listed below:

- Wounded Warrior Project (www.woundedwarrior-project.org)

- Paralympic Sports Clubs (www.findaclub .usparalympics.org)

- Disabled Sports USA (www.disabledsportsusa.org)

- Wheelchair and Ambulatory Sports USA (www .wasusa.org)

Inclusive sports are played by individuals with and without a disability. There are a large number of inclusive sports, and they can be found in many locations, including schools, rec centers, and sports clubs. Section 504 of the Rehabilitation Act of 1973 granted access to sports for all public school students.

---

adapted sports Sports played solely by people with a disability; also known as *adaptive sports*.

inclusive sports Sports played by individuals with and without a disability.

Fitness for Older Adults

LO **7** Describe common physical and mental changes associated with aging, and outline the guidelines for exercise for older adults.

The aging process results from a combination of genetics, environment, diet, and lifestyle factors (5, 27). Exercise is one of the lifestyle factors that can impact the aging process. For those age 65 and older, exercise is just as important as it is for younger adults. Everyone experiences a significant decline in VO_2 max with age regardless of their level of exercise participation. However, research has shown that

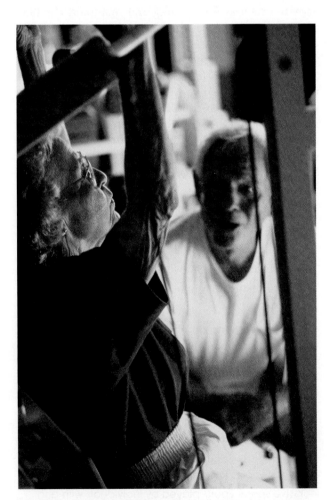

Exercise is beneficial for people of all ages.

older adults who engage in a regular, vigorous physical activity program can have levels of aerobic fitness that are similar to someone much younger (28). Thus, a 75-year-old male athlete can have an aerobic capacity similar to that of a 25-year-old sedentary man!

Physical and Mental Changes of Aging

As we age, we all experience a gradual decline in biological function. During youth, the organ systems in healthy bodies function at a higher level than is required for optimal function. Because of this, small, gradual age-related changes in organ systems do not impair their function. Over a longer period of time, the decline is more drastic and has a noticeable impact on functional ability. Most begin to notice age-related changes in their 30s and 40s (29).

The most common age-related changes are decreased cardiorespiratory function, increased body fat, and a more fragile musculoskeletal system (30). Approximately one-half of the decline in functional capacity results from a decrease in physical activity (29). Maintaining a regular exercise program can help you maintain a higher level of cardiovascular functioning as you age. Sedentary adults can improve cardiorespiratory function by beginning a regular exercise program (31), and regular exercise can help maintain a healthy body composition and the mineral content of bone.

Maximal heart rate decreases with age. (Recall that age is used in the equation to estimate maximal heart rate.) Because maximal heart rate decreases, maximal cardiac output also decreases. An additional cardiovascular change is a progressive buildup of fatty plaque in blood vessels, resulting in "hardening of the arteries," or the atherosclerotic process. These arterial changes can contribute to a gradual increase in blood pressure, resulting in age-related hypertension.

Bone and joint health are affected in the aging process. We gradually lose bone strength as a result of a decrease in bone mineral density (osteoporosis). These changes increase the risk for falls and fractures. We typically achieve peak bone mass in our early 20s, so developing adequate bone mass when we are young is important to prevent osteoporosis. Weight-bearing exercise and resistance training can help strengthen muscle and bone (32). The loss of bone mass in women is greatly accelerated after menopause because of the decline in estrogen. Aging also results in a loss of connective tissue between joints, which can result in arthritis, inflammation, and painful movement.

A loss of skeletal muscle mass and function, called **sarcopenia**, is a major age-related health problem for both men and women (30). Muscular strength lost during aging is directly related to loss of skeletal muscle mass. Total muscle mass declines by approximately

40% between the ages of 20 and 80. This is a significant issue because it results in reduced mobility and independence and increases the risk of falls. Skeletal muscles generate the force required to maintain bone mass, and loss of bone mass is associated with increased risk for falling and fractures. Thus, age-related loss of muscle results in a vicious cycle as it contributes to the loss of bone mass, as well.

Numerous other changes take place as we age, but we can slow some of the changes with our behaviors. Common age-related changes include the following:

▪ In the skin, oil production declines, connective tissue is lost, and pigmentation changes. As a result, the skin can appear dry, wrinkled, and blotchy.

▪ Many people experience changes in their vision around age 40. Inability to focus on close objects **(presbyopia),** impaired night vision, and a loss of depth perception are common changes.

▪ Changes in the cells on the tongue and in the nose lead to a decline in taste and smell. These changes can contribute to a loss of appetite.

▪ The brain and central nervous system also experience changes. There is a loss of brain cells (neurons) and a decrease in neurotransmitters. One of the more obvious changes in brain function is a gradual loss of memory.

▪ Hair begins to thin after about age 20. Also, as cells at the base of hair follicles age, they produce less pigment, so hair color fades and turns gray.

consider this! ////////////////

Studies have shown that mortality rates are 20% to 30% lower over a given time period among people who expend 1,000 kilocalories in physical activity per week.

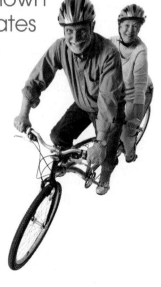

Exercise Prescription for Older Adults

Older adults can safely participate in aerobic, resistance, and flexibility exercises but might have to modify the exercise prescriptions presented earlier. An older adult who has exercised regularly her entire adult life may continue with the same exercise routine she followed during middle age. Keep in mind that exercise prescriptions are typically made relative to the individual's maximal capacity. The absolute levels of heart rate or resistance will change, but the prescription will still be based on a percentage of maximal heart rate or resistance.

An older person with a history of inactivity will likely have low cardiorespiratory functioning and weak muscles. For individuals with a lower level of functioning, a lower intensity than typically recommended can produce significant improvements (24). Older adults should consult with their health-care providers before beginning an exercise program and they should always consider issues of safety including the risk of falling and the amount of strength, balance, and coordination needed for an exercise. Using rate of perceived exertion or percentage of maximal heart rate to monitor exercise intensity is preferred when the person is taking medications that alter heart rate. Activities such as walking, cycling, swimming, and light weight training are generally recommended. Water exercises are a good choice for older adults beginning an exercise program (see the sample program at the end of this chapter).

The following guidelines outline some specific considerations for exercise after age 45 for men and after age 55 for women (24):

▪ Because the risk of heart disease increases with age, men over age 45 and women over age 55 should consult with a health-care provider to determine whether a physician-supervised, graded exercise stress test is needed before engaging in a vigorous physical fitness program.

▪ Non-weight-bearing exercises are recommended to reduce the risk of musculoskeletal problems. Weight-bearing exercises are beneficial but should be performed with balance support to avoid falls.

▪ Exercise intensity should be at the lower end of the target heart rate range.

sarcopenia Loss of skeletal muscle mass that occurs with aging.

presbyopia Farsightedness that results from weakening of the eye muscles due to aging.

- Exercise frequency limited to 3 to 4 days per week can reduce the risk of injury.
- Exercise duration should be modified to meet the needs (and abilities) of each individual.

MAKE SURE YOU **KNOW**...

- Aging is a slow, gradual decline in biological functions. The most common functional changes seen with both aging and inactivity are decreased cardiorespiratory function, increased body fat, and musculoskeletal fragility.
- Approximately one-half of the age-related decline in functional capacity is due to a decrease in physical activity.
- Exercise capacity decreases with age, but older adults who remain active can maintain a high level of cardiovascular functioning.
- Older adults who start an exercise program can improve their fitness levels and enjoy health benefits.

MasteringHealth™

Steps for Developing and Implementing a Wellness Plan

LO **8** List the steps involved in developing and implementing a wellness plan.

Recall from Chapter 1 that total wellness encompasses physical health plus emotional, intellectual, spiritual, social, environmental, occupational, and financial health. In the chapters that follow, you will go "in-depth" into many aspects of wellness that have a major impact on your health. Once you have covered the remaining chapters, you will be ready to put together a detailed wellness plan. Here we present four important steps that will help you achieve a higher level of wellness.

Step 1. Establish Your Goals

As with your fitness plan, this is the most important step. Without goals, any changes in behavior are likely to be temporary and yield little benefit. Writing down your goals and keeping them easily accessible (such as with sticky notes on your mirror or recorded in your phone) allows you to view them often as a reminder of what you are trying to accomplish. Remember from Chapter 1 that we encouraged the use of SMART goals: **S**pecific, **M**easureable, **A**ttainable, **R**ealistic, and **T**ime-framed. For example, if you decide to increase your physical activity by walking, a SMART goal is: "By the end of the month I will be walking 30 minutes per day, three days per week."

Step 2. Select Wellness Concepts that Are Appropriate for You

While many concepts of wellness play a part in your well-being, we have chosen the ones with the most significant potential impact on your health to discuss in upcoming chapters.

Diet In the absence of disease, diet and physical fitness are probably the most significant factors affecting your wellness. Bad dietary habits can lead to a host of negative effects such as obesity, cardiovascular disease, diabetes, and many more. Changing dietary habits can lead to significant improvements in health and wellness (see Chapters 8 and 9).

Stress Management Everyone has stress in their daily life, and it is important to learn how to cope with it to prevent long-term chronic effects (see Chapter 11).

Sexually Transmitted Infections Responsible sexual behavior requires asking questions of your potential partner, taking precautions, and educating yourself about the risks associated with sexual activity (see Chapter 14).

Addiction and Substance Abuse When a person cannot control his or her actions regarding a certain substance or behavior, he or she is addicted to that substance or action. The addiction may be to alcohol or other drugs, gambling, shopping, or video games. In contrast, substance abuse may or may not involve an addiction (see Chapter 15).

Health-Care Choices Making good decisions about managing your health care is another very important aspect of wellness. You must be a knowledgeable health-care consumer. This includes understanding your health insurance and making informed choices of health-care providers. Explore your options (see Examining the Evidence for information about potential providers and how to communicate with them).

hear it!

CASE STUDY

Should Eli pay for health care coverage? Listen to the online case study MasteringHealth™.

Step 3. Plan Your Behavior Changes

Now that you have learned the importance of setting goals and chosen the specific areas on which to focus your efforts, the next step is to plan how to change your behaviors. Two common examples of behavior change are quitting smoking and losing weight. (For guidance on behavior change, see Chapter 1. For information on quitting smoking, see Chapter 15. To learn more about a healthy diet and weight loss, see Chapters 8 and 9.)

EXAMINING THE EVIDENCE

Glossary of Medical Specialists

Everyone, regardless of age, needs a reliable health-care provider for common medical problems. Your primary care physician (PCP) will be familiar with your medical history, and you are more likely to develop a relationship that will make you more comfortable when discussing medical issues. In addition to general/family practitioners and internal medicine physicians, other medical professionals can serve as your PCP, such as nurse practitioners and OB/GYNs. Physician assistants also conduct routine tests and screenings.

In the United States, a licensed medical doctor holds either an MD (doctor of medicine) or DO (doctor of osteopathic medicine) degree. Medical specialists have received advanced training in a specific area of medicine and may be board-certified in their area of specialty. Medical specialists include those shown below:

Anesthesiologist Administers anesthesia during surgery and monitors the patient's immediate recovery following surgery.

Cardiologist Diagnoses and treats diseases of the heart and blood vessels.

Dermatologist Specializes in diagnosis and treatment of skin diseases.

Emergency room specialist Specializes in the care and treatment of trauma patients and acute illnesses.

Endocrinologist: Specializes in diseases of the endocrine system (such as diabetes, hypothyroidism, and other hormone-related conditions).

Gastroenterologist Diagnoses and treats diseases of the digestive system and liver.

Hematologist Specializes in disorders of the blood.

Internist Specializes in the nonsurgical treatment of adults. Major areas of medical interest may include heart disease, cancer, diabetes, and arthritis.

Neurologist Diagnoses and treats disorders of the brain and nervous system.

Neurosurgeon Specializes in surgical treatment of disorders of the brain and nervous system.

Obstetrician/Gynecologist An obstetrician specializes in the treatment of pregnant women and the delivery of babies. A gynecologist specializes in the treatment of the female reproductive system. Many practitioners are OB/GYNs and do both.

Oncologist Specializes in the treatment of cancer.

Orthopedist Specializes in treating injuries or diseases affecting the bones, muscles, joints, and ligaments.

Otorhinolaryngologist Specializes in diagnosis and treatment of problems in the ear, nose, and throat.

Pediatrician Specializes in the treatment of children.

Physiatrist Specializes in physical medicine and rehabilitation.

Psychiatrist Treats behavioral and mental health disorders using psychotherapy and medications. (Note that a psychologist holds an advanced degree in psychology or counseling but is not a medical doctor. Psychologists provide counseling but cannot prescribe drugs.)

Radiologist Specializes in the use of imaging technology to diagnose diseases and injuries.

Surgeon Performs surgery to diagnose and treat diseases. Surgeons specialize in specific types of procedures (such as cardiovascular, neurological, orthopedic, general, or plastic surgery).

Urologist Diagnoses and treats problems associated with the urinary tract in men and women, and in reproductive disorders in men.

Step 4. Monitor Your Progress

As with your fitness plan, a weekly log can be used to record your progress in accomplishing your behavior change goals. By doing this, you can see the obstacles you have overcome and your accomplishments. You can record your progress using a journal or a tracking app.

Tips for Success

Once you have your wellness plan in place, it's time to take action! You may find the following tips helpful as you work toward behavior change.

▪ **Start slow.** It takes some time for your body to adjust to changes. For example, if you try to lose weight too quickly by overly restricting calories, your body perceives this as starvation and your metabolism will slow to conserve energy (the opposite of the effect you want). Losing weight slowly makes it easier for you to develop new habits and allows your body to adjust and produce longer-lasting results.

▪ **Be consistent.** Small changes done consistently are more effective than making drastic changes in a short period of time.

see it!

ABC VIDEOS

Watch the "Yoga to Improve Posture at Your Desk" ABC News Video online at MasteringHealth™.

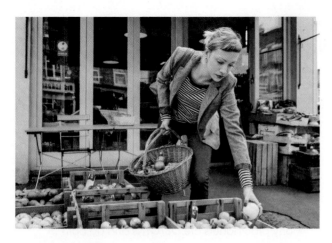

Choosing healthy foods at the grocery store will help you plan healthier meals.

- **Obtain support from friends.** If you have friends with similar behavior change goals, meeting and talking with them about their challenges and progress can be very helpful and motivating.

- **Incorporate variety into your plan.** Variety can make changes easier and even fun. For example, to distract yourself from an urge to smoke, you could go for a walk in a park or neighborhood you haven't visited before. If you like to cook, trying new recipes can be a fun part of a weight-loss plan.

- **Adapt to changing schedules.** As with your fitness plan, you need to allow for some flexibility in your schedule. How will social outings affect

your desire to smoke, drink, or eat? Anticipating special occasions or events and deciding ahead of time how you will deal with them will keep you on track.

- **Expect backsliding.** Backsliding is to be expected with any attempted behavior change. As previously discussed, don't let it get you down. Stressful situations will occur, and you may occasionally make unhealthy choices. You can see these times as learning experiences and move on.

MAKE SURE YOU **KNOW...**

- Behavior modification can be applied to many health-related behaviors, and a specific plan of action is essential in making positive changes.

- Choose to modify those aspects of wellness that are most affecting your health.

- Your goals for behavior change should be specific, measurable, attainable, realistic, and time-framed.

- Go slowly, be consistent, and incorporate variety in making changes to improve wellness and monitor your progress toward goals.

- Friends with similar goals can serve as a helpful support system.

- Backsliding can serve as a learning opportunity to help plan for future challenges.

MasteringHealth™

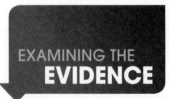

EXAMINING THE
EVIDENCE

Communicating Effectively with Your Health-Care Provider

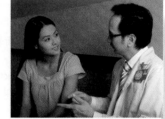

The relationship between patient and health-care provider plays an important role in the quality and effectiveness of medical care. Here are some guidelines for effective communication:

- Prepare for your appointment in advance. Studies show that 70% of correct medical diagnoses depend on what you tell the medical professional about your symptoms (17). Prior to your visit, write down a list of symptoms and concerns. Try not to leave anything out of your list, even if you think it seems minor.

- Make a list of all medications and supplements you are taking, and bring the list to your appointment. Include over-the-counter medications, supplements, and herbal treatments. You might think they are not important, but they can have side effects and can interact with medications.

- No question is a dumb question. Write out a list of questions before your appointment, and feel free to ask them. Let your provider know if you do not understand the answers or any other information you are given. If you are unclear about any part of your diagnosis and treatment options, ask for further explanation. If a provider dismisses your questions or acts as if they are not important, you may want to consider finding another doctor.

- If you want to know more about your condition, ask your doctor to recommend resources for additional information. Prior to leaving the doctor's office, make certain that you understand the next steps for your treatment (such as filling a prescription, a follow-up visit, or more tests).

Sample Programs for Fitness

Scan to plan your individualized program for fitness.

The following sample programs will help you plan your weekly exercise routine. Remember to choose a variety of activities you enjoy, and incorporate activities for enhanced cardiorespiratory endurance, muscular strength, and flexibility. Three sample plans follow: Beginner, Intermediate (someone who has completed 6–20 weeks of training), and Advanced (someone who has completed at least 20 weeks of training). Each includes an

option for a conventional workout and a second plan using HIIT. Refer to these samples as you plan your program in Laboratory 7.4.

It is very important to maintain an active lifestyle as we get older. Exercise recommendations for healthy older adults are not much different than those for young and middle-aged adults. One addition for older adults is the inclusion of exercises to improve balance and neuromuscular control. A sample program for healthy older adults is included.

Beginner Exercise Program (1–5 weeks of training)

This sample exercise program is designed for a beginner who is planning a weekly exercise routine. Before each exercise routine, warm up by performing 5–10 minutes of calisthenics or brisk walking. Cool down by engaging in 5–15 minutes of low-intensity exercise.

BEGINNER EXERCISE PROGRAM (1–5 weeks of training)

A - Conventional Training Plan

Activity	Mon	Tue	Wed	Thur	Fri	Sat
Cardiorespiratory	10–20 min walking, running, swimming, cycling		10–20 min walking, running, swimming, cycling		10–20 min walking, running, swimming, cycling	
Weight Training	1 set/15 reps/ 3 upper body and 3 lower body exercises		1 set/15 reps/ 3 upper body and 3 lower body exercises		1 set/15 reps/ 3 upper body and 3 lower body exercises	
Stretching		2 reps/15 sec each		2 reps/15 sec each		2 reps/15 sec each

B - HIIT Plan

Activity	Mon	Tue	Wed	Thur	Fri	Sat
Cardiorespiratory Intervals	Running or cycling 5 @ 60 sec (20 sec between at slow jog)		Running or cycling 5 @ 60 sec (20 sec between at slow jog)		Running or cycling 5 @ 60 sec (20 sec between at slow jog)	
Weight Training Intervals	1 set (10–15 rep max wt. to failure) 3 upper & 3 lower body exercises		1 set (10–15 rep max wt. to failure) 3 upper & 3 lower body exercises		1 set (10–15 rep max wt. to failure) 3 upper & 3 lower body exercises	
Stretching		2 reps/15 sec each		2 reps/15 sec each		2 reps/15 sec each

Intermediate Exercise Program (6–20 weeks of training)

This sample exercise program is designed for someone planning a weekly exercise routine who has completed at least 5 weeks of prior training. Before each exercise routine, warm up by performing 5–15 minutes of calisthenics or brisk walking. Cool down by engaging in 5–15 minutes of low-intensity exercise.

INTERMEDIATE EXERCISE PROGRAM (6–20 weeks of training)

A - Conventional Training Plan

Activity	Mon	Tue	Wed	Thur	Fri	Sat
Cardiorespiratory	20–40 min walking, running, swimming, cycling		20–40 min walking, running, swimming, cycling		20–40 min walking, running, swimming, cycling	20–40 min walking, running, swimming, cycling
Weight Training	2 sets/15 reps/ 3 upper body and 3 lower body exercises		2 sets/15 reps/ 3 upper body and 3 lower body exercises		2 sets/15 reps/ 3 upper body and 3 lower body exercises	2 sets/15 reps/ 3 upper body and 3 lower body exercises
Stretching		2 reps/15 sec each		2 reps/15 sec each		2 reps/15 sec each

B - HIIT Plan

Activity	Mon	Tue	Wed	Thur	Fri	Sat
Cardiorespiratory Intervals	Running or cycling 5 @ 60 sec (20 sec between at slow jog)		Running or cycling 5 @ 60 sec (20 sec between at slow jog)		Running or cycling 5 @ 60 sec (20 sec between at slow jog)	Running or cycling 5 @ 60 sec (20 sec between at slow jog)
Weight Training Intervals	2 sets (10–15 rep max wt. to failure) 3 upper & 3 lower body exercises		2 sets (10–15 rep max wt. to failure) 3 upper & 3 lower body exercises		2 sets (10–15 rep max wt. to failure) 3 upper & 3 lower body exercises	2 sets (10–15 rep max wt. to failure) 3 upper & 3 lower body exercises
Stretching	2 reps/15 sec each	2 reps/15 sec each		2 reps/15 sec each		2 reps/15 sec each

Advanced Exercise Program (20+ weeks of training)

This sample exercise program is designed for someone planning a weekly exercise routine who has completed at least 20 weeks of training. Before each exercise routine, warm up by performing 5–15 minutes of calisthenics or brisk walking. Cool down by engaging in 5–15 minutes of low-intensity exercise.

ADVANCED EXERCISE PROGRAM (20+ weeks of training)

A - Conventional Training Plan						
Activity	**Mon**	**Tue**	**Wed**	**Thur**	**Fri**	**Sat**
Cardiorespiratory	20–40 min walking, running, swimming, cycling	20–40 min walking, running, swimming, cycling	20–40 min walking, running, swimming, cycling	20–40 min walking, running, swimming, cycling	20–40 min walking, running, swimming, cycling	
Weight Training	3 sets/8 reps/ 6 upper body and 3 lower body exercises	3 sets/8 reps/ 6 upper body and 3 lower body exercises	3 sets/8 reps/ 6 upper body and 3 lower body exercises	3 sets/8 reps/ 6 upper body and 3 lower body exercises	3 sets/8 reps/ 6 upper body and 3 lower body exercises	
Stretching	3 reps/15 sec each	3 reps/15 sec each	3 reps/15 sec each	3 reps/15 sec each	3 reps/15 sec each	

B - HIIT Plan						
Activity	**Mon**	**Tue**	**Wed**	**Thur**	**Fri**	**Sat**
Cardiorespiratory Intervals	Running or cycling 10 @ 30 sec (30 sec between at slow jog)	Running or cycling 5 @ 60 sec (20 sec between at slow jog)	Running or cycling 12 @ 20 sec (40 sec between at slow jog)	Running or cycling 5 @ 60 sec (20 sec between at slow jog)	Running or cycling 8 @ 40 sec (30 sec between at slow jog)	
Weight Training Intervals	3 sets (10–15 rep max wt. to failure) 6 upper body exercises	3 sets (10–15 rep max wt. to failure) 6 lower body exercises	3 sets (10–15 rep max wt. to failure) 6 upper body exercises	3 sets (10–15 rep max wt. to failure) 6 lower body exercises	3 sets (10–15 rep max wt. to failure) 3 upper & 3 lower body exercises	
Stretching	3 reps/15 sec each	3 reps/15 sec each	3 reps/15 sec each	3 reps/15 sec each	3 reps/15 sec each	

Exercise Program for Healthy Older Adults

Below is a weekly exercise program for healthy older adults. Before each workout, warm up by performing 5–10 minutes of low-intensity activity, such as walking or riding a stationary cycle. Light stretching can be included in the warm-up. Cool down by engaging in 5 minutes of low-intensity activity.

Aerobic exercise should be at a moderate intensity. Moderate intensity is a 5–6 on a 0–10 point scale, with 0 being no effort and 10 being maximal effort. Moderate intensity using the talk test means you can engage in an intermittent conversation while exercising, but you are breathing harder than normal and your heart rate is slightly elevated.

Resistance exercises can include balance and stability exercises.

	Activity	Monday	Tuesday	Wed	Thursday	Friday	Saturday	Sun
Week 1	**Aerobic**	10–15 min			10–15 min		10–15 min	
	Resistance		2 sets/8–12 reps (1 set each for lower and upper body)			2 sets/8–12 reps (1 set each for lower and upper body)		
	Stretching	1–2 reps/ 15–20 sec each	1–2 reps/ 15–20 sec each		1–2 reps/15–20 sec each	1–2 reps/15–20 sec each	1–2 reps/15–20 sec each	

	Activity	Monday	Tuesday	Wed	Thursday	Friday	Saturday	Sun
Week 2	**Aerobic**	10–15 min			10–15 min		10–15 min	
	Resistance		2 sets/8–12 reps (1 set each for lower and upper body)			2 sets/8–12 reps (1 set each for lower and upper body)		
	Stretching	1–2 reps/ 15–20 sec each	1–2 reps/ 15–20 sec each		1–2 reps/ 15–20 sec each	1–2 reps/ 15–20 sec each	1–2 reps/ 15–20 sec each	
Week 3	**Aerobic**	15–20 min			15–20 min		15–20 min	
	Resistance		2 sets/8–12 reps (1 set each for lower and upper body)			2 sets/8–12 reps (1 set each for lower and upper body)		
	Stretching	1–2 reps/ 15–20 sec each	1–2 reps/ 15–20 sec each		1–2 reps/ 15–20 sec each	1–2 reps/ 15–20 sec each	1–2 reps/ 15–20 sec each	
Week 4	**Aerobic**	15–20 min			15–20 min		15–20 min	
	Resistance		2 sets/8–12 reps (1 set each for lower and upper body)			2 sets/8–12 reps (1 set each for lower and upper body)		
	Stretching	1–2 reps/ 15–20 sec each	1–2 reps/ 15–20 sec each		1–2 reps/ 15–20 sec each	1–2 reps/ 15–20 sec each	1–2 reps/ 15–20 sec each	
Week 5	**Aerobic**	20–25 min			20–25 min		20–25 min	
	Resistance		2 sets/8–12 reps (1 set each for lower and upper body)			2 sets/8–12 reps (1 set each for lower and upper body)		
	Stretching	2–3 reps/ 15–30 sec each	2–3 reps/ 15–30 sec each		2–3 reps/ 15–30 sec each	2–3 reps/ 15–30 sec each	2–3 reps/ 15–30 sec each	
Week 6	**Aerobic**	20–25 min			20–25 min		20–25 min	
	Resistance		2 sets/8–12 reps (1 set each for lower and upper body)			2 sets/8–12 reps (1 set each for lower and upper body)		
	Stretching	2–3 reps/ 15–30 sec each	2–3 reps/ 15–30 sec each		2–3 reps/ 15–30 sec each	2–3 reps/ 15–30 sec each	2–3 reps/ 15–30 sec each	
Week 7	**Aerobic**	25–30 min			25–30 min		25–30 min	
	Resistance		2 sets/8–12 reps (1 set each for lower and upper body)			2 sets/8–12 reps (1 set each for lower and upper body)		
	Stretching	2–4 reps/ 15–30 sec each	2–4 reps/ 15–30 sec each		2–4 reps/ 15–30 sec each	2–4 reps/ 15–30 sec each	2–4 reps/ 15–30 sec each	
Week 8	**Aerobic**	30 min			30 min		30 min	
	Resistance		2 sets/8–12 reps (1 set each for lower and upper body)			2 sets/8–12 reps (1 set each for lower and upper body)		
	Stretching	2–4 reps/ 15–30 sec each	2–4 reps/ 15–30 sec each		2–4 reps/ 15–30 sec each	2–4 reps/ 15–30 sec each	2–4 reps/ 15–30 sec each	

study plan

Customize your study plan—and master your health!—in the Study Area of **MasteringHealth.**

summary

 hear it! STUDY REVIEW

To hear an MP3 Chapter Summary, scan here or visit the Study Area in MasteringHealth™.

LO **1** ■ The four steps in building a personal fitness plan are to establish your goals, select your activities, plan your weekly routine, and monitor your progress.

■ A well-designed fitness program includes activities to improve cardiorespiratory fitness, muscular strength and endurance, and flexibility. The FITT principle provides a useful tool in planning your weekly fitness routine.

LO **2** ■ A realistic fitness program includes a variety of activities that you enjoy.

■ Strength training should involve alternating days or muscle groups (to avoid overtraining) and stretching exercises should be performed at least 2 days per week.

LO **3** ■ Your fitness action plan should be based on these guidelines: Adopt a gradual, consistent approach to exercise; exercise with friends (if you find it helpful); vary your activities and routine; get enough sleep; adapt to changing schedules; anticipate lapses; and combine exercise with other healthy behaviors.

LO **4** ■ Aging and other life changes will require adjustments in your fitness program.

■ Since rates of physical activity decrease with age, you should find activities that you can maintain as lifetime activities.

LO **5** ■ Approximately 30 minutes of exercise at a moderate intensity (RPE 12–14) is safe for healthy, pregnant women who are not experiencing complications. Pregnant women should avoid activities that require lying down or that put them at risk for trauma to the fetus.

LO **6** ■ Exercise is especially important in maintaining good health in people with disabilities.

■ There are two categories of sports for people with disabilities: adapted (adaptive) and inclusive.

LO **7** ■ Aging is a slow, gradual decline in biological functions that results in decreased cardiorespiratory function, increased body fat, and musculoskeletal fragility.

■ About one-half of the decline in functional capacity related to aging is due to a decrease in physical activity. If activity is maintained throughout life, a great deal of functional capacity can be retained.

LO **8** ■ Make sure your goals fitness goals are SMART: Specific, Measureable, Attainable, Realistic, and Time-framed.

■ Prioritize your goals. Focus first on changing behaviors that are placing your health most at risk.

■ Go slowly, be consistent, and monitor your progress toward goals.

study questions

review it! QUIZZES

Find more review questions online at MasteringHealth™.

LO **1** 1. The first and most important step in establishing a personal fitness plan is
a. selecting your activities.
b. creating a training log.
c. establishing goals.
d. planning your weekly fitness routine.

2. Most health benefits will occur with how many minutes of exercise per week?
a. 50–75
b. 80–100
c. 120–150
d. 200–250

3. Exercise training to improve muscular strength should be performed
a. 2–3 days per week.
b. 4–5 days per week.
c. 5–6 days per week.
d. 6–7 days per week.

4. List the four steps to developing a personal fitness plan.

5. Name the three major types of fitness goals and provide an example of each type.

6. What are the components of the FITT principle, and how do these apply to planning your weekly fitness routine?

LO ② 7. Why is it important to take your current fitness level into account when developing your exercise plan?

8. At a minimum, stretching should be performed at least
    a. 1 day per week.
    b. 2 days per week.
    c. 3 days per week.
    d. 4 days per week.

LO ③ 9. Explain why a gradual approach is the best way to implement an exercise program, especially for those who have not exercised regularly in the past.

LO ④ 10. Outline the key factors that play a role in maintaining a regular program of exercise over the lifespan.

LO ⑤ 11. Which is not a recommended exercise for pregnant women?
    a. water aerobics
    b. abdominal toning class performed on the floor
    c. walking on a treadmill
    d. light- or moderate-intensity resistance training

LO ⑥ 12. Name the two classes of sports for people with disabilities and explain how they differ.

LO ⑦ 13. Which of the following is not a change experienced during the aging process?
    a. decline in maximal heart rate
    b. decline in cardiorespiratory fitness
    c. decrease in muscle mass
    d. all of the above are changes that occur with aging

14. List three activities that are considered to be beneficial in promoting cardiorespiratory fitness for older individuals.

LO ⑧ 15. List the four steps to developing a wellness plan.

16. Your wellness action plan should
    a. begin quickly and progress as fast as you can.
    b. not include friends and family.
    c. not incorporate variety in your actions.
    d. adapt to changing schedules.

17. One aspect of being an informed health-care consumer is understanding
    a. the medical use of drugs.
    b. your health insurance.
    c. how foods are metabolized in the body.
    d. how to rid your life of stress.

suggested reading

Baechle, T., and R. Earle. *Essentials of Strength Training and Conditioning*. Champaign, IL: Human Kinetics, 2008.

Byrd, N. What gets measured is more likely to get done. *ACSM's Health and Fitness Journal* 15:26–29, 2011.

Donatelle, R. J. *My Health: An Outcomes Approach*. San Francisco: Benjamin Cummings, 2013.

Fieger, H. *Behavior Change*. New York: Morgan James, 2009.

Howley, E., and D. Thompson. *Fitness Professional's Handbook*. Champaign, IL: Human Kinetics, 2012.

Mayo Clinic Family Health Book, 4th ed. New York: Time, Inc. Home Entertainment, 2009.

Nieman, D. *Exercise Testing and Prescription*, 6th ed. St. Louis: McGraw-Hill, 2007.

Owen, N., P. Sparling, G. Healy, D. Dunstan, and C. Matthews. Sedentary behavior: Emerging evidence for a new health risk. *Mayo Clinic Proceedings* 85(12): 1138–1141.

Pate, R. Overcoming barriers to physical activity: Helping youth be more active. *ACSM's Health and Fitness Journal* 15:7–12, 2011.

Powers, S., and E. Howley. *Exercise Physiology: Theory and Application to Fitness and Performance*, 8th ed. New York: McGraw Hill, 2012.

Shumaker, S. A., J. K. Ockene, and K. A. Riekert. *The Handbook of Health Behavior Change*, 3rd ed. New York: Springer, 2008.

Turner, S. L., A. M. Thomas, and P. J. Wagner. A collaborative approach to wellness: Diet, exercise, and education to impact behavior change. *Journal of the American Academy of Nurse Practitioners* 20(6):339–344, 2008.

Volpe, S. L. Can dogs help with maintaining motivation? *ACSM's Health and Fitness Journal* 15:36–37, 2011.

Williamson, P. *Exercise for Special Populations*. Philadelphia: Lippincott Williams and Wilkins, 2011.

helpful weblinks

do it! WEBLINKS

For links to the organizations and websites listed, visit MasteringHealth™.

American College of Sports Medicine

Contains information about aging, exercise, health, and fitness. **www.acsm.org**

American Council on Exercise

Provides information on a variety of topics related to exercise and fitness. **www.acefitness.org**

Association for Applied Sport Psychology

Contains a wealth of information about goal-setting and adherence to exercise programs. **www.appliedsportpsych.org**

Behavior Change/Lifestyle Management Programs

University of California–Riverside provides programs and behavior change direction. **http://wellness.ucr.edu /behavior_change_programs.html**

Fit Pregnancy

Provides expert information for moms-to-be on prenatal nutrition and exercise. **www.fitpregnancy.com**

Guide to Behavior Change

National Heart, Lung, and Blood Institute's guide to changing behavior to improve heart health. **www.nhlbi.nih .gov/health/public/heart/obesity/lose_wt/behavior.htm**

Mayo Clinic

Contains information about a wide variety of diseases and medical issues. Also a good source for information about aging, nutrition, and choosing health-care providers. **www .mayoclinic.org**

National Center on Health, Physical Activity and Disability

Resource center on health promotion for people with disability. Includes information on physical and social activities, including fitness and aquatic activities, recreational and sports programs, adaptive equipment usage, and more. **www.nchpad.org/**

President's Council on Physical Fitness and Sports

Provides information concerning a wide range of subjects related to exercise and fitness. **www.fitness.gov**

WebMD

Information on a variety of health-related topics, including diet, exercise, and stress. **www.webmd.com**

laboratory 7.1

do it! LABS
Complete Lab 7.1 online in the
study area of **MasteringHealth.com**

Name _____ Date _____

Developing SMART Goals

SMART goals help promote achievement and success. A SMART goal defines what is expected and what measures are used to determine when the goal is achieved. A SMART goal is:

Specific: The goal should clearly state what you want to accomplish.

Measurable: The goal should be verifiable or measurable. How will you measure and evaluate your progress?

Attainable: The goal should be attainable and action-oriented (something that you can achieve).

Realistic: The goal should be reasonable for you. Certainly the goals should stretch or challenge your abilities, but they must be realistic in light of your circumstances and physical condition.

Time-framed: The goal should have a time frame, a set date by which you will achieve it. SMART goals can be short- or long-term.

Examples:

Not a SMART Goal	SMART Goal
I will lose weight.	By the end of April I will lose 5 pounds by walking 1 mile a day, 5 days a week.
I will go to the gym.	During the next 30 days I will increase my strength by weight training at the gym 3 days per week, 1 hour per day.

YOUR TURN:

Step 1: In the space below, write a behavior change goal you would like to accomplish.

_____

_____

_____

Step 2: Based on the above goal, answer the following questions:

1. **S**pecific: What are you going to do? How will it be accomplished? Why is it important?

_____

_____

_____

2. **M**easurable: How much, how often, how many? What will you measure to determine when your goal has been met? List at least two measurable indicators. These will help you monitor your progress.

_____

_____

3. **A**ttainable: What action is required to make the change you desire?

_____

_____

4. **R**ealistic: Do you have the necessary knowledge, skills, abilities, and resources to accomplish the goal, or do you need to modify it? Will meeting the goal challenge but not defeat you?

_____

_____

5. **T**ime-framed: How long will it take? When will you start and finish? The time frame for a short-term goal should be short enough to cause urgency, such as "I will start in 2 days and achieve my goal within 30 days." Unreasonably long time frames such as "Within the next two months I will ..." are less likely to motivate behavior change.

_____

_____

Use your responses to the previous questions and refine your initial goal into a more complete SMART goal.

_____

_____

_____

_____

_____

laboratory 7.2

do it! LABS
Complete Lab 7.2 online in the
study area of **MasteringHealth.com**

Name _____   Date _____

Personal Fitness Program Contract and Short-Term Fitness Goals

I, _____ (signature), am making a commitment to follow my personal fitness plan and achieve my established short-term goals.

My program will begin on _____ (date).

My short-term goals:

a. Performance goals:

_____

_____

_____

_____

b. Body composition goals:

_____

_____

_____

_____

c. Adherence goals:

_____

_____

_____

_____

Upon achievement of my goals, I will reward myself as follows:

a. _____ (goal #1) _____ (date) _____ (reward)

b. _____ (goal #2) _____ (date) _____ (reward)

c. _____ (goal #3) _____ (date) _____ (reward)

laboratory 7.3

do it! LABS
Complete Lab 7.3 online in the
study area of **MasteringHealth.com**

Name _____ Date _____

Personal Fitness Program Contract and Intermediate/Long-Term Fitness Goals

I, _____ (signature), am making a commitment to follow my personal fitness plan and achieve my established intermediate and long-term goals.

My intermediate goals:

a. Performance goals:

_____
_____
_____
_____

b. Body composition goals:

_____
_____
_____
_____

c. Adherence goals:

_____
_____
_____
_____

My long-term goals:

a. Performance goals:

_____
_____
_____
_____

b. Body composition goals:

_____
_____
_____
_____

c. Adherence goals:

_____
_____
_____
_____

Upon achievement of my intermediate goals, I will reward myself as follows:

a. _____ (goal #1) _____ (date) _____ (reward)

b. _____ (goal #2) _____ (date) _____ (reward)

c. _____ (goal #3) _____ (date) _____ (reward)

Upon achievement of my long-term goals, I will reward myself as follows:

a. _____ (goal #1) _____ (date) _____ (reward)

b. _____ (goal #2) _____ (date) _____ (reward)

c. _____ (goal #3) _____ (date) _____ (reward)

laboratory 7.4

do it! LABS
Complete Lab 7.4 online in the
study area of **MasteringHealth.com**

Name _____   Date _____

Planning a Personal Fitness Program

Use this lab to plan your personal fitness program. Record the appropriate information in the spaces provided below.

Activity	Intensity*	Duration (min/day)	Monday	Tuesday	Wednesday	Thursday	Friday	Saturday	Sunday
Cardiorespiratory endurance exercise									
Muscular strength/ endurance exercise									
Stretching exercises to improve flexibility									

*Establish intensity for your cardiorespiratory endurance exercise using heart rate or RPE (see Chapter 3)

8

Nutrition, Health, and Fitness

LEARNING OUTCOMES

1 Define the terms *nutrition* and *nutrient* and explain how nutrients are classified.

2 Describe the function of the four macronutrients in the body and list common dietary sources for each.

3 Explain what micronutrients are, which substances compose them, and why they are so important for health.

4 Outline the guidelines for a healthy diet.

5 List several resources that can be helpful in planning a healthy diet.

6 Explain why children, pregnant women, vegetarians, and those with food allergies or intolerances have special dietary needs and how these needs can be addressed.

7 Describe how rigorous exercise training alters a person's nutrition requirements.

8 List the pros and cons of dietary supplement use.

9 Describe the major issues of food safety and how changes in food technology affect the food we consume.

DIET IS A KEY FACTOR in achieving and maintaining wellness. A poor diet coupled with a sedentary lifestyle increases a person's risk for cardiovascular disease, stroke, hypertension, diabetes, and cancer (1). Together, these diseases contribute to more than 61% of all deaths in North America! In this chapter, you will learn about the importance of a healthy diet and how your body uses the food you eat. We'll discuss the classes of nutrients and their functions, the fundamental concepts of good nutrition, and guidelines for a healthy diet. We also explore how exercise training can modify nutritional requirements.

What Is Nutrition and Why Is It Important?

LO **1** Define the terms *nutrition* and *nutrient* and explain how nutrients are classified.

Nutrition is the study of food and nutrients—their digestion, absorption, metabolism, and their effect on health and disease. *Good nutrition* refers to a diet that supplies all of the essential nutrients required for the body to survive and thrive.

Nutrients are substances in food that provide nourishment; they are needed to support body function and maintain health. They serve three major functions in the body: providing energy, supporting growth and development, and regulating metabolism. Nutrients are categorized into two major groups, macronutrients and micronutrients (**FIGURE 8.1**).

Consuming too much or too little of any of the essential nutrients can lead to health problems. In the 19th and early 20th centuries, nutrient deficiencies were a major health problem. For example, inadequate vitamin C intake leads to scurvy, and insufficient iron intake results in anemia—both conditions were once prevalent among much of the world's population. Although these dietary deficiencies still exist today in some regions of the world, excess consumption of calories, leading to high levels of

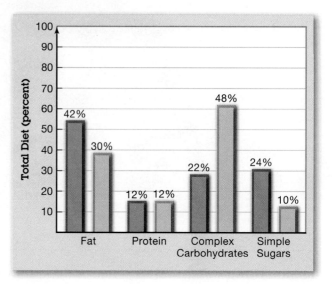

Key

▭ Typical Diet

▭ Recommended Diet

FIGURE 8.2 The recommended nutritionally balanced diet compared with the typical U.S. diet. The average American consumes too much fat and simple sugars and too few complex carbohydrates.
Source: Block, G. Junk foods account for 30% of caloric intake. *Journal of Food Composition and Analysis* 17:439–447, 2004.

body fat, is the current cause of most nutritionally linked health problems in the United States (**FIGURE 8.2**).

Diets high in calories, sugar, fat, and/or sodium increase the risk of health problems such as cardiovascular disease, cancer, obesity, and diabetes, which are the leading killers in the United States (1). In fact, over half of all U.S. deaths are associated with health problems related to poor nutrition (2). The good news is that by analyzing and modifying your diet, you can reduce your risk for these diseases and improve your quality of life. This is why a basic understanding of nutrition is important for everyone.

MAKE SURE YOU **KNOW...**

- Nutrition is the science of food and nutrients—their digestion, absorption, and metabolism and their effect on health and disease.

- Nutrients are the substances in foods that are required to support body function and maintain health.

MasteringHealth™

Macronutrients

LO **2** Describe the function of the four macronutrients in the body and list common dietary sources for each.

Nutrients that are required in relatively large amounts (more than a few grams per day) are **macronutrients**; this category includes carbohydrates, proteins, fats, and

---

Macronutrients
(present in large quantities)

Carbohydrates
Fat
Protein
Water

Micronutrients
(present in very small amounts)

Vitamins
Minerals

FIGURE 8.1 Types of nutrients in the human diet.

TABLE 8.1 ■ Food Sources of Macronutrients		
Carbohydrate (4 calories/gram)	Protein (4 calories/gram)	Fat (9 calories/gram)
Vegetables	Meat/Poultry	Butter
Fruits	Seafood	Oils
Grains and grain products	Eggs	Diary products (e.g., cheese)
Legumes (includes beans, peas, and peanuts)	Beans and peas	Animal fat (e.g., fatty red meats and pork)
Milk and dairy products	Nuts and seeds	Coconut
Foods containing sugar	Milk and dairy products	Margarine and shortening

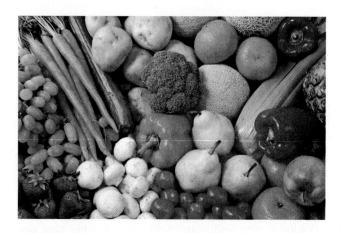

water. **TABLE 8.1** lists some of the major food sources of carbohydrates, proteins, and fats.

A major function of macronutrients is to provide energy for the body. Carbohydrates and fats provide the bulk of the energy required by your cells for normal function. Although proteins can also be used as fuel, their contribution to energy is small. The energy contained in foods is measured in **kilocalories** (commonly called *Calories* when referring to food energy). Carbohydrate and protein provide 4 calories per gram, and fat provides 9 calories per gram. The primary function of protein is to support growth and development of body tissues. Proteins serve as the building blocks for all cells.

Metabolism is defined as the sum total of all of the chemical events that occur in cells. This includes the process of converting the nutrients in food into usable energy and the breakdown and rebuilding of cellular proteins.

Carbohydrates

Carbohydrates exist in two forms, simple and complex, and serve several functions in the body. Simple carbohydrates are a primary source of energy during exercise. Moreover, your brain requires simple carbohydrates for normal function. Some complex carbohydrates (e.g., starch) can be used for energy. Others, such as fiber, serve different but important purposes.

Simple Carbohydrates Simple carbohydrates consist of chains of one or two simple sugars. Common simple sugars are glucose, fructose, and galactose. **Glucose** is a key simple sugar because it plays a major role as an energy source for the body. Glucose is stored in skeletal muscles and the liver as a complex carbohydrate called **glycogen**. However, to be used for fuel, glycogen must be broken down into glucose. When glucose is consumed in the diet, the amount not immediately used for energy or stored as glycogen will be stored as fat. On the other

hand, if you don't consume sufficient carbohydrates in food, your body will make glucose from protein. This is undesirable because it often results in the breakdown of body tissues such as muscle to provide the proteins for use as fuel. Therefore, dietary carbohydrates are important not only as a direct fuel source but also for their protein-sparing effect.

Complex Carbohydrates **Complex carbohydrates** exist in several forms and include glycogen, starches, and fiber. As noted previously, glycogen is the storage form of glucose; it is not consumed in the diet. Starches and fiber are found in the diet. **Starches** are long chains of glucose units that are the storage form of carbohydrates in plants.

nutrition The study of nutrients–their digestion, absorption, and metabolism and their effect on health and disease.

nutrients Substances in food that are necessary for survival and health.

macronutrients Carbohydrates, fats, proteins, and water; necessary for building and maintaining body tissues and providing energy.

kilocalorie Unit of measure used to quantify food energy or the energy expended by the body. Technically, the kilocalorie is the amount of energy necessary to raise the temperature of 1 kilogram of water 1°C. A kilocalorie is often called a *Calorie*.

carbohydrate Macronutrient that is a key energy source.

glucose A simple carbohydrate (sugar) that can be used as fuel.

glycogen Storage form of glucose; stored in the liver and skeletal muscles.

complex carbohydrates Long chains of sugar units linked together to form glycogen, starch, or fiber.

starches Long chains of glucose units; found in foods such as corn, grains, and potatoes.

Fiber is an undigestible carbohydrate found in plants. Because fiber is not digestible, it is not a fuel source but plays an important role in human health.

Dietary fiber provides bulk in the intestinal tract. This bulk aids in the formation and elimination of waste products, thus reducing the time necessary for waste to move through the digestive system. Importantly, adequate dietary fiber intake decreases the risk for colon cancer, cardiovascular disease, and type 2 diabetes by reducing the digestion and absorption of selected macronutrients and decreasing the contact time of cancer-causing agents (carcinogens) within the digestive system (3).

Broadly, there are two classifications of dietary fiber: 1) soluble fiber and 2) insoluble fiber. **Soluble fiber** dissolves in water; insoluble fiber does not. Soluble fiber is found in legumes, oats, psyllium, flaxseeds, and certain fruits and vegetables. Because soluble fiber attracts water and forms a gel, it delays stomach emptying, which makes you feel full. This effect may reduce appetite and assist with weight control. Slower stomach emptying may slow glucose absorption (helpful in managing diabetes) and also helps to lower blood cholesterol by interfering with cholesterol absorption.

Insoluble fiber adds bulk and passes through the gastrointestinal tract largely intact. This speeds up transit time, helping to maintain regularity of bowel movements and reducing the risk of colon cancer (3). Insoluble fiber is found in whole grains, nuts, seeds, and certain vegetables and fruits.

The recommended fiber intake is 25 to 38 grams per day for most people. High fiber intake can cause intestinal discomfort. However, excessive fiber intake does not appear to be a problem in the United States, as studies reveal that most Americans do not consume the recommended amounts (3). Your best bet for getting adequate dietary fiber is to eat sufficient amounts of vegetables and fruits (including the skin, when edible) every day. Individuals who can tolerate whole grains and legumes can include these as well. As you increase your fiber intake, be sure to drink plenty of water to prevent constipation.

see it!

ABC VIDEOS

Watch the "Grain Labels Do Not Reflect 'Whole' Truth" ABC News Video online at MasteringHealth™.

Carbohydrates in Foods The healthiest sources of carbohydrates are whole foods such as vegetables and fruits (see Table 8.1). Starch is plentiful in potatoes, corn, bread, and rice, and fiber is found in all plant-derived foods. Simple sugars found in foods include fructose, galactose, lactose, maltose, and sucrose. Fructose is found primarily in fruit, galactose and lactose are found in milk and dairy products, and maltose is found in some grains.

Sucrose, commonly known as table sugar, is present in a vast number of processed foods (not just in candy and other sweet foods).

Fats and Lipids

Although the terms *fats* and *lipids* are often used interchangeably, they are not the same. **Lipids** are a class of compounds that do not readily dissolve in water; these include fats, oils, and waxes. **Fats** are the most common types of lipids found in foods and in your body. Fat molecules contain the same structural elements as carbohydrates (carbon, hydrogen, and oxygen), but fats contain less oxygen.

Fats and lipids exist in several forms, and each type plays a different functional role in the body. For example, fats can be an important fuel source, and storage of this type of fat occurs in fat cells. Other types of fats and lipids play key structural roles in cells, and certain lipids form parts of important hormones such as cortisol, estrogen, and testosterone.

Types of Fats Several types of fats exist. The basic structure of most fats is the fatty acid. A **fatty acid** consists of a small chain of carbon, hydrogen, and a few oxygen atoms. The body stores fatty acids in fat cells as triglycerides. **Triglycerides** are composed of three fatty acids attached to a glycerol backbone. When the body needs fat as an energy source, triglycerides are broken down and fatty acids are released into the bloodstream. Circulating fatty acids can then be taken up into cells and used as fuel.

The structure of fatty acids provides the basis for the classification of fats and two major categories of fats exist: 1) saturated and 2) unsaturated. Fatty acids with no double bonds (connections) between carbon atoms are *saturated* fatty acids. Fatty acids with one or more double bonds are *unsaturated* fatty acids.

Unsaturated fatty acids include monounsaturated and polyunsaturated fatty acids. These fats are found in plants (including nuts, seeds, grains, and vegetable oils) and are liquid at room temperature. Unsaturated fats are deemed more heart-healthy because they do not increase blood cholesterol levels.

In fact, consumption of both monounsaturated and polyunsaturated fats has been shown to lower LDL ("bad") cholesterol and reduce the risk of heart disease. In particular, one polyunsaturated fatty acid, **omega-3 fatty acid**, has been reported to lower blood levels of both cholesterol and triglycerides. This fatty acid is found primarily in fish, especially mackerel, herring, sardines, tuna, and salmon. Because of this cholesterol-lowering effect, researchers have recommended one or two servings per week of fish containing omega-3 fatty acids to reduce the risk of heart disease (5). However, there is some concern about mercury content in certain types of fish, so consumers need to know how to choose high-quality, safe seafood (see the Consumer Corner box on page 215).

To maintain health, you must obtain two polyunsaturated fatty acids (linoleic acid and alpha-linoleic

How Do You Choose the Best and Safest Fish?

Seafood can be an important part of a healthy diet. Fish is low in fat and a great source of high-quality protein and other nutrients. However, some fish may contain toxins, particularly mercury, which can harm the nervous system and kidneys and cause birth defects in a developing fetus. Consumers need to know which types of fish carry the highest risk of containing methylmercury to be able to make safer, healthier choices.

Methylmercury, a toxin produced from inorganic mercury, enters waterways as runoff after the burning of wastes and fossil fuels. It enters the food chain when fish and other aquatic organisms acquire it from the water. When larger fish eat smaller fish, the methylmercury from the smaller fish accumulates in the larger fish's body. Thus older, larger fish have higher concentrations of methylmercury than smaller, younger fish. Some of the highest levels of methylmercury are found in large predatory fish, such as shark, swordfish, king mackerel, and tilefish, so it is best to avoid these species. However, eating less than 12 ounces per week of other species, such as certain wild-caught and farmed varieties, can safely provide protein, omega-3 fatty acid, and other nutrients.

An excellent source of information on safe seafood can be found at www.seafoodwatch.org. This resource (and free downloadable app) is sponsored by the Monterey Bay Aquarium's Seafood Watch program. This research-based program identifies seafood that has been caught or farmed responsibly and that provides significant health benefits.

Also, the U.S. Environmental Protection Agency (EPA) offers guidance on fish from local lakes and streams at http://water.epa.gov/scitech/swguidance/fishshellfish/fishadvisories. State and local health departments can also provide information.

---

acid) from your diet. These fatty acids are called essential fatty acids, and failure to consume adequate amounts can result in health problems that include itchy skin, diarrhea, and delayed wound healing.

Saturated fatty acids are solid at room temperature. These fatty acids are found in both animal (meat and dairy) and plant (coconut and palm oil) sources. Diets high in saturated fatty acids have been shown to increase blood levels of total cholesterol and LDL cholesterol, which can lead to heart disease (see Chapter 10).

Some food production processes convert unsaturated fatty acids into a dangerous mixture of saturated and unsaturated fatty acids known as **trans fatty acids** (trans fats). The primary sources of trans fats in the diet are fried foods, fast-food products, and processed snack foods and baked goods (**FIGURE 8.3**). Trans fats are unhealthy because they can increase blood levels of total cholesterol and LDL cholesterol, increasing heart disease risk. The U.S. Food and Drug Administration (FDA) has announced plans to remove artificial trans fats from the American food supply and is pushing the food industry to reformulate products that contain trans fats.

Other Major Types of Lipids In addition to fat, there are two other forms of lipids in the body: phospholipids and sterols. **Phospholipids** are vital components of cell membranes and play a key role in emulsification.

fiber Undigestible complex carbohydrate found in whole grains, vegetables, and fruits.

soluble fiber Viscous fiber that dissolves in water; slows stomach emptying.

insoluble fiber Fiber that does not dissolve in water; adds bulk and speeds elimination.

lipids Group of insoluble compounds that includes fats and cholesterol.

fats The most common types of lipids found in foods and in your body.

fatty acid Basic structural unit of triglycerides.

triglyceride Form of lipid that is broken down in the body and used to produce energy to power muscle contractions during exercise.

unsaturated fatty acid Type of fatty acid that comes primarily from plant sources and is liquid at room temperature.

omega-3 fatty acid Type of unsaturated fatty acid that lowers blood cholesterol and triglycerides and is found abundantly in some fish.

saturated fatty acid Type of fatty acid that comes primarily from animal sources and is solid at room temperature.

trans fatty acid Type of fatty acid that increases cholesterol in the blood and is a major contributor to heart disease.

phospholipid Type of lipid that contains phosphorus and is an important component of cell membranes.

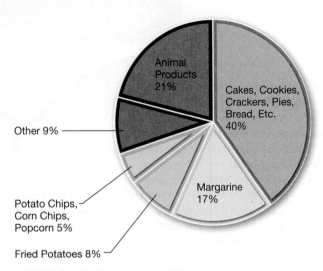

FIGURE 8.3 Major sources of trans fats in the diet.

Sources: National Cancer Institute. Sources of saturated fat in the diets of the U.S. population ages 2 years and older, NHANES 2005–2006; USDA and HHS. *Dietary Guidelines for Americans, 2010.* www.health.gov/dietaryguidelines.

Emulsifiers allow fat and water to mix, which aids in the digestion and absorption of dietary fats. **Sterols** are another important class of lipids with health implications. The most common sterol, **cholesterol**, is an important component of cells and is used to manufacture certain hormones, including male and female sex hormones.

Although cholesterol plays an essential role in the body, high blood cholesterol levels can increase the risk of heart disease. Cholesterol is transported in the blood in the form of **lipoproteins**, which are combinations of protein, triglycerides, and cholesterol. Lipoproteins exist in several forms; the two primary types are low-density lipoprotein (LDL) and high-density lipoprotein (HDL). LDL, or "bad," cholesterol consists of a limited amount of protein and triglycerides but contains large amounts of cholesterol. It is associated with promoting fatty plaque buildup in the arteries of the heart, which is the primary cause of heart disease. In contrast, HDL, or "good," cholesterol is primarily composed of protein, has limited amounts of cholesterol, and is associated with a low risk of heart disease (see Chapter 10).

Fats and Lipids in Foods Humans need very little fat in their diet to maintain health (4). You can find "good" fats, including the two essential fatty acids, in fish, seeds, nuts, and vegetable oils. Unhealthy saturated fats are found in fatty meats, butter, lard, fried foods, and many baked items such as cakes and doughnuts. These foods should be avoided or eaten only in limited amounts.

Dietary cholesterol is present in many foods from animal sources, including meats, shellfish, and dairy products. Although your body needs some cholesterol for

normal functioning, consuming cholesterol from foods is not required because your body can make all that it needs. In fact, diets high in saturated fats cause the body to produce more than normal amounts of cholesterol.

Plants do not produce cholesterol. When companies market a brand of vegetable oil as "cholesterol-free," they are trying to entice consumers to buy their product, but all vegetable oils are cholesterol-free. Plants do produce other sterols known collectively as *phytosterols.* Many phytosterols are reported to have positive health benefits and a diet high in phytosterols has been reported to lower blood cholesterol levels (5). Foods that are high in phytosterols include corn, wheat germ, rice bran, and peanuts.

Proteins

Aside from water, proteins form a major part of lean tissue, totaling about 17–20% of body weight. Thousands of substances in the body are made of proteins, but protein's primary role is to serve as the structural unit to build and repair body tissues, including muscle and connective tissue. Proteins are also important for the synthesis of enzymes, hormones, and antibodies; these compounds regulate metabolism and provide protection from disease.

As mentioned earlier, proteins are not usually a major fuel source. However, if your dietary intake of calories or carbohydrates is too low (such as during a very low-carbohydrate diet or fasting), proteins will be converted to glucose and used as fuel. If you consume adequate amounts of carbohydrates, excess calories from dietary protein are stored in adipose tissue as an energy reserve.

Protein Structure **Amino acids** are the basic structural units of proteins. There are 20 different amino acids, and they can be linked in various combinations to create different proteins with unique functions. Nine amino acids are **essential amino acids**, meaning that the body cannot make them and they must be consumed in the diet. The remaining 11 are **nonessential amino acids**, signifying that the body can synthesize them in adequate amounts.

Protein in Foods **Complete proteins** (also called whole proteins or high-quality proteins) contain all of the essential amino acids and are present only in animal foods and soy products. **Incomplete proteins** (also called low-quality proteins) are missing one or more of the essential amino acids and are present in numerous vegetable sources. Therefore, vegetarians must be careful to eat a variety of vegetables to ensure that they consume all of the essential amino acids. Plant sources of protein provide additional benefits because they often contain other important nutrients such as vitamin D, folate, iron, zinc, copper, and phytosterols.

Calculating Your Protein Needs	Example (Adult Female)
1. Determine your body weight	1. An adult female weighs 132 pounds.
2. Convert pounds (lb) to kilograms (kg) by dividing number of pounds by 2.2	2. 132 / 2.2 lb/kg = 60 kg
3. Multiply by 0.8 (adult females) or 0.9 (adult males) to get an RDA in grams/day	3. 60 kg × 0.8 g/kg = 48 g
	A 132 pound female needs to consume 48 grams of protein per day.

FIGURE 8.4 Estimated daily protein needs for adults. You can calculate the number of grams of protein you should consume daily.

Consuming sufficient protein is vital to maintain good health. Because of its role in building body tissue, protein is particularly important during periods of rapid growth, such as adolescence. Moreover, intense exercise training increases the body's protein requirements. Many American adults consume more protein than is required to maintain health and high amounts of protein in the diet may result in consuming too many calories. Protein-rich foods from animal sources fat (and high in calories), which can lead to heart disease, cancer, and obesity. See **FIGURE 8.4** to calculate your optimal protein intake.

Water

Although sometimes overlooked as a nutrient, water is the macronutrient needed in the highest quantity. Water makes up approximately 60% to 70% of total body weight and is important for numerous functions including temperature regulation, digestion, nutrient absorption, blood formation, and waste elimination (6). Adequate water consumption is especially important for physically active people and people who reside in hot climates. For example, a person engaging in vigorous exercise in a hot, humid environment can lose 1 to 3 liters of water per hour through sweating (6). Losing as little as 5% of body water causes fatigue, weakness, and the inability to concentrate; losing more than 15% can be fatal.

Most adults should consume 12 to 16 cups (2.7–3.7 liters) of water per day through foods and beverages (4). Since about 30% of our intake comes from food, and 10% is produced by metabolism, this means that adults should drink about 8 to 10 cups (1.8–2.3 liters) of water per day (**FIGURE 8.5**). Drinking water throughout the day and eating foods with high water content, such as fruits and vegetables, will allow you to meet this goal. People who experience diarrhea or vomiting need to replace lost fluids. Those who sweat excessively or exercise for a prolonged period in a hot environment will also need to increase their water intake (see Chapter 12). If you donate blood, your water needs that day will be higher than normal.

sterol Type of lipid that does not contain fatty acids; cholesterol is the most commonly known sterol.

Cholesterol A lipid that is necessary for cell and hormone synthesis. Found naturally in animal foods, but made in adequate amounts in the body.

lipoproteins Combinations of protein, triglycerides, and cholesterol in the blood that have an important role in influencing the risk of heart disease.

amino acids The building blocks of protein; 20 different amino acids can be linked in various combinations to create different proteins.

essential amino acids Nine amino acids that cannot be manufactured by the body and must be consumed in the diet.

nonessential amino acids Eleven amino acids that the body can make and are not necessary in the diet.

complete proteins Proteins containing all the essential amino acids.

incomplete proteins Proteins that are missing one or more of the essential amino acids.

Daily Water Balance in the Body

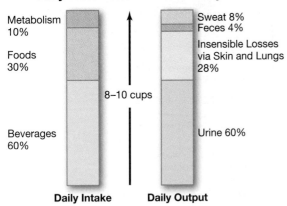

FIGURE 8.5 The amount of water you consume in food and beverages and that you produce during metabolism is about equal to the amount you excrete in urine, sweat, and feces and through exhalation and insensible water loss.

MAKE SURE YOU **KNOW...**

- The kilocalorie (commonly called a calorie) is a unit of measure for the energy in food or the energy expended by the body.

- The macronutrients are carbohydrates, fat, protein and water.

- Carbohydrates are the body's primary source of fuel. Glucose is the most important of the simple carbohydrates, and all other simple and complex carbohydrates must be converted to glucose before being used by the body. Starches and fiber are complex carbohydrates.

- Fats are the most common form of lipids in foods and in the body. All excess calories consumed will eventually be converted to fat for storage. Dietary cholesterol and trans fats are heart-unhealthy, and you should limit or avoid consumption of foods containing them.

- Proteins, made up of amino acids, are the key structural unit for building and repairing cells. Amino acids are either made by the body (nonessential amino acids) or must be consumed in the diet (essential amino acids).

MasteringHealth™

Micronutrients

LO **3** Explain what micronutrients are, which substances compose them, and why they are so important for health.

Nutrients that are required in small amounts (less than one gram) are called **micronutrients**; vitamins and minerals make up this category. Though needed in smaller

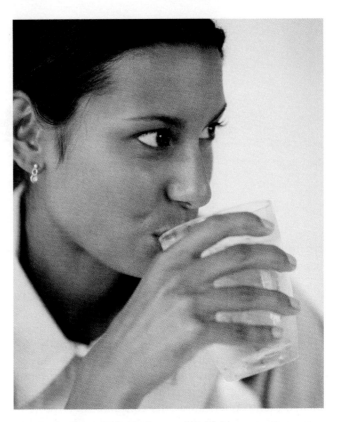

Water is a key ingredient in a healthy diet.

amounts, micronutrients are critical to body functions and are necessary in order to sustain life. They do not supply energy, but vitamins and minerals are very important in maintaining a healthy body.

Vitamins

Vitamins are essential organic (carbon-containing) substances that are required in the diet for normal function, growth, and maintenance of body tissues (5). Although vitamins do not provide energy, they play a key role in many body functions, including the regulation of growth and metabolism. Vitamins are essential in the human diet because they cannot be synthesized by the body in sufficient amounts to meet its needs.

Some vitamins are soluble in water; others are soluble in fat. Water-soluble vitamins include the B vitamins and vitamin C. With the exception of B_6 and B_{12}, water-soluble vitamins are not stored in the body and are eliminated by the kidneys. Vitamins A, D, E, and K are fat soluble. They are stored in body fat and can therefore accumulate in body tissue. Although a toxic effect from excessive intake of any vitamin is possible, vitamin A toxicity is the most likely to occur among Americans due to ingesting a supplement in large doses over a period of time. See **TABLE 8.2** on page 220 for details on the functions and dietary sources of selected vitamins.

Minerals

Minerals are chemical elements required by the body for normal functioning. There are two types: *major minerals* are those needed in higher amounts, and *trace minerals* are needed in very small quantities. Major minerals include calcium, phosphorus, potassium, sulfur, sodium, chloride, and magnesium. Trace minerals include iron, manganese, copper, zinc, iodine, fluoride, and selenium.

The functional role of minerals in the body varies widely. Some minerals act as cofactors with specialized proteins (enzymes) to regulate a chemical reaction in cells. Some minerals (such as iron) are key components of important molecules such as hemoglobin (transports oxygen) in red blood cells. Others play important roles in conducting nerve impulses, contracting muscles, and maintaining water balance. Minerals also serve a structural function. For example, calcium, phosphorus, and fluoride are components of bones and teeth.

Three key minerals that play important roles in the body are calcium, iron, and sodium. Calcium is important in bone formation. A deficiency contributes to the development of the bone disease called **osteoporosis**. A deficiency of dietary iron may lead to iron-deficiency **anemia**, which results in chronic fatigue. High sodium intake has been associated with hypertension, a major risk factor for heart disease. **TABLE 8.3** on page 221 summarizes several key minerals and their functions.

Micronutrients in the Diet

Though a few vitamins, including A, D, and K, can be made in the body, most must be consumed in foods (5). If you're eating a balanced diet with plenty of fresh fruits, vegetables, and whole grains, and some lean meat and poultry, you're likely getting all of the vitamins and minerals that you need. (See Tables 8.2 and 8.3 for specific food sources.) In general, the more brightly colored the fruit or vegetable, the higher its vitamin and mineral content. Note that some water-soluble vitamins can be destroyed during cooking or processing, so minimal cooking (such as by steaming, rather than boiling) and eating fresh fruits and vegetables rather than canned produce will provide higher amounts of micronutrients.

MAKE SURE YOU **KNOW...**

- Vitamins serve many important functions in the body, including facilitating metabolism. The B vitamins and vitamin C are water soluble and are not stored in the body. Vitamins A, D, E, and K are fat soluble and can be stored in the body.

- Minerals are chemical elements in foods that, like vitamins, play important roles in many body functions. Calcium is important for bone health, iron is important for healthy blood, and too much sodium can have a negative effect on heart health.

- Approximately 60% to 70% of body weight is water. To maintain adequate hydration, you should consume 8–10 cups of water each day in addition to the water contained in food.

— MasteringHealth™

What Are the Guidelines for a Healthy Diet?

LO **4** Outline the guidelines for a healthy diet.

Making healthy food choices is important to your health and wellness. In your lifetime, you will eat approximately 79,000 meals and consume 68 tons of food (5). While nutrition may seem like a complex subject, the basics of consuming a healthy diet are fairly simple:

- Consume an appropriate number of calories in light of calories expended.

- Eat a variety of healthy foods (especially vegetables and fruits).

- Consume less-healthy (processed and sugar-containing) foods rarely or in moderation.

Several national health agencies provide guidelines for healthy diets. The U.S. Department of Agriculture (USDA) recently released the *2015 Dietary Guidelines for Americans*. These guidelines emphasize two main concepts: First, individuals should maintain calorie balance over time to achieve and maintain a healthy weight. Second, individuals should focus on consuming nutrient-dense foods and beverages. *Nutrient-dense* means that a food or beverage provides a high number of nutrients

---

micronutrients Vitamins and minerals; they are involved in many body processes, including regulating cell function.

vitamins Micronutrients that play a key role in many body functions, including the regulation of growth and metabolism; classified as water-soluble or fat-soluble.

minerals Chemical elements required by the body in small amounts for normal functioning.

osteoporosis Bone disease in which the mineral content of bone is reduced, and the bone is weakened and at increased risk of fracture.

anemia Deficiency of red blood cells and/or hemoglobin that results in decreased oxygen-carrying capacity of the blood.

TABLE 8.2 ■ Selected Vitamins: Food Sources, Functions, and Deficiency and Toxicity Symptoms

Vitamin	Selected Food Sources	Selected Functions	Deficiency Symptoms	Toxicity Symptoms
Fat-soluble				
A	Liver, spinach, carrots, sweet potatoes; other orange and green leafy vegetables	Necessary for vision, bone growth, fertility	Night blindness, impaired immunity, infertility	Birth defects, loss of appetite, blurred vision, hair loss, liver damage
D	Fortified milk; produced in the skin under sunlight	Regulates blood calcium levels; bone health; cell differentiation	Rickets in children, bone weakness and increased fractures in adults	Hypercalcemia, calcium deposits in kidneys and liver
E	Vegetable oils, whole grains, nuts, seeds	Antioxidant; improves absorption of vitamin A	Anemia, impaired nerve transmission, muscle weakness	Inhibited blood clotting
K	Green leafy vegetables; cabbage, cauliflower	Helps with blood clotting	Reduced ability to form blood clots	No known symptoms
Water-soluble				
Thiamin (B_1)	Whole grains, organ meat, lean pork	Coenzyme in carbohydrate metabolism and some amino acid metabolism	Beriberi, weight loss, confusion, muscle weakness	No known symptoms
Riboflavin (B_2)	Dairy products, enriched breads and cereals, lean meats, poultry, fish	Coenzyme; helps maintain mucous membranes	Sore throat, swelling of the tongue, anemia	No known symptoms
Niacin (B_3)	Eggs, poultry, fish, milk, whole grains, nuts, enriched breads and cereals	Coenzyme in carbohydrate and fatty acid metabolism; plays role in DNA replication and repair and cell differentiation	Pellagra, rash, vomiting, constipation or diarrhea	Flushing, liver damage, glucose intolerance, blurred vision
Vitamin B_6	Eggs, poultry, fish, whole grains, liver, kidney, pork	Coenzyme involved in amino acid and carbohydrate metabolism; synthesis of blood cells	Dermatitis, anemia, convulsions	Skin lesions
Vitamin B_{12}	Meat, fish, poultry, fortified cereals	Coenzyme that assists with blood formation and nervous system function	Pernicious anemia, pale skin, fatigue, shortness of breath, dementia	No known symptoms
Folate	Green leafy vegetables, yeast, oranges, whole grains, legumes	Coenzyme involved in DNA synthesis and amino acid metabolism	Macrocytic anemia, weakness and fatigue, headache, neural tube defects in developing fetus	Masks symptoms of vitamin B_{12} deficiency; neurological damage
Vitamin C	Citrus fruits, peppers, spinach, strawberries, tomatoes, potatoes	Antioxidant; assists with collagen synthesis; enhances immune function; enhances iron absorption	Scurvy, bleeding gums and joints, loose teeth, depression, anemia	Nausea and diarrhea, nosebleeds, abdominal cramps

Source: Thompson, Janice; Manore, Melinda, *Nutrition: An Applied Approach, 3rd Ed.,* © 2012. Reprinted and Electronically reproduced by permission of Pearson Education, Inc., Upper Saddle River, New Jersey.

TABLE 8.3 ■ Selected Minerals: Food Sources, Functions, and Deficiency and Toxicity Symptoms

Mineral	Selected Food Sources	Selected Functions	Deficiency Symptoms	Toxicity Symptoms
Major minerals				
Calcium	Milk and milk products; sardines; dark green leafy vegetables; fortified orange juice	Builds bones and teeth; helps maintain acid–base balance; maintains normal nerve transmission	Osteoporosis, bone fractures, convulsions and muscle spasms, heart failure	Can interfere with the absorption of iron, zinc, and magnesium; shock, fatigue, kidney failure
Phosphorus	Meat, poultry, fish, eggs, milk, soft drinks	Maintains fluid balance; plays a role in bone formation	Muscle weakness or damage, bone pain, dizziness	Muscle spasms, convulsions, low blood calcium levels
Magnesium	Grains, legumes, nuts (especially almonds and cashews), seeds, soybeans	Essential component of bone tissue; bone growth; supports muscle contraction and blood clotting	Hypomagnesemia, resulting in low blood calcium levels, muscle cramps, spasms, or seizures; chronic diseases such as heart disease, high blood pressure, and osteoporosis	Diarrhea, nausea, abdominal cramps
Potassium	Potatoes, bananas, tomato juice, orange juice	Regulates muscle contraction and transmission of nerve impulses; maintains blood pressure	Muscle weakness, paralysis, confusion	Muscle weakness, irregular heartbeat, vomiting
Sodium	Salt, soy sauce, fast foods and processed foods	Maintains acid–base balance; assists with nerve transmission and muscle contraction	Muscle cramps, dizziness, fatigue, nausea, vomiting, mental confusion	Water retention; high blood pressure; may increase loss of calcium in urine
Trace minerals				
Iron	Meat and poultry; green leafy vegetables; fortified grain products	Assists with oxygen transport in blood and muscle; coenzyme for energy metabolism	Anemia, fatigue, depressed immune function, impaired memory	Nausea, vomiting, diarrhea, dizziness, rapid heartbeat, death
Zinc	Whole grains, meat, liver, seafood	Coenzyme for hemoglobin production; plays role in cell replication, protein synthesis	Growth retardation, diarrhea, delayed sexual maturation, hair loss	Intestinal pain, nausea, vomiting, loss of appetite, diarrhea; headache, depressed immune function
Iodine	Iodized salt, seafood, processed foods	Synthesis of thyroid hormones; temperature regulation	Goiter (enlargement of the thyroid gland), hypothyroidism; deficiency during pregnancy can cause birth defects	Goiter
Fluoride	Fluoridated water, tea, fish	Maintains health of bones and teeth	Dental cavities and tooth decay; lower bone density	Teeth fluorosis (staining and pitting of the teeth); skeletal fluorosis
Selenium	Organ meats, such as liver and kidney; pork; seafood	Antioxidant; immune function; assists in production of thyroid hormone	Keshan disease, impaired immune function, infertility, muscle pain	Brittle hair, skin rashes, weakness, cirrhosis of the liver

Source: Thompson, Janice; Manore, Melinda, *Nutrition: An Applied Approach*, 3rd Ed., © 2012. Reprinted and Electronically reproduced by permission of Pearson Education, Inc., Upper Saddle River, New Jersey.

in relation to its calorie content. The following is a list of recommendations related to these concepts:

- A well-balanced diet involves consuming a variety of foods achieved by a moderate intake of each food.
- A macronutrient-balanced diet is composed of approximately 58% carbohydrate, 30% fat, and 12% protein.
- Consume foods and drinks to meet, not exceed, calorie needs. Choose foods that contain limited saturated and trans (solid) fats, cholesterol, added sugars, salt, and alcohol.
- Maintain appropriate calorie balance during each stage of life.
- Engage in regular physical activity and avoid long periods of inactivity.
- Consume sufficient amounts of fruits, vegetables, and whole grains while staying within energy needs. Make half of your plate fruits and vegetables.
- Consume less than 10% of calories from saturated fats and less than 300 mg per day of cholesterol; consume as little trans fats as possible.
- Eat fiber-rich fruits, vegetables, and whole grains. Make at least half of your grains whole grains.
- Choose foods and beverages with little added sugars or caloric sweeteners.
- Consume less than 1 teaspoon of salt per day.
- If you choose to drink alcohol, do so only in moderation.
- Take proper food safety precautions.

Eat More Fruits, Vegetables, and Whole Grains

Choosing unprocessed (whole) foods that are modest in calories and low in fat and sodium is the best way to create a healthy diet. This means doing much of your grocery shopping in the produce aisle and buying whole-grain products. When you dine out with friends or family, try to keep your portions of fatty meats and high-sugar desserts small, and consume more fruits and vegetables. Further, when you need a midmorning or late-afternoon snack, reach for a banana or other fruit, raw veggies, nuts, or whole-grain crackers rather than a bag of chips or a chocolate bar. Individuals with food allergies or intolerances to substances such as gluten or dairy should focus on choices that avoid the offending foods and include a variety of fruits and vegetables.

Once you've adopted these healthy eating strategies, you will begin to reap the benefits of a good diet and you may even lose weight. Over the long term, you will have a lower risk for many chronic diseases and conditions.

coaching corner

Pack a healthy snack!

People report that they are more successful in making healthy eating choices when they plan ahead. Consider the following strategies.

- Plan your meal schedule. You may choose to eat something every 2–3 hours. This eating style is called "grazing" and involves 5–6 mini-meals each day. It may be helpful for some people in terms of losing weight and managing blood sugar. Others do well with three meals and one snack each day.
- To ensure that you eat at least 5 servings of fruits and vegetables during the day, think about fruits and vegetables you can easily take along with you. Make sure to pack your healthy snacks the night before or in the morning!
- Be aware of appropriate portion sizes, and be intentional about your food choices and the amounts you consume.
- Stay hydrated! Hydration is an important part of good nutrition. Fill your water bottle and keep it with you.

consider this! ////////////

The average American consumes more than 80 pounds of table sugar and 45 pounds of high fructose corn syrup each year.

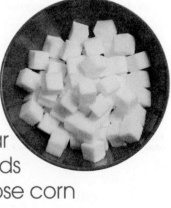

Manage Your Intake of Calories, Sugar, Alcohol, Fat, and Sodium

With the increase in overweight and obesity in the United States, it's clear that the balance of "calories in" versus "calories out" is a major issue for many individuals. Several factors are causing the increase in calorie consumption. For example, many people consume a large amount of simple sugars, often in the form of sucrose (table sugar) or high fructose corn syrup (a commercial sweetener used in numerous foods including baked goods, ice cream, and beverages). A key problem with foods that are high in simple sugars is that they contain many calories but few micronutrients (which is why they're called "empty calories"). It is estimated that half the dietary carbohydrate intake of the average U.S. citizen is in the form of simple sugars (5).

Another concern with consuming large amounts of simple carbohydrates is that fructose consumption does not suppress appetite and may promote overeating (4). Sugar in sweets also leads to tooth decay. Although brushing your teeth after eating sweets can prevent this problem, it will not solve the other problems related to overconsumption of sugar. One easy way to trim your sucrose intake is to use sugar substitutes instead of sugar to sweeten your foods or beverages. Artificial sweeteners such as saccharin®, aspartame®, or sucralose® add sweetness with little or no calories. However, the long-term health effects of artificial sweeteners remain largely unknown.

Alcohol, if consumed in excess, is another source of empty calories that can undermine an otherwise healthy diet. Chronic alcohol consumption can also lower the body's stores of some vitamins, possibly leading to severe deficiencies. Drinking too much alcohol can displace healthier foods in the diet by reducing the desire for solid food. Finally, consuming large amounts of alcohol significantly increases your risk of accidents and injury. When it comes to drinking alcohol, the best plan is to avoid it or, if you do drink, to do so only in moderation.

Another factor contributing to the rise in overweight and obesity in the United States is the high amount of fat in many people's diets. Foods high in fat are often high in cholesterol and contain over twice as many calories per gram as carbohydrate or protein (9 calories/gram versus 4 calories/gram). Limiting fat in the diet will lower your calorie intake and will also reduce your risk of heart disease, obesity, and certain cancers.

When cutting fat from your diet it is important to read food labels. Look for items that are low in fat or choose nonfat alternatives when available. Be aware that some products replace fat with sugar and other unhealthy ingredients, so it is best to avoid those. Also, consider how you prepare food. Compared to frying, baking, broiling, or steaming will reduce fat intake. Processed foods are often high in fat and sodium, and many dairy products are also high in fat. Heavy,

TABLE 8.4 ▪ Examples of Low or Nonfat Alternatives	
High-Fat Choice	Low or Nonfat Option
Whole milk	1% or skim milk
Whole-milk cheese	Part skim or fat-free cheese
Fried chicken with the skin	Skinless baked or broiled chicken
Creamy Italian or ranch dressing	Vinaigrette dressing
Mayonnaise	Mustard
Alfredo sauce	Marinara sauce
Shortening or butter	Cooking spray or olive oil

cream-based sauces and dressings can add fat to an otherwise healthy meal. **TABLE 8.4** provides guidelines to help you cut your dietary fat intake.

Although salt (sodium chloride) is a necessary micronutrient, the body's daily requirement is small (1.5 grams sodium and 2.3 grams chloride, approximately ¼ teaspoon of salt). Very active people who lose water and electrolytes due to sweating may need over 1½ teaspoons of salt per day (10). Many sedentary people consume much more sodium than required, which can increase their risk for developing high blood pressure (hypertension). You might be surprised just how much salt is in many foods you eat regularly. For example, **FIGURE 8.6** illustrates the "hidden" salt in an average pizza.

Too much sodium in the diet can be a complicating factor for people with high blood pressure. In countries where limited salt is added to foods, the incidence of high blood pressure is relatively low (8). Even if you don't have high blood pressure, you should limit salt intake to the minimal daily requirements.

see it!

ABC VIDEOS

Watch the "Coconut: How Healthy Is the Superfood?" ABC News Video online at MasteringHealth™.

live it!

ASSESS YOURSELF

Assess your fat intake with the *Cutting out the Fat* Take Charge of Your Health! Worksheet online at MasteringHealth™.

MAKE SURE YOU **KNOW...**

▪ Individuals should maintain calorie balance over time to achieve and maintain a healthy weight and focus on consuming nutrient-dense foods and beverages.

▪ The basic guidelines for a healthy diet are to eat adequate amounts of fruits, vegetables, and whole grains and to manage your intake of calories, sugar, fat, and sodium. If you choose to drink alcohol, do so only in moderation.

MasteringHealth™

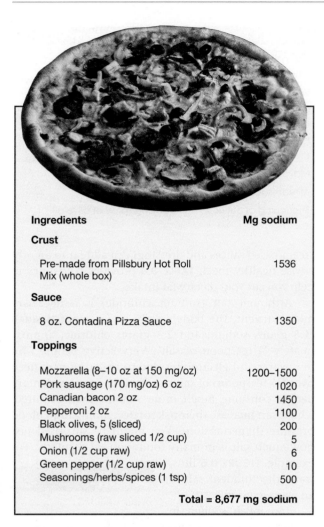

Ingredients	Mg sodium
Crust	
Pre-made from Pillsbury Hot Roll Mix (whole box)	1536
Sauce	
8 oz. Contadina Pizza Sauce	1350
Toppings	
Mozzarella (8–10 oz at 150 mg/oz)	1200–1500
Pork sausage (170 mg/oz) 6 oz	1020
Canadian bacon 2 oz	1450
Pepperoni 2 oz	1100
Black olives, 5 (sliced)	200
Mushrooms (raw sliced 1/2 cup)	5
Onion (1/2 cup raw)	6
Green pepper (1/2 cup raw)	10
Seasonings/herbs/spices (1 tsp)	500
Total = 8,677 mg sodium	

FIGURE 8.6 The amount of sodium in a typical medium pizza with "the works" will probably surprise you. Even if you eat only two slices, you are still likely consuming more than 1000 mg of sodium! Cutting back on the meat toppings and loading up on veggies will significantly lower the sodium.

Use Available Resources to Plan Healthy Meals

LO **5** List several resources that can be helpful in planning a healthy diet.

Several U.S. government agencies provide resources that can be of help in planning a healthy diet. The Institute of Medicine within the National Academy of Sciences has established guidelines for the quantity of each micronutrient required to meet the minimum needs of most individuals. These guidelines are the Dietary Reference Intakes (DRIs), which are a set of reference values used to plan the nutrient intake for healthy people (4). These values vary by age and gender and include the following standards:

1. *Recommended Dietary Allowance (RDA).* RDAs are the amount of nutrient that will meet the needs of

almost every healthy person within a specific age and gender group (see **TABLE 8.5** on pages 226–227).

2. *Adequate Intake (AI).* This value is an "educated guess." It is used when the RDA is not known because the scientific data aren't strong enough to produce a specific recommendation, yet there is enough evidence for a general guideline.

consider this! ///////////////////////

The average American consumes between 3 and 10 teaspoons of salt per day.

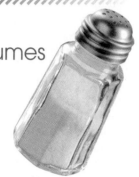

3. *Estimated Average Requirement (EAR).* This is the average daily amount of a nutrient that is estimated to satisfy the needs of 50% of people in a given age group.

4. *Tolerable Upper Intake Level (UL).* This is the highest average nutrient intake level that a person can consume without risking adverse health effects. Anything above this amount can result in toxicity.

Once you know the recommended daily allowances for nutrients, the key question becomes, "How do I choose foods to meet these goals?"

MyPlate

MyPlate is a visual guide developed by the U.S. Department of Agriculture (USDA) that depicts the proportions of each food group (fruits, vegetables, grains, protein, and dairy) that make up a healthy meal (**FIGURE 8.7**). Fruits and vegetables make up half the plate, which is consistent with the 2015 Dietary Guidelines. (People with a milk allergy or lactose intolerance, the inability to digest the form of sugar found in milk, can plan meals without a dairy component.) The website www.choosemyplate.gov includes sample food plans and the SuperTracker tool that allows you to plan, analyze, and track your daily diet and physical activity (see Laboratory 8.1 to analyze your dietary habits).

see it!
ABC VIDEOS
Watch the "Menu Calorie Counts" ABC News Video online at MasteringHealth™.

Food Labels

Food labels are required on almost all packaged foods (**FIGURE 8.8**). They include a list of ingredients in the food (shown in order by amount). The Nutrition Facts section of the label includes the number of calories per serving.

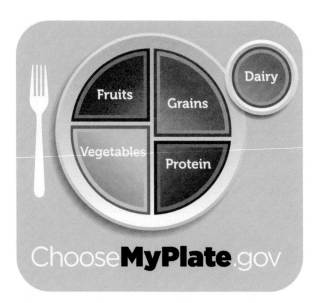

FIGURE 8.7 The USDA's MyPlate food guidance system reminds you to eat a varied diet with lots of nutrient-dense foods.

Source: www.choosemyplate.gov

It also shows the amount and the percent Daily Value (DV) of fat, carbohydrate, protein, sodium, and cholesterol in a single serving. Percent DVs are also shown for specific micronutrients.

Daily Values are a set of nutrition standards (based on a 2,000-calorie diet) established by the Food and Drug Administration for food labeling purposes. For example, if the label lists 20% DV for calcium, this means that one serving of the product provides 20% of the calcium you need each day.

Sample Meal Plan

Now that we have presented the guidelines for a healthy diet, let's put these principles into practice and construct a 1-day meal plan that provides all of the required macro- and micronutrients for a healthy adult.. You can refer to **TABLE 8.6** on page 228, which presents a sample meal plan for a college-age woman weighing 132 pounds (60 kg) who engages in light to moderate daily activities. To adapt this plan for yourself, adjust the quantities accordingly. An example of a balanced meal plan based on three meals (without the snacks shown in Table 8.6) follows.

- **Breakfast** A healthy breakfast might include 1/2 grapefruit, whole-grain cereal, skim milk, and a banana. This meal would provide two fruit servings, one grain serving, and one dairy serving. The breakfast is low in fat, cholesterol, and sodium. A quarter of the protein need is met, plus over 40% of calcium and iron needs. The fruits alone provide almost all of the recommended vitamin A and C intake for the day. You might also choose to include another low-calorie dairy product such as low-fat yogurt.

Sample Label for Macaroni and Cheese

(1) **Start Here**

Nutrition Facts

Serving Size 1 cup (228g)
Servings Per Container about 2

Amount Per Serving

Calories 250	**Calories from Fat 110**

	% Daily Value*
Total Fat 12g	**18%**
Saturated fat 3g	**15%**
Trans fat 1.5g	
Cholesterol 30mg	**10%**
Sodium 470mg	**20%**
Total Carbohydrate 31g	**10%**
Dietary Fiber 0g	**0%**
Sugars 5g	
Protein 5g	

Vitamin A	**4%**
Vitamin C	**2%**
Calcium	**20%**
Iron	**4%**

*Percent Daily Values are based on a 2,000 calorie diet. Your Daily Values may be higher or lower depending on your calorie needs:

	Calories:	2,000	2,500
Total Fat	Less than	65 g	80 g
Sat. Fat	Less than	20 g	25 g
Cholesterol	Less than	300 mg	300 mg
Sodium	Less than	2,400 mg	2,400 mg
Total Carbohydrate	Less than	300 g	375 g
Dietary Fiber		25 g	30 g

(2) **Limit These Nutrients**

(3) **Get Enough of These Nutrients**

FIGURE 8.8 Nutrition Facts on food labels can help you select foods that are low in fat, cholesterol, sodium, sugar, and calories and that are adequate in protein, carbohydrates, and selected micronutrients. The % Daily Value (DV) helps you determine how good a source a food is for a given nutrient. In general, foods with less than 5% of the DV are considered low in a nutrient, while those with more than 20% of the DV are considered high in that nutrient.

Source: U.S. Department of Agriculture. *Dietary Guidelines for Americans 2010.* Washington, DC: U.S. Government Printing Office.

- **Lunch** For lunch, a turkey sandwich (with low-sodium turkey) on whole-wheat bread and a handful of baby carrots will provide one serving of meat, two grain servings, and one vegetable. Adding lettuce and tomato to the sandwich will provide additional

see it!

ABC VIDEOS

Watch the "Changes Coming to Nutrition Labels" ABC News Video online at MasteringHealth™.

Daily Values Standard values for nutrient needs used as a reference on food labels; based on a 2,000-calorie/day diet.

TABLE 8.5 ■ Recommended Dietary Allowances of Micronutrients

Life Stage Group	Calcium (mg/d)	Phosphorus (mg/d)	Magnesium (mg/d)	Iron (mg/d)	Zinc (mg/d)	Selenium (mg/d)	Iodine (mg/d)	Copper (mg/d)	Manganese (mg/d)	Fluoride (mg/d)	Chromium (mg/d)	Molybdenum (mg/d)
Infants												
0 to 6 mo	200*	100*	30*	0.27*	2*	15*	110*	200*	0.003*	0.01*	0.2*	2*
6 to 12 mo	260*	275*	75*	11	3	20*	130*	220*	0.6*	0.5*	5.5*	3*
Children												
1–3 y	700	460	80	7	3	20	90	340	1.2*	0.7*	11*	17
4–8 y	1000	500	130	10	5	30	90	440	1.5*	1*	15*	22
Males												
9–13 y	1300	1250	240	8	8	40	120	700	1.9*	2*	25*	34
14–18 y	1300	1250	410	11	11	55	150	890	2.2*	3*	35*	43
19–30 y	1000	700	400	8	11	55	150	900	2.3*	4*	35*	45
31–50 y	1000	700	420	8	11	55	150	900	2.3*	4*	35*	45
51–70 y	1000	700	420	8	11	55	150	900	2.3*	4*	30*	45
>70 y	1200	700	420	8	11	55	150	900	2.3*	4*	30*	45
Females												
9–13 y	1300	1250	240	8	8	40	120	700	1.6*	2*	21*	34
14–18 y	1300	1250	360	15	9	55	150	890	1.6*	3*	24*	43
19–30 y	1000	700	310	18	8	55	150	900	1.8*	3*	25*	45
31–50 y	1000	700	320	18	8	55	150	900	1.8*	3*	25*	45
51–70 y	1200	700	320	8	8	55	150	900	1.8*	3*	20*	45
>70 y	1200	700	320	8	8	55	150	900	1.8*	3*	20*	45
Pregnancy												
14–18 y	1300	1250	400	27	12	60	220	1000	2.0*	3*	29*	50
19–30 y	1000	700	350	27	11	60	220	1000	2.0*	3*	30*	50
31–50 y	1000	700	360	27	11	60	220	1000	2.0*	3*	30*	50
Lactation												
14–18 y	1300	1250	360	10	13	70	290	1300	2.6*	3*	44*	50
19–30 y	1000	700	310	9	12	70	290	1300	2.6*	3*	45*	50
31–50 y	1000	700	320	9	12	70	290	1300	2.6*	3*	45*	50

vegetables with few calories and extra vitamins and minerals. This lunch provides a low-calorie meal with lots of protein, vitamin A, and iron.

■ **Dinner** Whole-wheat pasta with meatless tomato sauce and mushrooms adds more vegetables and whole grains. Broccoli and a fruit salad add vitamins A and C and calcium. The addition of a small serving of a lean meat such as chicken or lean ground beef would add a source of high-quality protein.

See Laboratory 8.2 to record your dietary goals and Laboratory 8.3 for help in planning a healthy diet.

Laboratory 8.4 will help you assess your current nutritional habits to determine if you need to make some adjustments.

MAKE SURE YOU **KNOW**...

■ Recommended Dietary Allowances and the USDA's MyPlate are tools you can use to plan a healthy diet.

■ Reading food labels will help you choose foods that are low in calories, fat, sodium, and sugar and that provide important nutrients your body needs.

MasteringHealth™

TABLE 8.5 ■ Recommended Dietary Allowances of Micronutrients

Life Stage Group	Vitamin A (mg/d)[a]	Vitamin D (mg/d)[b]	Vitamin E (mg/d)[c]	Vitamin K (mg/d)	Thiamin (mg/d)	Riboflavin (mg/d)	Niacin (mg/d)[d]	Pantothenic Acid (mg/d)	Biotin (µg/d)	Vitamin B6 (mg/d)	Folate (mg/d)[e]	Vitamin B12 (µg/d)	Vitamin C (mg/d)	Choline (mg/d)
Infants														
0 to 6 mo	400*	400*	4*	2.0*	0.2*	0.3*	2*	1.7*	5*	0.1*	65*	0.4*	40*	125*
6 to 12 mo	500*	400*	5*	2.5*	0.3*	0.4*	4*	1.8*	6*	0.3*	80*	0.5*	50*	150*
Children														
1–3 y	300	600	6	30*	0.5	0.5	6	2*	8*	0.5	150	0.9	15	200*
4–8 y	400	600	7	55*	0.6	0.6	8	3*	12*	0.6	200	1.2	25	250*
Males														
9–13 y	600	600	11	60*	0.9	0.9	12	4*	20*	1	300	1.8	45	375*
14–18 y	900	600	15	75*	1.2	1.3	16	5*	25*	1.3	400	2.4	75	550*
19–30 y	900	600	15	120*	1.2	1.3	16	5*	30*	1.3	400	2.4	90	550*
31–50 y	900	600	15	120*	1.2	1.3	16	5*	30*	1.3	400	2.4	90	550*
51–70 y	900	600	15	120*	1.2	1.3	16	5*	30*	1.7	400	2.4	90	550*
>70 y	900	700	15	120*	1.2	1.3	16	5*	30*	1.7	400	2.4	90	550*
Females														
9–13 y	600	600	11	60*	0.9	0.9	12	4*	20*	1	300	1.8	45	375*
14–18 y	700	600	15	75*	1	1	14	5*	25*	1.2	400	2.4	65	400*
19–30 y	700	600	15	90*	1.1	1.1	14	5*	30*	1.3	400	2.4	75	425*
31–50 y	700	600	15	90*	1.1	1.1	14	5*	30*	1.3	400	2.4	75	425*
51–70 y	700	600	15	90*	1.1	1.1	14	5*	30*	1.5	400	2.4	75	425*
>70 y	700	800	15	90*	1.1	1.1	14	5*	30*	1.5	400	2.4	75	425*
Pregnancy														
14–18 y	750	600	15	75*	1.4	1.4	18	6*	30*	1.9	600	2.6	80	450*
19–30 y	770	600	15	90*	1.4	1.4	18	6*	30*	1.9	600	2.6	85	450*
31–50 y	770	600	15	90*	1.4	1.4	18	6*	30*	1.9	600	2.6	85	450*
Lactation														
14–18 y	1200	600	19	75*	1.4	1.6	17	7*	35*	2	500	2.8	115	550*
19–30 y	1300	600	19	90*	1.4	1.6	17	7ᴧ	35*	2	500	2.8	120	550*
31–50 y	1300	600	19	90*	1.4	1.6	17	7*	35*	2	500	2.8	120	550*

Source: Thompson, Janice; Manore, Melinda, *Nutrition: An Applied Approach, 3rd Ed.*, © 2012. Reprinted and Electronically reproduced by permission of Pearson Education, Inc., Upper Saddle River, New Jersey.

Note: This table is adapted from the DRI reports; see www.nap.edu. It lists Recommended Dietary Allowances (RDAs), with Adequate Intakes (AIs) indicated by asterisks (*). RDAs and AIs may both be used as goals for individual intake. RDAs are set to meet the needs of almost all (97% to 98%) individuals in a group. For healthy breastfed infants, the AI is the mean intake. The AI for other life stage and gender groups is believed to cover the needs of all individuals in the group, but lack of data prevents being able to specify with confidence the percentage of individuals covered by this intake.

[a]Given as retinal activity equivalents (RAE).

[b]Also known as calciferol. The DRI values are based on the absence of adequate exposure to sunlight.

[c]Also known as α-tocopherol.

[d]Given as niacin equivalents (NE), except for infants 0–6 months, which are expressed as preformed niacin.

[e]Given as dietary folate equivalents (DFE).

TABLE 8.6 ■ Sample Diet for a College-Age Female Weighing 132 Pounds, Assuming Light to Moderate Daily Activities									
	kcal	Fat (g)	Cholesterol (mg)	Sodium (mg)	Carbohydrate (g)	Protein (g)	Vitamin A (RE)*	Vitamin C (mg)	Calcium (mg)
Breakfast									
½ grapefruit	41	0	0	0	10	1	59	44	15
Whole-grain cereal (1 cup)	114	0.5	0	207	29	2	155	16	104
Skim milk (1 cup)	83	0	5	103	12	8	149	0	299
1 banana	105	0	0	1	27	1	4	10	6
Snack									
Low-fat yogurt (4 oz.)	115	1	5	66	22	5	11	0	172
Almonds, dry roasted w/o salt added (1 oz.)	169	14	0	0	5	6	0	0	75
Lunch									
Turkey sandwich: whole-wheat bread with lettuce, tomato and mustard	199	1.6	19	446	27	15	67	7	81
Baby carrots (8)	33	0	0	55	8	1	668	5	26
Snack									
Trail mix with nuts, seeds, and dried fruit (½ cup)	176	7	0	2	13	6	0	0	30
Mozzarella string cheese stick, low sodium (1)	78	4.5	15	4	1	8	38	0	205
Dinner									
Whole-wheat pasta with meatless tomato sauce (1½ cups)	363	8	3	818	62	11	99	3	56
Mushrooms (½ cup)	22	0	0	2	4	2	0	3	5
Whole-wheat dinner rolls (2)	149	2.7	0	268	29	5	0	0	59
Broccoli (2 spears)	26	0	0	30	5	2	57	48	30
Fruit salad (1 cup)	93	0	0	2	24	1	28	26	14
Evening Snack									
Skim milk (1 cup)	83	0	0	103	12	8	149	0	299
Multigrain pretzels (½ cup)	76	0	0	2	16	2	0	0	6
Totals	1925	51	52	2110	302	85	1486	163	1481
RDA	1980	<30%	<300	<2300	<58%	48	700	75	1000
% of RDA	97	9	17	92	105	177	212	217	148

*RE = retinol equivalents

Special Dietary Considerations

 LO 6 Explain why children, pregnant women, vegetarians, and those with food allergies or intolerances have special dietary needs and how these needs can be addressed.

Some people have special dietary considerations that affect their needs for certain nutrients. For example, strict vegetarians need to manage their intake of protein, calcium, and certain vitamins, to ensure that they are getting adequate amounts. Children and pregnant women need to consume enough protein, iron, and other essential nutrients that promote growth. The following sections discuss some specific nutrient needs.

Vitamins: B_{12}, D, and Folate

Although most people do not need vitamin supplements if they are eating a healthy diet, people who have increased nutrient needs or special circumstances may benefit from enriched or fortified foods, a multivitamin, or a specific vitamin supplement. For example, strict vegetarians (vegans) who eat no animal foods need to be sure to get enough vitamin B_{12} (found primarily in animal sources) through fortified foods, such as cereals, or by taking a B$_{12}$ supplement. Vegetarians who do not get 15 to 30 minutes of exposure to sunlight every few days may also need to take a vitamin D supplement.

Pregnant women should monitor their folic acid intake to reduce the risk of birth defects. Some older adults have depressed appetites and may not consume enough food. They need to carefully monitor their nutrient intake to ensure that they are meeting their nutritional requirements.

Listed below are other groups that need to carefully monitor their nutrient intake:

- People with a chronic illness that depresses the appetite or limits the absorption of nutrients
- People on medications that affect appetite or digestion
- Athletes engaged in a rigorous exercise training program
- Lactating women
- Individuals on prolonged low-calorie diets

Minerals: Iron and Calcium

Iron is an essential component of red blood cells, which transport oxygen to all our tissues for energy production.

An iron deficiency can result in decreased oxygen transport to tissues, creating an energy crisis. Consuming sufficient iron can be a problem for women who are menstruating, pregnant, or nursing. Indeed, only half of all women of child-bearing age consume the necessary 15 mg of iron per day (5). According to the U.S. Centers for Disease Control and Prevention, approximately 9 percent of women between the ages of 12–49 suffer from iron-deficiency anemia. Although it is not advisable to take an iron supplement unless a physician prescribes it, people at risk for deficiency can modify their diets to ensure that they take in the RDA of iron. The following dietary modifications can help meet this requirement:

- Eat legumes, fresh fruits, whole-grain cereals, and broccoli (all are high in iron).
- Eat foods high in vitamin C, which assists in iron absorption.
- Eat lean red meats (high in iron) at least two or three times per week.
- Eat iron-rich organ meats such as liver once or twice per month.
- Don't drink tea with meals; it interferes with iron absorption.

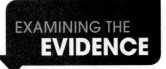

What Is the Glycemic Index and When Is It Helpful?

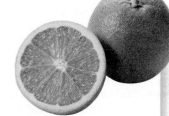

Low-carbohydrate diets are based on the notion that some carbohydrate-rich foods cause a dramatic increase in blood insulin level, which results in increased fat storage and a decrease in blood glucose that increases appetite. The diets are often based on the **glycemic index** (GI) of foods, a measure of the effect a given food will have on the amount of glucose in the blood. The concept is that eating foods with a low glycemic index results in less glucose fluctuation in the blood after a meal, which in turn stabilizes insulin levels and appetite. The typical reference for the GI is pure glucose, which has a GI of 100.

The GI of a food is not always easy to predict. Although some foods that contain simple sugars, such as candy, will logically have a higher GI, some foods with natural sugar, such as an apple (which is high in fructose), will have a lower GI. Additionally, the way the food is prepared and its fat and fiber content can affect its GI ranking. Instant mashed potatoes, white bread, and white rice have higher GIs than oat bran or kidney beans.

The glycemic index can be useful for some individuals, such as people with diabetes, to help them avoid fluctuations in blood glucose levels. In general, if you want to eat foods with lower, rather than higher, GIs, follow these guidelines:

- Eat breakfast cereals made of oats, barley, and bran.
- Eat dense, chewy breads made with whole seeds, not white bread.
- Choose brown rather than white rice.
- Enjoy all types of vegetables.
- Eat plenty of salad vegetables with vinaigrette dressing.
- Balance a meal containing high-GI foods with extra-low-GI foods.
- Add acidic foods (such as citrus fruits) to help slow stomach emptying and reduce the glycemic response.
- Consume fewer sugary foods and beverages.

Glycemic Index Range		
	Range	Example Foods
Low GI	0–55	Apples, oranges, bananas
Medium GI	56–69	White rice, ice cream
High GI	70–100	White bread, crispy rice cereal

The Truth about Gluten

Stories about gluten in the diet and potential health problems associated with gluten consumption are widespread in the media. In response to public concern, many food companies are now offering gluten-free versions of common foods. The market for gluten-free products is exploding, and the majority of food stores stock gluten-free products. So, what's the big deal with eating foods that contain gluten?

Gluten is a protein found in grains such as wheat, barley, and rye. Foods and beverages that may contain gluten are widespread and include beer, breads and other baked goods, cereals, soups, sauces, and many other packaged food products.

Gluten consumption poses a serious health problem for people with celiac disease. This condition, caused by an abnormal immune response to gluten, can damage the lining of the intestine. This damage prevents important nutrients from being absorbed. The incidence of celiac disease is estimated as about 1 percent of the U.S. population. A small number of people who do not have celiac disease also experience an allergic reaction to gluten or have gluten sensitivity.

For those with celiac disease or gluten sensitivity, consumption of gluten-free foods is essential to remain healthy. However, if you do not suffer from these conditions, is a gluten-free diet healthier than a diet that contains gluten? The short answer is no. Indeed, for people who are not allergic to gluten, a gluten-free diet has not been shown to be a healthier diet compared to diets containing gluten. A poorly balanced gluten-free diet can lack vitamins, minerals, and fiber. Therefore, unless you suffer from celiac disease or a gluten allergy problem, there is little reason to avoid gluten-rich foods.

Calcium is the most abundant mineral in the body and is essential for building bones and teeth and for normal nerve and muscle function. Consuming adequate calcium is especially important for pregnant or lactating women. Emerging evidence suggests that calcium may reduce the risk of both prostate and colon cancer (3).

The most recent RDAs call for a significant increase in calcium intake for both sexes beginning at age 9. Children between 9 and 18 years of age should consume 1,300 mg of calcium each day. Adequate calcium intake during childhood and adolescence may be important in preventing osteoporosis in later years, which strikes 1 in 2 women and 1 in 5 men over the age of 50 (4). Adults over age 18 should consume 1,000 mg of calcium per day.

The following recommendations can help you get the calcium you need:

- Add low-fat or nonfat dairy products to your diet.

- Choose other calcium-rich alternatives, such as canned fish (with bones, packed in water), turnip and mustard greens, and broccoli.

- Eat foods rich in vitamin C to boost calcium absorption.

- Use an acidic dressing, made with citrus juices or vinegar, to enhance calcium absorption from salad greens.

Vegetarian Diet

People choose a vegetarian diet for a variety of reasons including health, religion, or animal rights. Vegetarian diets can be healthy, but it is important to know how to plan meals that will meet the body's need for protein, iron, calcium, vitamin B_{12}, and other nutrients that are found in high quantities in animal sources. Because B_{12} is primarily found in animal sources, there may be a need for vegetarians to supplement this vitamin. Vegans need to ensure that their diet contains all the essential amino acids to avoid a loss of lean tissue (muscle, internal organs, etc.)

Food Allergies and Intolerances

A *food allergy* is an adverse immune reaction to a particular food, which can be life-threatening. According to the nonprofit organization Food Allergy Research and Education (FARE), about 15 million Americans have at least one food allergy. The CDC estimates that food allergies affect 4% to 6% of U.S. children under age 18 and reports that the incidence of food allergies among both children and adults is increasing. FARE reports the most common food allergens are milk, eggs, peanuts, tree nuts, soy, wheat, fish, and shellfish.

A *food intolerance* (also called food sensitivity) is an adverse reaction to a specific food that is not caused by the immune system. Intolerance/sensitivity can produce a wide range of symptoms, including headache and digestive problems. Food intolerance examples include lactose intolerance (reaction to the sugar in milk and dairy products) and gluten intolerance (reaction to gluten, a protein found in wheat and other grains).

People who suffer from a food allergy or intolerance can still achieve a balanced diet by replacing the offending foods with healthy choices that provide similar nutrients. It may be helpful for affected individuals to consult with a trained nutrition professional for assistance in planning healthy meals.

MAKE SURE YOU **KNOW...**

- Some people, including children and pregnant or lactating women, have special nutrient needs that may require increasing the intake of foods that provide certain nutrients and/or taking a vitamin or mineral supplement.

- It is important for those who choose a strict vegetarian (vegan) diet to make sure they consume the recommended amounts of macro- and micronutrients.

- People with food allergies or intolerances can achieve a balanced diet by replacing the offending foods with healthy choices that provide similar nutrients.

—MasteringHealth™

Does Exercise Alter Your Nutrition Requirements?

 LO 7 **Describe how rigorous exercise training alters a person's nutrition requirements.**

Exercise training requires stored carbohydrates and fat to provide the energy to support working muscles. Prolonged exercise results in a loss of body water and electrolytes due to the increased sweating required to cool the body during exertion. Therefore, important questions arise for active people. First, does rigorous exercise training alter the body's macro- and micronutrient requirements? If so, do athletes and other physically active people require dietary supplements (such as protein or vitamins) for optimal performance and health? We'll explore these questions in the sections that follow.

Nutrition for Exercise

Athletes and people who exercise regularly need to pay attention to the three Rs after exercise: rehydrate, replenish (body fuels, vitamins, and minerals), and repair (consume amino acids for muscle protein synthesis) (11). Good nutritional practices benefit athletes and physically active people in the following ways:

- Replacing body fluid and electrolytes lost during exercise

- Providing the needed fuel to perform exercise

- Promoting the optimal fitness gains from an exercise training program

- Providing enhanced recovery between workouts

- Achieving and maintaining a desired body composition

- Providing the many health benefits associated with a healthy diet

Because of differences in exercise training programs between individuals (variations in type of exercise, intensity, and duration), no single diet meets the needs of all active people. Getting the right amount of energy and nutrients to remain healthy and perform well is the key. Consuming too much energy (too many calories) will increase body fat, while not consuming enough will impede your ability to exercise. Beyond general guidelines for health, people engaged in rigorous exercise training have additional nutritional considerations that are important to optimize training and promote recovery between exercise sessions.

Does Exercise Increase Your Need for Carbohydrates and Fat?

Carbohydrates are the backbone of nutrition for many athletes and highly active individuals. However, carbohydrate consumption has become a widespread topic of debate because many popular diet books are based on low- and moderate-carbohydrate eating plans. Therefore, many active people are confused about the role of carbohydrates in the diet.

Although the recommendations for dietary carbohydrates have continued to evolve, the central idea that a diet rich in carbohydrates is important for active people has not changed. A carbohydrate-rich diet ensures that body stores of carbohydrates (glycogen in muscles and the liver) are adequate to meet the energy needs of exercise training. Sports nutritionists and exercise scientists often recommend that people participating in daily exercise programs should increase the complex carbohydrates in their diet from 58% to 70% of total calories consumed (fat intake is then reduced to 18% of total caloric intake) (7, 8).

The carbohydrate needs of active individuals are closely tied to the types of exercises performed and the daily training load (intensity and duration of exercise). So rather than ingesting a constant amount of carbohydrates every day, active individuals should vary their carbohydrate intake based on their fuel needs. Note that the intensity and duration of the exercise determines whether carbohydrates or fat are the predominant source of energy production (6, 7) For example, during prolonged (i.e., >30 minutes) low-intensity exercise (25% $\dot{V}O_2$ max) your body largely relies on

---

glycemic index Ranking system for carbohydrates based on a food's effect on blood glucose levels.

steps ▶ FOR BEHAVIOR CHANGE

Are you making the best choices when you eat out?

In almost any restaurant it is possible to make healthy food choices.
Take the following quiz to assess your current behavior.

Y N

☐ ☐ Do you typically order the largest size on the menu?

☐ ☐ Do you always order a fried entree or sandwich?

☐ ☐ Do you always order french fries?

☐ ☐ Is soda your default beverage?

☐ ☐ Are your sandwiches and salads typically loaded with mayonnaise, creamy dressings, or other high-fat sauces?

If you answered yes to more than two of these questions, you're probably consuming high amounts of fat and calories with every meal. Fortunately, there's a lot you can do to improve the nutritional quality of your meal by making better choices.

Tips for Eating Out

Tomorrow, you will:

☑ Review restaurant menus ahead of time (many are available online) to check the calorie and nutrient content of items you are likely to order.

☑ Select alternate items to replace any that do not fit with your healthier dietary plan.

Within the next 2 weeks, you will:

☑ Make healthier choices when eating out. For example, you can order small-sized items instead of large servings. Depending on the restaurant, a double cheeseburger may contain 600–700 calories, 30–40 grams of fat, 120–140 mg of cholesterol, and 1,000–1,200 mg of sodium! You'll be surprised how satisfied you'll be with a single burger and a salad or vegetable, and you'll save a ton of calories.

☑ Forgo sauces and creamy salad dressing. A typical tablespoon of tartar sauce contains about 20 grams of fat and 220 mg of sodium, and a tablespoon of mayonnaise adds 100 calories and 11 grams of fat.

☑ Order grilled meat instead of fried. Breaded chicken typically contains double the amount of fat as grilled.

☑ Choose healthier sides: Order a salad or steamed veggies instead of french fries, and fresh fruit instead of a heavy dessert.

☑ Skip the soda or milkshake. Drink water, nonfat milk, or 100% juice without added sugar with your meal.

By the end of the semester, you will:

☑ Decrease the number of times per week you eat in restaurants and consistently make healthy choices when you do dine out.

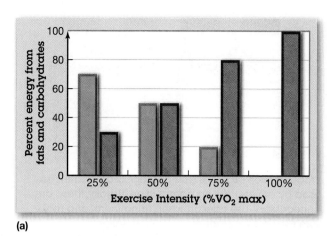

(a)

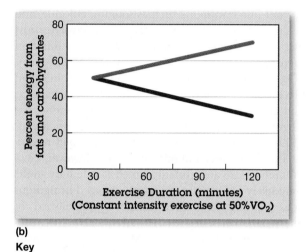

(b)

Key

▬ Fat

▬ Carbohydrate

FIGURE 8.9 The influence of exercise intensity and duration on fuel use. (A) The impact of exercise intensity on fat and carbohydrate use during exercise. Increasing intensity increases the reliance on carbohydrate as fuel. (B) The impact of exercise duration on fuel use during exercise. Increasing duration increases the reliance on fat as fuel.

TABLE 8.7 ■ Amount of Carbohydrate Needed to Sustain Daily Activity Levels		
Training Load	Type of Training	Carbohydrate Intake Target
Light	Low-intensity exercise (e.g., walking ~30 minutes/day)	3–5 grams per kilogram of body weight
Moderate	Moderate-intensity exercise (e.g., running, cycling, or resistance exercise 30–60 minutes/day)	5–7 grams per kilogram of body weight
High	High-intensity exercise (e.g., running, cycling, or swimming 1–3 hours/day)	6–10 grams per kilogram of body weight

Increasing the amount of complex carbohydrates in the diet and maintaining sufficient caloric intake can ensure that an adequate supply of energy from carbohydrates is stored in the muscles and liver to meet the needs of a rigorous exercise program. Therefore, individuals engaged in regular bouts of endurance exercise training (such as running or cycling) for more 30 minutes per day would likely benefit from a diet rich in complex carbohydrates. The target for carbohydrate intake depends upon your body size and your daily exercise intensity and duration (**TABLE 8.7**). For example, if your body weight is 70 kg (150 lb), and your daily exercise involves walking 30 minutes per day (low-intensity exercise), your diet should contain 210 to 250 grams of complex carbohydrates per day. Use Table 8.7 to determine how much carbohydrate you need to support your exercise routine.

Protein Needs Can Be Met Through Diet

Bodybuilders and others engaged in rigorous resistance training often consume large quantities of protein in the form of supplements in addition to the protein they consume in food, believing that this will promote the growth of muscle. Unfortunately, they're drinking protein shakes and eating protein bars largely in vain because research has shown that a well-balanced diet meets the protein requirements of most athletes (11–13).

How much protein is needed to maintain a healthy body and support exercise-induced muscle growth? Thousands of substances in the body are made of proteins, which make up about 17–20% of body weight. All cells undergo a continuous process of protein maintenance by removing damaged proteins and replacing them with new ones. The ability to manufacture these new proteins requires an ample supply of both nonessential and essential amino acids (the building blocks of proteins). The current RDA for protein in most adults is 0.8 grams per kilogram of body weight, so a 150-pound (70 kg) man would need about 56 grams of protein daily, and a 125-pound (57 kg)

fat as a fuel source, while carbohydrates are the dominant fuel source during higher-intensity exercise (75% $\dot{V}O_2$ max) (**FIGURE 8.9A**). During prolonged exercise at a moderate intensity (40–60% $\dot{V}O_2$ max), there is a progressive decrease in carbohydrate metabolism and an increasing reliance on fat as a fuel (**FIGURE 8.9B**). Although moderate-intensity exercise does require fat as a fuel source, there is no need to increase your intake of fat because your body has adequate fat stores to provide the needed energy.

In most cases, the energy you use during a workout comes from energy stored from meals eaten several hours before your exercise session. Hence, products such as sports drinks and carbohydrate gels are not necessary to provide energy during exercise training lasting less than 90 minutes.

woman would need about 46 grams per day. This level of protein intake can be met by a balanced dietary intake of meat, seafood, nuts, seeds, and vegetables.

Both endurance and resistance exercise training increase the rate of muscle protein synthesis and therefore, the RDA may not meet the protein needs of these individuals. Sports nutrition experts suggest that those engaged in rigorous resistance or endurance exercise training should consider increasing their daily protein intake above the RDA to 1.2 to 1.6 grams of protein per kilogram of body weight (11). This higher protein requirement can be easily achieved with protein-containing foods, without the need for protein supplementation.

Can a high-protein diet cause harm? In general, a diet that does not exceed 1.6 grams of protein per kilogram of body weight per day is not considered harmful (4). However, if a high-protein diet comes from meat sources that are high in saturated fats and cholesterol, this could increase the risk of heart disease. If a high-protein diet involves a reduced intake of fruits and vegetables, this puts a person at risk of not meeting daily requirements for some vitamins and minerals. A high-protein diet can also increase the work of the kidneys, so some nutritionists caution against protein intakes exceeding the recommended upper limits for active people. At present, it is not known if long-term consumption of a high-protein diet results in kidney damage in humans.

Consuming high-quality protein at each meal is important to ensure that the amino acids required for muscle protein synthesis are available throughout the day. Because protein synthesis is a continuous process, amino acids must be available at all times in order for cells to manufacture new proteins.

Research reveals that the timing of protein intake can optimize exercise-induced protein synthesis in skeletal muscles. For example, consuming approximately 20 grams of high-quality protein before exercise or within 30 to 60 minutes following exercise can increase protein synthesis in the exercised muscles (11). This can be achieved by consuming a milk protein (milk contains the high-quality proteins casein and whey). Note that consuming more than 20 grams of protein before or after exercise does not promote additional gains in muscle protein synthesis. The "extra" amino acids are used as fuel or stored as fat (11).

Water and Micronutrients

We have seen the important role that water plays in the body. Failure to adequately replace fluids throughout the day can lead to dehydration, which results in an elevated heart rate, fatigue, and an inability to cool the body. These symptoms increase as the level of dehydration becomes more severe.

Consuming water throughout the day is important because the body loses water in both urine and feces. Exercise results in increased water loss due to sweating. Because sweat contains electrolytes, the body also loses

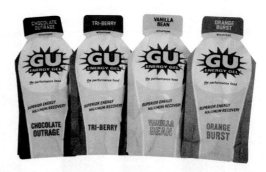

Products such as sports gels and drinks are sometimes used by athletes during competition. Usually, these are unnecessary. Use caution when using them, and make sure they are appropriate for your situation.

important micronutrients such as sodium, chloride, and potassium. The amount of water and electrolytes lost during exercise depends upon the intensity and duration of exercise and the environmental conditions. For example, high-intensity exercise generates more body heat and results in an increased sweat rate, as does exercise in a hot, humid environment. Also, the longer you exercise, the more you sweat, and the greater the loss of body water.

The Institute of Medicine (IOM) has issued recommendations for water and mineral intake; however, these recommendations are primarily aimed at sedentary adults and are likely inadequate for people engaged in rigorous exercise training. RDA values cannot be established for water intake because of the large variation in water needs across the population, so the IOM established adequate intake values of 16 cups (3.7 liters) of water per day for males and 12 cups (2.7 liters) of water for females (10). These numbers represent total water obtained in food and beverages. While these recommendations are adequate for sedentary individuals, these amounts may not meet the needs of active people.

Recall that the IOM recommendations for salt (sodium and chloride) for sedentary adults are 1.5 grams/day of sodium and 2.3 grams/day of chloride. The current recommendation for potassium is 4.7 grams/day. While these amounts are adequate for sedentary people, they are not enough to meet the needs of active individuals who lose a significant amount of sodium, chloride, and potassium in sweat.

So, what are the guidelines for replacing water and minerals for active people? Below are some practical tips for replacing water and electrolytes during periods of heavy exercise and profuse sweating (10):

- If you exercise daily, record your weight before and after each exercise session. The difference in weight before and after exercise will reflect the amount of body water loss due to sweating. Drink 3 cups of water (~0.7 liters) for every pound (i.e., ~0.5 kilogram) of weight loss during exercise.

- Consume water before, during, and immediately following exercise. Consuming 2 cups (0.5 liters) of water 30 to 60 minutes before exercise will help prevent dehydration.

▪ Weigh yourself each morning. If you notice that your body is a pound (~0.5 kg) lower than the previous morning, you may be dehydrated and need to increase your fluid intake during the day.

▪ A practical indicator of your hydration status is the color of urine. If the color of your urine in the morning is more like apple juice than lemonade, drink more water during the day. The goal is achieve urine that is the color of lemonade; this reflects an adequate state of hydration.

▪ Thirst is not always adequate to prompt you to drink enough to completely replace water lost during exercise.

▪ Salt your food to taste; this will assist in replacing sodium and chloride lost in sweat.

▪ For most people, sports drinks are not needed to replace water loss, but they can accelerate the rate of rehydration following exercise and assist in replacing electrolytes. Most sports drinks contain calories, which add to your daily calorie intake.

▪ While it is important to maintain adequate hydration, excessive fluid intake can, in extreme cases,

TABLE 8.8 ▪ Comparison of Popular Dietary Supplements

Supplement	Origin	Benefits Claimed	Evidence of Effectiveness
Caffeine	Compound found in coffee, cola, chocolate, candy, stimulants, weight-loss products.	Used to increase muscle fiber activation to increase strength, or to increase fat metabolism and endurance.	Increases endurance in events lasting more than 20 minutes. No consistent effects on strength.
Carbohydrates	Macronutrient found in most foods. Usually provided as a dietary supplement in the form of beverages or bars.	Increase in stored glucose in muscle and liver and increase in endurance.	Improves endurance in events longer than 90–120 minutes. Also helps restore glucose after exercise.
Protein	Macronutrient contained in many foods. Found as a dietary supplement in the form of beverages (shakes), powder, or bars.	Increase muscle protein synthesis	Consumption of high-quality protein immediately following exercise has been shown to promote small increases in muscle protein synthesis.
l-carnitine	Made by the body and ingested in meat products.	Increases transport of fat in cells, reduces lactate accumulation.	Carnitine is in adequate supply in the cells, and additional amounts provide no benefit before, during, or after exercise.
Chromium picolinate	Trace element found in several foods; picolinate is added to supplements to aid absorption.	Helps insulin action and is thought to aid glucose metabolism, blood fats, and have anabolic effects.	No good evidence for any benefits. *Side effects: Stomach upset, anemia, genetic damage, kidney damage.*
Coenzyme Q-10	Made by the body as a component of the biochemical pathway that makes adenosine triphosphate (ATP).	Enhances ATP production.	No evidence suggests a benefit during or after exercise.
Creatine	Made by the body and also found in meat products.	Decreases fatigue in short, intense exercise. Increases muscle size and strength.	Increases endurance in short, intense exercise. Causes water gain in muscle but not increases in strength.
Echinacea	Herbal supplement.	Reduces duration of colds, boosts immune system, heals wounds.	Some evidence suggests it may be beneficial for these conditions. *Side effects: Uncommon, but possible GI upset, chills, nausea.*
Ginkgo biloba	Extracts of dried leaves of *Ginkgo* plant.	Used for antioxidant properties and to improve blood flow and memory.	Does have antioxidant properties that may be beneficial in improving blood flow, improving neural function, and reducing production of stress hormones. *Side effects: Nausea, headache, dizziness, skin rash, hemorrhage if used with blood thinners.*
St. John's wort	Plant extract.	Used to treat depression and external wounds, burns, and muscle aches.	Some evidence suggests that it is beneficial for treating these conditions.

lead to a low sodium concentration (hyponatremia), which is a dangerous condition. Therefore, fluid replacement following exercise should approximate the volume of water lost in sweat.

High Vitamin Intake Does Not Improve Performance

Some supplement manufacturers promote the concept that mega-doses of vitamins can improve the exercise training response and exercise performance. This premise is based on the idea that exercise increases the need for energy and, because some vitamins are necessary for the breakdown of foods for energy, an extra load of vitamins (above the RDA) is required. There is no evidence to support this claim (also see next section), and the vitamin requirements of athletes and active people can be met by a well-balanced diet (8, 9). However, vitamin supplementation may be recommended by physicians or nutritionists for individuals with a clinically documented deficiency.

Mega-doses of vitamins can interfere with the delicate balance of other micronutrients and can also be toxic (4). For example, supplementation with very high levels of vitamin E can increase the time required for blood clotting (4). Therefore, indiscriminate supplementation with mega-doses of vitamins is unwise.

Antioxidants

Exercise results in increased production of free radicals in the working muscles. **Free radicals** (also referred to as radicals) are potentially harmful products that, if produced in large quantities, can damage cells (14). Fortunately, cells contain **antioxidants** that neutralize radicals and protect cellular components against radical-mediated damage (14). Antioxidants come in several forms. Some are proteins synthesized by cells, and many are found in the diet. Dietary antioxidants include vitamins C and E, beta-carotene (vitamin A precursor), and micronutrients such as copper, zinc, and selenium.

Because exercise increases the production of radicals, many supplement companies claim that active people can benefit from antioxidant supplementation. To date, there is no scientific evidence to support this idea (14). In fact, studies have shown that high doses (well above the RDA) of vitamins C and E may result in adverse effects such as blunting the exercise training response (14). Therefore, antioxidant supplementation is not recommended for people who consume a well-balanced diet.

MAKE SURE YOU **KNOW**...

- The amount of carbohydrate and fat used as fuel during exercise will vary according to the intensity of the exercise.
- Active people need to increase their carbohydrate intake to match the exercise demands.

- Consuming adequate protein with each meal is important to allow the body to replace and repair damaged proteins.
- Excess vitamin intake via supplements does not improve health or exercise performance.

— MasteringHealth™

Do Supplements Provide Improved Health or Performance?

LO **8** List the pros and cons of dietary supplement use.

The dietary supplement industry is large and growing. Over the past two decades, the use of nutritional and pharmaceutical supplements has become common. In 2014, American consumers spent more than $13 billion on these products. With their wide availability and so many marketing claims being made, it's important to understand both how this industry is regulated and when it may be appropriate to use supplements.

Regulation of Supplement Products

The U.S. Food and Drug Administration (FDA) estimates that over 25,000 products are available as dietary supplements. Many people assume that these products face the same rigorous FDA oversight as prescription drugs. Unfortunately, this is not the case due to a federal law in place since 1994. Manufacturers are required to attest that their products are safe in small quantities, but unlike prescription drugs, supplements are not tested by the FDA before they go to market. In fact, recent studies reveal that many over-the-counter supplements do not contain the ingredients shown on the label. For example, a study conducted by the International Olympic Committee tested more than 630 supplements from different companies around the world. Many products did not contain the contents specified on the label, and approximately 15% contained substances that would lead to a positive result in doping tests used during Olympic competition.

While the products themselves are not regulated by the FDA, the claims made on supplement labels are. Manufacturers are permitted to claim effects on the "structure or function" of the body, but they are not allowed to make claims concerning the prevention or cure of disease. For example, a company selling a calcium supplement can claim that consuming calcium "maintains healthy bones" without seeking FDA approval. In contrast, approval is required to claim that a calcium supplement will "prevent fragile bones in postmenopausal women." While manufacturers are required to document evidence for structure/function claims, be aware that the FDA does not examine the legitimacy of this documentation. Therefore, manufacturers must include on their labels a disclaimer stating that their product is not a drug and did not receive FDA approval.

Should You Use Supplements?

Although media, sports, and fitness celebrities often recommend specific dietary supplements to improve health, there is limited scientific evidence to validate the health or performance claims. Scientific reports on the use of supplements conclude that most offer no health benefits (14), and consuming mega-doses of certain supplements can pose a health risk (14–16). See **TABLE 8.8** on page 235 for an overview of some popular supplement products.

The indiscriminate use of dietary supplements can be expensive and even dangerous. But there are cases in which careful use of a supplement (such as vitamin D to correct a deficiency) can provide benefits. Since supplements are not tightly regulated in this country, the consumer is ultimately responsible for determining whether a specific product is necessary or safe (see the Consumer Corner box on page 238). It is often a good idea to consult with your health-care provider or a trained nutrition professional for help in deciding if a supplement product is right for you. If you elect to use a supplement, it is wise to choose a product that has been tested by an independent agency. Products with the USP Verified Dietary Supplement seal on their label have been verified by the U.S. Pharmacopeial Convention (USP), a nonprofit organization that has established standards for the identity and purity of supplements. These products have been submitted for testing by USP laboratories and their ingredients have been confirmed to contain the ingredients listed on the product label, to be consistent from batch to batch, and to meet acceptable limits for contamination.

MAKE SURE YOU **KNOW...**

- Supplements should never replace foods as major sources of dietary nutrients.
- Supplements are not tested or approved by the FDA, but the agency does have certain mandates in regard to claims made on product labels.
- Because dietary supplements are poorly regulated in the United States, consumers should be cautious when choosing and using these products.

MasteringHealth ™

Food Safety and Food Technology

LO ❾ Describe the major issues of food safety and how changes in food technology affect the food we consume.

Choosing a wide variety of healthy foods is essential to achieving a healthy diet. Ensuring that the food you eat is safe and free of contaminants is also very important.

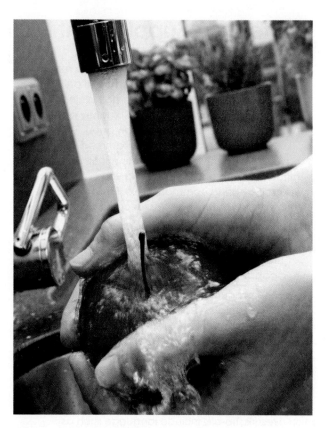

Washing fresh produce under running tap water will help you avoid foodborne illness.

Foodborne Illness

If a food carries a disease-causing microorganism, such as a bacterium, consuming the food can potentially make you sick. According to the U.S. Centers for Disease Control and Prevention, approximately 48 million cases of foodborne bacterial disease occur each year in the United States (17). These illnesses produce nausea, vomiting, and diarrhea from 12 hours to 5 days after infection. The severity of the illness depends on the microorganism ingested and the victim's overall health. Foodborne infections can be fatal in children, people with compromised immune systems, or other people in ill health.

You may have heard about *Salmonella* and *Escherichia coli (E. coli)* in news reports. The *Salmonella* bacterium is usually found in raw or undercooked chicken and eggs and in processed meats. A particular strain of the *Escherichia coli* bacterium,

see it!

ABC VIDEOS

Watch the "FDA Proposes New Food Safety Rules" ABC News Video online at MasteringHealth™.

free radicals Oxygen molecules that can potentially damage cells.

antioxidants Molecules that neutralize free radicals, preventing them from causing damage to cells.

Detecting Supplement Fraud

Most of the dietary supplements on the market today do not promote good health or improved exercise performance. They often do nothing more than cheat consumers out of their money and some products may do more harm than good.

How can you avoid being scammed? Marketers have sophisticated ways of making their products attractive to potential buyers, but you can protect yourself by using common sense. Beware of the following techniques, claims, or catch-phrases:

- **The product "does it all."** Be suspicious of any supplement that claims an extremely broad range of benefits. No one product is likely to be capable of such a wide range of effectiveness.

- **The product is supported by personal testimonials.** Testimonials are not necessarily true; sometimes they are complete fiction, or the person supporting the product has been paid for his or her statements. Because testimonials are difficult to prove, there is a possibility of fraud.

- **The product provides a "quick fix."** Be skeptical of products that claim to produce immediate results. Tip-offs include language such as, "Provides relief in days," or "You'll feel energized immediately." Legitimate products often take some time to produce an effect in the body.

- **The product is "natural."** The term *natural* suggests that the product is safer than conventional treatments. Any product—synthetic or natural—that is potent enough to produce a significant physiological effect is potent enough to cause side effects.

- **The product is "a new, breakthrough treatment."** Be suspicious of any product that claims to be based on "cutting edge" research you haven't heard about. If a "new discovery" were really so revolutionary, it would be widely reported in the media and prescribed by health professionals, not featured in obscure ads.

- **Your "satisfaction is guaranteed."** Money-back guarantees are often empty promises. The makers of this claim know that most people won't go to the trouble of returning a product for a refund.

- **Ads contain meaningless medical jargon.** The use of scientific-sounding terms such as "aerobic enzyme booster" may seem impressive and may even contain an element of truth, but these terms likely cover up a lack of scientific data concerning the product.

Always ask yourself, "Does this claim seem too good to be true?" If it does, then the product is probably a fraud. If you're still not sure, talk to your health-care provider or a trained nutrition professional. The Better Business Bureau or your state attorney general's office can tell you whether other consumers have lodged complaints about a product or company; if there have been many complaints, proceed with caution. The Federal Trade Commission provides information on fraudulent products and health-related scams at http://www.consumer.ftc.gov/health.

O157:H7, is sometimes found in contaminated raw or undercooked ground beef and can lead to bloody diarrhea, among other symptoms.

To reduce your risk of foodborne illness, follow these guidelines:

- Select foods that are clean and fresh.
- Wash produce thoroughly with running water; use a vegetable brush on firm fruits and vegetables.
- Drink only pasteurized milk and juices.
- Don't eat raw eggs.
- When storing perishable foods, keep them cold or frozen to prevent bacterial growth.
- Cook all meat products thoroughly (using a meat thermometer ensures safety). When dining out, order meats cooked to at least medium doneness.
- Cook all shellfish thoroughly.
- Avoid raw fish; it may contain parasitic round-worms. Cook fresh fish within two days or freeze it for later use.
- Use separate sets of cutting boards and knives for meat and produce; chopping raw meat and vegetables with the same knife, without washing it thoroughly first, can lead to cross-contamination.
- Wash utensils, plates, cutting boards, knives, and other cooking tools in hot water and dish detergent after each use.

See the Consumer Corner box on page 239 for more about minimizing your risk for foodborne illness.

Keep Hot Foods Hot and Cold Foods Cold to Avoid Foodborne Illness

Whether from restaurants, supermarkets, or other establishments, take-out foods have become part of our way of life. But to avoid foodborne illnesses, you must keep these foods at the appropriate temperature. The next time you order take-out or bring food to a party or family function, keep the following recommendations in mind.

food in a microwave oven—cover and rotate—and then let it stand for 2 minutes to ensure thorough, even heating.

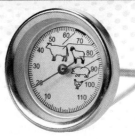

For Hot Foods

- Keep hot foods above 140°F. You can cover food with foil (to keep it moist) and keep it warm—140°F or above—in the oven (check the food's temperature with a meat thermometer). Using a slow cooker is another option for some foods. It's best to eat food within 2 hours of preparation.

- If the food won't be eaten for more than 2 hours, refrigerate it in shallow, covered containers. Before serving, reheat it in an oven to 165°F or until it's hot and steaming. If you prefer, reheat

For Cold Foods

- Keep cold foods at 40°F or below.

- If cold foods are not eaten right away, refrigerate them as soon as possible.

- Discard any foods kept at room temperature for more than 2 hours. If conditions are warmer than 90°F, toss the food after only 1 hour.

- Transport and store cold foods in chilled insulated coolers.

- If you're going to serve a platter of deli meats, place it on ice to keep it cool.

Source: USDA Food Safety and Inspection Service. *Cooking for Groups: A Volunteer's Guide to Food Safety.* Item #604H, Pueblo, CO 81009.

Food Additives

Food additives are used by manufacturers for a variety of reasons: to improve nutritional quality, as a preservative to maintain freshness or increase shelf life, to improve taste or color, or to make it more appealing in some other way. Among the most commonly used additives are sugar, salt, and corn syrup. Other additives, such as monosodium glutamate (MSG) and sulfites, may cause a reaction in people who are sensitive to them. Nitrites, which are found in bacon, sausages, deli meats, and other processed foods, may also form cancer-causing agents (nitrosamines) in the body. If you are sensitive to a particular food additive, read labels carefully and avoid foods that contain additives to which you are likely to have a reaction.

Organically Grown Foods

As consumers become more aware of the quality of the foods they eat, they are buying increasing quantities of **organic** foods. *Organic* refers to foods grown without the use of pesticides, hormones, antibiotics, or chemical fertilizers. The United States, European Union, Japan, and many other countries require producers to obtain

certification before marketing a food as organic.

USDA-certified organic products display a symbol on product packaging (**FIGURE 8.10**). Organic produce in supermarkets is identified with a sticker code that starts with the number 9. Produce sold at local farmers' markets is not marked with these stickers, but you can ask farmers about their growing practices.

For consumers who buy conventionally grown produce, the Environmental Working Group (www.ewg.org) publishes an annual shopper's guide to pesticides, each year naming the Dirty Dozen (containing the most pesticide residue) and the Clean 15 (containing the least).

Animals raised on factory farms live in close quarters and are often treated with antibiotics to prevent infections. Though there is little evidence at this time, some people are concerned that consuming meat or dairy products

see it!

ABC VIDEOS

Watch the "Organic Produce" ABC News Video online at MasteringHealth™.

organic Plant or animal foods that are grown without the use of pesticides, chemical fertilizers, antibiotics, or hormones.

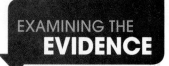

Are Organic Foods Healthier than Conventional Foods?

The U.S. market for organic foods has grown rapidly over the past two decades, and organic products are now widely available in specialty food stores, supermarkets, and online. Public interest largely stems from consumers' desire to improve their diets and the belief that organic foods offer health advantages over conventional foods.

Organic farms grow crops and raise livestock in ways that avoid the use of synthetic chemicals, hormones, antibiotics, genetically modified crops, and irradiation (1). The U.S. Department of Agriculture (USDA) has established standards that include specific requirements for both crops and livestock. For example, to qualify as organic, crops must be produced on farms that have not used pesticides, herbicides, or fertilizer for three years before harvest (1). Organic livestock must have access to the outdoors and are raised without the use of antibiotics and hormones. Organic farmers apply for government certification, pass a test, and agree to annual inspections to ensure compliance with USDA standards.

Are organic foods healthier than conventional foods? A complete answer to this question is not yet available because there are not enough human studies that investigate whether organic diets result in less disease than diets composed of conventional foods (1, 2). However, studies comparing the nutritional differences between organic and conventional foods provide some insights (2):

- Current evidence suggests that conventional foods (vegetables and animal products) contain similar nutrient levels when compared to organic foods.

- Organic produce contains fewer pesticide residues than conventional produce and therefore, consuming a diet of organic produce should reduce your exposure to pesticides.

- No differences exist between organic and conventional foods (vegetables and animal

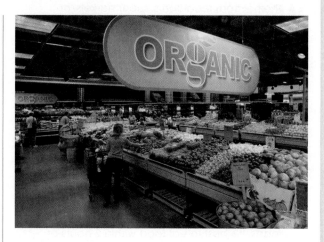

products) regarding the risk of bacterial contamination.

- Conventional chicken and pork products have a higher risk for contamination with bacteria that are resistant to antibiotics compared to organic alternatives.

In summary, current evidence indicates that consuming organic foods should reduce your risk of pesticide exposure and could lower your contact with antibiotic-resistant bacteria. While organic foods appear to provide some health benefits over conventional foods, additional studies are required to determine if a lifetime consumption of organic foods will reduce the risk of disease and increase human lifespan. Stay tuned!

References

1. Forman, J. and J. Silverman: Organic Foods: Health and Environmental Advantages and Disadvantages. American Academy of Pediatrics. 2012. E1406-E1415.

2. Smith-Spangler, C. et al. Are organic foods safer or healthier than conventional alternatives?: A systematic Review. Ann. Internal Med. 2012. 157:348–366.

from these animals could lead to the development of antibiotic-resistant bacteria in humans.

Some farmers use hormones in animals to increase meat and milk production. Recombinant bovine growth hormone (rBGH), also known as recombinant bovine somatotropin, is used to increase milk production in dairy cows. Some consumers fear that hormones in food may cause health problems in humans (such as increased cancer risk), so many supermarket chains are restricting

the sale of milk containing these hormones. Producers whose dairy products do not contain rBGH will state that on the carton or label.

Many people choose to eat organic foods for health or environmental reasons. Presently, there is limited evidence to support the idea that organic foods are nutritionally superior to their nonorganic counterparts, but research is continuing (see Examining the Evidence, above). Organic foods tend to be more expensive, but as consumer demand increases, prices may move closer to that of non-organic food. Buying organic produce in-season through farmers' markets or community co-ops is sometimes no more expensive than conventional produce.

Irradiated and Bioengineered Foods

Irradiation is sometimes used to kill microorganisms in foods and to prolong the shelf life of the food (17). Irradiated food can be stored for years in sealed containers at room temperature without spoiling. In addition, irradiation can delay the sprouting of vegetables such as potatoes and onions and delay the ripening of fruits such as bananas, tomatoes, and avocados. This can result in significant cost savings.

Are these irradiated foods safe to eat? Currently, most research indicates that these foods are safe and that the nutritional content is maintained (17). Irradiated foods must be identified with a symbol on product packaging (**FIGURE 8.11**).

Another practice that has become controversial is the use of bioengineered foods, known as genetically modified (GM) foods, which are produced from genetically modified organisms (GMOs). Bioengineering involves inserting the genes from one plant or animal species into another plant or animal's DNA to achieve a desired trait. Crops such as corn and tomatoes have been bioengineered to improve yields, pest resistance, and longevity (which improves their ability to be shipped long distances). Although there are benefits from bioengineering, the practice is considered by some countries to be unproven and possibly unsafe.

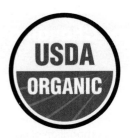

FIGURE 8.10 Organic food symbol

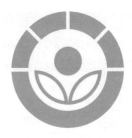

FIGURE 8.11 Irradiated food symbol

MAKE SURE YOU **KNOW...**

- Proper food storage and preparation are essential in preventing foodborne illness.
- The use of the word *organic* on food labels is strictly regulated; organic foods are grown without the use of pesticides, hormones, antibiotics, or chemical fertilizers.
- Irradiation and bioengineering are two forms of food technology that are used to enhance food safety and increase yields and pest resistance. Both techniques remain somewhat controversial in terms of long-term safety for humans.

MasteringHealth™

irradiation The use of radiation to kill microorganisms that grow on or in food.

Sample Program for Changing Daily Caloric Intake

Scan to plan your individualized program for nutrition.

The plan below is for an individual who needs to change the composition of daily caloric intake and reduce the overall caloric intake. (Also consider the recommendations from the MyPlate.gov dietary analysis in Laboratory 8.1.) Specific recommendations for weight loss, weight gain, or change due to an increase in physical activity will vary. Note that the plan presented does not eliminate all "bad foods," but makes recommendations for allowing sweets or higher-fat foods in moderation. Maintain the changes each week and incorporate the new changes until the recommendations from Myplate.gov are met.

You can eliminate empty calories by cutting down on soda and candy and replacing sugary beverages with water or lower-sugar options.

	Food Category	Monday	Tuesday	Wednesday	Thursday	Friday	Saturday	Sunday
Week 1	Caloric Intake	Eliminate at least 150 "empty calories"	Eliminate at least 150 "empty calories"			Eliminate at least 150 "empty calories"	Eliminate at least 150 "empty calories"	
	Beverages and Alcohol	Replace beverages with water or lower-fat options	Replace beverages with water or lower-fat options	Replace beverages with water or lower-fat options	Replace beverages with water or lower-fat options	(1) Replace beverages with water or lower-fat options (2) If you drink alcohol, limit to 1–2 drinks	Replace beverages with water or lower-fat options	Replace beverages with water or lower-fat options
	Fruits and Vegetables							
	Carbohydrates							
	Protein							
	Fats			Substitute a low-fat option for a high-fat food	Substitute a low-fat option for a high-fat food			Substitute a low-fat option for a high-fat food
	Reward							Allow a splurge of one serving of a food you enjoy

	Food Category	Monday	Tuesday	Wednesday	Thursday	Friday	Saturday	Sunday
Week 2	**Caloric Intake**							
	Beverages and Alcohol							
	Fruits and Vegetables	Increase fruit and vegetable intake, and eat a variety of fruits and vegetables		Increase fruit and vegetable intake, and eat a variety of fruits and vegetables		Increase fruit and vegetable intake, and eat a variety of fruits and vegetables	Increase fruit and vegetable intake, and eat a variety of fruits and vegetables	
	Carbohydrates		Replace refined carbo-hydrate choices with whole grains		Replace refined carbo-hydrate choices with whole grains			
	Protein	Reduce protein intake		Reduce protein intake		Reduce protein intake	Reduce protein intake	
	Fats							
	Reward							Allow a splurge of one serving of a food you enjoy
Week 3	**Caloric Intake**							
	Beverages and Alcohol	Consume water or low-fat/low-sugar beverages	Consume water or low-fat/low-sugar beverages	Consume water or low-fat/low-sugar beverages	Consume water or low-fat/low-sugar beverages	(1) Consume water or low-fat/low-sugar beverages (2) If you drink alcohol, limit to 1–2 drinks	(1) Consume water or low-fat/low-sugar beverages (2) If you drink alcohol, limit to 1–2 drinks	Consume water or low-fat/low-sugar beverages
	Fruits and Vegetables	Increase fruit and vegetable intake, and eat a variety of fruits and vegetables	Increase fruit and vegetable intake, and eat a variety of fruits and vegetables	Increase fruit and vegetable intake, and eat a variety of fruits and vegetables	Increase fruit and vegetable intake, and eat a variety of fruits and vegetables	Increase fruit and vegetable intake, and eat a variety of fruits and vegetables	Increase fruit and vegetable intake, and eat a variety of fruits and vegetables	Increase fruit and vegetable intake, and eat a variety of fruits and vegetables
	Carbohydrates	Replace refined carbohydrate choices with whole grains	Replace refined carbohydrate choices with whole grains	Replace refined carbohydrate choices with whole grains	Replace refined carbohydrate choices with whole grains	Replace refined carbohydrate choices with whole grains	Replace refined carbohydrate choices with whole grains	Replace refined carbohydrate choices with whole grains
	Protein	Replace high-fat protein sources with a lower-fat protein source	Replace high-fat protein sources with a lower-fat protein source	Replace high-fat protein sources with a lower-fat protein source	Replace high-fat protein sources with a lower-fat protein source	Replace high-fat protein sources with a lower-fat protein source	Replace high-fat protein sources with a lower-fat protein source	Replace high-fat protein sources with a lower-fat protein source
	Fats							
	Reward							Allow a splurge of one serving of a food you enjoy

summary

hear it! STUDY REVIEW

To hear an MP3 Chapter Summary, scan here or visit the Study Area in MasteringHealth™.

LO **1** ■ Nutrition is the science of food and nutrients; their digestion, absorption, metabolism, and their effect on health and disease.

■ Nutrients are substances that are required to support body function and maintain health. They provide energy, support growth and development, and regulate metabolism. Nutrients are classified into two major categories: macronutrients and micronutrients.

LO **2** ■ Macronutrients include carbohydrates, fats, proteins, and water.

■ Carbohydrates and fats are the major energy source for cells. They exist in two major forms: simple and complex carbohydrates. Glycogen is the major storage form of carbohydrates in the body and is the major fuel source for skeletal muscle during many types of exercise.

■ Fats are a subclass of lipids and exist in several forms in the body. Fatty acids are small chains of carbon, hydrogen, and a few carbon atoms; they are a major source of energy and are stored as triglycerides in fat cells.

■ Proteins form a major part of lean tissue and comprise about 17–20% of total body weight. Amino acids are the building blocks of proteins. Twenty different amino acids exist; nine are essential (must be contained in the diet) and the remaining amino acids are nonessential (can be synthesized in the body).

■ Foods containing all of the essential amino acids are called complete proteins (e.g., red meat). Foods that are missing one or more of the essential amino acids are called incomplete proteins (e.g., some vegetables).

■ Water is an essential macronutrient and is required for numerous body functions including temperature regulation, digestion, nutrient absorption, blood formation, and waste elimination.

LO **3** ■ Vitamins and minerals are micronutrients. Vitamins are essential and must be contained in the diet to maintain health. Although vitamins do not provide energy, they play a key role in body functions that include the regulation of growth and metabolism.

■ Minerals serve numerous functional roles in the body. Some act as cofactors with specialized proteins (enzymes), and others play important roles in regulating functions such as nerve impulse conduction, muscle contraction, and maintaining body water balance.

LO **4** ■ The components of a healthy diet are straightforward: consume high-quality protein with every meal, eat a variety of foods, including abundant fruits and vegetables, and consume less-healthy foods rarely or in moderation.

■ Other important guidelines are to carefully manage your intake of fat and sodium and limit the amount of sugar and alcohol in the diet.

LO **5** ■ Use available resources, including RDAs, MyPlate guidelines, and food labels to plan healthy meals.

LO **6** ■ Certain people such as children, pregnant women, and those with food allergies or intolerances have special dietary needs. It is possible to create a healthy diet even when avoiding specific foods by making sure that nutrient and energy needs are being met.

LO **7** ■ People engaging in regular exercise should adhere to the three Rs after a workout: rehydrate (replace lost fluids), replenish (replace body fuels, vitamins, and minerals), and repair (consume amino acids for muscle protein synthesis).

■ Rigorous exercise training programs increase your need for dietary carbohydrates and proteins. Those engaged in regular endurance exercise training should increase their intake of complex carbohydrates. The amount needed depends upon the intensity and duration of exercise training sessions.

■ Intense exercise increases the need for protein intake. Those engaged in rigorous regular exercise training (resistance and endurance) should increase their daily protein intake beyond the RDA to 1.2 to 1.6 grams of protein per kilogram of body weight. This can be achieved with a healthy diet.

■ For individuals who consume a healthy and well-balanced diet, rigorous exercise training does not create a need for antioxidant, protein, or vitamin supplements.

LO **8** ■ Use of any dietary supplement should be approached with caution because supplements are not regulated by the FDA.

LO ⑨ ▪ The most common type of foodborne illness occurs from consuming food contaminated with bacteria. The risk of foodborne illness is reduced by purchasing fresh foods, washing produce thoroughly, and not consuming raw eggs, meat, or fish.

▪ Food additives are used by manufacturers to improve nutritional quality, to preserve foods

for longer shelf life, and to improve the appearance of foods.

▪ Organic foods are produced without the use of pesticides, hormones, antibiotics, or chemical fertilizers. There is limited evidence to support the concept that organic foods are nutritionally superior to nonorganic foods, but they do reduce the risk of exposure to harmful toxins.

study questions

review it! QUIZZES

Find more review questions online at MasteringHealth™.

LO ① 1. Explain the function of nutrients in the body.

LO ② 2. What is the major role of carbohydrates in the diet?
   a. building tissue
   b. providing energy
   c. forming hormones
   d. forming enzymes

3. The primary role of protein in the diet is to
   a. provide energy.
   b. provide hydration.
   c. build tissues.
   d. regulate hormones.

4. Water is important for
   a. providing energy.
   b. building bones.
   c. forming blood.
   d. building protein.

5. What approximate percentages of carbohydrate, fat, and protein are recommended to be consumed in the daily diet?
   a. 60, 20, 20   c. 40, 20, 40
   b. 58, 22, 20   d. 58, 30, 12

6. Name the subcategories of carbohydrates and list the main food sources of dietary carbohydrates.

7. Define *triglycerides* and describe their function in the body.

8. How do saturated and unsaturated fatty acids differ?

9. What are trans fatty acids?

10. How do essential and nonessential amino acids differ?

11. Which of the following nutrients is classified as a macronutrient?
   a. protein   c. iron
   b. calcium   d. vitamin C

LO ③ 12. What are the classes of vitamins, and what role do vitamins play in body functions?

13. Explain the role that minerals play in body functions.

LO ④ 14. How many calories are contained in 1 gram of carbohydrate, fat, and protein, respectively?

LO ⑤ 15. Explain how MyPlate and the RDAs can be used to assist in planning a healthy diet.

LO ⑥ 16. Which vitamin found primarily in animal sources might need to be added as a supplement by those who follow a vegan diet?
   a. vitamin D   c. vitamin B_{12}
   b. vitamin B_6 d. vitamin C

LO ⑦ 17. Why is fluid replacement of such importance for active people? What are the guidelines for proper fluid replacement?

18. Why is consuming both carbohydrates and protein important for people who exercise regularly?

LO ⑧ 19. Explain the structure/function rule in regard to the marketing of dietary supplements.

LO ⑨ 20. Which of the following is one of the most common causes of foodborne illness?
   a. parasites
   b. food past expiration date
   c. bacteria
   d. overcooked or burned food

suggested readings

Centers for Disease Control and Prevention. Foodborne illness. http://www.cdc.gov/foodsafety/facts.html 2015.

Forman, J., and J. Silverman: Organic foods: Health and environmental advantages and disadvantages. *American Academy of Pediatrics* E1406–E1415, 2012.

Powers, S. K., and E. T. Howley. *Exercise Physiology*. New York: McGraw-Hill, 2015.

Powers, S. K, and K. J. Sollanek. Endurance exercise and antioxidant supplementation: Sense or nonsense? Part 1. *Sports Science Exchange* 27(137): 1–4, 2014.

Powers, S. K., and K. J. Sollanek. Endurance exercise and antioxidant supplementation: Sense or nonsense? Part 2. *Sports Science Exchange* 27(138): 1–4, 2014.

Smith-Spangler, C., et al. Are organic foods safer or healthier than conventional alternatives? A systematic review. *Annals of Internal Medicine* 157:348–366, 2012.

Wardlaw G., and Smith, A.: *Contemporary Nutrition: A Functional Approach*. New York: McGraw Hill, 2014.

helpful weblinks

do it! WEBLINKS

For links to the organizations and websites listed, visit MasteringHealth™.

Academy of Nutrition and Dietetics

Presents nutritional resources, FAQs, links, and more. **www.eatright.org**

Ask the Dietician

Presents sound nutritional advice on many diet-related questions. Includes an excellent "Healthy Body Calculator" for formulating diet and exercise programs. **www.dietitian.com**

Food and Drug Administration

Home page for the FDA office dealing with food and supplement regulations. Great information on food safety and supplements. The FDA provides key information and updates about regulatory actions related to food labeling, nutrition, and dietary supplements, as well as educational materials and important announcements. **www.fda.gov**

FoodSafety

Gateway to government food safety information. Includes news and safety alerts, consumer advice, national food safety programs, and foodborne pathogens. **www.foodsafety.gov**

MedlinePlus Health Information: Vitamin and Mineral Supplements

A service of the National Library of Medicine, National Institutes of Health, that provides information on health topics, including vitamin and mineral supplements. **www.nlm.nih.gov/medlineplus/vitamins.html** and **www.nlm.nih.gov/medlineplus/dietarysupplements.html** and **www.nlm.nih.gov/medlineplus/dietarysupplements.html**

MyPlate

Home page for the USDA's food guidance system, which includes SuperTracker to help you track your diet and physical activity. **www.choosemyplate.gov**

Nutrition.gov

A federal resource that provides easy access to all online federal government information on nutrition. **www.nutrition.gov**

Nutrition: MedlinePlus—National Library of Medicine

www.nlm.nih.gov/medlineplus/nutrition.html

Nutrition and Healthy Eating, Tools & Resources, NHLBI, NIH

www.nhlbi.nih.gov/health/educational/wecan/tools-resources/nutrition.htm

USDA Center for Nutrition Policy and Promotion

Provides guidelines for diets. **www.cnpp.usda.gov**

USDA Food Safety Publications

Contains articles about all aspects of safety in food preparation, storage, and handling. **www.fsis.usda.gov/Factsheets/index.asp**

laboratory 8.1

do it! LABS
Complete Lab 8.1 online in the
study area of **MasteringHealth.com**

Name _____ Date _____

Analyzing Your Diet

The purpose of this assessment is to analyze your eating habits. For a 3-day period (two weekdays and one weekend day), eat the foods that typically constitute your normal diet. Use the SuperTracker feature on ChooseMyPlate.gov (select "Food Tracker" under "Track Food & Activity") to chart the foods you ate that day and the amounts of each food. You can enter your food or search for the items you ate during the day. After you record your food intake, you can use the dietary analysis features to determine the nutrients in each food, the daily totals, and the average for the 3 days. The nutrient recommendations are based on the information you entered for your age, weight, sex, and activity level.

Select the "Food Details" report and click the "Select All" box under "Nutrients" to see the nutrient totals for each day. This report will provide nutrient values for each item that you consumed per day. Next, select the "Nutrients Report" for the average of your calorie and nutrient values over the 3-day period. When you create your profile, your data will be saved in SuperTracker. You can use the site to monitor your diet as you make healthy modifications. You can also print your report or save it to your computer for reference.

Compare your average intake for each of the nutrients with the recommended values based on your age, sex, and activity level. (Remember that this analysis is only as representative of your normal diet as the foods you eat over the 3-day period.) Then answer the following questions:

1. How did you do on calories? Are you taking in more or fewer calories than you should be for your sex, age, and activity level?

   _____

2. Was your fat, sodium, cholesterol, and empty calorie intake higher than it should be?

   _____

3. What nutrients did you eat in inadequate amounts?

   _____

4. What are three substitutions you could have made that would improve the quality of your diet?

   _____

RECOMMENDED DIETARY ALLOWANCES*

- Kcal total (total daily energy expenditure) equals body weight multiplied by kcal per pound per day:

  _____ × _____ = _____
  Body weight in lb   kcal per lb per day   **kcal total (total daily**
                         (from Table 9.1 on page 257)   **energy expenditure)**

- Kcal from fat should be no more than 30% of total calories per day:

  _____ × _____ = _____
  30% (0.3)   kcal per day   **recommended MAXIMUM kcal from fat**

- Protein intake should be 12% of total calories per day, or 0.8 to 0.9 gram per kilogram (0.36 g per pound) of body weight. (Pregnant women should add 15 g, and lactating women should add 20 g.):

  _____ × _____ = _____
  0.36 g   body weight in lb   **recommended protein intake**

- Carbohydrate intake should be approximately 58% of total calories per day:

  _____ × _____ = _____
  58% (0.58)   kcal per day   **recommended carbohydrate intake**

  Fat <30% of diet; fiber ~30% of diet; saturated fat <10% of diet; cholesterol <300 mg; sodium <3000 mg.

*See Table 8.5 on pages 226–227 for vitamin and mineral RDA values.

laboratory 8.2

do it! LABS
Complete Lab 8.2 online in the
study area of **MasteringHealth.com**

Name _____   Date _____

Setting Goals for a Healthy Diet

What are your three worst dietary habits? (Use your Nutrient Report from Laboratory 8.1 to help identify problems areas with your dietary habits.)

1. _____
2. _____
3. _____

Check the appropriate boxes in the table below to indicate the changes that you think you need to make to improve your diet.

	Increase	Decrease	Keep the Same
Calories			
Carbohydrates			
Fat			
Protein			
Vitamins			
Minerals			

Based on your selections above, list two short-term and two long-term SMART goals for improving your diet:

Short-term goal 1

_____

_____

Short-term goal 2

_____

_____

Long-term goal 1

_____

_____

Long-term goal 2

_____

_____

do it! LABS
Complete Lab 8.3 online in the
study area of **MasteringHealth.com**

Name _____ Date _____

Planning a New Diet

The purpose of this exercise is to plan a new diet using the principles outlined in this chapter. You can also use the My Plan tool of SuperTracker. This feature will provide general recommendations, and then you can select specific foods to meet those recommendations. After completing Laboratory 8.1, you should have a general idea of how your diet may need modification. Follow the example given in Table 8.6 on page 228 and the discussion in the text to choose foods to build a new diet that meets the recommended dietary goals presented in this chapter. Fill in the chart below with the requested information obtained from Food-A-Pedia on SuperTracker or from package labels. Use the totals for each column and the RDA for each nutrient in Laboratory 8.1 or Table 8.5 on pages 226–227 to determine your percentage of RDA for each nutrient.

	Kcal (g)	Protein (g)	Sat. Fat (g)	Chol. (mg)	Sod. (mg)	Carb. (g)	Vit. A (IU)	Vit. C (mg)	Ca (mg)	Iron (mg)	GI
Breakfast											
Lunch											
Dinner											
Totals											
RDA	*	<30%†	<10%	<300	3000	>58%	1000	60	1200	12	‡
% of RDA											

*See Table 9.1 in Chapter 9 (page 257) for determination of kcal requirements.

†Protein intake should be 0.8 g/kg of body weight (0.36 g/lb). Pregnant women should add 15 g, and lactating women should add 20 g.

‡For a complete list of the glycemic index of various foods, visit www.glycemicindex.com

laboratory 8.4

do it! LABS
Complete Lab 8.4 online in the
study area of **MasteringHealth.com**

Name _____   Date _____

Assessing Nutritional Habits

Read the following scenarios and select which option applies to you. Score your answers according to the instructions at the end.

1. You don't have time to make dinner, so you run out to get "fast food." What do you get?
   a. grilled chicken breast sandwich
   b. supersized burger

2. You go to a movie, find yourself hungry, and cannot resist a snack. Which do you buy?
   a. unbuttered popcorn
   b. candy

3. You're late for work and realize you forgot breakfast. You decide to stop and grab something to eat. What do you pick up?
   a. a banana
   b. a sausage biscuit

4. You decide to go out for a nice dinner at an Italian restaurant. What do you order?
   a. spaghetti with red sauce
   b. five-cheese lasagna

5. It's 3:00 P.M., and you didn't have much lunch and need an afternoon snack. What do you reach for?
   a. an apple
   b. M&Ms

6. You stop for ice cream. Which do you pick?
   a. a fruit sorbet
   b. regular ice cream

7. What kind of dessert would you normally choose to eat?
   a. a bowl of mixed berries with a sprinkling of sugar
   b. chocolate cake with frosting

8. What do you use to stir fry vegetables?
   a. olive oil
   b. margarine

9. Which of the following salty snacks would you prefer?
   a. pretzels
   b. potato chips

10. You want cereal for breakfast. Which would you choose?
    a. whole-grain flakes
    b. peanut butter puffs

INTERPRETATION

If you answered "b" to any of the above questions, you chose foods that are high in calories, fat, or sugar. Follow the advice in this chapter and the MyPlate food guidance system to improve your food choices.

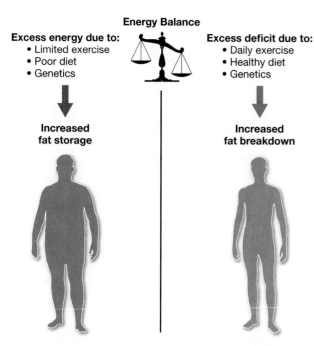

FIGURE 9.1 Factors that regulate energy balance in the body. Consuming more calories than you expend results in a positive energy balance and increased body fat storage. Expending more calories than you consume results in a negative energy balance and increased breakdown of body fat stores.

energy expenditure exceeds energy intake. This is known as the **energy balance** concept, which is often simplified as "calories in versus calories out." Taking in more calories than you expend results in a "positive energy balance," and your fat stores (body weight) will increase. If you expend more calories than you consume, this results in a "negative energy balance," and you will lose weight (**FIGURE 9.1**). If you consume the same amount of energy that you expend each day, your body weight and amount of body fat will remain relatively constant. While this basic concept is easy to understand, the factors that regulate energy balance in the body are complex.

Daily Energy Expenditure

The total amount of energy expended each day is the sum of energy expended at rest and energy expended during physical activity. The three components of total daily energy expenditure are resting metabolic rate, physical activity/exercise, and the thermic effect of food (**FIGURE 9.2**).

Recall from Chapter 4 that *resting metabolic rate (RMR)* is the amount of energy expended during sedentary activities, including the energy required to maintain necessary body functions (the basal metabolic rate) plus the energy required to perform activities such as sitting. In most people, the RMR represents 60% to 75% of the total daily energy expenditure (5). Resting metabolic rate is influenced by several factors, including genetics, age, gender, and the amount of lean body mass an individual

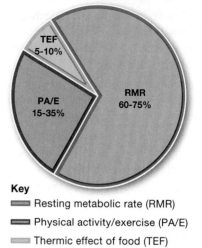

Key
▬ Resting metabolic rate (RMR)
▬ Physical activity/exercise (PA/E)
▬ Thermic effect of food (TEF)

FIGURE 9.2 The three components that make up total daily energy expenditure: The sum of your resting metabolic rate, the amount of energy expended each day due to physical activity/exercise, and the amount of energy expended during the digestion and storage of food.

possesses. For example, RMR (expressed per pound of body weight) is higher in growing children than in adults, and it declines with age. Men often have a higher RMR than women, and RMR is higher in lean individuals with a high percentage of muscle mass compared to those with more body fat. This is because the energy needed to maintain muscle tissue is greater than the energy required to maintain fat tissue (8).

Physical activity/exercise (PA/E) represents the energy expenditure during any form of physical activity (such as walking or doing chores) and during exercise. In sedentary individuals, PA/E constitutes only 15% of the total daily energy expenditure. In active people, PA/E accounts for 20% to 35% of the total daily energy expenditure (6, 7), and the energy used during exercise can be 6 to 20 times higher than RMR (8). Therefore, daily exercise increases the PA/E and is an important factor in all weight-loss plans.

see it!
ABC VIDEOS
Watch the "TV and Movies May Lead to More Snacking" ABC News Video online at MasteringHealth™.

A small amount of energy is required each day to digest and store the nutrients consumed in food. This energy expenditure is known as the thermic effect of food (TEF) and accounts for 5% to 10% of the total daily energy requirement.

energy balance The state of consuming a number of calories that is equal to the number expended.

physical activity/exercise (PA/E) Amount of energy expended during any form of physical activity or exercise.

MAKE SURE YOU **KNOW...**

▪ The amount of fat stored in the body is determined by the rate that fat is synthesized and stored and the rate that it is broken down in fat cells and used for energy (metabolized).

▪ To maintain a constant body weight, caloric intake must equal caloric expenditure; this results in a state of energy balance.

▪ Consuming more calories than expended results in weight gain, and consuming fewer calories than expended results in weight loss.

MasteringHealth™

Factors that Influence Weight Management

LO **3** List and describe four key factors that influence weight management.

Having too much body fat results from both internal and external factors. Internally, our hormones and genes influence appetite and resting metabolic rate. Externally, lifestyle factors, including dietary choices and your environment, and the amount and type of physical activity and exercise you engage in, play major roles in determining whether you gain or lose body fat.

Hormonal Control of Appetite

The appetite control center is located in a region of the brain called the hypothalamus. One section of this control center is responsible for stimulating appetite, and a different section promotes satiety (a sense of feeling full and satisfied after eating). Circulating hormones influence our desire to eat and our sense of when to stop. **Ghrelin** is the primary hormone that stimulates appetite, producing the desire for food. Other circulating hormones such as **leptin** and **peptide YY** act to suppress appetite (**FIGURE 9.3**). Numerous factors regulate the levels of these appetite-controlling hormones.

Heredity

Genetic makeup has a significant influence on a person's tendency to gain weight and on how fat is stored in the body. Genes provide the instructions for cells to make proteins that control metabolism. Humans possess about 25,000 genes, and several hundred can influence energy balance and body composition (9). It is estimated that genes are responsible for 40% to 70% of how and why people store body fat (9). Genetics impact body fat stores in two important ways. First, genes can influence energy balance by regulating the appetite control center in the brain. For example, certain genes increase the blood levels of appetite-stimulating hormones such as ghrelin, while others promote increases in hormones that depress appetite such

Regulation of Appetite and Food Intake

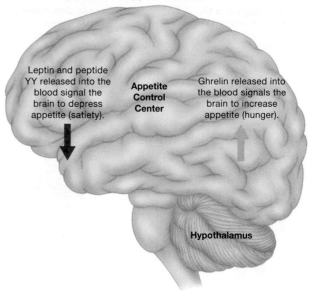

FIGURE 9.3 The hypothalamus is the body's appetite control center. This brain region responds to hormones and regulates our feelings of hunger and satiety.

as leptin and peptide YY (10). Second, genes also play a key role in regulating resting metabolic rate. Some people are genetically predisposed toward a high resting metabolic rate and others toward a lower-than-average RMR (9).

While experts agree that the current obesity epidemic is primarily due to lifestyle factors, there are a few rare genetic conditions that account for extreme obesity in about 1% of the population (10). These genetic disorders are present at birth, and affected individuals develop obesity early in life.

Lifestyle and Environment

We know that today's obesity epidemic can be largely attributed to lifestyle and behavior (11). These factors remain the primary focus for many health professionals in designing weight-loss programs for overweight and obese individuals.

Understanding what triggers the desire to eat is an important first step in weight management. Some people eat in response to emotional stressors, both good and bad. Think about how your family celebrates an important occasion such as a birthday, anniversary, or graduation. Food is often at the center of these celebrations. Negative stressors can also influence your food intake. When facing negative feelings such as depression, loneliness, or boredom, many people turn to food for comfort.

The increase in the number of fast food restaurants has had a negative influence on the dietary habits of many Americans. Convenience, low cost, high caloric content, and large portion sizes have made fast food a major contributor to the obesity epidemic. The restaurant industry overall has also increased portion sizes to meet market demand. In fact, serving sizes have increased over the last 20 years to the point that the average person does not realize what a normal serving size should be and ends up consuming more food (and calories) than needed to maintain body weight.

Ingrained eating habits may be difficult to change. Nonetheless, like other habits we seek to change, eating habits can be modified when we are motivated and equipped with an appropriate plan for behavior change. Do you know what situations or events affect your eating habits? See the Steps for Behavior Change box on page 256 to identify your food triggers.

Physical Activity and Exercise

Physical activity and exercise increase your daily energy expenditure and are key to effective weight management. FIGURE 9.4 illustrates the effect that increased physical activity has on total daily energy expenditure. This illustration compares the total energy expenditure (kcal/day) of three college-age males, each weighing 154 pounds (70 kilograms). John is very active and walks a lot each day. He also performs 60 minutes of vigorous exercise on a daily basis. Bill is less active but performs 30 minutes of exercise each day. Henry is sedentary,

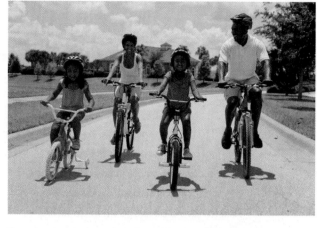

Exercise is a key component to any weight-loss program. Family and friends can help support exercise and healthy behaviors.

engaging in limited physical activity and no regular exercise. Notice the large differences in daily energy expenditure: John expends 2,600 kcal/day, Bill expends 2,160, and Henry only 1,900. It follows that if all three consume an average of 2,600 kcal/day, John will maintain a constant body weight, but both Bill and Henry will likely increase their fat storage and gain weight.

MAKE SURE YOU KNOW...

■ Internal factors (hormones and genetics) and external factors (diet and lifestyle as well as physical activity and exercise) influence weight management.

—— MasteringHealth™

Designing a Successful Weight-Loss Program

LO **4** Explain why lifelong weight management is important, and outline four essential steps involved in designing a successful weight-loss program.

We have established that if you consume more calories than you expend, you will gain body fat, and if you expend more calories than you consume, you will lose fat weight. Healthy weight-loss programs include both a reduction in caloric intake and an increase in caloric expenditure achieved through exercise (8, 12).

ghrelin Hormone that stimulates appetite.

leptin Hormone that depresses appetite.

peptide YY Hormone that depresses appetite.

Key
- Physical activity/exercise
- Sleeping/sitting
- Thermic effect of food

FIGURE 9.4 The effect of daily physical activity and exercise on total caloric expenditure.

Bar chart – Energy Expenditure (kcal/day):
- John (very active): 2600 calories/day
- Bill (active): 2160 calories/day
- Henry (sedentary): 1900 calories/day

What triggers your eating?

Take the following quiz to help assess some of the cues that cause you to eat.

Y   N

☐   ☐   I need to have a snack and a beverage when I study.

☐   ☐   I cannot watch television or sit through a movie without a snack.

☐   ☐   I would order the small portion at a fast food restaurant, but I get more for my money if I order the largest size.

☐   ☐   Leaving food on my plate is wasteful.

☐   ☐   I like to have a beverage when I'm driving.

If you answered yes to more than one of these questions, you're likely eating out of habit or because of your environment. This behavior could lead to weight gain.

Tips to Curb Your Calorie Consumption

Tomorrow, you will:

☑ Drink water instead of soda while studying, and if you get hungry, stop for a break and go get a piece of fruit for a snack.

☑ Visit friends or go for a walk in the evening instead of watching television. You'll eat less and work in some physical activity.

Within the next 2 weeks, you will:

☑ Order only small sandwiches and fries when eating fast food or, better yet, order no fries and a side salad instead.

☑ Pay attention to your body's signals and eat only until you feel full. Despite what our families may have taught us, cleaning your plate is not a good idea because it leads to overeating. Put less on your plate to begin with (you can always have seconds if you are still hungry) or, if dining out, get a doggie bag for the extra food.

By the end of the semester, you will:

☑ Opt for a reusable water bottle in your car, and use that to stay hydrated during road trips. The calories in sodas and sugar- and milk-laden coffee drinks quickly add up.

Estimating your daily energy expenditure is the first step in planning a weight-loss program and adjusting the energy balance equation. One of the simplest ways to estimate your daily caloric expenditure is to determine your activity level and use it to calculate the average number of calories you expend in a 24-hour period (**TABLE 9.1**). For example, let's calculate the daily energy expenditure for a moderately active college-age female who weighs 120 pounds. Using Table 9.1, you can see that she expends 15 calories per pound per day. Her estimated daily caloric expenditure is calculated by multiplying 120 (body weight in pounds) by 15 (calories expended per pound per day):

$$\text{Daily caloric expenditure} = 120 \text{ pounds} \times 15 \text{ calories/pound/day}$$

$$= 1,800 \text{ calories/day}$$

If this woman takes in an average of 2,000 calories per day, those extra 200 calories put her on the road to

weight gain. Use the table and Laboratory 9.2 to calculate your daily caloric expenditure. Do you think your daily expenditure is equal to or higher than the amount of calories you take in each day?

live it!

ASSESS YOURSELF

Assess your dietary habits with the *Out of Control or Overcontrol?* Take Charge of Your Health! Worksheet online at MasteringHealth™.

Expending more calories than you consume requires changes in both your diet and level of physical activity that must be sustainable over the long term. The maximum recommended rate for weight loss is 1 to 2 pounds per week. Diets resulting in a weight loss of more than 2 pounds per week are associated with a significant loss of lean body mass and are not recommended.

The energy deficit required to lose 1 pound per week is approximately 3,500 calories. Thus, a negative energy balance of 500 calories per day (3,500 calories

TABLE 9.1 ■ Estimating Daily Caloric Expenditure

To compute your estimated daily caloric expenditure, multiply your body weight in pounds by the calories per pound corresponding to your activity level.

Activity Level	Description	Calories per Pound of Body Weight Expended during 24-Hour Period
1 Very sedentary	Very limited daily movement; primary activities include lying down and sitting (e.g., working at a desk, playing video games or watching TV)	13
2 Sedentary	Job or activities that involve limited walking but sitting most of the day	14
3 Moderate activity	Some daily physical activity and weekend recreation	15
4 Very physically active	Daily physical activity and exercise at least 3–4 times/week (30–60 minutes/day)	16
5 Competitive athlete	Daily physical activity and daily vigorous exercise training (>60 minutes)	17–18

per week divided by 7 days per week = 500 calories per day) would theoretically result in a loss of 1 pound of fat per week.

The rate of loss during the first several days or weeks will be greater than the rate later on. At the onset of a weight-loss program, you lose not only fat, but also carbohydrate and water stores (8). You may also lose some lean tissue, such as muscle, at the beginning, so you will often lose more than 1 pound during the first 3,500-calorie-deficit period. However, as you continue with your plan, you will lose weight at a slower rate. Don't be discouraged if the rate of weight loss levels off after the first 2 to 4 weeks. The weight you lose later will come primarily from fat stores, and sticking with your plan will result in a significant fat loss over time.

Lifetime Weight Management

Weight management should not be a short-term goal. Maintaining a healthy body weight over the long term is important for good health and requires an ongoing commitment to a healthy diet and regular exercise. If you improve your habits and lose weight but then slip into unhealthy behaviors such as overeating or being sedentary once the weight has come off, you will undo your efforts. And you may even gain more weight than you

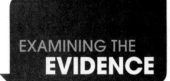

EXAMINING THE EVIDENCE

Focus on Fructose and Weight-Loss Supplements

Does Fructose Promote Weight Gain?

It is widely believed that the ingestion of sugars is one of the contributory factors to the obesity epidemic (13–16). Both cane sugar and high-fructose corn syrup contain glucose and fructose. Compared to glucose, fructose has been shown to increase the synthesis of fat, and consuming large amounts is predicted to increase body fat storage. Even worse, growing evidence suggests that excessive intake of fructose (750 grams or more per day) may be linked to an increased risk of hypertension and diabetes (15, 17).

High-fructose corn syrup is used to sweeten many beverages including soft drinks, juices, and sports drinks. Given that U.S. soft drink consumption has tripled in recent decades, paralleling the dramatic increase in obesity, this has led to speculation that consumption of fructose-sweetened soft drinks is a major contributory factor to the rising obesity crisis. Although studies indicate that fructose-sweetened soft drinks cause weight gain, it seems unlikely that soft drink consumption alone is the sole cause in the obesity crisis (16).

Can Dietary Supplements Promote Weight Loss?

Hundreds of weight-loss supplements are on the market, and it is estimated that more than 45 million Americans use diet supplements in an effort to lose weight. Unfortunately, the large majority have not been proven to promote weight loss (18, 19). Supplements called "fat burners" claim to increase fat metabolism. Often these supplements contain a number of ingredients including caffeine, green tea extracts, chromium, conjugated linoleic acid, and kelp. However, only caffeine and green tea have scientific evidence to back up the claim of increased fat metabolism (20). Further, this increase in fat metabolism is extremely small and is likely of limited benefit to weight loss (20).

There is limited evidence to support the benefit of most over-the-counter weight-loss products and few live up to their claims. Remember that dietary supplements are not regulated by the FDA and therefore, most products have not undergone quality testing. Just because a supplement is on the market does not mean that it is safe, and most medical and nutrition experts do not recommend the use of these weight-loss products (19, 20).

initially lost. This is the reason that fad diets are typically unsuccessful.

The key factors in long-term weight management are a positive attitude, regular exercise, and a personal commitment to maintaining a desired body composition. Like many other facets of life, weight control has its ups and downs. Be prepared for occasional setbacks. For instance, many people gain weight during holiday periods. If this happens, don't criticize yourself, just reestablish your commitment to a weight-loss goal. You will already know which habits you need to change.

The importance of family and friends in lifetime weight management is significant. Their encouragement and support can help you maintain healthy eating habits and sustain a commitment to exercise. Losing weight is much easier if the people close to you support your goals rather than tempt you into unhealthy behaviors. Encourage others to join you in exercising and exploring new ways to prepare healthy foods. You may become the role model they need to make positive changes!

To lose weight and keep it off, you need to implement four basic steps:

1. Establish a realistic goal for weight loss.

2. Analyze your diet and determine how you can reduce your caloric intake while still consuming the nutrients you need for health.

3. Decide which physical activities and types of exercise you will engage in to increase your daily caloric expenditure and build (or maintain) muscle mass. Choose activities that you enjoy and are likely to do long-term.

4. Modify your lifestyle to support your weight-loss goal and prevent future weight gain.

Set a Realistic Goal The first step in setting a realistic weight loss goal is to decide where your percentage of body fat should fall within the optimal healthy range (8%–19% for men, 21%–32% for women). Establishing a long-term goal that will place you in the middle of the optimal weight range (13%–15% for men, 24%–26% for women) is a good place to start. After setting your long-term goal, it is useful to establish short-term goals—the number of pounds you want to lose per week. Keep in mind that 1–2 pounds per week is realistic and healthy. Attempting a goal such as losing 5 pounds per week is not realistic or healthy and will set you up for failure. See Laboratory 9.3 for a worksheet you can use to help set short- and long-term goals.

Assess and Modify Your Diet A key to losing weight successfully is to identify the healthy and less-healthy dietary choices you're making on a daily basis. If you're eating fast food regularly, you are likely consuming too many high-fat, high-calorie foods that are impeding your ability to lose weight. If you can't remember the last time you ate a fresh fruit or vegetable, you may be getting too few nutrients. A balanced, healthy diet can lead to weight loss, and once you know what can be improved, you can work on making changes.

The first step is to determine how many calories you are consuming each day. Most people underestimate the amount of food they consume. Keeping a food diary for as few as 3 days (see Laboratory 8.1) can help you determine your total calorie intake and make you more aware of your food choices.

When considering how to modify your diet to lose weight, be aware that many diets promoted in books, on TV, and online often do not provide balanced nutrition and may be difficult to sustain (see Examining the Evidence). When you are assessing potential diet plans, a general rule is to avoid fad diets that promise fast and easy weight loss. If you have concerns about the safety or effectiveness of a particular diet, you can seek help from a trained nutrition professional (for a directory of registered dietician nutritionists see www.eatright.org).

Any safe and nutritionally sound diet should adhere to the following guidelines (2, 18, 19):

- Should be low in calories but provide all the essential nutrients the body requires. It should be balanced with foods that provide adequate vitamins and minerals on a daily basis.

consider this! //////////////////////

Approximately 90% of fat loss occurs in the body regions with the highest fat storage, generally the thighs and hips in women and the abdominal region in men.

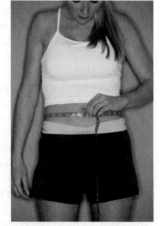

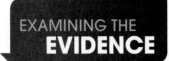

Popular Diet Plans

Many diet plans exist, and although some popular diets are based on long-standing nutritional and medical advice, others deviate from mainstream nutritional guidelines (21–24). The most popular diet plans fall into one of four general categories:

Very low-carbohydrate: These diets recommend that carbohydrates make up less than 30% of your total calorie consumption, resulting in a high intake of proteins and fats. The Atkins diet is the most popular very low-carbohydrate diet plan. Most such plans are structured in 3–4 phases. The first phase limits carbohydrate intake to very low levels (less than 100 calories per day). In subsequent phases, the amount of carbohydrates consumed typically increases to 20%–30% of total caloric intake.

Proponents of very low-carbohydrate diets argue that they have two major advantages over conventional diet plans. First, eating high-carbohydrate foods reduces the rate of fat metabolism. The evidence to support this claim is that consuming high-carbohydrate foods increases the release of the hormone insulin. High insulin levels can be counterproductive to weight loss because insulin stimulates both fat storage and reduces the use of fat as a body fuel (13).

The second argument is that high-carbohydrate foods are less effective in decreasing hunger than foods containing high levels of proteins (13). Therefore, low-carbohydrate diets may promote satiety, reduce overall caloric intake, and assist in achieving a negative caloric balance.

Based on these assumed advantages, these plans are often promoted as diets on which "you never feel hungry" and "you will lose weight fast." Both claims can be misleading. Not everyone experiences appetite suppression while on a very low-carbohydrate diet. Further, the initial weight loss is often temporary, due to loss of body water rather than of fat. Consequently, as the individual resumes a normal diet, the body regains the water and the initial weight loss is eliminated (8).

Low-carbohydrate: This class of diets advocates a prescribed ratio of calories from macronutrients (carbohydrates, proteins, and fats). One of the most popular diets in this category is called the Zone Diet. This diet program centers on a 40:30:30 ratio of calories obtained from carbohydrates, proteins, and fats. The Zone Diet is a restricted-carbohydrate diet because it limits the consumption of carbohydrates to 40% of the total caloric intake, and it also regulates the types of carbohydrates consumed by limiting the intake of carbohydrates with a high glycemic index.

Low-fat: Low-fat diets limit the number of calories consumed from fats. Some low-fat diets are vegetarian diets, while others simply limit protein intake from red meat (red meat contains high levels of fat).

Advocates of low-fat diets argue that limiting fat intake is an advantage for two major reasons. First, foods rich in fat are also high-calorie foods. Second, consumption of a diet high in fat is often associated with increased risk for cardiovascular disease because high-fat diets often promote elevated blood cholesterol (21–24).

One of the best-known low-fat diets is the Ornish Diet, a vegetarian plan that concentrates on removing fats and cholesterol from your diet by adding whole grains, legumes, fruits, and vegetables. The Ornish Diet recommends a 70:20:10 ratio of daily calories obtained from carbohydrates, proteins, and fats.

Nutritionally balanced diet with restricted calories: The Academy of Nutrition and Dietetics recommends that any diet designed to lose weight should be guided by the MyPlate food guidance system (see Chapter 8). This system is based on national nutritional guidelines and, when followed, results in a diet that is low in fat and high in carbohydrates. It is based on long-standing nutritional guidelines and achieves weight loss by restricting caloric intake by limiting food portion sizes.

Two well-known diets that use this approach are the Weight Watchers plan and the LEARN diet. Weight Watchers uses a point system for tracking and focuses on eating healthy and getting more exercise. The LEARN (Lifestyle, Exercise, Attitudes, Relationships, and Nutrition) diet recommends that you consume a 60:30:10 ratio of daily calories obtained from carbohydrates, proteins, and fats. Similar to the Ornish Diet, the LEARN diet is classified as a balanced but low-fat diet.

So what is the bottom-line recommendation? In short, research indicates that a reduced-calorie diet will result in weight loss regardless of which macro-nutrient is emphasized (24). Therefore, based on recommendations from the Academy of Nutrition and Dietetics, a nutritionally balanced reduced-calorie diet is the most desirable for weight loss. This diet contains a balance of macro- and micronutrients and can be sustained over the long term.

- Should be low in fat (less than 30% of total calories) and high in complex carbohydrates.

- Should involve a variety of foods to appeal to your tastes and ensure adequate nutrient intake.

- Should be compatible with your lifestyle, and the foods should be easily obtainable.

- Should be a plan that can be followed over the long term. This will greatly increase your chances of keeping weight off once you've lost it.

In addition to these diet guidelines, here are some helpful reminders for planning a healthy, balanced diet:

- Focus on whole foods, not processed foods. Avoid high-calorie, low-nutrient foods such as those high in sugar (e.g., candy bars, cookies, soft drinks, and alcohol). Instead, select lower-calorie, nutrient-dense foods such as lean protein, fruits, and vegetables.

- Reduce the amount of saturated fat in your diet and avoid trans fats (sometimes found in processed foods and baked goods). High-fat foods are high in calories, and eating too much saturated fat can also increase your risk for heart disease. For example, choose lean meats such as lean cuts of beef, chicken, and fish. Avoid fried foods; choose high-quality, low-fat dairy products, such as milk, yogurt, and cottage cheese.

- Select fresh fruits and vegetables whenever possible; the next best are frozen. Avoid canned fruits in heavy syrup.

- Drink fewer alcoholic beverages, which are low in nutrients and high in calories.

- Eat to satisfy hunger, not due to boredom or other emotional reasons. Remember that a negative energy balance of 500 calories per day will result in a weight loss of approximately 1 pound per week. The key to maintaining this caloric deficit is careful meal planning and accurate calorie-counting.

Plan Your Physical Activity Physical activity and exercise play a key role in weight loss for several reasons. Increased physical activity elevates your daily caloric expenditure, and regular cardiorespiratory exercise improves the ability of skeletal muscles to burn fat as energy (8). Further, regular resistance exercise (such as weight training) can reduce the loss of muscle that occurs during dieting (8). This is important because your primary goal during weight loss is to lose fat, not muscle mass. Increasing your muscle mass via resistance training will elevate your resting metabolic rate, which further aids weight loss by increasing your daily energy expenditure (8). Finally, evidence suggests that regular exercise training can diminish hunger and reduce food intake (25, 26).

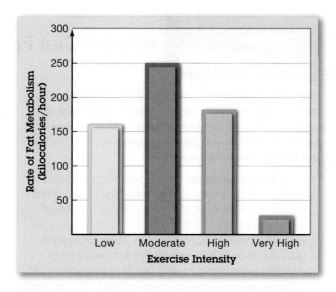

FIGURE 9.5 Illustration of the rates of fat metabolism during low-intensity exercise (20% $\dot{V}O_2$ max), moderate-intensity exercise (50% $\dot{V}O_2$ max), high-intensity exercise (80% $\dot{V}O_2$ max), and very-high-intensity exercise (90% $\dot{V}O_2$ max). While this figure is not intended to promote the "ideal" exercise intensity for all people, it indicates that moderate-intensity exercise is often optimal for maximizing the amount of fat metabolized during physical activity.

Many people assume that aerobic exercise (running, cycling, etc.) must be maintained at a low intensity if fat is to be burned as fuel. It is true that fat is a primary fuel source during low-intensity exercise. The total amount of fat burned during exercise varies with the intensity of exercise, and for a given exercise duration, more total fat is metabolized during moderate-intensity exercise (**FIGURE 9.5**). Therefore, moderate-intensity exercise (approximately 50% $\dot{V}O_2$ max or 70% maximum heart rate) is typically the optimal intensity for burning the most fat during an endurance exercise workout. If you are overweight or your fitness level is low, start with a low-intensity workout (25% $\dot{V}O_2$ max or 50% maximum heart rate) until you improve your cardiorespiratory fitness enough to support a moderate-intensity workout.

How much exercise must you perform during a weight-loss program? In general, exercise sessions designed to promote weight loss should expend more than 250 calories (8). By doing this, the negative caloric balance can be achieved equally by exercise and diet. An individual who is aiming for a 500-calorie-per-day deficit could increase exercise energy expenditure by 250 calories by walking for 45 to 60 minutes and then also reduce caloric intake by 250 calories.

While exercise intensity is an important factor in improving cardiorespiratory fitness, it is the total amounts of energy expended and fat burned that are important in weight loss. Some authors have argued that low-intensity, prolonged exercise is better than short-term, high-intensity exercise in burning fat and promoting weight loss (27). However, evidence clearly demonstrates that both high- and low-intensity exercise can promote fat loss (28).

For a sedentary, obese individual, low-intensity exercise is the best choice because it can be performed for longer periods of time and increases the ability of skeletal muscle to metabolize fat for energy (28). The initial goal of the exercise program should not be to improve cardio-vascular fitness, but rather to increase voluntary energy expenditure and to establish a regular exercise routine. It is often advisable that obese individuals beginning an exercise program work with a fitness professional, at least at the outset, to create a realistic program and avoid injury.

The number of calories burned during exercise varies by the type of activity and its duration. For example, walking (17 minutes per mile) burns about 5.5 calories per minute, while running (8 minutes per mile) burns about 12.5 calories per minute. Playing golf (without a golf cart) burns less than 4 calories per minute, while playing tennis (singles) burns 7 calories per minute. You can measure your caloric expenditure in a number of ways. Phone apps are available that calculate your caloric expenditure during various activities. Fitness equipment such as stationary bicycles, treadmills, and ellipticals usually includes a monitor that tracks calories burned during an exercise session.

Focus on Behavior Modification   Research demonstrates that behavior modification plays a key role in achieving short-term weight loss and maintaining weight loss over the long term (29, 30). Most behaviors are learned and therefore can be modified. For example, many people eat popcorn and candy at the movie theater, and a nightly television habit often includes unhealthy snacks such as chips and soda. Since these behaviors are learned, they can also be "unlearned." In regard to weight control, behavior modification is used primarily to reduce or (ideally) eliminate social or environmental stimuli that promote overeating.

The first step in modifying behavior is to identify factors that act as triggers for overeating. You can do this by keeping a written record of daily activities for 1 or 2 weeks to identify people and situations associated with consuming too many calories and making unhealthy food choices (**FIGURE 9.6**). How many of the factors shown occur in your activity diary?

After identifying problematic behaviors, you can design a plan for modifying those behaviors. The following techniques will make weight loss easier (30):

- *Make a personal commitment to losing weight.*
  Establishing realistic short-term and long-term

coaching corner

Log exercise in daily journal!

Many myths and misconceptions exist about weight loss diets. When designing your nutritional plan to lose body fat, consider the following:

- Research does not support the concept that low-carbohydrate diets are more effective in producing long-term weight loss when compared to a nutritionally balanced, low-calorie diet (24).

- Limited evidence exists to support the idea that major commercial weight loss programs are effective in maintaining long-term weight loss.

- When creating your weight-loss plan, remember that interventions based on a reduced-calorie diet plus exercise are more effective in maintaining weight loss than a low-calorie diet alone (see Clark (2015), and Franz et al. (2007) in Suggested Reading section).

weight-loss goals helps you maintain a lifelong commitment to weight management.

- *Develop healthy, low-calorie eating patterns.* Avoid eating when you are not hungry. Practice eating slowly, chewing thoroughly, and only while sitting at the table. Reduce portion sizes to stay within your caloric guidelines.

- *Avoid social settings where you are likely to overeat or consume too many liquid calories.* If you go to parties where high-calorie foods are served, don't show up hungry. Eat a low-calorie meal beforehand. Avoid social situations where you are encouraged to drink more than one alcoholic drink. Research shows that alcohol consumed before or after meals tends to increase food intake (31).

- *Exercise daily.* Regular exercise that uses large-muscle groups can play an important role in increasing your daily caloric expenditure.

- *Reward yourself with nonfood rewards.*
  Positive feedback is an important part of behavior modification, and it doesn't have to relate to food to be effective. For example, after reaching your first short-term weight-loss goal, do something that you consider a special treat, such as buying a new item of clothing or going to a concert.

- *Think positively.* Positive thinking about your ability to lose weight promotes confidence and maintains the enthusiasm necessary for a lifetime of successful weight management.

1. *Activities.* You may find a correlation between specific types of activities, such as watching TV and eating snacks.

2. *Emotional behavior before or during eating.* Many people overeat when they are depressed or under stress.

3. *Location of meals.* Do you eat your meals in front of the television? Do you associate specific rooms with snacking?

4. *Time of day and level of hunger.* Do you eat at specific times of the day? Do you eat even if you are not hungry?

5. *People involved.* Are specific people associated with periods of overeating?

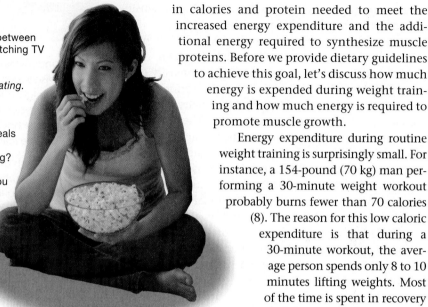

FIGURE 9.6 Do you overeat because of any of these social or environmental influences?

MAKE SURE YOU **KNOW...**

- Estimating your daily caloric expenditure is the first step in planning a weight loss program.

- A safe rate of weight loss is 1 to 2 pounds per week. Losing 1 pound per week will require a caloric deficit of 3,500 calories during the week (i.e., a caloric deficit of 500 calories per day).

- There are four basic steps to designing a successful weight loss program: 1) Set realistic goals; 2) assess and modify your diet; 3) plan regular exercise; and 4) avoid activities and situations that will derail your efforts.

MasteringHealth™

Exercise and Diet Programs to Gain Weight

LO **5** Describe the components of a diet and exercise program designed to gain lean body weight.

Thus far, this chapter has focused on how to lose body fat. But some people have the opposite problem—being underweight—and they may need to implement a program to gain lean body weight. You can achieve weight gain by creating a positive energy balance (taking in more calories than you expend). When increasing body weight, you'll want to aim to increase muscle mass, rather than fat mass, for the sake of your health.

The key to gaining muscle mass is a program of rigorous weight training combined with the increase in calories and protein needed to meet the increased energy expenditure and the additional energy required to synthesize muscle proteins. Before we provide dietary guidelines to achieve this goal, let's discuss how much energy is expended during weight training and how much energy is required to promote muscle growth.

Energy expenditure during routine weight training is surprisingly small. For instance, a 154-pound (70 kg) man performing a 30-minute weight workout probably burns fewer than 70 calories (8). The reason for this low caloric expenditure is that during a 30-minute workout, the average person spends only 8 to 10 minutes lifting weights. Most of the time is spent in recovery periods between sets.

Current estimates are that approximately 2,500 calories are needed to synthesize 1 pound of muscle mass, of which about 400 calories (100 grams) must be protein (32). To compute the additional calories required to produce an increase in muscle mass, you must first estimate your rate of muscular growth. This is difficult because the rate of muscular growth during weight training varies widely among people. Although relatively large muscle mass gains are possible in some individuals, studies have shown that most men and women rarely gain more than a quarter pound of muscle per week during a 20-week weight-training program (3 days per week, 30 minutes per day). If we assume that the average muscle gain is a quarter pound per week and that 2,500 calories are required to synthesize 1 pound of muscle, a positive caloric balance of fewer than 100 calories per day is needed to promote muscle growth. This estimate was computed as follows:

$$0.25 \text{ pound per week} \times 2,500 \text{ calories per pound} = 625 \text{ calories per week}$$

Therefore, 625 calories per week ÷ 7 days per week = 90 calories per day.

You can use the MyPlate food guidance system (see Chapter 8) to increase your caloric intake. This will ensure that your diet meets the criteria for healthful living and provides adequate protein for building muscle. Be sure to avoid high-fat foods, and limit your positive caloric balance to approximately 90 calories per day. Increasing your positive caloric balance above this level will not promote a faster rate of muscular growth but will increase body fat. Finally, if you discontinue your weight-training program, be sure to lower your caloric intake to match your reduced daily energy expenditure because a failure to do so will result in fat gain.

Extreme Measures for Weight Loss

 6 Describe several extreme medical measures used for weight loss when other options haven't worked.

Most people can attain a healthy body weight through diet and exercise, but for some extremely obese individuals, these may not be enough. In such cases, surgical procedures or prescription medications may be recommended by a health-care provider.

Surgery

According to the American Society for Bariatric Surgery, surgical procedures may be recommended for weight loss in severely obese individuals (BMI >40). The surgery is considered a last resort for individuals who have tried and failed at losing weight and whose obesity poses a serious health risk. There are three basic types of weight-loss surgery: restrictive, malabsorptive, and combined restrictive/malabsorptive procedures. Restrictive procedures, such as gastric banding, work by decreasing the amount of food that can be consumed at one time. Reduced stomach capacity, along with behavioral changes, can result in lower caloric intake and consistent weight loss. Malabsorptive procedures alter digestion by bypassing the small intestine, thus limiting the absorption of calories. One of the most common bariatric surgeries is a combination of restrictive and malabsorptive procedures. The combination helps patients lose weight quickly and continue to lose weight for an extended period after the surgery (33).

All of these weight-loss procedures are considered major surgery and are associated with significant health risks, including surgical complications, bowel obstruction, blood clots, vitamin or other nutritional deficiencies, and potential psychological problems following surgery. Anyone considering a bariatric procedure should investigate these potential problems and discuss the risks with your surgeon.

Prescription Medications

For some people, prescription weight-control drugs are deemed appropriate by their health-care provider. Unlike diet pills, which are typically ineffective, several prescription medications have been scientifically shown to help achieve weight loss. In general, these medications work by either preventing food absorption or depressing appetite. Orlistat (brand name Xenical®) is a popular weight-loss drug that works by preventing about one-third of ingested fat from being absorbed in the digestive tract. The undigested fat is eliminated as waste, so side effects may include oily stool. Orlistat is the only FDA-approved weight-loss drug that acts to block fat absorption. The relatively new prescription drug Belviq® (lorcaserin HCl) suppresses appetite by increasing serotonin levels in the brain. Orlistat and Belviq® are two of three weight-loss medications approved for longer-term use in significantly obese people; however, their safety and long-term effectiveness remain unclear.

What Is Disordered Eating?

 7 Name and describe three common eating disorders and explain their associated health risks.

Although attaining a healthy body weight is a highly desirable goal, for some people the social pressures to be thin and/or muscular can lead to a negative body image and an unhealthy relationship with food. Women may feel like they need to emulate the often unattainably thin figures of popular actresses and models, and men may wish to achieve the muscular appearance of professional athletes. *Disordered eating* is a term used to describe a variety of abnormal eating behaviors. Three common forms of disordered eating that affect young adults are anorexia nervosa, bulimia nervosa, and binge eating disorder. While losing weight can be important for health and self-esteem, disordered eating is not the way to achieve weight loss. If you or any of your friends exhibit one or more of the symptoms described in the following sections, please seek professional help.

Anorexia Nervosa

Anorexia nervosa is an eating disorder in which the individual severely limits caloric intake, eventually resulting in a state of starvation. As the condition advances, the individual becomes emaciated. The psychological cause of anorexia nervosa is unclear, but it seems to be linked to an unfounded fear of fatness that may be related to familial or societal pressures to be thin (34).

Although the condition occurs in both men and women, rates of anorexia nervosa are particularly high among adolescent girls, and as many as 1 out of every

---

anorexia nervosa Eating disorder in which a person severely restricts caloric intake because of an intense fear of gaining weight.

100 adolescent girls may suffer from this condition. In females, the average age of onset is between 14 and 18 years (34). Once this eating disorder has developed, it may continue into adulthood. Evidence indicates that upper-middle-class young women who are extremely self-critical of their appearance have the highest probability of developing anorexia nervosa (34).

consider this! ///////////////

The average "female" store mannequin is 6 feet tall with a 23-inch waist, while the average woman is 5 feet, 4 inches tall with a 30-inch waist.

People suffering from anorexia nervosa may use a variety of techniques to remain thin, including starvation, excessive exercise, and laxatives. The effects include excessive weight loss, cessation of menstruation, and, in extreme cases, death. Because the condition is a serious mental and physical disorder, treatment by a team of health-care professionals (physician, psychologist or psychiatrist, and nutritionist) is needed. Treatment may require long-term psychological counseling and nutritional guidance.

The first step in seeking treatment for anorexia nervosa is recognizing that a problem exists. The following common symptoms may indicate anorexia nervosa:

- An intense fear of gaining weight
- The feeling that one is fat even at normal or below-normal body fatness because of a highly distorted body image
- In women, the absence of three or more menstrual cycles
- The development of odd behaviors concerning food; for example, preparing elaborate meals for others but only a few low-calorie foods for one's own consumption

Bulimia Nervosa

Bulimia nervosa is characterized by cycles of binge eating and purging. People with bulimia nervosa may repeatedly ingest large quantities of food and then force themselves to vomit to prevent weight gain. The frequent vomiting can damage the teeth and the esophagus due to exposure to stomach acids. Like anorexia nervosa, bulimia nervosa is most common in young women, has a psychological origin, and requires professional treatment when diagnosed. Bulimia affects approximately 1% to 3% of U.S. adolescents. The illness usually begins in late adolescence or early adult life (34).

People with bulimia nervosa may look "normal" and be of normal weight. However, even when their bodies are slender, their stomachs may protrude because they have been stretched by frequent eating binges. Other common symptoms include:

- Recurrent binge eating
- Lack of control over eating behavior
- Regular self-induced vomiting and/or use of diuretics or laxatives
- Strict fasting or use of vigorous exercise to prevent weight gain
- Averaging two or more binge eating episodes per week over a 2- to 3-month period
- Excessive concern with body shape and weight

Binge Eating Disorder

A disordered eating pattern that has recently begun to attract attention from the medical community is **binge eating disorder**, a condition in which an individual consumes mass quantities of food but does not purge after binging. The person may feel embarrassed and ashamed about gorging and resolve to stop, but the compulsion continues. The end result is weight gain and persistent feelings of shame and guilt about the out-of-control eating. The cause of binge eating is unknown, and only a very small percentage of overweight and obese individuals engage in it.

MAKE SURE YOU **KNOW...**

- Eating disorders such as anorexia nervosa, bulimia nervosa, and binge eating disorder involve patterns of severe calorie restriction, bingeing and purging, or bingeing without purging.
- Severe and prolonged eating disorders can result in an unhealthy body weight, poor health, and even death.

MasteringHealth™

bulimia nervosa Eating disorder that involves overeating (binge eating) followed by vomiting (purging).

binge eating disorder A compulsive need to gorge on food without purging.

summary

hear it! STUDY REVIEW

To hear an MP3 Chapter Summary, scan here or visit the Study Area in MasteringHealth™.

LO 1 ■ The optimal body composition for health and fitness for men ranges from 8%–19% body fat, and the optimal range for women is 21%–32% body fat.

LO 2 ■ Energy balance is achieved when the number of calories you take in through food and beverages equals the number of calories you expend through physical activity and normal body processes.

■ Total daily energy expenditure is the sum of resting metabolic rate, the energy expended to digest and store food (thermic effect of food), and the physical activity/exercise energy expenditure.

LO 3 ■ Both internal factors (hormones and genetics) and external factors (diet and lifestyle as well as physical activity and exercise) influence weight management.

LO 4 ■ The four basic components of a comprehensive weight-control program are setting realistic goals for weight loss, assessing and modifying your diet, planning physical activity, and modifying behaviors that contribute to weight gain.

■ Weight-loss goals should include both short-term and long-term goals. Losing 1 to 2 pounds per week is considered a safe rate of weight loss.

■ Research indicates that a reduced calorie diet will result in weight loss regardless of which macronutrient is emphasized. Therefore, a low-carbohydrate or low-fat diet is not superior to any other diet that results in a similar caloric deficit.

■ It is widely accepted that a nutritionally balanced but reduced calorie diet is the most desired diet for weight loss because it contains a healthy balance of nutrients and can be sustained for the long-term.

LO 5 ■ People seeking to gain weight need to take in more calories than they expend. They should seek to gain muscle mass (rather than fat) by engaging in an appropriate strength-training program.

LO 6 ■ Weight-loss options for extremely obese individuals whose weight creates health risks include prescription medications and bariatric surgery.

LO 7 ■ The eating disorders anorexia nervosa, bulimia nervosa, and binge eating disorder are serious medical conditions that require professional treatment.

study questions

review it! QUIZZES

Find more review questions online at MasteringHealth™.

LO 1 1. The optimal percentage of body fat for men and women is
   a. 5%–15% for men and 10%–20% for women.
   b. 8%–19% for men and 21%–32% for women.
   c. 15%–25% for men and 20%–30% for women.
   d. 20%–30% for men and 25%–35% for women.

2. What is optimal body weight, and how is it calculated?

LO 2 3. Identify the true statement regarding energy balance:
   a. To maintain a constant body composition, caloric intake should equal caloric expenditure.
   b. Weight gain occurs when caloric intake exceeds caloric expenditure.
   c. Weight loss occurs when caloric expenditure exceeds caloric intake.
   d. All of the above statements are true.

4. Compare exercise metabolic rate with resting metabolic rate.

5. Explain the roles of resting metabolic rate and physical activity/exercise metabolic rate in determining total caloric expenditure. Which is more important in total daily caloric expenditure in most people?

LO 3 6. Hormones that play a role in appetite include which of the following?
   a. glucagon
   b. ghrelin
   c. leptin
   d. estrogen
   e. both (a) and (d) are correct
   f. both (b) and (c) are correct

LO ④ 7. Which of the following types of exercise would be most beneficial in increasing energy expenditure?
   a. Pilates
   b. yoga
   c. strength training and cardiorespiratory endurance training
   d. table tennis

8. To lose one pound of fat tissue requires a negative caloric balance (caloric deficit) of approximately
   a. 1,000 kilocalories
   b. 1,500 kilocalories
   c. 2,500 kilocalories
   d. 3,500 kilocalories

9. Outline a simple method for computing your daily caloric expenditure and provide an example.

10. List the four major components of a weight-loss program.

11. Explain the role of behavior modification in weight loss.

12. List and describe the four major categories of weight loss diets. Which of these diet plans is recommended by the Academy of Nutrition and Dietetics for weight loss?

LO ⑤ 13. For people who need to gain weight, describe the best strategy for gaining lean muscle mass.

LO ⑥ 14. Name three types of bariatric surgery and explain how each type assists in weight loss.

LO ⑦ 15. Compare and contrast the symptoms of anorexia nervosa, bulimia nervosa, and binge eating disorder.

suggested reading

Centers for Disease Control. Healthy weight-It's not a diet, it's a lifestyle. 2015. http://www.cdc.gov/healthyweight/index.html

Clark, J. E. Diet, exercise or diet with exercise: Comparing the effectiveness of treatment options for weight loss and changes in fitness for adults (18–65 years old) who are overfat or obese: Systematic review and meta-analysis. *Journal of Diabetes and Metabolic Disorders* 13:31–11, 2015.

Donnelly, J., S. Blair, J. Jakicic, M. Manore, J. Rankin, and B. Smith. ACSM position stand: Appropriate physical activity intervention strategies for weight loss and prevention of weight regain for adults. *Medicine and Science in Sports and Exercise* 41:459–471, 2009.

Franz, M., J. VanWormer, A. Crain, J. Boucher, T. Histon, W. Caplan, J. Bowman, and N. Pronk. Weight-loss outcomes: A systematic review and meta-analysis of weight-loss clinical trials with a minimum 1-year follow-up. *Journal of American Dietary Association* 107: 1755–1767, 2007.

Powers, S., and E. Howley. *Exercise Physiology: Theory and Application to Fitness and Performance*, 9th ed. New York: McGraw-Hill, 2015.

Sherer, E., and J. Sherer. Examining the most popular weight-loss diets: How effective are they? *Journal of the American Academy of Physician Assistants* 21:31–34, 2008.

helpful weblinks

do it! WEBLINKS

For links to the organizations and websites listed, visit MasteringHealth™.

Academy of Nutrition and Dietetics

Contains articles about nutrition and weight-loss and a directory of registered dietician nutritionists. **www.eatright.org**

Centers for Disease Control and Prevention: Obesity at a Glance

Discusses the obesity epidemic and the health consequences of obesity. **www.cdc.gov/chronicdisease/resources/publications/aag/obesity.htm**

ChooseMyPlate.gov

Walks you through the advice illustrated in the MyPlate food guidance system. **www.choosemyplate.gov**

National Eating Disorders Association

Provides information and resources on eating disorders and a toll-free confidential helpline. **www.nationaleatingdisorders.org**

laboratory 9.1

do it! LABS
Complete Lab 9.1 online in the
study area of **MasteringHealth.com**

Name _____ Date _____

Determining Ideal Body Weight Using Percent Body Fat and the Body Mass Index

There are several different ways to compute an ideal body weight. Method A of this laboratory enables you to compute and record your ideal body weight using skinfold measurements, and Method B enables you to calculate and record your ideal body weight using the body mass index (BMI) procedure (see Chapter 6). Choose one of these techniques, and complete the appropriate section.

METHOD A: COMPUTING IDEAL BODY WEIGHT USING PERCENT BODY FAT

STEP 1: Calculate fat-free weight

100% − _____% (your percent body fat estimated from skinfold measurements) = _____% fat-free weight

Therefore,

_____ (your fat-free weight expressed as a decimal) × _____ (your body weight in pounds)
= _____ pounds of fat-free weight

STEP 2: Calculate optimal weight

Remember: Optimal body fat ranges are 8%–19% for men and 21%–32% for women. Optimal weight = pounds of fat-free weight ÷ (1.00 − optimal % fat), with optimal % fat expressed as a decimal. Therefore, the low and high optimal weights in the range for your gender are as follows:

For low end of % fat range: Optimal weight = _____ pounds

For high end of % fat range: Optimal weight = _____ pounds

METHOD B: COMPUTING IDEAL BODY WEIGHT USING BODY MASS INDEX (BMI)

The BMI uses the metric system. Therefore, you must express your weight in kilograms (1 kilogram = 2.2 pounds) and your height in meters (1 inch = 0.0254 meter).

STEP 1: Compute your BMI

$$\text{BMI} = \text{body weight(kilograms)} \div (\text{height in meters})^2$$

Your BMI = _____

STEP 2: Calculate your ideal body weight based on BMI

The ideal BMI for both men and women is often cited as between 18.5 and 24.9. The formula for computing ideal body weight using BMI is

$$\text{Ideal body weight(kilograms)} = \text{Desired BMI} \times (\text{height in meters})^2$$

The following example illustrates the computation of ideal body weight using the BMI. A young man who weighs 60 kilograms (132 pounds) and is 1.5 meters tall computes his BMI to be 26.7. His ideal BMI is between 18.5 and 24.9; therefore, his ideal body weight range is as follows:

Ideal body weight (low end of range): $18.5 \times 2.25 = 41.6$ kilograms (91.5 pounds)

Ideal body weight (high end of range): $24.9 \times 2.25 = 56.0$ kilograms or (123 pounds)

Now complete this calculation using your values for BMI.

My ideal body weight range using the BMI method is _____ to _____ kilograms or _____ to _____ pounds.

Note: BMI may not be a good method to determine ideal body weight for a highly muscular individual.

laboratory 9.2

do it! LABS
Complete Lab 9.2 online in the
study area of **MasteringHealth.com**

Name _____   Date _____

Estimating Daily Caloric Expenditure and the Caloric Deficit Required to Lose 1 Pound of Fat per Week

PART A: ESTIMATING YOUR DAILY CALORIC EXPENDITURE

Using the table below, compute your estimated daily caloric expenditure.

Estimated daily caloric expenditure = _____ calories/day

Note: To maintain current body weight, your caloric intake should equal your daily caloric expenditure.

To compute your estimated daily caloric expenditure, multiply your body weight in pounds by the calories per pound corresponding to your activity level.

Activity Level	Description	Calories per Pound of Body Weight Expended during 24-Hour Period
1 Very sedentary	Very limited daily movement; primary activities include lying down and sitting (e.g., working at a desk, playing video games or watching TV)	13
2 Sedentary	Job or activities that involve limited walking but sitting most of the day	14
3 Moderate activity	Some daily physical activity and weekend recreation	15
4 Very physically active	Daily physical activity and exercise at least 3–4 times/week (30–60 minutes/day)	16
5 Competitive athlete	Daily physical activity and daily vigorous exercise training (>60 minutes)	17–18

PART B: CALCULATING CALORIC INTAKE REQUIRED TO PROMOTE 1 POUND PER WEEK OF WEIGHT LOSS

Recall that 1 pound of fat contains approximately 3,500 calories. Therefore, a negative caloric balance of 500 calories per day will result in a weight loss of 1 pound per week. Use the following formula to compute your daily caloric intake to result in a daily caloric deficit of 500 calories.

Estimated daily caloric expenditure − 500 calories (deficit) = Daily caloric intake needed to produce a 500-calorie deficit

In the space provided, compute your daily caloric intake needed to produce 1 pound per week of weight loss.

_____ (estimated caloric expenditure) − 500 (caloric deficit) = _____ (target daily caloric intake)

Note: To increase body weight by 1–2 pounds per week, increase daily caloric intake by 90–180 calories per day.

laboratory 9.3

do it! LABS
Complete Lab 9.3 online in the
study area of **MasteringHealth.com**

Name _____ Date _____

Weight-Loss Goals and Progress Report

In the spaces provided, record your short-term and long-term weight-loss goals. Then keep a record of your progress.

Ideal body weight (range): _____

Short-term weight loss goal: ___1–2___ (pounds/week)

Long-term weight loss goal: _____ pounds

Week No.	Body Weight	Date	Weight Loss
1			
2			
3			
4			
5			
6			
7			
8			
9			
10			
11			
12			
13			
14			
15			

laboratory 9.4

do it! LABS
Complete Lab 9.4 online in the
study area of **MasteringHealth.com**

Name _____ Date _____

Assessing Body Image

Respond to the questions below.

1. Where do you get your ideas about the "ideal body"? If more than one applies, how do they rank?
    a. TV/movies
    b. friends (including partners)
    c. parents and family
    d. professional athletes

2. What other sources contribute to your image of the "ideal body"?

    _____

    _____

Fill in the blanks to complete the following statements about your body image. Use extra paper if needed.

3. The thing I like most about my body is

    _____

    _____

4. The thing I like least about my body is

    _____

    _____

5. When I eat a big meal, I feel

    _____

    _____

6. When I look in the mirror, I see

    _____

    _____

7. I like/dislike (choose one) shopping for clothes because

    _____

    _____

8. I feel self-conscious when

    _____

    _____

9. Compared to others, I feel my body is

    _____

    _____

10. In the presence of someone I find attractive, I feel

    _____

    _____

11. I feel that my appearance is

    _____

    _____

12. One word to describe my body is

    _____

INTERPRETATION

Review your answers and think about whether they are positive or negative. To improve a negative body image, keep the following strategies in mind:

- Focus on good physical health. Engage in physical activities that you enjoy.
- Remember that your self-worth is not dependent on how you look.
- Avoid fad diets and chronic, restrictive dieting.
- Recognize that there is much more to you than your body. Think about the qualities that you like best about yourself, and be sure to appreciate them.

laboratory 9.5

do it! LABS
Complete Lab 9.5 online in the
study area of **MasteringHealth.com**

Name _____   Date _____

What Triggers Your Eating?

By identifying the triggers that cause you to overeat, you can develop a strategy to counter those habits. Use the questions below to determine your motivation for eating. For each statement, check yes or no.

EMOTIONAL TRIGGERS

Yes	No	
_____	_____	I cannot lose weight and keep it off.
_____	_____	My eating is out of control.
_____	_____	Even if I'm not hungry, I eat.
_____	_____	I eat when I am stressed or upset.
_____	_____	Food gives me great pleasure and I use it as a reward.
_____	_____	Eating is usually on my mind.
_____	_____	My eating causes problems with weight management.
_____	_____	I go on eating binges or find myself eating constantly.
_____	_____	My eating habits cause me embarrassment.
_____	_____	I use food to help me cope with feelings.

SOCIAL TRIGGERS

Yes	No	
_____	_____	I eat whenever others around me are eating.
_____	_____	If anyone offers food, I take it.
_____	_____	When I am in a stressful social situation, I want to eat.
_____	_____	When I am in a relaxed social situation, I want to eat.
_____	_____	I eat more in a social setting than when I am alone.
_____	_____	I eat less when others are around to see me.
_____	_____	In a social setting, the amount of food I eat depends on the group of people.
_____	_____	I eat different foods in a social setting than when I am alone.

ENVIRONMENTAL TRIGGERS

Yes	No	
_____	_____	I eat more at restaurants than I do at home.
_____	_____	I eat less at restaurants than I do at home.
_____	_____	If I smell or see food, I can't resist the urge to eat.
_____	_____	If I walk by a restaurant or bakery, I can't resist the urge to eat.
_____	_____	I like to eat while reading or watching TV.
_____	_____	I find food comforting in various environmental conditions, such as on a rainy day or in cold weather.
_____	_____	I find food comforting when I am in unfamiliar surroundings.
_____	_____	If I am outdoors, I feel like I can eat more.

INTERPRETATION

Insignificant influence: If you answered "Yes" to 1 question within a section or fewer than 6 questions total, weight management is probably relatively easy for you.

Some influence: If you answered "Yes" to 2 questions within a section or 6 to 9 questions total, there are issues complicating your weight management. It might help to talk with a health-care professional while developing a weight-management plan.

Significant influence: If you answered "Yes" to 3 questions within a section or 10 to 13 questions total, there are several issues affecting your weight-management plan. Speaking with a health-care professional or counselor can help you deal with issues that trigger your eating.

Severe influence: If you answered "Yes" to 4 or more questions within a section or 14 or more questions total, there are many issues that complicate your weight management. Counseling and speaking with a health-care professional will help you develop a weight-management plan.

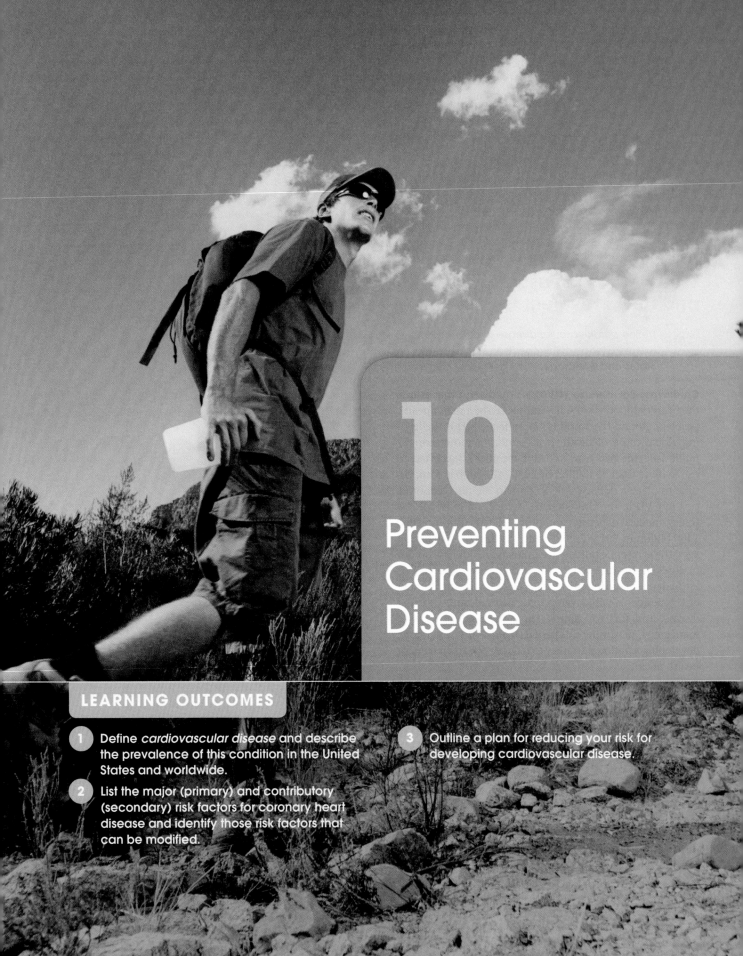

10

Preventing Cardiovascular Disease

LEARNING OUTCOMES

1 Define *cardiovascular disease* and describe the prevalence of this condition in the United States and worldwide.

2 List the major (primary) and contributory (secondary) risk factors for coronary heart disease and identify those risk factors that can be modified.

3 Outline a plan for reducing your risk for developing cardiovascular disease.

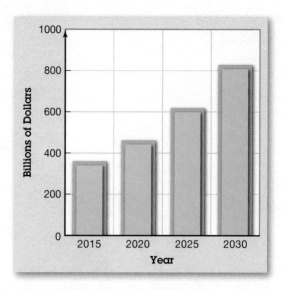

NEARLY EVERY FAMILY has been touched by heart disease, and each year millions of people worldwide die or are permanently injured due to heart attack or stroke. Although genetics plays a role in the development of cardiovascular disease in some people, everyone can reduce the risk by adopting a healthy lifestyle. In this chapter, we'll explore the factors involved in the risk of developing cardiovascular disease. A major focus will be on lifestyle changes (such as exercise and diet) that can reduce your risk of developing this dangerous disease.

What Is Cardiovascular Disease and How Prevalent Is It?

 LO Define *cardiovascular disease* and describe the prevalence of this condition in the United States and worldwide.

Cardiovascular disease (CVD) is any disease that affects the heart or blood vessels. It continues to be a major health problem around the world (1, 2). In fact, CVD is the leading global cause of death. It accounts for more than 17 million deaths per year, and this number is expected to rise to more than 23 million by 2030. Although it is impossible to place a dollar value on human life, the economic cost of CVD in the United States is great. Estimates of lost wages, medical expenses, and other related costs exceeded $480 billion in 2015 (2, 3). Further, as the U.S. population ages, the economic burden of cardiovascular disease on our nation's health-care system will become even greater. It is estimated that during the next 15 years, a growing number of U.S. residents will develop some form of cardiovascular disease, and this will almost triple the medical costs of managing CVD during this period (**FIGURE 10.1**). Therefore, developing a national strategy to reduce CVD risk is a major health priority.

Cardiovascular Disease in the United States

Although public awareness is often more focused on diseases such as cancer, cardiovascular disease remains the number-one cause of death in the United States, accounting for nearly one of every three deaths. In fact, CVD claims more lives than all forms of cancer combined (1). About 86 million Americans currently have one or more forms of CVD, and approximately 787,000 people die annually from cardiovascular disorders (1). The incidence of CVD varies among ethnic groups and is particularly high in African Americans; nearly half of all African-American adults have some form of the disease (1). See the Appreciating Diversity box on page 280 to learn more about ethnicity and CVD risk.

FIGURE 10.1 Projections of the increase in health-care cost of cardiovascular disease in the United States from 2010 to 2030.

consider this! ////////////////////////

Each day, more than 2,100 Americans die from CVD—one death every 40 seconds!

Types of Cardiovascular Disease

There are hundreds of diseases that can impair normal cardiovascular function. The four most common are arteriosclerosis, coronary heart disease, stroke, and hypertension. Let's look at each of these in more depth.

Arteriosclerosis **Arteriosclerosis** is a group of diseases characterized by a narrowing, or "hardening," of the arteries. The end result of any form of arteriosclerosis is a progressive blockage of one or more arteries, which eventually impedes blood flow to vital organs. **Atherosclerosis** is a special type of arteriosclerosis that results in arterial blockage due to buildup of a fatty deposit inside the blood vessel (**FIGURE 10.2**). This plaque deposit is typically composed of cholesterol, cellular debris, fibrin (a clotting material in the blood), and calcium. Atherosclerosis is a progressive disease that begins in childhood, with symptoms appearing later in life. The disease occurs in varying degrees, with some arteries exhibiting little blockage and others exhibiting major obstruction. Development of severe atherosclerosis within arteries that supply blood to the heart is the cause of almost all heart attacks.

Coronary Heart Disease **Coronary heart disease (CHD)** is also known as coronary artery disease. It is the result of atherosclerotic plaque blocking one or more of the blood vessels that supply the heart. CHD begins in childhood and advances as a person ages (1). Therefore, it is vital to reduce your risk of developing plaque in your coronary arteries early in life. When a major coronary artery becomes more than 75% blocked, the restriction of blood flow to the heart muscle causes chest pain. This type of chest pain, called *angina pectoris,* occurs most frequently during exercise or emotional stress, when the heart rate increases and the heart works harder than normal (4, 5). The elevated work requires an increase in blood flow to the heart muscle to provide both oxygen and nutrients. Blockage of coronary blood vessels by atherosclerotic plaque prevents the necessary increase in blood flow to the heart, and pain results.

If coronary arteries are severely blocked, a blood clot can form around the layer of plaque. If the resulting blockage completely impedes blood flow to the heart, a **heart attack** can occur (**FIGURE 10.3**). A heart attack results in the death of heart muscle cells in the left

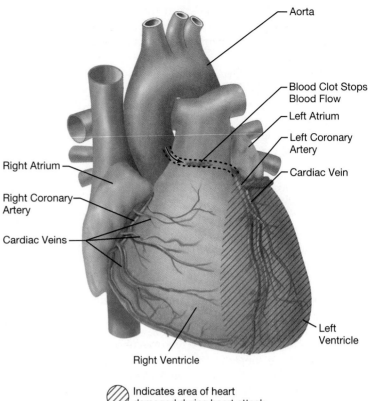

FIGURE 10.3 If the coronary arteries become blocked, the lack of oxygen due to restricted bloodflow will lead to damaged muscle tissue.

ventricle, and the severity of the heart attack is determined by how many heart muscle cells are damaged (5). A "mild" heart attack may damage only a small portion of the heart, whereas a "major" heart attack may destroy a large number of heart muscle cells. Because the number of cells destroyed during a heart attack determines the patient's chances of recovery, recognizing the symptoms

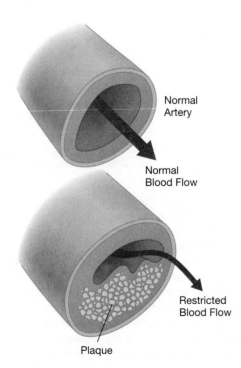

FIGURE 10.2 As plaque builds up in an artery, blood flow is restricted.

cardiovascular disease (CVD) Any disease that affects the heart or blood vessels.

arteriosclerosis Group of diseases characterized by a narrowing, or "hardening," of the arteries.

atherosclerosis Type of arteriosclerosis that results in arterial blockage due to buildup of a fatty deposit (*atherosclerotic plaque*) inside the blood vessel.

coronary heart disease (CHD) Disease that results from atherosclerotic plaque blocking one or more coronary arteries (blood vessels supplying the heart); also called *coronary artery disease.*

heart attack Stoppage of blood flow to the heart, resulting in the death of heart cells; also called *myocardial infarction.*

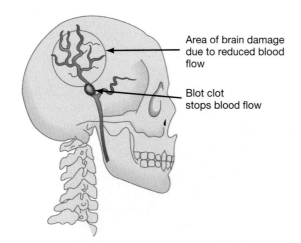

Area of brain damage due to reduced blood flow

Blot clot stops blood flow

FIGURE 10.4 A blocked artery in the brain can result in a stroke.

of a heart attack and getting prompt medical attention are crucial (see the Examining the Evidence box).

Stroke A **stroke** (also called a cerebrovascular accident) occurs when blood supply to the brain is cut off for more than a few minutes. Each year, an estimated 795,000 Americans suffer a stroke, killing nearly 129,000 (1). A common cause of stroke is blockage (due to atherosclerosis) of arteries leading to the brain (**FIGURE 10.4**). However, strokes can also occur due to a blood clot or when a blood vessel in the brain ruptures and disturbs normal blood flow to that region of the brain.

Similar to a heart attack, which results in death of heart cells, a stroke results in death of brain cells. The severity of the stroke may vary from slight to severe, depending on the location and the number of brain cells damaged. Minor strokes may involve a loss of memory, speech problems, disturbed vision, and/or mild paralysis in the extremities. Severe strokes may result in major paralysis or death.

consider this! ////////////////////

Every year more than 766,000 Americans have a heart attack, and 40% die within the first hour.

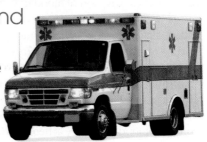

Hypertension Blood pressure is the force that blood exerts against the artery walls. **Hypertension** is abnormally high blood pressure. When the heart contracts, blood pressure increases; it follows that blood pressure decreases when the heart relaxes between beats. Blood pressure is measured in millimeters of mercury (mm Hg)

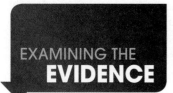

EXAMINING THE EVIDENCE

During a Heart Attack, Every Second Counts

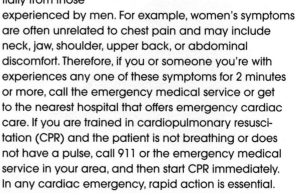

If you ever witness someone having a heart attack, or have one yourself, recognizing the symptoms and taking appropriate emergency action could mean the difference between life and death.

Here are the common signs of a heart attack (5):

- Mild to moderate pain in the chest that may spread to the shoulders, neck, or arms
- Uncomfortable pressure or sensation of fullness in the chest
- Severe pain in the chest
- Dizziness, fainting, sweating, nausea, or shortness of breath

Note that not all of these symptoms occur in every heart attack, and symptoms may differ between individuals. Symptoms in women can differ substantially from those experienced by men. For example, women's symptoms are often unrelated to chest pain and may include neck, jaw, shoulder, upper back, or abdominal discomfort. Therefore, if you or someone you're with experiences any one of these symptoms for 2 minutes or more, call the emergency medical service or get to the nearest hospital that offers emergency cardiac care. If you are trained in cardiopulmonary resuscitation (CPR) and the patient is not breathing or does not have a pulse, call 911 or the emergency medical service in your area, and then start CPR immediately. In any cardiac emergency, rapid action is essential.

and is expressed as the systolic blood pressure (pressure when your heart contracts) and the diastolic blood pressure (pressure when your heart relaxes). Normal resting systolic blood pressure is typically 120 mm Hg, and normal diastolic is 80 mm Hg. Hypertension is defined as a resting blood pressure over 140 mm Hg systolic and a diastolic pressure of 90 mm Hg or higher (5).

Your blood pressure increases during exercise. This increase is maintained while you are exercising, and blood pressure returns to resting levels soon after the exercise session ends (4). This type of short-term increase in blood pressure does not cause damage to the heart or blood vessels. However, longer-term, chronic hypertension can lead to significant health problems. Chronic high blood pressure increases the workload on the heart, which may eventually damage heart muscle and reduce the heart's ability to pump blood effectively throughout the body (5). It also damages the lining of arteries, resulting in atherosclerosis and increasing the risk of CHD and stroke (5).

Several factors can increase your risk of hypertension, including lack of regular exercise, a high-salt diet, obesity, chronic stress, family history of hypertension, gender (men have a greater risk than women), and race (African Americans have a greater risk than other groups). You can control some of these risk factors, but you cannot control others.

The prevalence of hypertension in the United States is remarkably high (**FIGURE 10.5**). The American Heart Association estimates that approximately one of every three people suffers from hypertension (1). Unfortunately, the symptoms of hypertension, such as severe headaches or dizziness, don't show up in everyone, and many people are unaware that they are hypertensive. Without annual medical checkups or blood pressure screenings, hypertension may go undiagnosed for years. For this reason, hypertension is often called the "silent killer."

MAKE SURE YOU **KNOW...**

- *Cardiovascular disease* refers to any disease that affects the heart or blood vessels; it remains the number-one cause of death in the United States and the world.

- The four major cardiovascular diseases are arteriosclerosis, coronary heart disease, stroke, and hypertension.

—MasteringHealth™

What Risk Factors Are Associated with Coronary Heart Disease?

LO **2** List the major (primary) and contributory (secondary) risk factors for coronary heart disease and identify those risk factors that can be modified.

Because CHD is the leading contributor to heart attacks, researchers are focused on understanding its causes and developing strategies for prevention. They have identified a number of major and contributory risk factors that increase the chance of developing both CHD and stroke. Major risk factors (also called *primary risk factors*) are directly related to the development of CHD and stroke. Contributory risk factors (or *secondary risk factors*) are those that increase the risk of CHD, but their direct contribution to the disease process has not been precisely determined (**FIGURE 10.6** on page 280).

Major Risk Factors

Each year the American Heart Association publishes new information concerning the major risk factors associated with the development of CHD and stroke. The most recent list includes tobacco smoking,

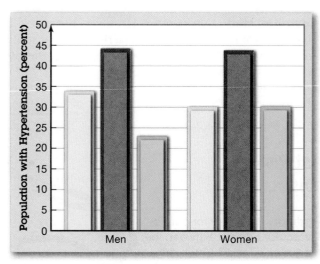

Key

░ White

▓ African American

▒ Mexican American

FIGURE 10.5 One in three Americans will develop hypertension.

stroke Brain damage that occurs when the blood supply to the brain is reduced for a prolonged period of time.

hypertension High blood pressure.

Cardiovascular Disease Risk Factors

Primary (Major) Risk Factors
Cannot be controlled:
- Heredity
- Gender
- Increasing age

Can be controlled:
- Tobacco use
- High blood pressure
- High cholesterol
- Sedentary lifestyle
- Overweight and obesity
- Diabetes

Secondary (Contributory) Risk Factors
Can be controlled:
- Stress
- Diet and nutrition
- Alcohol consumption

FIGURE 10.6 Primary and secondary risk factors for cardiovascular disease.

consider this! ///////////////////////

Within 10 years of quitting smoking, a person's risk of death from CHD is reduced to a level equal to that of someone who has never smoked.

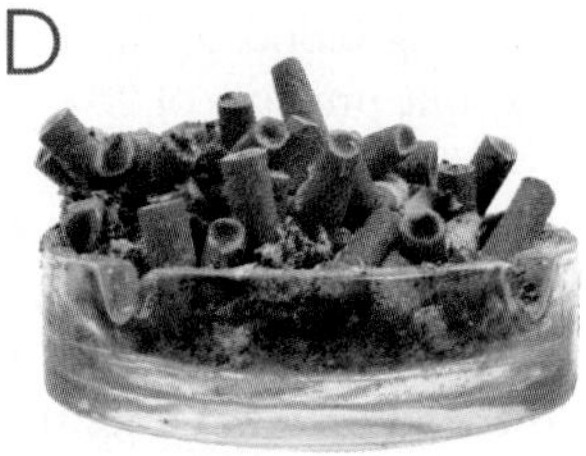

hypertension, high blood cholesterol levels, physical inactivity, obesity and being overweight, diabetes mellitus, heredity, gender, and increasing age (1). The greater the number of risk factors an individual has, the greater the likelihood that he or she will develop CHD. However, it is important to note that of the nine major risk factors, you can modify, treat, or control six of them (see Figure 10.6).

Smoking A smoker's risk of developing CHD is more than twice that of a nonsmoker (1). Smoking is also considered the biggest risk factor for sudden death due to cardiac arrest, a heart attack, or irregular heartbeats (**arrhythmias**). Smoking promotes the development of atherosclerosis in peripheral blood vessels (such as in the arms or legs), which can lead to hypertension and increased risk of stroke. And smokers who have a heart attack are more likely to die within an hour after the attack than are nonsmokers. Studies have also concluded that passive inhalation of cigarette smoke (secondhand smoke) can increase the risk of both cardiovascular and lung disease (6). Both the American Heart Association and the American Cancer Society report that breathing secondhand smoke can be as dangerous to your health as direct inhalation.

Cigarette smoking can affect your risk for CHD in at least four ways. First, the nicotine in the smoke increases both heart rate and blood pressure. Second, smoking increases the stickiness of the platelets in your blood, increasing the likelihood of clotting and raising the risk of heart attack. Third, nicotine influences the way your heart functions, leading to arrhythmias and potentially, sudden cardiac death. Finally, smoking increases your chance of developing atherosclerosis by elevating the amount of cholesterol in the blood and promoting fat deposits in arterial walls (6). Women who both smoke and take birth control pills are at an even higher risk for developing CHD (1).

Hypertension Hypertension is unique because it is both a disease in its own right and a risk factor for stroke and CHD. It contributes to CHD by accelerating the rate of atherosclerosis development (5, 7).

A diet high in sodium (such as from processed foods and fast food) increases the risk of developing

APPRECIATING DIVERSITY **Who Is at Greatest Risk for Cardiovascular Disease?**

Ethnicity, gender, age, and socioeconomic status can all affect an individual's risk of developing cardiovascular disease, and these factors explain why CVD is more prevalent in certain segments of the U.S. population. African Americans, for example, are at greater risk of developing hypertension compared to the U.S. population as a whole. Similarly, Native Americans and people of Latino heritage have higher prevalence of diabetes, an important primary risk factor for cardiovascular disease. Between the ages of 20 and 50, men are at greater risk than women for developing cardiovascular disease. Finally, individuals with low incomes experience higher incidences of both heart disease and obesity (a primary risk factor for heart disease).

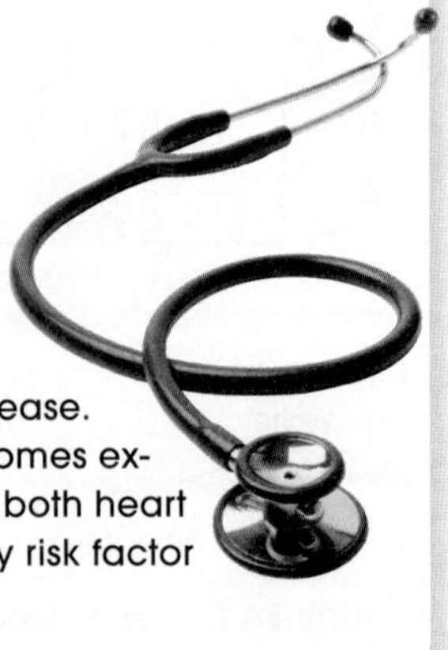

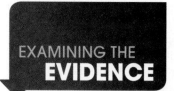

What Additional Factors Contribute to Atherosclerosis and Heart Attacks?

Clearly, an unfavorable ratio of LDL and HDL cholesterol in the blood increases your risk of both atherosclerosis and heart attack. Yet research reveals that half of heart attack victims have normal blood cholesterol levels (5). This finding indicates that factors other than cholesterol contribute to your level of risk. Two other factors that increase the rate of atherosclerosis are high blood levels of homocysteine and chronic inflammation.

Homocysteine is an amino acid that normally does not accumulate in high levels in the blood because the body can eliminate it via chemical reactions that require B vitamins (folate, B6, and B12). However, a diet low in B vitamins can cause homocysteine levels to rise in the blood. Plus, some people have a genetic predisposition toward developing high blood homocysteine levels, which can damage blood vessels and promote atherosclerosis (5). Although the American Heart Association has not classified high levels of homocysteine as a major risk factor, they recommend screening for high blood homocysteine levels in patients with a family history of heart disease.

Inflammation is a protective response by the body's immune system involving certain cells and blood vessels that work to eliminate the cause of tissue injury or infection. Normally, acute inflammation is tightly regulated by the body as part of this response. Prolonged inflammation (called chronic inflammation) is an abnormal immune response that can lead to health problems such as atherosclerosis (5). Because chronic inflammation has been shown to increase the risk of both atherosclerosis and heart attacks, the FDA has approved the measurement of a blood marker of inflammation called C-reactive protein as an independent biomarker of CVD risk. C-reactive protein is a blood protein that increases in the presence of chronic inflammation. People with elevated levels of C-reactive protein have a two-fold increase in risk of having a heart attack than individuals with normal blood levels. The risk of heart attack is even greater in individuals with both elevated C-reactive protein and unfavorable cholesterol levels, resulting in a nine-fold increase in risk!

---

hypertension. High plasma levels of sodium expand the blood volume and thereby increase blood pressure. Although sodium is a required micronutrient, the daily requirement for most people is small (1,500 mg/day). Some individuals are more sensitive to sodium than others, and sodium-sensitive individuals with hypertension can often lower their blood pressure by reducing their salt intake. For example, sodium-sensitive people who ingest less than 1,500 mg of sodium each day typically do not develop hypertension. In contrast, sodium-sensitive people who consume more than 1 teaspoon of salt per day (about 2,300 mg of sodium) are at risk for hypertension.

Even athletes or outdoor workers who lose large amounts of water and electrolytes via sweat rarely require more than 3,000 mg of sodium per day. Currently, many U.S. citizens consume more than 5,000 mg every day; clearly, this level of sodium intake is beyond the amount needed for normal body function.

The key to lowering your sodium intake is avoiding foods that are high in salt, primarily processed food and beverages and items from fast-food chains. Take the time to read labels and learn which foods contain a lot of sodium, and limit your intake to less than 1,500 mg per day. Because of the link between hypertension and salt intake, the National Institutes of Health has developed a Dietary Approach to Stop Hypertension (called DASH). This DASH eating plan is recognized as an excellent approach to prevent and lower hypertension.

High Blood Cholesterol Levels Cholesterol is a type of lipid that can either be consumed in foods or be synthesized in the body, and it is a primary risk factor for CHD. The risk of CHD increases as blood cholesterol increases. As described in Chapter 8, triglycerides are another type of fat that when combined with cholesterol can increase your risk of developing CHD.

Because cholesterol is not soluble in blood, it is combined with proteins in the liver so it can be transported in the bloodstream. This combination of cholesterol, triglycerides, and protein results in two major forms of cholesterol: **low-density lipoprotein (LDL)** and **high-density lipoprotein (HDL)**. The association between

---

arrhythmia Irregular heartbeat.

low-density lipoprotein (LDL) A combination of protein, fat, and cholesterol in the blood, composed of relatively large amounts of cholesterol. LDLs promote the fatty plaque accumulation in the coronary arteries that leads to heart disease; also called "bad cholesterol."

high-density lipoprotein (HDL) A combination of protein, fat, and cholesterol in the blood, composed of relatively large amounts of protein. Protects against the fatty plaque accumulation in the coronary arteries that leads to heart disease; also called "good cholesterol."

elevated blood cholesterol and CHD is due primarily to LDL. Individuals with high blood LDL levels have an increased risk of CHD, whereas those with high levels of HDL have a decreased risk of CHD (1, 7–9). Because of these relationships, LDL has been called "bad cholesterol" and HDL has been called "good cholesterol." Although the exact role that triglycerides play in the development of CHD remains under investigation, people with high blood triglyceride levels often have high blood levels of LDL and low blood levels of HDL.

Even though the risk of developing CHD is best predicted from LDL and HDL levels in the blood, measurement of total blood cholesterol (the sum of all types of cholesterol) also provides a good indication of CHD risk (1, 4, 10). A total blood cholesterol concentration of less than 200 mg/dL (milligrams per deciliter) indicates a low risk of developing CHD, whereas a concentration greater than 240 mg/dL indicates a high CHD risk (10). Unfortunately, due to lifestyle factors, more than 43% of adults in the United States have total blood cholesterol levels above 240 mg/dL (1).

The National Institutes of Health released new guidelines for assessing CHD risks using blood levels of LDL and HDL. For a brief overview of these guidelines, see the Examining the Evidence box. Other factors also contribute to the risk of atherosclerosis and heart attacks; see Examining the Evidence box on page 281.

Physical Inactivity The first evidence that physical activity reduces the risk of heart disease emerged more than 60 years ago. Since this initial research, studies have consistently concluded that regular physical activity reduces the risk of developing CHD (12, 13). Moreover, research shows that while some physical activity is better than none, additional heart health benefits occur as physical activity increases (12).

Although it is well known that exercise reduces the risk of CHD, the mechanism by which this works is unclear. Possible explanations include improvements in body weight, blood pressure, and blood lipid profile, and the reduced risk of diabetes (8–10), all of which are associated with regular exercise. Collectively, these changes can greatly reduce the overall risk of developing CHD.

Diabetes Mellitus Diabetes is a disease that results in elevated blood sugar levels due to the body's inability to use blood sugar properly. Diabetes occurs most often in middle age and is common in people who are overweight. The link between diabetes and CHD is well established, as approximately 75% of all individuals with diabetes die from some form of cardiovascular disease. The role that diabetes plays in increasing the risk of CHD could be linked to the fact that people with diabetes are often inactive, have unfavorable blood cholesterol levels, and suffer from hypertension (10).

Overweight and Obesity Compared to individuals who maintain their ideal body weight, overweight and obese individuals are more likely to develop CHD, even if they have no other major risk factors (11). However,

---

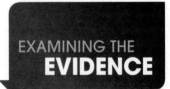

Blood Cholesterol Guidelines from the National Institutes of Health

In response to studies conclusively showing that lowering blood LDL ("bad cholesterol") levels can reduce the risk of heart disease by 40% (10), the National Institutes of Health (NIH) has released guidelines for optimal blood levels of LDL and HDL. Even though the major focus of the guidelines is to provide recommendations for managing blood LDL levels, NIH included recommendations for blood levels of HDL ("good cholesterol") because HDL can carry cholesterol away from arteries and back to the liver. The guidelines are summarized in the table.

In short, the guidelines consider LDL levels under 100 mg/dL to be optimal for reducing the risk of developing CHD, whereas LDL levels above 159 mg/dL are considered indicative of a high risk for CHD. Because the presence of HDL can lower LDL levels, low blood levels of HDL can indicate an increased risk of developing CHD.

Accordingly, the guidelines consider blood HDL levels below 40 mg/dL to be low and undesirable in terms of CHD risk.

Cholesterol Concentration (mg/dL)	Classification
LDL	
<100	Optimal
100–129	Near optimal
130–159	Borderline high
160–189	High
>189	Very high
HDL	
<40	Low (undesirable)
>60	High (very desirable)

obese individuals more commonly will exhibit multiple major risk factors for CHD such as problematic blood cholesterol levels and hypertension (11).

Of particular interest is the fact that a person's fat distribution pattern affects the risk of CHD. Waist-to-hip circumference ratios greater than 1.0 for men and 0.8 for women indicate a significant risk for development of CHD. The precise physiological reason for the link between CHD and regional fat distribution is unclear, but excess abdominal fat is often associated with numerous CHD risk factors, including low blood levels of HDL, inflammation, and type 2 diabetes.

Possible causes of hypertension in obese individuals include high sodium intake, which elevates blood pressure, and increased vascular resistance, which results in the need for higher pressure to pump blood to the tissues (4).

Heredity Children of parents with CHD are more likely to develop CHD than are children of parents who do not have CHD (1, 3, 5). Evidence suggests that the familial risk for CHD may be linked to factors such as blood cholesterol, hypertension, diabetes, and obesity. People with a family history of CHD are not doomed to develop this disease, but in order to reduce their risk they must adopt a lifestyle that includes maintaining a healthy weight, eating a healthy diet, and engaging in regular exercise.

Gender Up to age 55, men have a greater risk of developing CHD and stroke than do women. Much of the protection against CHD in women is linked to the female sex hormone estrogen, which may elevate HDL cholesterol. Although the risk of CHD increases markedly in women after menopause, it never becomes as great as for men (3).

Increasing Age As we age, our risk for developing CHD increases. This is partly due to the fact that the buildup of arterial plaque is an ongoing process; the longer one lives, the greater the buildup. More than 80% of people who die of CHD are age 65 or older (1). Increasing age also increases your risk of stroke. Most people who have strokes are over 55, and the risk of stroke increases with age (1).

Contributory Risk Factors

Contributory (secondary) risk factors are those that increase your risk of developing a major risk factor. The American Heart Association recognizes stress, alcohol, and diet as contributory risk factors for CHD.

Stress Stress contributes to the development of several major CHD risk factors. For example, people under stress may start smoking in an effort to relax, or stress could influence smokers to smoke more than they normally would. Stress increases the risk of developing both hypertension and an unfavorable blood cholesterol profile. The physiological connection appears to be that stress induces the release of hormones that elevate blood pressure.

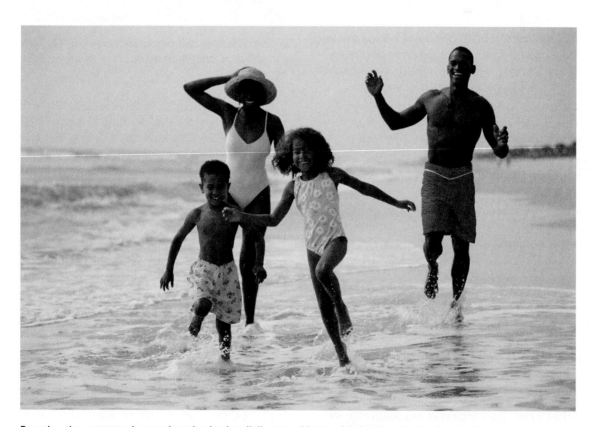

People who engage in regular physical activity are at lower risk for developing heart disease.

Alcohol Consumption Although there is some evidence that moderate alcohol consumption (one drink per day for women and two drinks per day for men) may lower risk for heart disease, drinking too much alcohol raises risk. People who drink too much alcohol are more likely to experience high blood pressure, heart failure, and stroke. Excessive alcohol consumption can also contribute to high triglycerides, cancer, and liver disease. The American Heart Association recommends that nondrinkers continue to abstain and that moderate drinkers should not increase their alcohol consumption.

Diet A healthy diet can reduce your risk of developing cardiovascular disease. The food you eat (and the amount) can affect several controllable risk factors including blood cholesterol levels, blood pressure, diabetes, and being overweight or obese. Therefore, consuming nutrient-rich foods that are high in vitamins, minerals, fiber, and other nutrients but are low in calories and fat can reduce the chances that you develop major risk factors for cardiovascular diseases.

see it!

ABC VIDEO

Watch the "Importance of Heart Health in Your Youth" ABC News video online at MasteringHealth™.

MAKE SURE YOU **KNOW**...

- Researchers have identified major (primary) and contributory (secondary) risk factors that increase the chance of developing coronary heart disease (CHD) and stroke.

- Major risk factors for CHD and stroke include smoking, hypertension, unfavorable blood cholesterol levels, physical inactivity, diabetes mellitus, overweight and obesity, heredity, gender, and increasing age.

- Tobacco use, blood pressure, blood cholesterol levels, activity level, overweight/obesity and diabetes are factors that can be controlled.

- Risk factors that cannot be controlled are heredity, gender, and increasing age.

- Contributory risk factors for CHD and stroke include stress, overconsumption of alcohol, and poor diet. All of these can be controlled by lifestyle changes.

MasteringHealth™

How Can You Reduce Your Risk of Heart Disease?

LO ③ Outline a plan for reducing your risk for developing cardiovascular disease.

Although cardiovascular disease remains the number-one killer in the United States, incidence has declined in recent years (1). This drop has occurred primarily because people

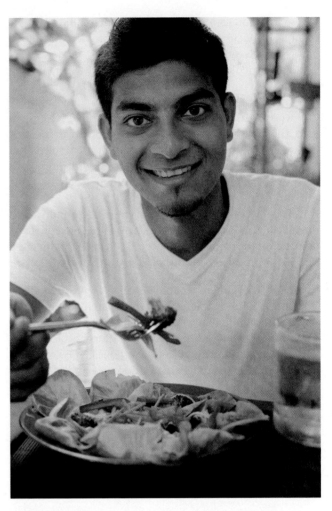

Eating a healthy diet, particularly one that's low in sodium, saturated fat, and cholesterol, can reduce your risk for heart disease.

have reduced their risk factors for CHD. Nonetheless, a recent study reveals that more than half of college-age students (18–24 years) have at least one major CHD risk factor, and nearly one-quarter of these students have advanced atherosclerotic lesions (plaque buildup in arteries) (14). Remember, the majority (70%) of risk factors can be modified by changes in behavior.

Don't Smoke

As soon as a smoker quits, CHD risk begins to decline. If you don't currently smoke, the best advice is not to start. If you do smoke, you need to stop. Unfortunately, for most people, smoking is a difficult habit to break. Major behavior modification is needed to stop smoking and to remain smoke-free for the rest of your life.

Lower Your Blood Pressure

Hypertension can be combated in several ways. In some instances, medication may be required to control high blood pressure. However, in many cases, exercise and a

Coronary heart disease (CHD) is our nation's greatest threat to life expectancy, and physical inactivity is a major risk factor. You can reduce your risk by becoming physically active and following the American Heart Association's recommendations for exercise to improve your overall cardiovascular health:

- Perform at least 30 minutes of moderate-intensity aerobic activity 5 days per week (150 minutes total)

Or

- Perform at least 25 minutes of vigorous aerobic activity at least 3 days per week (75 minutes total)

Plus

- Perform moderate-to high-intensity resistance exercise training at least 2 days per week for additional health benefits.

- For adults with high blood pressure or high cholesterol, the recommendation is 40 minutes of aerobic exercise at a moderate intensity 3–4 days per week to lower your risk of heart attack and stroke.

healthy diet low in sodium can assist in lowering blood pressure. Finding ways to successfully manage stress is also important.

Reduce Blood Cholesterol Levels

High blood cholesterol levels are a major factor in risk for CHD, and the best way to improve your lipid profile is through diet and exercise. Decreasing your intake of cholesterol can often reduce your blood cholesterol levels. Saturated fats stimulate cholesterol synthesis in the liver and therefore contribute to elevated blood cholesterol. Saturated fats are found mostly in meat and dairy products, so avoid a high intake of these foods. If diet and exercise are not effective in lowering blood lipid levels to a desirable range, cholesterol-lowering drugs (called statins) are available (15, 16).

Be Physically Active

Regular exercise has been shown to improve blood lipid profiles in most people. In addition, regular aerobic exercise has been shown to modify other CHD risk factors by positively influencing blood pressure, body composition, and insulin resistance. Even modest levels of exercise (see Coaching Corner) can reduce the risk of developing CHD due to physical inactivity (1).

Although small amounts of exercise can provide some protection against CHD, studies reveal that the risk of death from CHD decreases as the total physical activity energy expenditure increases from 500 to 3,500 kilocalories per week (12). Further, while total energy expenditure from exercise is important in preventing CHD, the intensity of exercise is also important. Studies reveal that individuals engaged in regular vigorous exercise (50% $\dot{V}O_2$ max or higher) were better protected against CHD than people exercising at much lower levels (12, 13).

Remember, regular endurance exercise (3 or more days per week) is the key. Sporadic bouts of exercise (3–5 days per month) will not reduce your risk, and completely stopping exercise will result in a loss of exercise-induced protection from heart disease. Make a commitment to a consistent, lifelong exercise program today. Your heart will love you for it!

see it!
ABC VIDEO
Watch the "Mediterranean Diet Could Help Reduce Heart Disease" ABC News video online at MasteringHealth™.

Reduce Your Stress Level

Relaxation techniques can help counteract the effects of a stressful lifestyle and reduce the risk of developing

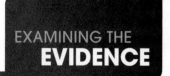

EXAMINING THE EVIDENCE

Are Some People at Risk for Sudden Cardiac Death During Exercise?

While regular physical activity reduces the risk of developing CHD, vigorous exercise can acutely increase the risk of both sudden cardiac death and heart attacks in susceptible persons (17). For example, people with advanced heart disease might have an increased risk for sudden death during exercise because of blockage in a major coronary artery. Individuals with hereditary cardiac abnormalities may also be at risk during exercise (17). If problems are suspected, a medical history and physical exam by a qualified physician can detect hidden heart disease that could pose a risk for participating in regular exercise.

CHD. Everyone's life contains stressful elements. For example, college students often face stress related to studying for exams and completing course assignments on time. If you are stressed about school-related issues, try exercising later in the day to reduce tension. If you find yourself getting angry or hostile easily, consider scheduling sessions with a school counselor trained in anger management.

hear it!

CASE STUDY

How can Keisha reduce her risk of heart disease? Listen to the online case study at MasteringHealth™.

MAKE SURE YOU **KNOW...**

- Although heart disease remains the number-one killer in the United States, its incidence has declined in recent years. This reduction has likely occurred because people have modified their behavior to reduce their risk factors.

- You can reduce your risk of developing CHD by not smoking, controlling your blood pressure, eating a healthy diet, being physically active, and reducing your stress level.

—MasteringHealth™

steps ▶ FOR BEHAVIOR CHANGE

What's your risk for cardiovascular disease?

Although you may not be able to imagine the day when you'll have high blood pressure or diabetes, you do have a chance of developing one or both of these conditions during your lifetime. Take this quiz to determine whether your current habits put you at higher risk for developing CVD.

Y N

☐ ☐ Do you get up and move around often enough to accumulate 30 minutes of physical activity per day?

☐ ☐ Do you usually avoid eating high-fat foods?

☐ ☐ Do you watch your sodium intake and refrain from using too much salt during cooking and at the table?

☐ ☐ Do you monitor your stress level and practice stress management when necessary?

☐ ☐ Do you avoid smoking cigarettes and using other tobacco products?

If you answered yes to three or more of these questions, congratulations! You are on your way to developing a lifetime of healthy habits. If you answered no to most of these questions, you may already be at increased risk for CVD.

Tips to Lower Your CVD Risk

Tomorrow, you will:

☑ Start an exercise program. Even a half hour per day a few days a week will go a long way in improving heart health. You'll look and feel better, too.

Within the next 2 weeks, you will:

☑ Watch your diet. Although the occasional fast food meal isn't the end of the world, in general, you should eat whole foods, such as fruits, vegetables, and whole grains, and avoid deep-fried or other high-fat foods.

☑ Eat less salt. Sodium is an essential nutrient for several body processes, but you actually need very little to be healthy, and too much sodium has been linked to high blood pressure.

By the end of the semester, you will:

☑ De-stress. Too much stress is linked not only to increased risk of CVD, but also to high blood pressure. (See Chapter 11.)

☑ Establish a plan to quit smoking. Tobacco use leads to numerous health problems. If you don't smoke, don't start. If you smoke, take steps to stop.

study plan

Customize your study plan—and master your health!—
in the Study Area of **MasteringHealth.**

summary

hear it! STUDY REVIEW

To hear an MP3 Chapter Summary, scan here or visit
the Study Area in MasteringHealth™.

LO ① ■ Cardiovascular disease (CVD) is the number-one
cause of death in the United States, and its
incidence is expected to rise over the next two
decades.

■ Cardiovascular disease refers to any disease that
affects the heart and blood vessels. Common
CVDs are atherosclerosis, coronary heart disease,
stroke, and hypertension.

LO ② ■ Primary (major) risk factors for coronary heart
disease (CHD) are those that directly increase
the risk of disease. Secondary (contributory) risk

factors may increase your chance of developing
CHD by promoting the development of a major
risk factor.

■ Primary risk factors for developing CHD include
smoking, hypertension, unfavorable blood
cholesterol levels, physical inactivity, diabetes
mellitus, overweight and obesity, heredity,
gender, and increasing age.

■ Secondary risk factors include stress, poor diet,
and overconsumption of alcohol.

LO ③ ■ You can reduce your risk of developing CHD
by not smoking, eating a healthy diet, being
physically active, maintaining a healthy
body weight and optimal blood pressure,
and reducing stress.

study questions

review it! QUIZZES

Find more review questions online at MasteringHealth™.

LO ① 1. The leading cause of death in the United States is
   a. AIDS.
   b. cancer.
   c. cardiovascular disease.
   d. accidents.

  2. Define the following terms:
   a. cardiovascular disease
   b. coronary heart disease
   c. stroke
   d. hypertension

  3. Which of the following blood pressure measurements would be considered hypertension?
   a. 100/80   c. 130/80
   b. 110/80   d. 140/90

LO ② 4. Which of the following is *not* a major risk factor
for CHD?
   a. smoking
   b. hypertension
   c. unfavorable blood cholesterol
   d. high resting pulse rate

LO ③ 5. Which of the following risk factors for CHD
cannot be modified by a change in behavior?
   a. obesity
   b. heredity
   c. hypertension
   d. stress

  6. Explain the difference between major (primary)
and contributory (secondary) risk factors for developing coronary heart disease and list factors that
fall under each category.

  7. Why are high-density lipoproteins known as
"good" cholesterol? Conversely, why are low-density lipoproteins labeled "bad" cholesterol?

  8. How does a high-sodium diet contribute to
hypertension?

  9. How does smoking increase the risk of developing
cardiovascular disease?

  10. Summarize the American Heart Association's
recommendations for exercise to reduce your
risk of heart disease.

suggested reading

American Heart Association. Heart disease and stroke statistics—2012 update. *Circulation* 125:e2–e220, 2012.

Franklin, B., and C. Lavie. Triggers of acute cardiovascular events and potential strategies: Prophylactic role of regular exercise. *Physician and Sports Medicine* 39:11–21, 2011.

Löllgen, H., A. Böckenhoff, and G. Knapp. Physical activity and all-cause mortality: An updated meta-analysis with different intensity categories. *International Journal of Sports Medicine* 30:213–224, 2009.

Powers, S., and E. Howley. *Exercise Physiology: Theory and Application to Fitness and Performance*, 9th ed. New York: McGraw-Hill, 2015.

Trogdon, P., O. Khavjou, J. Butler, K. Dracup, M. Ezekowitz, et al. Forecasting the future of cardiovascular disease in the United States: A policy statement from the American Heart Association. *Circulation* 123:933–944, 2011.

Waisted: Abdominal obesity and your health. *Harvard Men's Health Watch* 13:1–6, 2009.

helpful weblinks

do it! WEBLINKS

For links to the organizations and websites listed, visit MasteringHealth™.

American Heart Association

Contains information about a variety of topics related to both heart disease and stroke. **www.heart.org**

American Medical Association

Offers many sources of information about a wide variety of medical problems, including heart disease. **www.ama-assn.org**

Lowering Your Blood Pressure with DASH

A guide to the DASH eating plan from the National Heart, Lung and Blood Institute. **www.nhlbi.nih.gov/health/public/heart/hbp/dash/new_dash.pdf**

Mayo Clinic

Contains wide-ranging information about diet, fitness, and health. **www.mayoclinic.org**

WebMD

Presents information about a wide variety of diseases and medical problems, including heart disease. **www.webmd.com**

STEP 2: DETERMINE IF YOU NEED A TREATMENT PLAN

If your overall CHD risk indicates that you need to lower your LDL cholesterol level, you can do this by making lifestyle changes. In some cases, medication may also be prescribed. Locate your CHD risk in the chart below. This risk is based on the 10-year heart attack risk that you just calculated, as well as your overall CHD risk factors.

If you are at moderate to high risk, make an appointment with your health-care provider now to establish a treatment plan.

CHD RISK GROUPS

Very High

1. Ten-year heart attack risk of 20% or more *or*

2. History of coronary heart disease, diabetes, peripheral artery disease, carotid artery disease, or aortic aneurysm

High

1. Ten-year heart attack risk of 10% to 20% *and*

2. Two or more major coronary risk factors[†]

Moderately High

1. Ten-year heart attack risk under 10% *and*

2. Two or more major coronary risk factors[†]

Low to Moderate

1. One or no major coronary risk factors[†]

[†] Major coronary risk factors includes tobacco smoking, hypertension, high blood cholesterol levels, physical inactivity, obesity and being overweight, diabetes mellitus, heredity, gender, and increasing age.

laboratory 10.2

do it! LABS
Complete Lab 10.2 online in the
study area of **MasteringHealth.com**

Name _____ Date _____

Understanding Your Risk for Cardiovascular Disease

Each of us has a unique level of risk for various diseases. You can take action to change some of these risks; others are risks that you need to consider as you plan a lifelong strategy for overall risk reduction. Answer each of the following questions, and total your points in each section. If you score between 1 and 5 in any section, consider your risk: The higher the number, the greater your risk. If you answered "Don't know" to any question, talk to your parents or other family members as soon as possible to find out whether you have any unknown risks.

PART I: ASSESS YOUR FAMILY RISK FOR CVD

1. Do any of your primary relatives (mother, father, grandparents, siblings) have a history of heart disease or stroke?

   Yes _____ (1 point)   No _____ (0 points)   Don't know _____

2. Do any of your primary relatives (mother, father, grandparents, siblings) have diabetes?

   Yes _____ (1 point)   No _____ (0 points)   Don't know _____

3. Do any of your primary relatives (mother, father, grandparents, siblings) have high blood pressure?

   Yes _____ (1 point)   No _____ (0 points)   Don't know _____

4. Do any of your primary relatives (mother, father, grandparents, siblings) have a history of high cholesterol?

   Yes _____ (1 point)   No _____ (0 points)   Don't know _____

5. Would you say that your family consumed a high-fat diet (lots of red meat, dairy products, butter or margarine) during your time spent at home?

   Yes _____ (1 point)   No _____ (0 points)   Don't know _____

Total points _____

PART II: ASSESS YOUR LIFESTYLE RISK FOR CVD

1. Is your total cholesterol level higher than it should be?

   Yes _____ (1 point)   No _____ (0 points)   Don't know _____

2. Do you have high blood pressure?

   Yes _____ (1 point)   No _____ (0 points)   Don't know _____

3. Have you been diagnosed as prediabetic or diabetic?

   Yes _____ (1 point)   No _____ (0 points)   Don't know _____

4. Do you smoke?

   Yes _____ (1 point)   No _____ (0 points)   Don't know _____

5. Would you describe your life as being highly stressful?

   Yes _____ (1 point)   No _____ (0 points)   Don't know _____

Total points _____

PART III: ASSESS YOUR ADDITIONAL RISKS FOR CVD

1. How would you best describe your current weight?

    a. Lower than what it should be for my height and weight. (0 points)
    b. About what it should be for my height and weight. (0 points)
    c. Higher than it should be for my height and weight. (1 point)

2. How would you describe the level of exercise that you get each day?

    a. Less than what I should be exercising each day. (1 point)
    b. About what I should be exercising each day. (0 points)
    c. More than what I should be exercising each day. (0 points)

3. How would you describe your typical caloric intake?

    a. About the recommended number of calories each day. (0 points)
    b. Less than the recommended number of calories each day. (0 points)
    c. More than the recommended number of calories each day. (1 point)

4. Which of the following best describes your typical dietary behavior?

    a. I select from each of the major food groups and try to eat the recommended amounts of fruits and vegetables. (0 points)
    b. I eat high amounts of saturated fat from red meat and dairy products each day. (1 point)
    c. Whenever possible, I try to substitute olive oil or canola oil for other forms of dietary fat. (0 points)

5. Do you have a history of *Chlamydia* infection?

    a. Yes. (1 point)
    b. No. (0 points)

Total points _____

laboratory 10.3

do it! LABS
Complete Lab 10.3 online in the
study area of **MasteringHealth.com**

Name _____   Date _____

Assessing Your Genetic Predisposition
for Cardiovascular Disease

Following is a family tree that allows you to fill in risk factors for heart disease in your family members. Remember that heart disease has a genetic component, so examining your relatives' health and lifestyles will provide insight into your future susceptibility to heart disease. Write in risk factors related to heart disease for each family member. Examples include hypertension, high blood cholesterol, diabetes, stroke, obesity, and heart attack.

Your Family History of Heart Disease

Grandparents   Grandparents

_____   _____
_____   _____
_____   _____

Aunts/Uncles   Mother ————————— Father   Aunts/Uncles

_____   _____   _____   _____
_____   _____   _____   _____
_____   _____   _____   _____

Sisters   You   Brothers

_____   _____   _____
_____   _____   _____
_____   _____   _____

In the space below, list any additional diet, behavior, or lifestyle risks in your life that may contribute to heart disease. Examples include high stress level, poor diet, physical inactivity, or high sodium intake.

_____

_____

_____

_____

INTERPRETATION

Inherited traits can increase your risk of cardiovascular disease. Discovering that you have a family history of CHD risk factors is a good first step in reducing your own risk. You are not necessarily destined to develop any of the conditions present in your relatives. Lifestyle changes that include moderate exercise and proper diet can reduce your risk of developing cardiovascular disease. Being aware of health concerns and problems within your family that may be passed on genetically will make you a more informed, health-conscious individual.

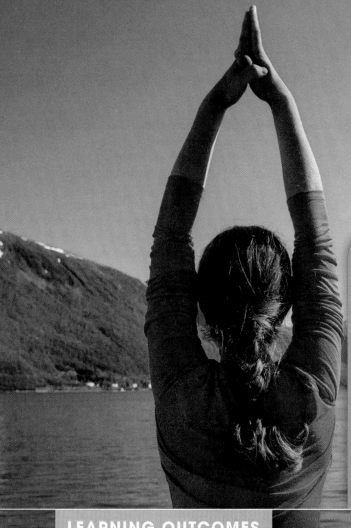

11
Stress Management

LEARNING OUTCOMES

1. Define *stress* and describe the physiological stress response.

2. List three factors that can affect your stress level.

3. Explain how stress can affect your health.

4. Describe three effective strategies for managing stress and explain why they work.

DO YOU TEND to get sick during finals or have difficulty sleeping when an important assignment is due? Does a disagreement leave you unfocused? Do you feel muscle tension while sitting in rush-hour traffic? These familiar everyday situations often lead to stress and the associated negative physical symptoms. However, some stress can be good. For example, you may have noticed that feeling some stress before a test, competition, or performance pushes you to do your best. Remember, the goal is not to eliminate all stress, but to manage it so it does not negatively affect your health and performance.

What Is Stress and the Stress Response?

LO **1** Define *stress* and describe the physiological stress response.

When stressed, the body is in a state of mental and physical tension, because the balance (homeostasis) of the body's systems is disrupted. **Stress** is caused by different types of **stressors**, including physical (such as an injury) or mental (such as a deadline or personal conflict). Under any type of stress the body's physiological and emotional responses usually cause feelings of tension and anxiety. The body's reaction to stress, called the **stress response**, prepares us to deal with stressors so homeostasis can be restored.

Stressors can be acute (such as the death of a loved one), cumulative (such as a series of events that lead to the breakup of a committed relationship), or chronic (such as daily job- or school-related pressures). Although it is clear that chronic or extreme stress is unhealthy, some degree of stress is required to maximize performance. For any type of "performance" activity there is an optimal level of stress that pushes us to perform and excel. This level is specific to each individual, and it is motivating and energizing. Stress that is positive and associated with improved performance is called **eustress**.

Too much stress or poorly managed stress can have a negative impact on health and lead to poor performance and impaired judgment. Negative stress is called **distress**. Regular exercise can be described as a positive stressor. However, regular exercise at very high frequency or intensity increases the risk of injury and emotional tension; it can be considered a negative stressor because performance often suffers. Distress results from negative situations, ranging from frustrations such as a computer crash to life-changing events such as divorce or serious illness.

Physiological Changes Caused by the Stress Response

Imagine you are driving home, and a car runs a stop sign and barely misses your car. Your body has a set of predictable responses to this acute stressor. For instance, your heart rate increases, your palms become sweaty, your senses heighten, and **endorphins** are released. These reactions are part of the stress response. The body's responses to stress are mediated by an area in the brain called the *hypothalamus* and are initiated when the hormones **epinephrine**, **norepinephrine**, and **cortisol** are released into the bloodstream. The hormones cause a number of physiological changes (some are shown in **FIGURE 11.1**). The two body systems primarily responsible for the changes that occur during the stress response are the **nervous system** and the **endocrine system**.

The nervous system controls both voluntary movements (such as your raising your hand) and involuntary body processes (such as your heart rate and digestion). Involuntary actions are controlled by the **autonomic nervous system**, of which there are two branches: the **parasympathetic branch** and the **sympathetic branch**. The parasympathetic branch is in control of body processes and functions when you are relaxed or

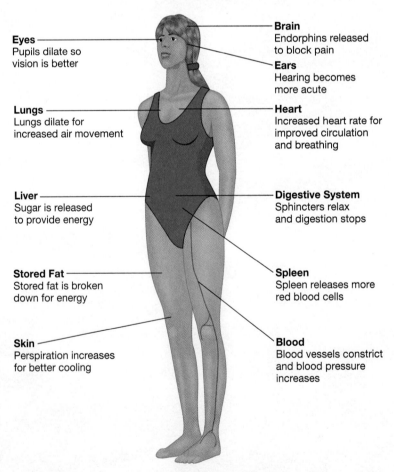

Eyes
Pupils dilate so vision is better

Lungs
Lungs dilate for increased air movement

Liver
Sugar is released to provide energy

Stored Fat
Stored fat is broken down for energy

Skin
Perspiration increases for better cooling

Brain
Endorphins released to block pain

Ears
Hearing becomes more acute

Heart
Increased heart rate for improved circulation and breathing

Digestive System
Sphincters relax and digestion stops

Spleen
Spleen releases more red blood cells

Blood
Blood vessels constrict and blood pressure increases

FIGURE 11.1 The body's physiological responses to stress.

resting. Maintaining resting heart rate and blood pressure, growth, digestion, and energy storage are controlled by the parasympathetic nervous system.

The sympathetic branch is the excitatory part of the autonomic nervous system. This branch is activated when you need to react and produce energy. Activation responses of the sympathetic division include increases in heart rate, respiration, and perspiration, along with an initial release of epinephrine.

In response to stressors, the sympathetic nervous system activates the endocrine system, which in turn releases hormones. Cortisol, the main stress hormone, is predominant during periods of distress and under prolonged stress. Functions of cortisol include aiding in glucose formation, breaking down fat for energy, increasing production of epinephrine and norepinephrine, and suppressing the immune response.

see it!

ABC VIDEOS

Watch the "Generation Stress: Tips for Millenials to Reduce Stress" ABC News Video online at MasteringHealth™.

The Fight-or-Flight Response

The **fight-or-flight response** occurs when the autonomic nervous system and the endocrine system responses are combined. This initial response to stress was first discovered by Harvard physiologist Walter Canon (1) and later elaborated on by the biologist Hans Selye (2). Canon described the stress response as an inborn, automatic, and primitive response designed to prepare individuals to face (fight) or run away from (flight) any type of perceived threat or challenge to survival. According to Canon, once a person perceives a threat, the brain initiates a sequence of physiological and physical changes that ready the body for action. The challenge does not have to be a matter of life or death; the stressors we face in everyday life can cause the fight-or-flight response.

Your body has "activation" responses to enable you to fight or flee (see Figure 11.1). As part of these changes, blood is directed away from the digestive tract and into the muscles to provide extra energy for fighting or running away. You will have an increased awareness of your surroundings, quickened impulses, and diminished pain perception. Your body physically and mentally prepares to "battle" the stressor. After you successfully cope with your stressor or no longer perceive it as threatening, the body returns to homeostasis. However, if the situation is not resolved, you will stay in this aroused state.

During the fight-or-flight response, people are in an "attack mode" and are focused on short-term "survival." Primitive people were required to exert themselves

---

stress State of physical and mental tension in response to an actual or perceived threat or challenge.

stressor Factor that produces stress.

stress response Physiological and behavioral changes that occur in reaction to a stressor.

eustress Stress that results in improved performance; also called *positive stress*.

distress Negative stress that is harmful to performance.

endorphins Group of hormones released during the stress response.

epinephrine Hormone secreted by the inner core (medulla) of the adrenal gland; also called *adrenaline*.

norepinephrine Hormone secreted by the inner core (medulla) of the adrenal gland.

cortisol Hormone secreted by the outer layer (cortex) of the adrenal gland.

nervous system The brain, spinal cord, and nerves of the body.

endocrine system Group of glands and tissues that secrete hormones to regulate body processes.

autonomic nervous system Branch of the nervous system that controls basic body functions that do not require conscious thought; consists of the parasympathetic and sympathetic branches.

parasympathetic branch Division of the autonomic nervous system that is dominant at rest and controls energy conservation and restoration processes.

sympathetic branch Division of the autonomic nervous system that is in control when we need to react or respond to challenges; the excitatory branch.

fight-or-flight response Series of physiological reactions that prepare a person to combat a real or perceived threat.

consider this! //////////////////////

About one-third of students who responded to the 2013 National College Health Assessment reported that their stress levels had negatively affected their academic performance.

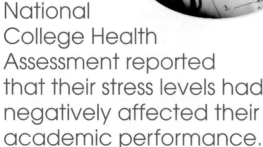

physically while fighting or fleeing from wild animals, and this exertion would rid the body of excess levels of stress hormones, allowing it to return to homeostasis. But today's common stressors, such as traffic congestion, being late for an appointment, too many emails or deadlines, or having an argument with your significant other, do not typically require physical exertion. Many people are in a state of chronic stress, experiencing some level of arousal from stress almost constantly. There is often no release in the form of physical exertion, and over time the stress hormones accumulate in the body, causing illness and chronic disease.

MAKE SURE YOU KNOW...

- Stress is a mental and physical response to situations we perceive as challenges or threats. It can be positive (eustress) or negative (distress).
- Stressors can come from many sources.
- Some degree of stress is required to maximize performance.
- The autonomic nervous system and the endocrine system are responsible for changes that occur during the stress response. The parasympathetic branch of the autonomic nervous system is in control at rest, and the sympathetic branch is activated when you need to react. Cortisol is the main stress hormone produced by the endocrine system.
- Changes that occur during the stress response that prepare the body to either fight or flee are collectively referred to as the fight-or-flight response.

MasteringHealth™

What Factors Affect Your Stress Level?

LO **2** List three factors that can affect your stress level.

Although everyone feels stress, life events and situations do not affect everyone the same way. Our personalities, past experiences, and gender all influence how we perceive situations and cope with stress. For example, your grandmother who recently recovered from a hip fracture might experience stress when she enters a setting with a lot of stairs and uneven terrain. However, as a healthy young adult, you do not find that environment threatening. On the other hand, you might

live it!

ASSESS YOURSELF

Assess your stress levels the *Stress* Take Charge of Your Health! Worksheet online MasteringHealth™.

have a tendency to freak out during finals, while your roommate remains calm.

Personality Behavior Patterns

Different reactions to the same stressful situation can be due to personality differences and how people have learned to respond.

There are many different ways to describe personalities and behavior patterns. Note that although there is no one specific (or completely reliable) way of identifying a stress-prone personality, a common classification method describes individuals as having characteristics that fit mainly into one of four behavior patterns: Type A, Type B, Type C, and Type D (**TABLE 11.1**). You can assess your behavior patterns using Laboratory 11.1.

People who exhibit Type A behavior pattern (TABP) are highly motivated, time-conscious, hard-driving, impatient, and sometimes hostile, cynical, and angry. They have a heightened response to stress, and their hostility and anger, especially if repressed, place them at greater risk for heart disease (3, 4). Individuals with Type B behavior pattern are easygoing, nonaggressive, and patient, and they are not prone to hostile episodes. People with Type B behavior pattern are less likely to perceive everyday annoyances as significant stressors and are at low risk for heart disease from stress.

Most people have heard of Type A and Type B behavior patterns, but you might not be familiar with the other two types. People with Type C behavior pattern have many of the positive qualities of TABP. They are confident, highly motivated, and

live it!

ASSESS YOURSELF

Assess your anger with the *Anger Log Test* Take Charge of Your Health! Worksheet online MasteringHealth™.

TABLE 11.1 ■ Personality Behavior Patterns and Their Risks for Heart Disease		
Personality Behavior Pattern	Qualities	Risk for Heart Disease
A	Impatient, competitive, aggressive, highly motivated, sometimes hostile	High
B	Patient, nonaggressive, easygoing	Low
C	Competitive, highly motivated, highly confident, able to maintain a constant level of emotional control	Low
D	Negative, anxious, worried, socially inhibited	High

competitive. However, individuals with Type C behavior pattern typically do not express the hostility and anger seen with TABP, and they use their personality characteristics to maintain a constant level of emotional control and to channel their ambition into creative directions. Because people with Type C behavior pattern do not express negative emotions and feelings in the same manner as those with TABP, they experience the same low risk for stress-related heart disease as do those with Type B behavior pattern. However, a person with Type C behavior pattern can face a higher risk for heart disease due to keeping emotions inside rather than expressing them.

Individuals with Type D behavior pattern also are considered to be at greater risk for stress-related disease. These individuals are prone to worry and anxiety and also tend to be inhibited and uneasy when interacting with others. Their social clumsiness results in a chronic state of anxiety, which places them at greater risk for heart disease (5, 6).

Past Experiences

We must keep in mind that ultimately, it is our perception of a stressor and the way we react to it that determine any resulting health effects. We learn from our experiences, and what we learn can help us respond more positively in future situations. For example, finals time is a common stressor. You would expect a person with TABP to be extremely stressed during the time leading up to finals. But a person with TABP who has learned that too much stress leads to unfocused study time and poor grades might plan structured study time weeks ahead of the final to reduce last-minute stress. Likewise, a student with Type B behavior who performed poorly in the past because she was too relaxed and did not prepare well might learn to prepare more diligently to improve her future exam performance.

Gender

Gender can influence the way we react to stressors. There are no sex differences in the physiological responses to stress, but gender can affect the way we perceive situations and how we react to stressors. For example, our society has traditionally deemed it more acceptable for women to express their emotions openly. Thus, a woman might feel more comfortable discussing stressors and be better able to cope with them than a man who has been socialized to "keep his feelings in." Conversely, a woman might have been taught that certain responses, such as anger, are not "ladylike" and so will refrain

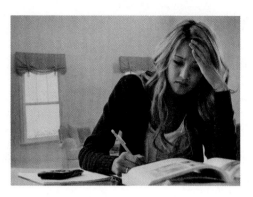

College life comes with stressors from many sources.

from expressing her anger, leading to greater stress. Participating in activities outside traditional gender roles also has the potential to produce stress. A man who decides to be a stay-at-home dad or work from home so his wife can pursue her career, for example, might experience higher levels of stress because his choice does not fit with societal norms. Gender-related reactions to stress also vary across cultures.

Regardless of your personality characteristics, past experiences, and gender, you can learn ways to deal effectively with the stress in your life. The first step is to examine your current stress level using Laboratory 11.2. If the results suggest that you are experiencing unhealthy levels of stress, you should implement stress management techniques.

Common Causes of Stress

Recognizing the everyday life situations that contribute to your stress level is important in managing stress. The pressure of performing well in classes, along with competing deadlines for papers, projects, and tests, can be a source of stress, especially if you do not have strong time-management skills. Choosing a major and planning for your future after graduation are also stressful processes. Making use of career counseling services and talking with your professors and faculty advisors can help you find the best options in light of your strengths and interests.

Interpersonal relationships often change when you enter college. If you relocate to attend college, getting connected within the college community and developing new relationships can be stressful. Leaving family and friends can also be a challenge. Even if you did not relocate, your existing relationships still might be affected

consider this! /////////////////////

College students who use Facebook report studying

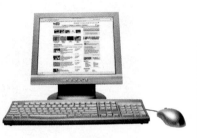

1 to 5 hours per week and have lower GPAs compared to nonusers, who studied 11 to 15 hours per week.

as you balance school, work, friends, family, and other responsibilities.

Financial responsibilities can be a source of stress during many stages of life. Costs associated with tuition, fees, and books are high, and you may have to rely on loans to assist with college expenses. Work-study arrangements or other jobs can relieve some of the financial burden, but they place additional demands on your already limited time. Work demands can be a significant source of stress because they affect relationships, time, and schoolwork. Also, when selecting your major, you have to consider the job opportunities and earning potential of the career paths that interest you. The need to attend graduate school or take low-paying or nonpaying internships can further add to financial strain and stress. Learning financial management skills can help reduce stress. Budgeting and planning for expenses are important skills to develop. Avoiding credit card debt also reduces the stress of the financial burden of college.

Other common college stressors include traffic, parking on campus, and adjusting to college life. Students with families have the combined stresses of balancing work and family responsibilities with the demands of school. Nontraditional students may feel out of place and experience stress related to those feelings. Students with disabilities may face stressors in trying to navigate a campus that might not adequately accommodate their specific situation.

In addition to balancing the demands of school, work, and relationships, some students engage in activities, such as spending too much time online, that negatively affect productivity and, in turn, may lead to stress. Excessive online game playing or social media interactions can increase stress levels by interfering with effective time management. A relatively new source of stress is cyberbullying, in which a student is threatened or

humiliated via electronic communication (see Examining the Evidence).

MAKE SURE YOU **KNOW...**

- Personality can impact the way we perceive situations and respond to stress. Type A and Type D behavior patterns are associated with higher risk for heart disease.
- Past experiences and gender also influence our reactions to stressful situations.
- College life can present many stressors. Some of the most common include academic responsibilities, time management, relationships, finances and interpersonal issues such as bullying.

— MasteringHealth™

Stress and Health

LO **3** **Explain how stress can affect your health.**

Chronic (persistent) stress is related to some of the most significant health problems in the United States. Heart disease, depression, and migraines are all associated with stress and have significant direct and indirect health-care costs. Stress is a risk factor for depression and anxiety, and up to 25% of the U.S. adult population suffers from these and other mental health problems every year (7). Approximately 75% to 90% of all physician visits are for stress-related complaints, and millions of people take medication for stress-related illnesses (8). From a medical standpoint, stress can affect both emotional and physical health. Chronic stress has been linked to elevated blood pressure, heart disease, hormonal imbalances, reduced resistance to disease, and emotional disorders (9, 10, 11) (**FIGURE 11.2**).

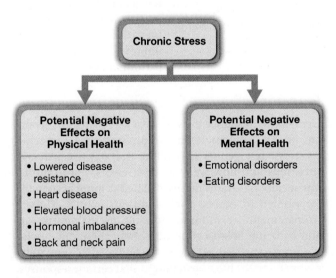

FIGURE 11.2 Chronic stress can have negative effects on both physical and mental health.

EXAMINING THE EVIDENCE: Bullying on College Campuses

Bullying is defined as aggressive behavior such as humiliating or intimidating a weaker person. While most of us think of this occurring among children, bullying occurs among adults as well. In many cases, high school bullies continue their behavior and become college bullies, and workplace bullying is a serious problem. Bullying can include verbal, physical, and electronic assaults. Much of the bullying that college students experience revolves around relationship issues.

Cyberbullying takes place using electronic technology. Examples include mean or threatening text messages or emails, rumors or embarrassing photos or videos spread via email or social networking sites, and fake websites or profiles. Bullies may use both face-to-face contact and electronic means to intimidate their victims. Cyberbullying among college students is a growing problem:

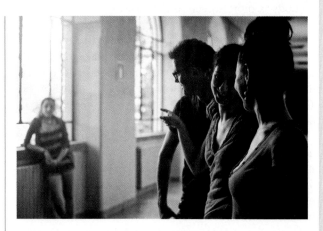

- 18.5% of college students reported having been bullied by another student at least once.

- 22% reported being a victim of cyberbullying.

- 42% said they had witnessed someone being bullied by another student.

Why does bullying occur? College women may bully to climb the social ladder or to intimidate another student due to romantic jealousy. Males bully other males to exert their dominance. Males also bully women who have rejected their advances or ended a relationship.

College students living away from family and friends must cope with bullying on their own. It may be difficult to escape the bully, especially if he or she is a roommate or classmate. Feelings of being alone and isolated are especially difficult for college students, and many victims never tell anyone that they are being bullied. They may keep silent due to embarrassment or believing that they should be able to handle the situation on their own. Consequently, significant health and psychological issues can develop, including anxiety disorders, depression, low self-esteem, and poor academic performance. In severe cases, suicidal thoughts and behavior can result.

What to Do About Bullying

- Break the silence. Staying silent empowers bullies and allows their behavior to continue unchecked.

- Become familiar with your campus security and campus and local police resources, and contact them to report threatening behavior.

- Victims should talk to someone they trust such as a resident advisor, faculty member, academic advisor, health services counselor, or a close friend or family member.

- Friends or other students who witness bullying can also contact a campus or police representative.

Sources: Chapell, M., D. Casey, C. De la Cruz, J. Ferrell, J. Forman, R. Lipkin, M. Newsham, M. Sterling, & S. Whittaker. Bullying in college by students and teachers. Adolescence. 39:153, 53–64, 2004; Chappell, M., S. Hasselman, T. Kitchin, S. Lomon, K. MacIver & P. Sarullo. Bullying in elementary school, high school, and college. Adolescence. 41:164, 633–648, 2006; Selkie E., K. Rajitha, C. Ya-Fen, and M. Megan. *Cyberpsychology, Behavior, and Social Networking.* February 2015, 18(2): 79–86. doi:10.1089/cyber.2014.0371; Stopbullying.gov. Site managed by the *U.S. Department of Health and Human Services.*

Stress-related problems cost businesses and government billions of dollars every year in the form of employee absenteeism and health-care costs. Stress can suppress the immune system, making a person more susceptible to illness. Acute stress can also impact productivity. Headaches and tension might cause a person to miss work or class or be less focused. Therefore, stress is a major health problem that affects individual lives and the economy as a whole.

Hans Selye developed one of the earliest scientific theories to explain the relationship between stress and disease. Selye proposed that humans adapt to stress in a response he termed the **general adaptation syndrome**, which involves three stages: an alarm stage, a resistance stage, and an exhaustion stage (2).

---

general adaptation syndrome Pattern of responses to stress that consists of an alarm stage, a resistance stage, and an exhaustion stage.

During the alarm stage, the fight-or-flight response occurs. Stress hormones are released, and their effects on the body can cause anxiety, headaches, and disrupted patterns of sleeping and eating (2). During this phase, the body is more susceptible to disease and more prone to injury.

With continued exposure to stress, the individual reaches the resistance stage. During this stage, the body's resistance to stress is higher than normal, and mechanisms are activated that allow the body to resist disease effectively. In short, the resistance stage represents an improved ability to cope with stress (2).

Selye proposed that when the stress persists, the individual reaches the exhaustion stage. Note that "exhaustion" in this sense refers to a depletion of the physical and psychological resources to cope with stress that occurs with chronic exposure. Selye suggested that the body is vulnerable to disease during this stage because of this depletion of resources. During this phase, physical symptoms that appeared in the alarm stage can reappear, but they now are more serious and can sometimes compromise health.

Although Selye's model of adaptation to stress is still viewed as an important contribution to our understanding of the stress response, newer research findings have improved our understanding of the relationship between stress and disease. We now know that the underlying cause of many stress-related diseases is the body's inability to respond to stress in the normal way. When facing long-term exposure to stress, the repeated and/or prolonged stress response results in the continual activation of the nervous, endocrine, and immune systems, including the continual release of stress hormones, including cortisol.

The concepts of **allostasis** and **allostatic load** are better explanations of the relationship between stress and disease. Allostasis refers to the body's ability to change and adapt to stressful situations. Under long-term stress, the body does not adapt as well. The allostatic load is the point at which the high level of stress exceeds the system's stress response (12). The continued or repeated activation causes the stress response to become inefficient.

One's risk of developing a stress-related illness increases because, over time, high levels of cortisol in the blood impair the immune system's ability to fight infections (12, 13, 14). As you have realized by now, prolonged stress places an individual at greater risk for illness and other problems. Understanding how stress

coaching corner

Will this stressor matter later?

Stress is omnipresent in college. As you become aware of how you respond to demands, managing stress becomes more practical. Each time you have an emotional or stressful reaction, ask yourself the following questions:

- Are my perceptions of this situation correct, or do I need more information to make a decision or plan of action? Many times we do not have enough information to make the best decision. When in doubt, seek more information.

- Is it possible to negotiate the deadline that is causing increased stress? Although most people will not accommodate procrastination, many are open to negotiating due dates if upfront communication occurs. The key is to be honest and ask well before a deadline is looming.

- Will this matter to me tomorrow, 2 weeks from now, or a year from now? In many cases you can reduce anxiety or stress simply by considering the long-term impact of a situation. If it won't matter beyond the 2-week mark, it may not be that important.

affects you and learning effective stress-management skills are important for maintaining a high level of wellness.

MAKE SURE YOU **KNOW...**

- Depression and anxiety have a significant impact on the U.S. adult population, and stress is a risk factor for both conditions.

- General adaptation syndrome, which includes the alarm, resistance, and exhaustion stages, was one of the first theories proposed about the relationship between stress and disease.

- The concept of the allostatic load is that repeated, long-term exposure to stress and the continual activation of the stress response compromise health.

—————— MasteringHealth™

How Can You Manage Stress?

LO **4** Describe three effective strategies for managing stress and explain why they work.

There are two general steps to managing stress: Reduce the amount of stress in your life, and cope with stress by improving your ability to relax (15). A sample program for stress management is presented on pages 309–310.

steps ▶ FOR BEHAVIOR CHANGE

How well do you manage your time?

Take the quiz below to find out whether you are a good time manager.

Y   N
☐ ☐ Do you procrastinate?
☐ ☐ Do you take on more responsibilities than you can handle?
☐ ☐ Are you consistently late for class, appointments, or work?
☐ ☐ Do you need more hours in the day to accomplish all of your daily tasks?
☐ ☐ Do you have little time for fun with friends or family?

If you answered "Yes" to most or all of these questions, you can probably use some tips for better time management.

Tips to Improve Your Time Management Skills, Reduce Stress, and Increase Productivity

Tomorrow, you will:

☑ **Plan ahead.** Plan your day by using your cell phone or daily planner to organize tasks. Make a realistic schedule and allow time for unscheduled events and delays.

☑ **Evaluate how you spend your time.** Determine how you can make adjustments in your day to increase or better use your free time (e.g., cut back on TV time, texting, or using social media).

Within the next 2 weeks, you will:

☑ **Establish goals.** Create a list of short- and long-term SMART goals.

☑ **Prioritize.** List your tasks in order of importance (high priority to low priority), and then follow that list. Establish a daily goal of accomplishing the three most important tasks on your list.

☑ **Schedule time for you.** Find time each day to relax and do something you enjoy. Regularly evaluate your ratio of work time to home and leisure time, and make sure you maintain balance.

By the end of the semester, you will:

☑ **Delegate responsibility.** If you are involved with clubs or group projects, share and delegate responsibility. Learn to say no to activities that prevent you from achieving your goals. Before accepting a new responsibility, complete your current task or eliminate an unnecessary project.

☑ **Re-evaluate your progress and goals** to make any necessary adjustments.

People who experience chronic stress or very high levels of stress and its associated feelings of anxiety can experience **burnout** (16). The first significant way to lower the impact of stress on your life is to reduce the number of stressors you encounter. Although you will not be able to avoid all sources of stress, you can eliminate many unnecessary forms. The first step is to recognize those factors that produce daily stress. Use Laboratory 11.2 to assess your stressors and to help determine which ones you can most readily work to eliminate, avoid, or better manage. Getting adequate amounts of rest and sleep and exercising regularly are also important factors in managing your stress levels.

One example of a stressor that you can eliminate is over commitment, a frequent cause of stress in college students. If you plan your time carefully and prioritize your activities, you can avoid feeling overwhelmed by having too much to do and not enough time to do it. You can plan a daily schedule that allows you to accomplish the things you need to without being distracted by

---

allostasis The ability to maintain homeostasis through change.

allostatic load A continual stress level that causes the inability to respond appropriately to stress; leads to compromised health.

burnout Loss of physical, emotional, and mental energy.

less-important activities. Be aware of activities that steal your time. The increasing number of social networking websites can use more of your time than you realize (see Examining the Evidence). The Steps for Behavior Change box on page 306 and Laboratory 11.3 can help you take steps to better manage your time.

Another common stressor that you may be able to better manage is financial pressure. You cannot eliminate the costs associated with tuition, rent (or room and board), or course fees and materials, but you can prioritize your spending and make sure you budget for essential expenses. For example, you can wait to purchase the newest smart phone or trendy boots until after buying your books. And make it a habit to pay off credit cards every month or save until you have the money for a purchase. Working to minimize debt from student loans and credit cards can reduce both present and future financial stress. Avoiding overuse of credit cards and developing a budget are two very important strategies. Look for ways to reduce your everyday expenses, and do not buy expensive clothes or gadgets if you do not have the money to pay for them now.

Rest and Sleep

One of the most effective means of reducing stress is to get adequate sleep. How much sleep do you need? Although individual needs vary greatly, adults typically need 7 to 9 hours of restful sleep per night. Because of the body's natural hormonal rhythms, you should also try to go to bed at approximately the same time every night. See the Steps for Behavior Change box on page 306 to determine whether you're getting enough sleep and **TABLE 11.2** for some helpful apps.

In addition to a good night's sleep, 15 to 30 minutes of rest during the day can help reduce stress. You

TABLE 11.2 ■ Overview of Selected Stress Management Apps			
App	Cost	Features	Compatible Devices
Sleep Bug www.sleepbug.net	Free (24 scenes) Sleep Bug Pro: $1.99 (includes additional scenes)	Sleep aid that acts as a white noise machine. Choose from a variety of scenes with sounds and/or music. Can customize and add your own. Features a custom timer.	Requires iOS 7.0 or later. Compatible with iPhone, iPad, and iPod touch. Optimized for iPhone 5. Requires Android 4.1 and up.
Sleep Cycle Alarm Clock www.sleepcycle.com	$.99 for iPhone $1.69 for Android	Select the time you want to wake up, place your phone face down on the bed, and the app will wake you up within a 30-minute window when you are in your lightest sleep. Pinpoints REM cycles so it doesn't wake you from a deep sleep.	Requires iOS 7.0 or later. Compatible with iPhone, iPad, and iPod touch. Optimized for iPhone 5, iPhone 6, and iPhone 6 Plus. Requires Android 4.0 and up.
Twilight https://play.google.com/store/apps/details?id=com.urbandroid.lux&hl=en	Free	Before bed, blue light emanating from the screens of devices can disrupt sleep cycles. Twilight slowly removes the blue light from your phone when the sun starts to set outside.	Android requirements vary with device.
Calm www.calm.com	$9.99/month	Daily sessions of guided meditation that focus on releasing anxiety, building compassion, and feeling more confident. Can choose session lengths from 2 to 20 minutes.	Requires iOS 7.0 or later. Compatible with iPhone, iPad, and iPod touch. Optimized for iPhone 5, iPhone 6, and iPhone 6 Plus. Requires Android 2.3.3 and up.
Headspace www.headspace.com	$12.95/month or discounted annual rate	Guided 10-minute meditations.	Requires iOS 7.0 or later. Compatible with iPhone, iPad, and iPod touch. Optimized for iPhone 5, iPhone 6, and iPhone 6 Plus. Requires Android 3.0 and up.

EXAMINING THE EVIDENCE

How Many "Friends" Do You Have?

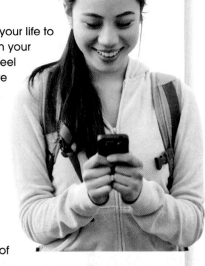

Having a strong or large support network is typically associated with better stress management and mental health. But what is the effect if the social network is mostly or all online? As more social networking websites have emerged, adolescents and young adults are developing large online networks. Does having a network of 500 or more "friends" really mean one has a stronger support network? Texting and the use of social media are not necessarily problematic, but they can be for some people. How and why you choose to use these sites can affect the impact that use has on social relationships and health.

It appears that extroverts use social networking sites to enhance their social relationships and interactions, while introverts use them for social compensation. Studies have shown that higher amounts of time spent using these sites is associated with depression, psychological distress, and lower self-esteem. Furthermore, some might experience increases in anxiety when the use of social media is limited or stopped. How do you know whether your texting or use of social media is problematic? If you have multiple "Yes" answers to the following questions, you might want to re-evaluate your use of social media and texting.

- Do you spend less time in face-to-face interactions than you do in online interactions? Or have your online "friends" replaced people in your life?

- Do you experience symptoms of stress or anxiety when you are unable to text, update your status, or interact online?

- Do you frequently text or use social media at times that are considered inappropriate (e.g., while in class, at work or church, or on a date)?

- Do you compare your life to the lives of those in your network? Do you feel bad or inadequate when you make comparisons?

- Have your texting and social media habits had a negative impact on your relationships, grades, work performance, or any other aspect of your life?

- Does the time spent texting and using social media impact your time management?

Sources: Chou, H., and N. Edge. "They are happier and having better lives than I am": The impact of using Facebook on perceptions of others' lives. *Cyberpsychology, Behavior and Social Networking* 15(2):117–121, 2012; Durocher, J., K. Lufkin, M. King, and J. Carter. Social technology restriction alters state-anxiety but not autonomic activity in humans. *American Journal of Physiology: Regulatory, Integrative and Comparative Physiology* 301(6):R1773–1778, 2011; Kujath, C. Facebook and MySpace: Complement or substitute for face-to-face interaction? *Cyberpsychology, Behavior and Social Networking* 14(1–2):75–78, 2011; Kuss, D., and M. Griffiths. Online social networking and addiction: A review of the psychological literature. *International Journal of Environmental Research and Public Health* 8(9):3528–3552, 2011; Mango, A., T. Taylor, and P. Greenfield. Me and my 400 friends: The anatomy of college students' Facebook networks, their communication patterns, and well-being. *Developmental Psychology* 48(2):369–390, 2012; O'Dea, B., and A. Campbell. Online social networking amongst teens: Friend or foe? *Studies in Health Technology and Informatics* 167:133–138, 2011; Wilson, K., S. Fornasier, and K. White. Psychological predictors of young adults' use of social networking sites. *Cyberpsychology, Behavior and Social Networking* 13(2):173–177, 2010.

live it!

ASSESS YOURSELF

Assess your sleep with the *Sleep Inventory* Take Charge of Your Health! Worksheet online at MasteringHealth™.

can get this rest by finding a quiet location, putting your feet up, and closing your eyes as a short break from constant activity. A well-rested body is the best protection against stress and fatigue.

Exercise

Light to moderate exercise can reduce many types of stress and anxiety. Even if you are not an experienced exerciser, you can benefit from the calm feeling that comes after an exercise session. The recommended types of exercise for optimal stress reduction are low- to

moderate-intensity aerobic exercises, such as brisk walking, swimming, and cycling. Yoga, tai-chi, and Pilates are other popular types of exercise that help you relax and reduce stress. Many gyms and health clubs offer classes in these forms of exercise.

Studies have shown that exercise is very effective for stress reduction (17, 18, 19). **FIGURE 11.3** compares the effects of a 30-minute session of exercise (running) to two other common forms of stress reduction: reading while resting and meditation. In this study, meditation provided the greatest stress reduction, with exercise finishing a close second (17). Other studies have shown that exercise reduces stress about as much as other types of relaxation techniques (20). Also, the relaxing effects of exercise can last for hours after a workout (16).

steps ▶ FOR BEHAVIOR CHANGE

Are you getting enough sleep?

Making sure that you get enough sleep will help you effectively deal with your daily stressors and may also help improve your grades. Answer these questions to find out whether you are getting enough sleep.

Y N

☐ ☐ Do you fall asleep as soon as your head hits the pillow?

☐ ☐ Do you find yourself dozing in class or at other inappropriate times of the day?

☐ ☐ Do you frequently take naps during the day?

☐ ☐ Do you have an irregular bedtime?

☐ ☐ Do you "binge" sleep on the weekend?

☐ ☐ Do you have difficulty waking in the morning?

If you answered "Yes" to more than two of the above questions, you may not be getting enough sleep at night.

Tips to Help You Get Consistent, Restful Sleep

Tomorrow, you will:

☑ Establish a bedtime and a set wake-up time that can be maintained on a regular basis.

☑ Sleep in a comfortable environment. A cool, dark room with little noise is recommended for a good night of sleep.

☑ Use bright light in the morning to help you wake up.

Within the next 2 weeks, you will:

☑ Not drink caffeinated beverages after 4:00 p.m.

☑ Avoid stimulating reading material, television shows, or movies in the evening. Instead, try meditating or listening to soothing music to help you unwind and relax.

By the end of the semester, you will:

☑ Avoid disrupting your regular sleep pattern. Long naps during the day and using the weekend to play "catch up" on sleep missed during the week can disrupt sleep patterns.

☑ Be well rested and ready for finals!

Although we consistently see that people feel more relaxed after exercise, we do not know exactly how exercise reduces stress. Several ideas have been proposed. One theory is that exercise causes the brain to release several natural tranquilizers (endorphins), which can produce a calming effect (21). Another theory is that exercise may be a diversion or break from your stressors and worries. The improved physical fitness and self-image that you enjoy as a result of regular exercise also increase your resistance to stress. A final possibility is that all of these factors may contribute to the beneficial effects of exercise. The next time you feel stressed, try exercising; you will feel and look better as a result.

Use Relaxation Techniques

Stress management techniques can help reduce the potentially harmful effects of stress. Most of these are designed to relax you and thereby reduce your stress level. When trying to relax, ask yourself two questions: What prevents me from relaxing? What am I not doing that could help me relax? (9). Your answers can help you determine how and where to focus your efforts. Lowering your levels of stress and practicing effective stress management techniques will increase your overall level of wellness (14). Following are some of the more common approaches used in stress management.

Progressive Relaxation Progressive relaxation is a technique that uses exercises to reduce muscle tension. (Muscle tension is a common symptom of stress.) You practice the technique while sitting quietly or lying down. First you contract muscle groups and then relax them one at a time, beginning with your feet and moving up your body to your hands, neck, and face until you achieve a complete state of muscle relaxation (see the Examining the Evidence box).

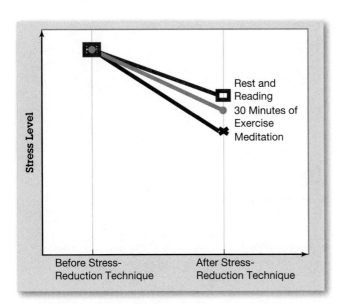

FIGURE 11.3 Rest, exercise, and meditation are all techniques you can use to reduce your stress level.

Proponents of progressive relaxation techniques say that relaxing the muscles in this manner will also relax the mind and thereby relieve stress. The theory behind this concept is that an anxious (stressed) mind cannot exist in a relaxed body.

see it!
ABC VIDEOS
Watch the "Meditation Becoming More Popular Among Teens" ABC News Video online at MasteringHealth™.

Breathing Exercises Breathing exercises can also help you relax. The following is a sample step-by-step breathing exercise for reducing stress:

1. In a quiet room, assume a comfortable position (sitting or lying down) with your eyes closed.
2. Begin to slowly inhale and exhale. Count from 1 to 3 during each inhalation and each exhalation to maintain a slow and regular breathing pattern.

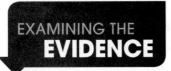 **Progressive Relaxation Training**

There are many types of progressive relaxation training methods, and over 200 different exercises have been described. The basic technique involves contracting and relaxing muscle groups, starting in your lower body and moving upward. The following technique is one of the many forms that you can use.

1. Find a quiet, comfortable, and private place. Remove your shoes. Wear loose, comfortable clothing, or loosen any tight clothing. The first few times, you can expect emerging thoughts and emotions to distract you from your attempts to relax. After some practice, you will be able to block distractions. Listening to soothing music can help you relax and filter distractions; there are many relaxation music CDs and MP3s available. You may also read the instructions into a recorder and use them to guide you through your relaxation session. This strategy will avoid your having to remember the steps involved.

2. Assume a relaxed position (sitting or lying down). Close your eyes, and begin by focusing on your breathing. Become aware of how it feels to breathe in and breathe out. Breathe deeply and slowly through your nose, and imagine that you are breathing in good, healing air and breathing out stress and muscle tension. You may find it useful to inhale to a count of 7—1-2-3-4-5-6-7—and exhale to the same count. Breathe this way for several minutes before starting your progressive relaxation exercise.

3. Without speaking, focus on relaxing each part of your body, beginning with your feet. You are consciously "telling" each part of your body to relax.

Contracting the muscles in each body part first and then relaxing them can help you to feel the difference, because sometimes we are not aware of tension we carry in our muscles. Do not move on to the next area until you have relaxed the part you are focusing on.

Proceed in the following order:

a. Toes of left foot	m. Chest
b. Toes of right foot	n. Left shoulder
c. Left foot	o. Right shoulder
d. Right foot	p. Left arm
e. Left ankle	q. Left hand
f. Right ankle	r. Left fingers
g. Lower left leg	s. Right arm
h. Lower right leg	t. Right hand
i. Left thigh	u. Right fingers
j. Right thigh	v. Neck
k. Buttocks	w. Face
l. Abdomen	

4. Now you should be completely relaxed. Continue slow, deep breathing for the next few minutes. Try not to let your mind wander—remain in this relaxed state.

5. At the end of your session, take a deep breath. Slowly bring yourself out of your relaxed state. Stand up and stretch. You should feel renewed and refreshed.

3. Next, combine stretching and breathing to provide greater relaxation and stress reduction. For example, stretch your arms toward the ceiling as you inhale, then lower your arms as you exhale.

Try this exercise for 5 to 15 minutes.

Meditation Meditation has been practiced for ages to help people relax and achieve inner peace. There are many types of meditation, and there is no scientific evidence that one form is superior to another. Most types of meditation have the same common elements: sitting quietly for at least 15 to 20 minutes twice a day, concentrating on a single word or image or on the breath, and breathing slowly and regularly. The goal is to achieve a complete state of physical and mental relaxation.

Some people find it easier to begin a meditation program with the help of an experienced meditation or yoga instructor. Also, there are many meditation CDs, online downloads, and apps available (see Table 11.2 for examples). Some online aids feature guided meditation and others provide music that is appropriate for meditation. You can start on your own using the following overview of one technique:

1. First, choose a word or sound, called a *mantra*, to repeat during the meditation. The idea of using a mantra is that this word or sound should become your symbol of complete relaxation. Choose a mantra that has little emotional significance for you.

2. Next, find a quiet area and sit comfortably with your eyes closed. Take several deep breaths and concentrate on relaxing; let your body go limp.

3. Concentrate on your mantra as you inhale and exhale. Try not to hear or think about anything else. Repeat your mantra over and over in your mind or out loud, and relax. As distracting thoughts come up, let them go and refocus on the mantra.

4. After 15 to 20 minutes, open your eyes. End the session by making a fist with both hands and then relax. You will feel both alert and refreshed.

Visualization Visualization (sometimes called *imagery*) uses mental pictures to reduce stress. The idea is to create an appealing mental image (such as a quiet mountain setting) that promotes relaxation and reduces stress. To practice visualization, follow the instructions presented for meditation, but substitute a relaxing mental scene for the mantra. If you fail to reach a complete state of relaxation after your first several sessions, do not be discouraged. Achieving complete relaxation with this technique may require some additional practice.

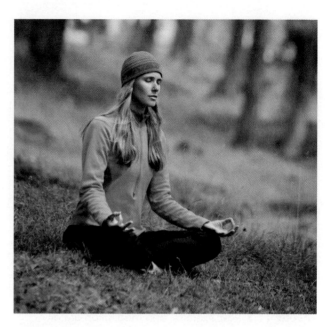

Assuming a relaxed position in a quiet setting is central to several relaxation techniques.

Develop Spiritual Wellness

Spiritual wellness is associated with better recovery from illness and improved mental health (as discussed in Chapter 1). Spiritual wellness can provide a sense of peace. People who report high levels of spiritual wellness often engage in behaviors such as prayer, meditation, and enjoying the beauty of nature to reduce stress and anxiety.

Develop a Support Network

Having a network of friends and family to help you cope with stressors can help to reduce or eliminate stress. Sometimes just talking through your stressful situation can help you think more clearly and develop an effective plan for addressing the issue. Others who have your best interest at heart will likely help you with a plan for stress management. When you are dealing with stressors that cannot be eliminated, your network will be there for support while you work through difficult times.

Avoid Counterproductive Behaviors

Some people make poor health choices, such as smoking cigarettes or drinking alcohol, in an attempt to manage stress. However, these behaviors are counterproductive and can lead to more cumulative stress in the long term.

Using Tobacco Many people say that they smoke cigarettes "to relax," but the nicotine in cigarettes and other tobacco products is actually a stimulant that

Can Nutritional Supplements Reduce Emotional Stress?

Currently, there is no scientific evidence that any specific nutritional supplement, including megadoses of vitamins, will reduce stress. According to researchers at the University of Texas Southwestern Medical Center at Dallas, most "stress formulas" on the market contain B vitamins, such as niacin and riboflavin, which are meant to aid in recovery from physical stress (e.g., injuries), not emotional stress.

B vitamins are sometimes used as a supplement for people recovering from surgery. Emotional stress does not cause the body to require increased energy or nutrients.

Getting plenty of rest and exercising regularly, along with eating a healthy diet, are the best ways to deal with emotional stress. Combining healthy lifestyle practices with stress management techniques such as those offered in this chapter can help you effectively deal with life's stressors.

---

produces responses similar to the fight-or-flight response. Additionally, nicotine is an addictive substance that has serious long-term effects. Smoking is the leading cause of preventable death, increasing the risk for lung and other types of cancer and for heart disease. Smoking and tobacco use are also very costly habits.

Using Alcohol or Other Drugs Using alcohol or other substances might make you briefly forget about problems or stressors, but these behaviors do not eliminate or reduce the stressor. Alcohol (especially binge drinking) or drug use can affect your sleep patterns and productivity, which results in more stress. Using alcohol or other substances to cope with your problems can lead to abuse. Even legal substances, such as caffeine, can cause problems such as interfering with restful sleep.

Disordered Eating Patterns *Disordered eating patterns* are eating patterns that are not healthy, but that do not meet the clinical definitions for eating disorders. These patterns can lead to the development of an eating disorder. Undereating or overeating can be disordered eating. Skipping meals will result in lack of nutrients and energy, which can affect how well you can focus and cope with stressors. Overeating, binge eating, or using "comfort foods" to cope with stress can lead to weight gain and health problems. Also, blood glucose levels can be affected, resulting in fluctuations in your energy level and decreased ability to deal with stress.

MAKE SURE YOU **KNOW**...

- The two steps usually involved in stress management are reducing the sources of stress and using relaxation techniques to help you cope with stress.

- Getting more rest and sleep; engaging in exercise; and practicing progressive muscle relaxation, breathing exercises, meditation, and visualization are some of the many techniques that can help you cope with stress.

- Developing spiritual and social wellness can be very important in managing stress.

- Using unhealthy behaviors to relax, such as smoking, drinking alcohol, or taking drugs, actually leads to higher levels of stress in the long term.

— MasteringHealth™

---

meditation Relaxation technique that involves sitting quietly, focusing on a word, image, or the breath, and breathing slowly and rhythmically.

visualization Relaxation technique that uses appealing mental images to promote relaxation and reduce stress; also called *imagery*.

Sample Program for Stress Management

Stress Relief in the Moment
Everyone has the power to reduce the effects of stress. Learning to reduce stress will take self-exploration and practice. The first step is recognizing when you are stressed. If you do not feel calm, alert, and focused most of the time, then too much stress could be your problem. Some of the strategies discussed in this chapter require practice for you to attain proficiency and maximize their

benefits. The techniques below will require some trial and error to find those that work best for you.

Sleep is a great stress reliever. Every night, try to sleep 7–8 hours. Remember that the effects of stress are cumulative and you should practice stress-relief techniques daily. Identifying which stress management techniques work best for you and practicing them at the first sign of stress will help you cope with life's challenges and remain healthy.

Step 1: Recognize Your Stress

Breathing: Learn to pay attention to your breathing. Is your breath shallow? Are you "forgetting" to breathe? Check out your breathing by placing one hand on your chest and the other over your stomach. Watch the rise and fall of your hands as you breathe. Does your breathing seem shallow?

Muscles: Pay attention to your muscles. Are your hands and/or jaw clenched? Do your muscles feel tense? Are you feeling tension in the back of your neck and shoulders?

Step 2: Identify Your Stress Response

Internally we respond to stress in the same way. However, externally our response to stress can vary in a variety of ways. The most common external responses to climbing levels of stress include becoming angry and agitated; becoming depressed, spaced-out, or withdrawn; and becoming stuck (frozen) or shutting down.

Knowing how you respond to stress can help you choose the most effective stress reduction techniques. If you are someone who becomes angry, agitated, or keyed up when stressed then you should choose stress relief techniques that calm you down. Those who become depressed, withdrawn, or spaced-out under stress need techniques that stimulate and energize.

Those who become stuck or freeze when under stress can react by speeding up or slowing down. For those who speed up under stress, stress reduction techniques aimed at slowing you down will be most effective; for those who slow down, choose techniques that energize and invigorate.

Listed below are a variety of things that can help you de-stress. Your job is to find the ones that will work best for you. Remember, you will not be an expert at first; keep trying because the results are worth your effort.

Step 3: Ways to De-Stress

Talking through your stress with someone who is calm and a good listener can be helpful. Supportive friends and family members can be effective helpers when you are under stress. Remember that not everyone is a good listener, so it may take time for you to identify those in your network who are both trustworthy and helpful.

Our five senses can be useful allies in our fight to reduce the effects of stress on our body. The table below shows ways we can use our senses to help us lower our stress levels.

Identify an image, specific type of sound, or type of movement that will be an effective stress reliever for you. The right image, sound, or movement should instantly lift and relax you.

Stress relief using: Sight	Stress relief using: Sound	Stress relief using: Smell	Stress relief using: Taste	Stress relief using: Movement
Closing your eyes and imagining your perfect relaxation place; Photos or mementos; Plants or flowers in your home or workspace; Sitting in a garden; Going to the beach or a lake or scenes displayed in your home or workspace; Visiting a park; Creating a relaxing workspace with colors you enjoy.	Sing or hum your favorite tune; Listen to uplifting music; Listen to nature sound tracks with sounds you find relaxing such as rustling leaves, crashing waves, and bird or whale songs; Buy a small fountain for your home or workspace; Hang wind chimes where you can easily hear them; Practice using positive self-talk with phrases such as: My breathing is slowing down. I feel my heart rate decreasing. My anxiety is dropping. I have the power to calm myself. I will get through this. Nothing lasts forever. Develop some phrases of your own.	If stress agitates you, use comforting and calming scents; If stress depresses you, use energizing and invigorating scents; Light an appropriately scented candle or use incense at home or work; Scent your bed sheets with lavender to help you relax and sleep; Smell highly scented flowers like lilies or roses; Visit a beach and smell the air; Use scented oils and fragrances on your clothes or in the air; Soak in a scented bath.	Chew a piece of sugarless gum; Eat a piece of ripe fruit; Eat a small piece of dark chocolate; Sip on a cup of coffee or tea (jasmine and other scented teas relieve stress through both smell and taste); Eat something crunchy.	Run in place; Jump up and down; Stretch your neck and roll your head in alternating circles; Squeeze a stress ball; Play with play dough or modeling clay; Color or doodle; Go for a brisk walk or run; Walk and meditate: As you take 4 steps forward breathe in deeply; exhale as you walk 4 more steps. Repeat at least 3 times. You can increase the number of repetitions you do and/or the number of steps you take as you breathe; You can also do the exercise above sitting down—raising your arms as you inhale and lowering them as you exhale;

Sources: Davis,M., E. Eshelman, & M. McKay. (2008). The Relaxation and Stress Reduction Workbook (6th Ed). New Harbinger Publications; Oakland; White, D. (2013). Quick Stress Relief Tips Through Your 5 Senses. *Psych Central.* Retrieved on April 29, 2015, from http://psychcentral.com/blog/archives/2013/07/23/quick-stress-relief-tips-through-your-5-senses/; Scott, E. (2014). Free Positive Affirmations for Stress Relief. *About Health.* Retrieved on April 29, 2015 from http://stress.about.com/od/optimismspirituality/a/freeaffirmation.htm.

study plan

summary

hear it! STUDY REVIEW
To hear an MP3 Chapter Summary, scan here or visit the Study Area in MasteringHealth™.

LO 1
- Stress is defined as a physiological and mental response to things in our environment that we perceive as threatening. Any factor that produces stress is called a stressor.

- The autonomic nervous system consists of the parasympathetic and sympathetic branches and works with the endocrine system to produce the stress response. The combined physiological responses of these systems result in the fight-or-flight response, which prepares the body to fight or flee.

LO 2
- Personality factors, past experiences, and gender can affect the way we perceive situations and behave in response to stressors.

- Common stressors for college students include academic and financial responsibilities, managing interpersonal relationships, and everyday life hassles.

LO 3
- Excessive stress or poorly managed stress can lead to headaches, digestive problems, heart disease, and mental health problems.

- General adaptation syndrome is a pattern of stress responses consisting of the alarm, resistance, and exhaustion stages.

- The allostatic load represents the point at which chronic stress leads to health problems.

LO 4
- Two important steps in managing stress are to reduce stressors and to better cope with stress by improving your ability to relax.

- Exercise, adequate rest and sleep, and avoiding unhealthy habits are essential to stress management.

- Common relaxation techniques include progressive relaxation, breathing exercises, meditation, and visualization.

- Developing spiritual wellness and a social network also helps in managing stress.

study questions

review it! QUIZZES

Find more review questions online MasteringHealth™.

LO 1

1. Define *stress* and *stressor*, and list at least three common stressors.

2. Which of the following is a physical symptom of stress?
   a. muscle tension
   b. headaches
   c. anxiety
   d. all of the above

3. Positive stress associated with optimal performance is called ____.
   a. distress
   b. visualization
   c. eustress
   d. productive stress

4. Which of the following is not a hormone that is part of the stress response?
   a. dopamine
   b. cortisol
   c. epinephrine
   d. norepinephrine

5. Differentiate between *eustress* and *distress*.

LO 2

6. Common stressors include ____.
   a. financial responsibilities
   b. interpersonal relationship problems
   c. academic pressures
   d. all of the above

7. List three factors that affect how an individual responds to stress.

LO 3

8. Name and describe the three stages of the general adaptation syndrome.

9. List four health consequences of chronic stress.

LO 10. Which of the following is not a healthy way to cope with stress?
   a. exercise
   b. alcohol
   c. meditation
   d. progressive muscle relaxation

11. List at least four steps you can take to manage stress.

12. Describe four common relaxation techniques.

13. Explain why exercise and effective time management are helpful in reducing stress.

suggested reading

Atkinson, D. *Live Right! Beating Stress in College and Beyond.* San Francisco: Benjamin Cummings, 2008.

Barrett, S., W. London, R. S. Baratz, and M. Kroeger. *Consumer Health: A Guide to Intelligent Decisions*, 8th ed. New York: McGraw-Hill, 2006.

Benson, H. *The Relaxation Response.* New York: Avon, Wholecare, 2000.

Daniel, E. (Ed.). *Annual Editions: Health*, 25th ed. Guilford, CT: McGraw-Hill, 2004.

Donatelle, R. *Health: The Basics*, 10th ed. San Francisco: Pearson Education, 2013.

Fraser, A. *The Healing Power of Meditation: Leading Experts on Buddhism, Psychology, and Medicine Explore the Health Benefits of Contemplative Practice.* Shambhala Publications, 2013.

Greenberg, J. *Comprehensive Stress Management*, 10th ed. Dubuque, IA: McGraw-Hill, 2006.

helpful weblinks

do it! WEBLINKS

For links to the organizations and websites listed, visit MasteringHealth™.

American College Counseling Association

Offers information related to counseling and college students. **www.collegecounseling.org**

American College Health Association (ACHA)

Offers health-related information for college students. **www.acha.org**

American Psychological Association

Provides information on stress management and psychological disorders. **www.apa.org**

Mayo Clinic

Contains information about stress, diet, fitness, and mental health. **www.mayoclinic.org**

National Institute of Mental Health

Working to improve mental health through biomedical research on mind, brain, and behavior. **www.nimh.nih.gov**

WebMD: Stress Management Health Center

Contains information about stress management and stress and health. **www.webmd.com**

Weil Lifestyle

Provides a wide range of wellness information. **www.drweil.com**

laboratory 11.1

do it! LABS
Complete Lab 11.1 online in the
study area of **MasteringHealth.com**

Name _____   Date _____

Assessing Your Personality Behavior Pattern

Select the position that you feel best reflects your typical behavior in the situations described.

Extreme Type A Behavior Pattern						Extreme Type B Behavior Pattern
Fast at doing things	1	2	3	4	5	Slow at doing things (eating, talking, walking)
Unable to wait patiently	1	2	3	4	5	Able to wait patiently
Never late	1	2	3	4	5	Unconcerned about being on time
Very competitive	1	2	3	4	5	Not competitive
Poor listener (I finish other people's sentences for them)	1	2	3	4	5	Good listener
Always in a hurry	1	2	3	4	5	Never in a hurry
Always do two or more things at once	1	2	3	4	5	Take one thing at a time
Speak quickly and forcefully	1	2	3	4	5	Speak slowly and deliberately
Need recognition from others	1	2	3	4	5	Don't worry about what others think
Push myself (and others) hard	1	2	3	4	5	Easygoing
Don't express feelings	1	2	3	4	5	Good at expressing feelings
Few interests outside of school or work	1	2	3	4	5	Many hobbies and interests
Very ambitious	1	2	3	4	5	Not ambitious
Eager to get things done	1	2	3	4	5	Deadlines don't bother me

INTERPRETATION

- If the majority of your responses are 1s, then you fall in the **Extreme Type A Behavior Pattern**. This personality behavior pattern is described as extremely competitive, highly committed to work, with an extreme sense of time urgency. Such individuals are extremely goal oriented and can become hostile if someone gets between them and a goal they have established.

- If the majority of your responses are 2s with a few 1s, then you fall in the **Type A Behavior Pattern**. Type A behavior pattern is characterized by the traits listed for Extreme Type A behavior pattern, but they are moderated somewhat. People who exhibit this behavior pattern are ambitious, competitive, and goal oriented, with a sense of time urgency.

- If your responses are a mixture of the behavior patterns, you are described as a **Balanced Personality**. People with this type of personality get things done, but not at all costs. They can compete but do not feel they have to. They are more laid-back and inclined to give people the benefit of the doubt. They balance leisure time and work time.

- If the majority of your responses are 4s with some 5s, then you fall in the **Type B Behavior Pattern**. People with Type B behavior pattern are easygoing and lack a strong sense of time urgency. They don't like to compete and won't let deadlines interfere with vacation or leisure time. It is not that they are less ambitious than those with Type A behavior pattern; they are just more relaxed.

- If the majority of your responses are 5s, then you fall in the **Extreme Type B Behavior Pattern.** This personality behavior pattern is very relaxed, with no sense of time urgency. In fact, Extreme Type Bs typically don't wear a watch. They try to avoid competition at all costs and never mix leisure time and work time.

REMEMBER

This inventory is only one aspect of your personality. If your responses indicate Type A tendencies, you may want to assess your lifestyle and address some of the more stressful areas.

Knowing your behavior pattern will help you understand the types of stressors that affect you the most. For example, individuals with a Type B personality may find their lack of urgency causes them to wait until the last minute to finish assignments. Knowing this tendency, these individuals can work on better time management as part of their semester plan. Type A personalities may procrastinate because they love the adrenaline rush when working under pressure. These individuals may need to make an effort to incorporate recreational activities into their schedule and to engage in less competitive activities when they are experiencing higher levels of stress. Personality types do not change. However, we can recognize our stressors and our typical responses and take steps to manage stress in healthy ways.

laboratory 11.2

do it! LABS
Complete Lab 11.2 online in the
study area of **MasteringHealth.com**

Name _____ Date _____

Stress Index Questionnaire

The purpose of this stress index questionnaire is to increase your awareness of stress in your life. Answer "Yes" or "No" to each of the following questions.

Yes	No	1.	I have frequent arguments.
Yes	No	2.	I often get upset at work.
Yes	No	3.	I often have neck and/or shoulder pain due to anxiety/stress.
Yes	No	4.	I often get upset when I stand in long lines.
Yes	No	5.	I often get angry when I listen to the local, national, or world news or read the newspaper.
Yes	No	6.	I do not have enough money for my needs.
Yes	No	7.	I often get upset when driving.
Yes	No	8.	At the end of a workday I often feel stress-related fatigue.
Yes	No	9.	I have at least one constant source of stress/anxiety in my life (e.g., conflict with boss, neighbor, mother-in-law).
Yes	No	10.	I often have stress-related headaches.
Yes	No	11.	I do not practice stress management techniques.
Yes	No	12.	I rarely take time for myself.
Yes	No	13.	I have difficulty in keeping my feelings of anger and hostility under control.
Yes	No	14.	I have difficulty in managing time wisely.
Yes	No	15.	I often have difficulty sleeping.
Yes	No	16.	I am generally in a hurry.
Yes	No	17.	I usually feel that there is not enough time in the day to accomplish what I need to do.
Yes	No	18.	I often feel that I am being mistreated by friends or associates.
Yes	No	19.	I do not regularly perform physical activity.
Yes	No	20.	I rarely get 7 to 9 hours of sleep per night.

SCORING AND INTERPRETATION

Answering "Yes" to any of the questions means that you need to use some form of stress management technique. Count your "Yes" answers, and use the following scale to evaluate the level of stress in your life.

Number of "Yes" Answers	Stress Category
6–20	High stress
3–5	Average stress
0–2	Low stress

1. Are you satisfied with your score? If not, name the areas you could target to reduce your level of stress.

_____

_____

_____

2. If you named areas you want to target in the previous question or you are in the high-stress category, what techniques will you employ to help lower your stress level? Write out a specific plan for how you will attempt to use at least of one of the stress management strategies for a specific stressor that you face.

_____

_____

_____

_____

laboratory 11.3

do it! LABS
Complete Lab 11.3 online in the
study area of **MasteringHealth.com**

Name _____   Date _____

Managing Time and Establishing Priorities

Many people feel that there are not enough hours in the day, and they never seem to get around to all the things they plan to do. They think they will find time in the future, but as more and more things are put off, some are never even started, let alone completed. If this sounds like you, use the following time management tool to help you set your priorities and budget your time.

STEP 1: ESTABLISH PRIORITIES

Rank each priority that applies to you in the list below. Use 1 for the highest priority, 2 for the second highest, and so on. You may add priorities as necessary.

Priority	Rank	Priority	Rank
More time with family		More time for exercise and physical activity	
More time with friends		More time to relax	
More time for work and professional pursuits		More time to study	
More time for leisure and recreation		More time for myself	
More time with boyfriend/girlfriend/spouse		Other: _____	

STEP 2: MONITOR YOUR CURRENT TIME USE

Pick one day of the week, and track what you do each hour of the day.

Time	Activity
5:00 A.M.	
6:00	
7:00	
8:00	
9:00	
10:00	
11:00	
12:00 P.M.	
1:00	
2:00	
3:00	
4:00	
5:00	
6:00	
7:00	
8:00	
9:00	
10:00	
11:00	
12:00 A.M.	

STEP 3: ANALYZE YOUR CURRENT TIME USE

1. During which activities did you use stress reduction techniques? Did they help? Why or why not?

   _____

   _____

   _____

   _____

2. In which activity did you spend the most time? The least time? For example, did you watch TV for 3 hours? Did you spend 10 minutes on exercise?

   _____

   _____

   _____

   _____

3. Did the amount of time you spent on these activities reflect the priorities you indicated earlier? Why or why not?

   _____

   _____

   _____

4. Which activities will you spend less time in? Which will require increased time?

   _____

   _____

   _____

   _____

5. During which hours can you spend time doing activities that are important to you? How can you replace current activities with those on your prioritized list?

   _____

   _____

   _____

   _____

6. Based on your priorities, what changes will you make in your daily schedule?

   _____

   _____

   _____

   _____

STEP 4: MAKE A SCHEDULE

Write in your planned activities for the next day, and try to stick to this schedule as much as possible.

Time	Activity
5:00 A.M.	
6:00	
7:00	
8:00	
9:00	
10:00	
11:00	
12:00 P.M.	
1:00	
2:00	
3:00	
4:00	
5:00	
6:00	
7:00	
8:00	
9:00	
10:00	
11:00	
12:00 A.M.	

Were you able to modify your schedule to find time for your priorities? If not, state how you will modify your plan to accommodate your priority activities.

_____

_____

_____

_____

12

Special Considerations Related to Exercise and Injury Prevention

1. List and describe injuries that can occur as a result of exercising in heat or cold and explain how they can be prevented. Describe how the body acclimates to hot and cold environments.

2. Explain the primary challenge to the body when exercising at high altitude and the precautions that must be taken to avoid problems.

3. Name the air pollutants that can cause harm when exercising outdoors, and summarize the long-term effects of exercising in a polluted environment.

4. Explain the risks associated with increasing the amount and/or intensity of exercise and how to prevent injury while increasing fitness.

5. Name common injuries associated with exercise training, list their causes and treatments, and describe how each can be prevented.

6. Explain the principle of injury treatment and how the cryokinetics procedure is used in rehabilitation.

7. Differentiate between *unintentional injury* and *accident*. List common unintentional injuries and describe how you can reduce your risk for each.

319

A **NUMBER OF** special considerations need to be taken into account when beginning an exercise program. These can be grouped into two categories: environmental concerns and injury prevention.

Have you ever had a hard time catching your breath after a run on a hot day? Or felt woozy after just a few minutes of hiking in the mountains? You probably know that your environment affects your exercise performance and safety. But do you know why and how? In this chapter, we discuss common environmental hazards and outline ways to cope with environmental stress, particularly in regard to heat, humidity, cold, high altitude, and air pollution. Once you have completed the chapter, you can check your knowledge of environmental hazards using Laboratory 12.1.

Many physical and recreational activities that Americans enjoy involve some risk of injury. Each year, about 20 million weekend athletes and another 10 million school children experience sports injuries (1). Among runners, the incidence of injuries ranges from 25% to 75%.

In addition to exercise-related injuries, Americans are also at risk of unintentional injuries. As of 2013, unintentional injuries were the leading cause of death in people between the ages of 1 and 44 (2). As with exercise-related injuries, most can easily be prevented.

Exercising in Hot or Cold Environments

 List and describe injuries that can occur as a result of exercising in heat or cold and explain how they can be prevented. Describe how the body acclimates to hot and cold environments.

Air temperature matters during exercise because humans are **homeotherms**; that is, our body temperature is regulated to remain close to a set point—98.6°F (37°C). If body temperature falls too far below or rises too far above this normal temperature, serious injury can result (**FIGURE 12.1**). The body must maintain precise temperature control to avoid a life-threatening situation.

During exercise, your muscles produce heat as a byproduct of muscular contractions. High-intensity exercise using large-muscle groups produces more body heat than low-intensity exercise involving small-muscle groups. Thus, when large-muscle groups are vigorously exercised under hot conditions, the body produces excess heat that it must release in order to prevent a dangerous rise in body temperature. If the body cannot eliminate enough heat to keep its temperature below 105°F (41°C), then heat injury can ensue (3). There are several types of heat injury, and their symptoms can include cramps, dizziness, nausea, clammy skin, rapid heartbeat, lack of sweating, seizures, and hot, dry skin.

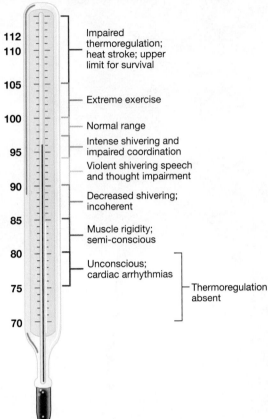

Range of Body Temperatures (°F)

- 112, 110 — Impaired thermoregulation; heat stroke; upper limit for survival
- 105 — Extreme exercise
- 100 — Normal range
- 95 — Intense shivering and impaired coordination
- 90 — Violent shivering speech and thought impairment
- — Decreased shivering; incoherent
- 85 — Muscle rigidity; semi-conscious
- 80 — Unconscious; cardiac arrhythmias
- 75 — Thermoregulation absent
- 70

FIGURE 12.1 A scale representing the range of temperatures for human survival and bodily injury.

Heat Loss During Exercise

There are two primary means of heat loss during exercise: convection and evaporation. The body loses heat by **convection** when air or water moves around the body. Convective heat loss occurs only when the air or water molecules moving over the surface of the body are cooler than skin temperature; the faster the flow of cool air or water around the body, the greater the heat loss. Minimal convective cooling occurs during exercise in a hot environment where there is limited air movement (such as when riding a stationary exercise bicycle). In contrast, bicycling outdoors on a cold day or swimming in cool water results in a large amount of convective cooling.

During **evaporation**, the body releases heat when sweat on the skin is converted to a gas (water vapor). On a warm day with limited air movement around the body, evaporation is the most important means of body heat loss (4). The evaporation of sweat on the skin's surface removes heat from the body, even if the air temperature is higher than body temperature, as long as the air is dry. However, if the air temperature is high and the **humidity** is also high (i.e., the air is relatively saturated with water), then evaporation is limited and the body

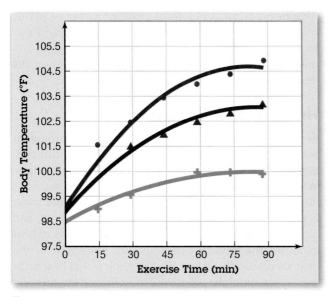

Key

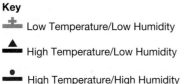 Low Temperature/Low Humidity

▲ High Temperature/Low Humidity

● High Temperature/High Humidity

FIGURE 12.2 Body temperature responses to prolonged exercise under three different environmental conditions.

Category	Heat Index	General Effect of Heat Index on People in Higher Risk Groups
1	130° or higher	Heat/sunstroke highly likely with continued exposure
2	105°–130°	Sunstroke, heat cramps, or heat exhaustion likely and heatstroke possible with prolonged exposure and/or physical activity
3	90°–105°	Sunstroke, heat cramps, and heat exhaustion possible with prolonged exposure and/or physical activity
4	Below 90°	Fatigue possible with prolonged exposure and/or physical activity

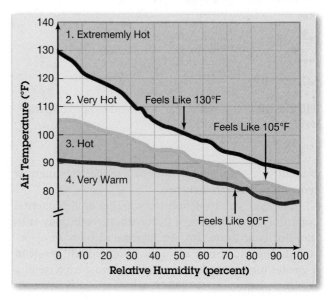

FIGURE 12.3 The concept of "heat index" or "effective" temperature.

cannot release as much heat. Under these conditions, the body retains the heat produced by the contracting muscles, and body temperature increases gradually throughout the exercise session. Prolonged exercise in a hot and humid environment can result in a dangerous increase in body temperature. **FIGURE 12.2** illustrates the differences in body temperature rise during exercise in a high-temperature/high-humidity environment, a high-temperature/low-humidity environment, and a low-temperature/low-humidity environment.

Short-term exposure (30–60 min) to an extremely hot environment is sufficient to cause heat injury in some people (4), especially those at high risk. (Older adults and people with low cardiovascular fitness levels are most susceptible.) Even individuals who are physically fit and accustomed to heat are at risk if they exercise in a hot environment.

In addition to air temperature, humidity can also be a significant factor during heat stress (**FIGURE 12.3**). The higher the humidity, the higher the "effective" temperature or heat index—the temperature that the body senses (see chart below and Figure 12.3). At high levels of humidity, sweat on the skin cannot readily evaporate into the air, impairing the body's ability to release heat. This causes body temperature to increase above what it would be on a less humid day at the same air temperature.

Looking at Figure 12.3, you can see that exercise at 100°F and 52% humidity makes you feel like you are

exercising at 130°F! This is an extremely hot environment and therefore very dangerous. It may not be obvious, but the body undergoes the same heat stress at only 88°F when the relative humidity approaches 100%. In both cases, it feels like the temperature is 130°F. Thus, high

---

homeotherm Animal that regulates body temperature to remain close to a set point.

convection Heat loss by the movement of air or water over the surface of the body

evaporation Conversion of water (sweat) to a gas (water vapor); the most important means of releasing heat from the body during exercise.

humidity The amount of water vapor in the air.

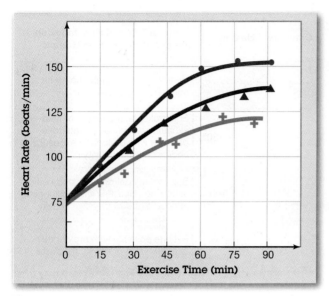

Key

+ Low Temperature/Low Humidity

▲ High Temperature/Low Humidity

● High Temperature/High Humidity

FIGURE 12.4 Changes in heart rate during prolonged exercise.

humidity causes the body to sense a moderately high air temperature as extremely hot.

The best way to determine whether environmental conditions are imposing a heat load on your body is to monitor your heart rate. An increase in body temperature during exercise in a hot environment will result in a greater increase in heart rate than during exercise in a cooler environment. **FIGURE 12.4** shows the differences in how exercise heart rates respond to three different environmental conditions. A temperature-induced increase in exercise heart rate is significant because it makes staying within your target heart rate zone more difficult.

Exercise Attire for Hot Environments

You can reduce your risk of heat injury during exercise in a hot environment by wearing the proper clothing (5). The first rule is to minimize the amount of clothing to maximize the exposed body surface area for evaporation. Clothing should be lightweight and made from materials that readily absorb moisture and allow air to move through them freely, features that promote both evaporative and convective cooling. Cottons and linens are best for these purposes.

You also don't necessarily want to switch to dry clothing when your initial clothing becomes saturated with sweat, because wet clothing promotes heat exchange better than dry clothing. Thus, switching to dry clothing delays the resumption of evaporative cooling. Don't

wear heavy fabrics or clothing made of rubber or plastic because they trap humid air next to the skin and also impair evaporative heat loss. Finally, wearing light-colored clothing when exercising outdoors will lessen the amount of radiant heat you absorb from the sun.

Heat Acclimatization

Exercise in a hot—or even a moderately hot—environment will cause the body to adapt, or **acclimatize**, to this condition, thereby decreasing the likelihood of heat injury. When the body is in a hot environment and needs to dissipate more heat, sweating begins earlier, more sweat is produced (to facilitate more evaporative cooling), and blood volume increases (5). Within 10 to 12 days of heat exposure, the physiological responses to exercise in the heat are drastically altered (5). The result is that heat acclimatization promotes a decrease in exercise heart rate and in body temperature.

Heat injury can occur when the exercise heat load exceeds the body's ability to regulate body temperature. It is a serious condition and can result in damage to the nervous system and, in extreme cases, death. The following are the most common types of heat injury.

- **Heat cramps** are characterized by muscle spasms or twitching of the limbs. They usually occur in people who are not acclimatized to the heat. Anyone with these symptoms should be moved to a cool place, laid down, and given 1 to 2 glasses of water with ½ teaspoon of salt added to each glass.

- **Heat exhaustion** results in general weakness, fatigue, a possible drop in blood pressure, blurred vision, occasionally a loss of consciousness, and profuse sweating from pale, clammy skin. Heat exhaustion can occur in an acclimatized individual. First aid should consist of moving the victim to a cool place, removing the clothing, applying cold water or ice, and giving 1 cup of water containing ½ teaspoon of salt every 15 minutes for 1 hour.

- **Heat stroke** is a life-threatening emergency. A person experiencing heat stroke stops sweating, and the skin becomes hot and red. Muscles are limp. Signs include involuntary limb movement, seizures, diarrhea, vomiting, and a rapid, strong heartbeat. The individual may hallucinate and eventually lapse into a coma. Any of these signs should be taken very seriously. Seek emergency medical assistance immediately, and administer first aid by moving the victim to a cool place, removing clothing, and lowering body temperature as rapidly as possible (by giving liquids, immersing in water or ice, and/or fanning).

Each of these conditions is initiated by heat exposure and involves significant loss of water and electrolytes. The body also stores additional heat, as indicated by a high core temperature. Note that you can minimize water loss

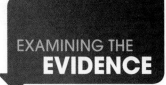

Guidelines for Managing Dehydration and Fluid Intake during Exercise in a Hot Environment

Exercise in the heat can be extremely dangerous, depending on exercise intensity, ambient temperature, relative humidity, clothing, and state of hydration. Because the sweat you lose during exercise is replaced with water from the blood, the ultimate danger during prolonged exercise in the heat is **dehydration** and decreased blood volume. The loss of body weight during exercise in heat is due to water loss through sweating. Thus, prolonged, profuse sweating is the first warning signal of impending dehydration.

The best strategy for preventing a decrease in blood volume is maintaining a regular schedule of fluid intake during exercise. You cannot rely on thirst as an indicator for when additional fluid is necessary, because the thirst mechanism lags behind fluid loss. Your body does not recognize a need for fluid until after a significant change in blood composition. Therefore, you should start to take fluids within 10 to 20 minutes after beginning exercise, before a fluid deficit accumulates (6). The following guidelines for fluid replacement will help you meet your body's need for water during exercise.

Drink approximately 16 ounces (2 cups) of fluid about 2 hours prior to the workout.

Drink approximately 4 to 8 ounces (½ to 1 cup) every 10 to 20 minutes during exercise, regardless of whether you feel thirsty.

The drink should

- be low in sugar (generally less than 8 grams per 100 milliliters {3.5 oz} of water),
- contain only a small amount of electrolytes (sodium and potassium), and
- be free of alcohol.

Water is the best fluid to drink during short-duration exercise. For longer or more intense exercise sessions, an electrolyte-containing sport drink may be beneficial. Alcoholic beverages can impair performance and should be avoided for 24 hours before exercise.

In general, you should consume 30 milliliters (about 1 ounce) of fluid for every minute of exercise performed. Another means to estimate how much fluid you need is to weigh yourself before exercising and immediately after your cool-down. The difference in body weight is a measure of how much fluid you lost via sweating, and you should replace more than that amount. Each ounce of body weight lost due to sweating is equivalent to 1 fluid ounce. For example, a body weight difference of 1 pound indicates that your body lost 16 ounces of sweat during exercise. Therefore, you would need to consume more than 16 ounces (2 cups) of fluid to replenish body fluid stores (6).

by drinking plenty of fluids whenever it's hot. Inattention to any of the signs of heat injury can lead to heat stroke and finally to death. Do not take these symptoms lightly!

You can exercise in hot and/or humid conditions, but be sure to keep the following in mind:

- Start exercising slowly, and keep your exercise session relatively short (15 to 20 minutes).
- Monitor your heart rate often, and keep your exercise intensity low to stay within your target heart rate zone.
- Wear appropriate clothing.
- To avoid dehydration, drink plenty of fluids before, during, and after the exercise session (see Examining the Evidence).
- Exercise in the morning or evening, when outside air temperatures are cooler because there is less radiant heat from the sun. If you must exercise during the heat of the day, try to find a shaded area. This might mean exercising indoors or hiking or jogging in a wooded area.

Maintaining Body Temperature in a Cold Environment

If you do not retain enough body heat in extremely cold temperatures, you are more likely to experience **hypothermia**, which can be life-threatening (7).

---

acclimatize To undergo physiological adaptations that help the body adjust to environmental extremes.

heat injury Injury that occurs when the heat load exceeds the body's ability to regulate body temperature. Also called *heat illness*.

dehydration Loss of too much body water, resulting in impaired function.

hypothermia Significant decline in body temperature due to exposure to cold.

Advances in Cold-Weather Clothing

Even though wearing several layers of clothing is beneficial while exercising in the cold (because the air trapped between layers provides great insulation), exercising in the cold can be extremely dangerous if the clothing gets wet from perspiration. Thus, materials that help remove moisture from the skin are better worn next to the skin than are materials that absorb moisture, such as cotton.

New high-tech fabrics combine several layers to provide insulation, breathability, and water resistance. One example is the ComforMaxTM fabric. The polyester fiberfill in the center of the fabric traps pockets of warm air, providing insulation, while the nonwoven membrane retains and reflects the body's own radiant heat. The open-pore structure of the membrane allows perspiration to pass out of the fabric and evaporate easily. An outer shell provides additional protection from both wind and water. Materials like ComforMaxTM are used in many types of active wear that require warmth, insulation, and weather resistance without excessive bulk.

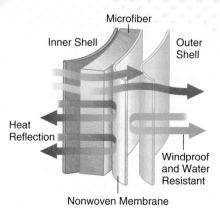

Exercising in the cold for long periods (e.g., 1–4 hours) or swimming in cold water may overwhelm the body's ability to prevent heat loss, resulting in hypothermia. Severe hypothermia can result in a loss of judgment, which increases the risk of further cold injury. Hypothermia can be avoided by limiting the duration of exercise in a cold environment, dressing appropriately, and staying out of cold water (if you're in water that makes you shiver, then it's too cold).

Contrary to popular belief, exercising in the cold will not damage your lungs. Research suggests that exercise in temperatures between 15°F and 32°F does not present a major risk to lung tissues (7). Inhaled cold air is rapidly warmed by the nasal passages and airways, so that by the time it reaches the lungs, it is close to normal body temperature.

Exercise Attire for Cold Environments

The key to exercising in the cold is to wear the proper clothing—that is, clothing that traps just enough of the heat produced during exercise to maintain normal body temperature, but not enough to overheat the body. The ideal clothing permits sweat to be transferred from the skin to the outer surface of the clothing, so that it does not evaporate from your skin and cause too much heat loss.

The best way to trap heat is to wear multiple layers of clothing so that air, an excellent insulator, is trapped between the layers. The thicker the zone of trapped air between the body and the outside of the clothing, the more effective the insulation; thus, several layers of lightweight clothing provide much greater insulation than a single bulky coat.

Dressing the upper body in layers is critical to maintaining the body's core temperature. The base layer (underwear) should remove moisture from your skin and move it to the next layer (wicking). This is critical because wet clothing can lose its insulating properties.

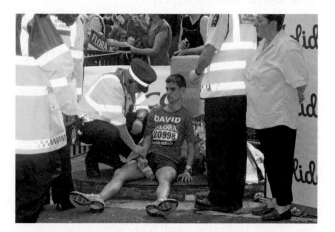

Be aware of the signs of heat injury. Distance runners and athletes who exercise vigorously in hot conditions are especially prone to the serious effects of heat injury.

Be sure to avoid cotton clothing for the base layer, because cotton will get wet and stay wet when you perspire, making you colder.

The primary purpose of the middle layer is to further insulate the body while still wicking moisture outward. Middle layers are often a bit heavier than the base layer. They should be used only in very cold conditions and should fit loosely over the base layer. The middle layer should be easy to remove for changing environmental conditions. Suggested fabrics include Polartec, Thermax, and fleece.

The outer layer should protect you from wind and water. The wind makes the "effective" temperature colder than the actual air temperature (the wind-chill effect; see **FIGURE 12.5**). Water causes virtually the same effect by conducting heat away from the body more rapidly than air. Thus, the outer layer should be a light-weight, microfiber, well-ventilated, windproof jacket. This type of material will protect you against cold, wind, rain, or snow while still allowing perspiration to evaporate. The final layer of clothing should be a hat, scarf, and gloves that protect your extremities from frostbite and keep heat from escaping through your head and neck.

consider this! ///////////////////

You lose 30% to 40% of your body heat through the head, so wearing a hat is important when exercising in the cold.

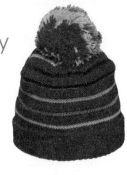

The proper amount of clothing to provide comfort during exercise varies with the temperature, the wind speed, and the intensity and duration of exercise. If you wear too little clothing, your body will lose too much heat. Too much clothing, in contrast, can limit your free-dom of movement and, even more important, can trap so much heat that you sweat. If you sweat during extreme

Calm

Wind (mph)	40	35	30	25	20	15	10	5	0	-5	-10	-15	-20	-25	-30	-35	-40	-45
5	36	31	25	19	13	7	1	-5	-11	-16	-22	-28	-34	-40	-46	-52	-57	-63
10	34	27	21	15	9	3	-4	-10	-16	-22	-28	-35	-41	-47	-53	-59	-66	-72
15	32	25	19	13	6	0	-7	-13	-19	-26	-32	-39	-45	-51	-58	-64	-71	-77
20	30	24	17	11	4	-2	-9	-15	-22	-29	-35	-42	-48	-55	-61	-68	-74	-81
25	29	23	16	9	3	-4	-11	-17	-24	-31	-37	-44	-51	-58	-64	-71	-78	-84
30	28	22	15	8	1	-5	-12	-19	-26	-33	-39	-46	-53	-60	-67	-73	-80	-87
35	28	21	14	7	0	-7	-14	-21	-27	-34	-41	-48	-55	-62	-69	-76	-82	-89
40	27	20	13	6	-1	-8	-15	-22	-29	-36	-43	-50	-57	-64	-71	-78	-84	-91
45	26	19	12	5	-2	-9	-16	-23	-30	-37	-44	-51	-58	-65	-72	-79	-86	-93
50	26	19	12	4	-3	-10	-17	-24	-31	-38	-45	-52	-60	-67	-74	-81	-88	-95
55	25	18	11	4	-3	-11	-18	-25	-32	-39	-46	-54	-61	-68	-75	-82	-89	-97
60	25	17	10	3	-4	-11	-19	-26	-33	-40	-48	-55	-62	-69	-76	-84	-91	-98

Temperature (°F)

Key: Frostbite Times

◻ 30 minutes

◼ 10 minutes

◼ 5 minutes

FIGURE 12.5 The "wind-chill" index.

Source: NOAA National Weather Service. NWS Wind-chill chart. **www.nws.noaa.gov/om/windchill**.

cold, the loss of body heat can lead to hypothermia, which can be fatal (7).

MAKE SURE YOU **KNOW...**

- Evaporation is the most important means of heat loss during exercise in a hot environment.

- Heat acclimatization occurs after several days of exposure to a hot environment. It increases the body's ability to cool itself, reducing the likelihood of heat injury.

- Heat cramps, heat exhaustion, and heat stroke can all result from the body's failure to release enough heat during exercise; each of these conditions is potentially serious and needs to be treated immediately.

- You can exercise safely in a hot environment as long as you follow safety guidelines, such as wearing loose, light-colored clothing and drinking plenty of fluids.

- Exercise in the cold can be safe and enjoyable, provided that the necessary precautions are taken to maintain heat balance and avoid hypothermia: Limit the duration of exercise, avoid cold water, and dress in appropriate layers of clothing.

MasteringHealth™

Exercising at High Altitudes

 LO **2** Explain the primary challenge to the body when exercising at high altitude and the precautions that must be taken to avoid problems.

The number of people going to high altitudes for hiking, skiing, camping, mountain climbing, and other activities is growing yearly. In fact, according to the National Ski Area Association, over 57 million visits are made to ski slopes alone each year. How does the body respond to exercise at high altitudes, and how can you adjust your exercise prescription?

The primary concern with exercise at high altitude is that the lower barometric pressure limits the amount of oxygen transported in blood (5). As a result, less oxygen reaches the exercising muscles, and therefore both exercise tolerance and $\dot{V}O_2$ max are reduced (**FIGURE 12.6**).

To cope with this decrease in oxygen delivery to the exercising muscles, the body makes several physiological adjustments (**FIGURE 12.7**). Breathing becomes deeper and faster in an attempt to maximize oxygen transfer from the lungs to the blood. Exercise heart rate rises to increase blood flow and oxygen delivery to the exercising muscles. To stay within your target heart rate zone during exercise at high altitude, it is necessary to lower your exercise intensity to less than your normal level. In general, there is little need to alter your duration or frequency of training during a

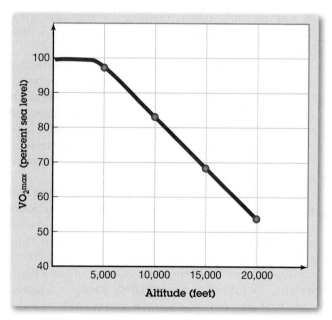

FIGURE 12.6 The effects of altitude on maximal exercise capacity.

brief stay at high altitude. However, the air is very dry at high altitudes, so your body loses more water during breathing (5). In addition, the body decreases its water content as a way of coping with the stress of altitude exposure. Be sure to drink plenty of fluids during and after exercise.

A problem associated with recreation at very high altitude (above 8,000 ft) is *acute mountain sickness (AMS)*. This occurs in about 20% of people going above this altitude and may occur in as many as 80% of those who fly into areas with elevations of 12,000 feet or above. AMS is characterized by severe headaches, nausea, weakness,

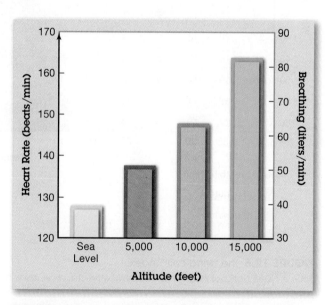

FIGURE 12.7 The effect of elevation on heart rate and ventilation during moderate exercise.

and dizziness, which, if not corrected, can cause fluid to collect in the brain or lungs, a life-threatening condition. The major cause of AMS is going too high too fast, with the result that your body doesn't have time to adjust the rate and depth of breathing.

To reduce the likelihood of AMS, try these strategies during your next trip to the mountains:

■ Ascend slowly. (Hiking is best; if you drive, spread the trip over several days; if you fly in, wait at least 24 hours before engaging in exercise.)

■ If you go above 10,000 feet, increase your altitude by no more than 1,000 feet per day.

■ Sleep at the lowest elevation possible.

■ If you feel the onset of AMS, don't go higher—if symptoms get worse, get off the mountain.

■ Drink plenty of water. Mountain air is typically dry, and you can dehydrate without sweating (make sure urine output is normal and clear).

■ Avoid alcohol and other depressants because they decrease your rate of breathing.

■ Eat a high-carbohydrate diet.

■ If you know you get AMS, see your doctor. There are medications that can help with acclimatization.

MAKE SURE YOU **KNOW...**

■ Exercise at high altitudes reduces the amount of oxygen in the blood, which in turn reduces oxygen transport to the working muscles and lowers both $\dot{V}O_2$ max and exercise tolerance.

■ At high altitudes, it is necessary to reduce the intensity of exercise to stay within your target heart rate range. There is little need to reduce the duration or frequency of exercise training during brief stays.

■ If possible, make your ascent to high altitudes gradually, so your body can adjust to the lower air pressure.

MasteringHealth™

Exercise and Air Pollution

LO ③ Name the air pollutants that can cause harm when exercising outdoors, and summarize the long-term effects of exercising in a polluted environment.

Air pollution is a growing problem in many parts of the world. Particulate matter in the air can lead to respiratory problems. The increase in rate and depth of breathing during exercise increases the exposure of your lungs to polluted air. If you exercise outdoors in a polluted environment, you should take measures to minimize pollution's effects.

Major Forms of Air Pollution

Two major pollutants that affect exercise performance are ozone and carbon monoxide (8). **Ozone** is a gas produced primarily by a chemical reaction between sunlight and the hydrocarbons emitted from car exhaust. This form of pollution is extremely irritating to the lungs and airways, causing tightness in the chest, coughing, headaches, nausea, throat and eye irritation, and, worst of all, bronchoconstriction (8). In fact, exposure to ozone can trigger an asthma attack.

Many cities monitor air quality and issue health alerts when it is poor. Stage 1 health alerts are issued when ozone reaches 0.2 ppm (parts per million), and stage 2 alerts are issued at 0.35 ppm. These alerts suggest that anyone with lung problems should not exercise outdoors. Many large metropolitan areas now have stage 1 alerts on more than 100 days out of the year. Although the long-term effects of ozone exposure are not clear, research suggests that chronic exposure to ozone diminishes lung function.

Carbon monoxide is a gas produced during the burning of fossil fuels, such as gasoline and coal, and it is also present in cigarette smoke. This pollutant binds to hemoglobin in the blood and thus reduces the blood's oxygen-carrying capacity. High levels of carbon monoxide can impair exercise performance by reducing oxygen delivery to the exercising muscles (8). In cities where traffic is heavy and congested, carbon monoxide can be a serious deterrent to exercise. For example, research suggests that runners in large metropolitan areas exhibit carbon monoxide levels in the blood that are twice the level necessary to negatively affect exercise performance (8).

live it!

ASSESS YOURSELF

Assess your health risk for asthma with *the Check Your Asthma I.Q.* Take Charge of Your Health! Worksheet online MasteringHealth™.

Coping with Air Pollution

The best way to minimize the effects of air pollution during exercise is to avoid exercising when ozone or carbon monoxide levels are highest. On hot summer days, ozone levels are highest at midday (11:00 a.m. to 3:00 p.m.) when the sun's ultraviolet rays are strongest. Avoid exercising during these times and when automobile

---

ozone Gas produced by a chemical reaction between sunlight and the hydrocarbons emitted from car exhaust.

carbon monoxide Gas produced during the burning of fossil fuels such as gasoline and coal; also present in cigarette smoke.

traffic is heavy. Carbon monoxide levels reach approximately 35 ppm in moving traffic and can exceed 100 ppm in slow and congested conditions (8). Because these levels can extend 20 to 30 yards away from traffic, exercisers should avoid heavily traveled roads and stay at least 30 yards away from the road if possible. Exposure to carbon monoxide (from sitting in traffic with the windows down or being in a smoke-filled room) can be detrimental before exercise, as well, because carbon monoxide leaves the blood slowly. In fact, the body may need more than 6 hours to remove significant amounts of carbon monoxide from the blood (8).

Air pollution is not always visible. Therefore, you must be aware of the times of day at which various pollutants are in highest concentrations and avoid exercising then. Pollutants not only affect exercise performance, but also, with chronic exposure, are hazardous to your health. In addition to doing what you can to avoid pollution, you can also take action to reduce pollution in your local area. Whenever possible, walk or take public transportation rather than driving. Recycle waste, and don't burn leaves or garbage.

MAKE SURE YOU **KNOW...**

- Ozone is produced by a chemical reaction between sunlight and automobile exhaust. Carbon monoxide is produced by the burning of fossil fuels. Both forms of air pollution can impair exercise tolerance.

- Avoid exercising during the times of day when ozone or carbon monoxide levels are highest. Ozone levels are highest during midday on hot summer days. Carbon monoxide levels are highest when automobile traffic is heavy.

MasteringHealth™

Risks Associated with Increased Physical Activity

 LO **4** Explain the risks associated with increasing the amount and/or intensity of exercise and how to prevent injury while increasing fitness.

Unfortunately, the more you exercise, the more likely you are to suffer from an exercise-related injury. Although many factors have been blamed for the injuries that recreational and competitive athletes experience, the majority (two-thirds) result from improper training techniques (9).

One result of improper training can be **overtraining syndrome**, a major cause of exercise-related injuries.

Overtraining is associated with too much exercise and not enough recovery time between workouts. The signs and symptoms may include increased resting heart rate, reduced appetite, weight loss, irritability, disturbed sleep, elevated blood pressure, frequent injuries, increased incidence of colds and flu, and chronic fatigue.

To prevent overtraining, a good rule of thumb is to increase your exercise intensity or duration by no more than 10% over a 2-week period. In addition, listen to your body. If you notice any signs or symptoms of overtraining, reduce your intensity and/or duration, and increase the frequency and/or length of your rest intervals. By avoiding overtraining, you can greatly reduce your chance of injury and maintain a positive attitude about fitness.

Two other common causes of exercise-related injuries are alignment problems in the legs or feet and inappropriate footwear. Although little can be done about alignment abnormalities, a change of shoes can help prevent injury in many cases. Approximately one-third of runners experience a decrease in injuries after changing to proper shoes because of the increased cushioning and support for the arch of the foot. Using shoes specially designed for such activities as tennis or aerobic dance can also reduce injuries.

Programs such as low-impact aerobics, step aerobics, and certain dance aerobics carry an increased risk for injury. Approximately one-half of all participants in traditional dance classes (e.g., ballet, tap, etc.) report

TABLE 12.1 ■ Risk Factors for Sports Injuries	
Intrinsic Risk Factors	**Extrinsic Risk Factors**
Age. Risk increases with age. As you age, soft tissues become less elastic, and injuries are more likely.	*Environmental factors (terrain, surface, weather).* Rough terrain or poor weather conditions increase risk for injury.
Body size and composition (weight, body fat). More weight puts more stress on joints, bones, and connective tissue, thereby increasing risk of injury.	*Equipment (footwear, clothing).* Improper shoes can lead to joint injuries in the leg, and inadequate or inappropriate clothing can lead to overheating in the summer or hypothermia in the winter.
Physical fitness. Risk is greater in unfit individuals. As you become more fit, bones and muscles get stronger and more resistant to damage.	*Type of activity.* Competitive activities are more likely to result in injury than are leisure activities.
Bone density and structure. Less dense or weaker bones are more prone to fracture and break.	*Intensity and amount of activity.* Intense activity and fatigue cause more injuries.
Gender (sex hormones, menarche). Women are at greater risk of injury than men. Hormonal differences may cause women to be at higher risk of lower leg injuries during exercise.	*Warm-up.* Some evidence suggests that a warm-up before exercise decreases risk
Muscle flexibility and strength. Less flexibility and strength predispose you to risk.	

Source: Based on Murphy, D. F., D. A. Connolly, and B. D. Beynnon. Risk factors for lower extremity injury: A review of the literature. *British Journal of Sports Medicine* 37(1):13–29.

injuries (10), which occur at a rate of approximately one injury per 100 hours of dancing. One study found that more than three sessions per week, improper shoes, and nonresilient surfaces were the primary causes of injury (10).

Excessive distance or duration may cause wear to tissues, such as connective tissue in joints. Drastic changes in training routines may put greater stress on tissues and can result in torn tissues. See **TABLE 12.1** for additional risk factors for injury during physical activity.

MAKE SURE YOU **KNOW...**

- The factors most closely associated with exercise-related injuries are improper training techniques, inadequate shoes, and alignment problems in the legs and feet.

- The one factor most likely to cause exercise-related injury is overtraining.

- Factors associated with injuries in aerobic dance are participating in more than three sessions per week, improper shoes, and nonresilient surfaces.

—MasteringHealth™

Common Conditions and Injuries

LO ⑤ Name common injuries associated with exercise training, list their causes and treatments, and describe how each can be prevented.

Although many injuries can result from overtraining, some are more common than others. This section discusses the cause and prevention of many general types of injuries and conditions associated with exercise training.

Back Pain

One of the most common complaints among athletes and nonathletes alike is back pain, especially in the lower back. Back pain can range from a vague ache to a searing, sharp pain that shoots up the spine. As with other injuries, there are mild and severe forms, and the degree to which back pain interferes with your physical activity can vary.

Cause One important cause of back pain is inadequate muscle strength in the abdomen and lower back. For someone experiencing back pain, exercise may be extremely helpful or extremely harmful. For example, exercise has been effectively used in pain clinics for treating back pain (11) and can sometimes prevent or correct back problems by strengthening weak muscles and stretching the stronger ones (see Chapter 5). However, if you have any type of back pain, you should attempt to find the cause with the help of a health-care provider or physical therapist before starting or continuing an exercise program. Certain types of exercise may compound the problem and thus should be avoided.

Prevention Exercises to increase flexibility and strength, reduce body fat, improve balance between the abdominal and back muscles, and prevent osteoporosis can decrease your risk of developing back problems (11).

---

overtraining syndrome Phenomenon in which too much exercise and not enough recovery time between workouts result in exercise-related injuries.

In addition, these exercises can help alleviate back pain that you may already be experiencing. See Laboratory 12.2 to assess your risk.

Use the following guidelines to help prevent back problems from getting worse or to prevent the onset of back pain:

- Maintain a healthy body weight and body composition. Obesity puts great strain on the lower back.
- Warm up before engaging in any physical activity.
- Do exercises to strengthen the abdominal muscles.
- Do exercises to stretch the lower back and hamstring muscles.
- When lying down, lie on your side with your knees and hips bent. Try to avoid lying on your back, but if you do, place a pillow under your knees.
- During prolonged standing, take the strain off of the lower back by propping one foot on an object such as a rail, step, or box, bending the leg at the hip and knee. Alternate legs occasionally.
- Avoid quick, jerking movements of the spine.
- Do not overextend the neck or lower back or overflex the neck.
- Avoid stretching the long or weak muscles, especially the abdominal muscles.
- Be especially careful when being passively stretched by another person. Avoid passive back or neck stretches or any ballistic passive stretches.
- Avoid movements that place force on spinal disks, such as extending and rotating the spine simultaneously, trunk and neck circling, and double leg lifts.
- Avoid forceful hyperextension and flexion of the spine.
- Avoid improper lifting. Squat to lift any object, and never bend at the waist.

Acute Muscle Soreness

Acute muscle soreness is not an injury but a form of fatigue, and it is common among athletes who train vigorously. Once exercise ceases, the athlete is left with a temporary feeling of weakness and stiffness.

Cause Acute muscle soreness may develop during or immediately following an exercise session that has been too long or too intense. If you are exercising to improve your fitness, you should not train so hard as to cause acute soreness. If you do feel local muscle weakness or stiffness after a workout, this may be a sign that your workout was a bit more strenuous than anticipated. Despite popular belief, lactic acid is not the cause of this type of soreness (12). Instead, it is more likely caused by other alterations in the chemical balance within muscle, increased fluid accumulation in muscle, or injury to muscle tissue.

Prevention Abnormally strenuous or prolonged exercise is likely to cause acute muscle soreness. Novice exercisers should be particularly cautious to not overdo it when beginning an exercise training program. Muscle soreness can be further prevented by not abruptly beginning or ending each exercise session. All exercise sessions should begin with a warm-up period of 5 to 15 minutes to allow muscles to increase their internal temperature slowly to avoid damage during the more stressful exercise training session. Finally, a post-exercise cool-down is important to allow the muscles to return to their normal, pre-exercise condition.

Delayed-Onset Muscle Soreness

Delayed-onset muscle soreness (DOMS), as the name implies, does not occur immediately after exercise, but rather 1–2 days after the exercise session. Acute muscle soreness is likely to be present as well, but the causes of the two are different.

Cause DOMS can develop after a bout of exercise that is excessive in duration or intensity (13). It is also common following new or unique physical activities that use muscle groups unaccustomed to exercise. For example, it is not unusual for a runner to experience soreness in the upper body after beginning a weight-training program.

DOMS is likely caused by microscopic tears in the muscle (13), leading to swelling and pain. Many investigators believe that this type of injury occurs primarily during the lengthening phase (the eccentric portion) of muscular contraction. The damage apparently is due to the greater force placed on the muscle during this phase of the contraction. For example, an individual who runs downhill (which emphasizes such contractions) and is not accustomed to this type of exercise will generally experience soreness in the leg muscles afterward. Similarly, DOMS is likely to occur in people unaccustomed to walking up and down steps if they begin a program that involves this form of exercise.

Prevention As with acute muscle soreness, DOMS can be prevented by refraining from exercise that is more strenuous or more prolonged than normal. Start with a warm-up, and limit both the intensity and duration of the first several workouts. Remember that eccentric contractions are more likely to result in muscle damage than are concentric (shortening) contractions. Therefore, in the beginning stages of an exercise program, try to avoid heavy weights for exercises that involve large amounts of eccentric contractions (e.g., walking down steps, running downhill, and performing certain movements during weight lifting).

Muscle Strains

Commonly referred to as a "pulled muscle," a muscle **strain** can occur with any type of unfamiliar movement involving a load that is abnormally high. Strains occur fairly frequently among weight lifters and other people engaged in activities that involve lifting heavy loads. Depending on the severity of the damage, recovery can take from a few days to many weeks.

Cause If a muscle is overstretched or forced to shorten against an extremely heavy weight (such as when lifting a heavy box), muscle fibers may be damaged. The resulting strain can range from minor to major damage to the muscle (14). There are three degrees of muscle strain:

- **First-degree strain.** Only a few muscle fibers are stretched or torn. Movement is painful, but a full range of motion is still possible.

- **Second-degree strain.** Many muscle fibers are torn, and movement is extremely painful and limited. The torn area may be apparent as a soft, sunken area in the muscle. Swelling may occur around the tear as a result of hemorrhage (bleeding).

- **Third-degree strain.** The muscle is torn completely (**FIGURE 12.8**). The tear can be in the belly of the muscle, in the tendon, or at the point where the tendon attaches to the bone. Movement is generally

impossible. Initial pain is intense but quickly subsides because nerve fibers are also damaged. Surgery is usually necessary for repair.

Prevention Because strains occur when muscles must generate excessive force, it follows that strains can be prevented by limiting the amount of stress placed on muscles. But note that it is not possible to predict just how much force is needed to cause muscle damage; moreover, warm muscles are more pliable (more easily stretched and less likely to tear) than cold muscles. Therefore, before lifting a heavy object or engaging in any activity that requires quick, jerking movements, warm up thoroughly for 5 to 15 minutes. Though a good warm-up should prevent muscle strains, remember that muscle contractions that are more strenuous than normal may result in DOMS.

Tendonitis

Tendonitis, the inflammation or swelling of a tendon, is one of the most common exercise-related injuries (14). Because tendons are located around joints, activities that stress the joints, such as tennis or jogging, are often the culprit behind these injuries.

Cause As muscles shorten and pull on tendons, the tendons move across other tendons, muscles, and soft tissue. This movement, if unfamiliar, can cause irritation and swelling in the tendon. Once tendonitis develops, pain associated with movement is the first symptom. Swelling, redness, and warmth generally follow. Tendonitis can occur in a number of areas, such as the elbow and shoulder. It is a common injury in weight lifters as well as in runners and tennis players.

Prevention Tendonitis is generally caused by strenuous, prolonged muscle contractions to which an individual is unaccustomed. Therefore, the best prevention of tendonitis is to avoid overuse. If you feel tendon pain or discomfort during a workout, stop exercising. This will prevent further irritation and reduce the severity of tendon damage. If you cannot stop using the muscle and tendon causing the pain, follow the guidelines for managing injuries provided later in this chapter.

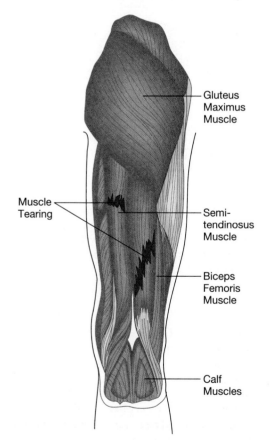

FIGURE 12.8 A third-degree muscle strain involves a complete tear of the muscle and loss of function. Surgery may be necessary to repair this degree of muscle strain.
Source: Karren, Keith J.; Hafen, Brent Q.; Limmer, Daniel J.; Mistovich, Joseph J., *First Aid for Colleges and Universities*, 9th Ed., © 2008. Reprinted and Electronically reproduced by permission of Pearson Education, Inc., Upper Saddle River, New Jersey.

Labels in figure: Gluteus Maximus Muscle; Muscle Tearing; Semi-tendinosus Muscle; Biceps Femoris Muscle; Calf Muscles

---

acute muscle soreness Muscle discomfort or pain that develops during or immediately following an exercise session that has been too long or too intense.

delayed-onset muscle soreness (DOMS) Muscle discomfort or pain that develops within 24 to 48 hours after an exercise session that is excessive in duration or intensity.

strain Damage to a muscle that can range from a minor separation of fibers to a complete tearing of the muscle.

tendonitis Inflammation or swelling of a tendon.

Ligament Sprains

A **sprain** is caused by damage to a ligament (14). Recall that ligaments connect the bones, provide joint support, and determine the direction and range of motion of joints.

Cause Ligament damage can occur if excessive force is applied to a joint. One of the most common sites of ligament damage is the ankle. When walking or running on an uneven surface, it is easy to "turn" the ankle, which means that the ankle joint is rotated such that much of the body weight is placed on the side of the foot. Because the ankle joint is not designed to rotate to that degree, the stress on the joint damages the ligaments. There are three degrees of ligament damage:

- **First-degree sprain**: Stretching and separation of a limited number of ligament fibers, resulting in minor instability of the joint (**FIGURE 12.9A**). Minor pain and swelling are the likely result.

- **Second-degree sprain**: Tearing and separation of a significant number of ligament fibers (**FIGURE 12.9B**). Moderate instability of the joint, with definite pain, swelling, and stiffness, occurs.

- **Third-degree sprain**: Total tearing or separation of the ligament, causing major instability of the joint (**FIGURE 12.9C**). Nerves may be damaged, and pain may subside quickly. Considerable swelling generally occurs.

Prevention Lightweight metal braces can provide added support to joints and therefore some protection from ligament damage. These braces are commonly used in football, a sport recognized for inducing knee damage. Without these expensive, high-tech devices, the best protection against torn ligaments is to refrain from activities that may subject a joint to high stress, including tennis, soccer, racquetball, and basketball. In addition, if you have a particular joint that has been injured previously or is weak, work to maintain maximum strength in the muscles surrounding the joint because strong muscles provide additional support.

Torn Cartilage

Cartilage on the end of bones in certain joints, such as the elbow, knee, and ankle, acts as a shock absorber to cushion the weight of one bone on another and to protect the bones from the friction due to joint movement. Torn cartilage does not commonly result from a fitness program, but swelling and pain can indicate that damage has been done.

Cause Unusually high forces or unusual movements can tear cartilage, resulting in joint pain. This is usually seen in athletes who undergo high-force activities while

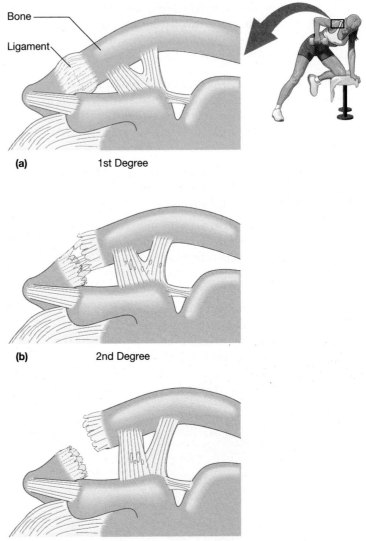

FIGURE 12.9 The extent of damage in the three categories of sprains, which involve damage to the ligaments that support the joint. **(a)** First-degree sprain at the shoulder, with minimal disruption of ligament. **(b)** Second-degree sprain with severe tearing and loss of joint stability. **(c)** Complete separation.

a joint is stretched. Damaged cartilage can also result from abnormal wear of misaligned bones or from excess wear due to weak musculature around a joint. This type of injury, like severe ligament damage, normally requires surgical correction.

Prevention The good news is that you don't need to incorporate activities that put you at high risk for torn cartilage in a general fitness program. Walking, swimming, and biking are examples of activities that don't put much force on joints and do not usually result in torn cartilage. To avoid cartilage injury, limit activities that produce excess stress on the joint or forceful movements that take the joint outside its normal range of motion.

Patellofemoral Pain Syndrome

Patellofemoral pain syndrome (PFPS) is a common exercise-induced injury that manifests as pain behind the patella, or kneecap (14). Also known as "runner's knee," PFPS may account for as much as 10% of all visits to sports injury clinics and 20%–40% of all knee problems (14).

Cause   PFPS results when the patella gets "off track," which causes excessive wear of the patella, leading to pain. Among the factors that predispose an individual to PFPS are misalignments of the thigh muscles that extend the knee, overuse or prolonged immobilization of the muscles, acute trauma, obesity, and genetics.

When any of these factors are present, the increased forces and repetitive movements of exercise result in pain and possibly also in cracking and popping sounds during movement. Over time and with increased use, the articular (joint) cartilage may begin to degenerate, which eventually may lead to osteoarthritis.

Prevention   You can prevent PFPS by avoiding stress on the knee due to excessive amounts of running, jumping, aerobic dancing, and stair climbing. Further, you can reduce your chances of developing PFPS by strengthening the front thigh muscles (quadriceps); this improves the tracking of the patella and reduces wear on the patellar surface.

The two best exercises seem to be knee extension exercises over the last 20 degrees of extension and/or isometric contractions of the quadriceps muscles with the leg fully extended (try to press the back of the knee to the floor while lying on your back) (14). Remember to avoid unnecessary stresses on the knee, such as squatting.

Finally, PFPS is one injury that may be prevented by using the proper athletic footwear. If you develop any of the symptoms of PFPS, see your physician or a podiatrist (foot specialist) to determine whether footwear may be contributing to the problem.

Treatment   An aggressive rehabilitation program that includes quadriceps exercises, rest, and anti-inflammatory drugs has proved beneficial for most PFPS patients. Although ice neither prevents PFPS nor rehabilitates the joint, it (like anti-inflammatory agents) may provide some relief from the pain and inflammation.

Shin Splints

Shin splints refers to pain associated with injuries to the front of the lower leg (14). The condition is common among runners, particularly distance runners, and can be quite painful.

Cause   Three of the most common injuries that cause shin splints are strain and irritation of one or several muscles and tendons located in the lower leg (**FIGURE 12.10**);

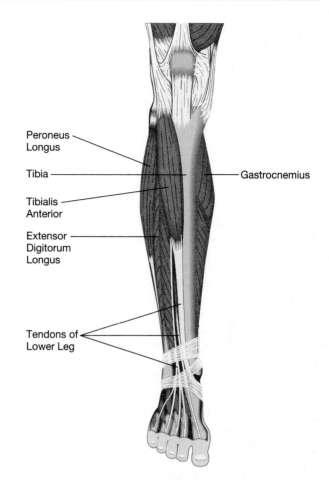

Peroneus Longus

Tibia

Tibialis Anterior

Extensor Digitorum Longus

Tendons of Lower Leg

Gastrocnemius

FIGURE 12.10 Muscles and tendons that are often irritated in shin splints.

inflammation of tissue connecting the two bones of the lower leg, the tibia and the fibula; and microscopic breaks (stress fractures, discussed next) in either the tibia or the fibula.

Prevention   Shin splints can be avoided by running on soft surfaces; by wearing well-padded, shock-absorbing shoes; and by slowly increasing exercise intensity from walking to running. If shin pain develops, it could be due to a fracture or break of a bone and therefore should not be regarded lightly. High-impact activities such as running should be stopped and replaced with low-impact activities such as cycling or swimming. Stretching muscles in the front and back of the lower leg may help prevent the problem.

---

sprain Damage to a ligament that occurs when excessive force is applied to a joint.

patellofemoral pain syndrome (PFPS) Common exercise-induced injury, sometimes called "runner's knee," that manifests as pain behind the kneecap (patella).

shin splints Term referring to pain associated with injuries to the front of the lower leg.

Stress Fractures

Stress fractures are tiny cracks or breaks in bone. Although stress fractures can occur in any leg bone, the long bones of the foot extending from the bones in the heel to the toes (the metatarsal bones) are especially susceptible (**FIGURE 12.11**). In fact, these are the most common sites of stress fractures in the body.

Cause Stress fractures result from excessive force applied to the leg and foot during running or other types of weight-bearing activities (15). The most likely candidates for this injury are individuals who have high arches or poor flexibility in the lower body and who increase training intensity or duration too rapidly.

Prevention People with high arches should seek exercise advice from their physician or a podiatrist, who might prescribe arch supports to help prevent a stress-related problem. A key factor in preventing stress fractures is to avoid overtraining by increasing your training load gradually (no more than 5%–10% per week). Often, lack of flexibility in the hips and the back of the legs causes the body's weight to shift such that some bones become chronically overloaded and predisposed to fracture. Thus, maintaining flexibility in the hips and back of the legs will reduce your chances of developing a stress fracture. If pain in the foot or leg makes you suspect a stress fracture, stop activities that involve the injured area. See your physician for an X-ray examination. If a stress fracture is present, only rest can assist the healing process.

While recognizing and understanding the injuries we've discussed so far is important, the best strategy is to reduce your risk of sustaining them. To assess your exercise program in regard to its potential risks of injury, see Laboratory 12.3.

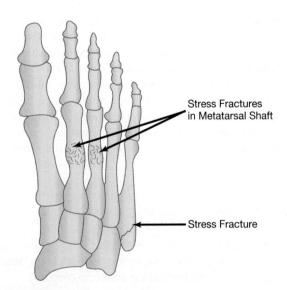

FIGURE 12.11 Metatarsal stress fractures can result in pain during any weight-bearing movement.

Stress Fractures in Metatarsal Shaft

Stress Fracture

MAKE SURE YOU **KNOW...**

- Exercise can play an important role in preventing back pain and in rehabilitating back problems.

- Acute muscle soreness, which occurs during or immediately after exercise, may be due to muscle damage, accumulation of fluid within the muscle, and/or chemical imbalances within the muscle itself.

- Delayed-onset muscle soreness (DOMS) usually occurs 24 to 48 hours after an exercise session. Eccentric exercise is a common cause of DOMS.

- When muscle is forced to contract against excessive resistance, the resulting damage to muscle fibers is called a strain. Such damage can range from a minor separation of fibers to a complete tear in the muscle.

- A sprain is caused by damage to a ligament.

- Tendonitis is a common overuse injury associated with physical activity; torn cartilage is not common but can be extremely painful when it does occur.

- PFPS occurs when the articular cartilage on the back of the kneecap (patella) is damaged by chronic use during exercise.

- Shin splints refer to various injuries to the front of the lower leg.

- Stress fractures are microscopic breaks in the bone.

- To reduce your risk of developing an exercise-related injury, engage in a program of muscle-strengthening exercises to maintain balance in strength around joints; warm up before and cool down after each workout; use proper equipment and proper footwear; increase exercise intensity and duration slowly; maintain the proper rest-to-exercise ratio; and do not overtrain.

MasteringHealth™

Managing Injuries

LO **Explain the principle of injury treatment and how the cryokinetics procedure is used in rehabilitation.**

As noted earlier, almost everyone who engages in regular physical activity will experience some type of injury. In the following sections we discuss injury treatment and provide an overview of the rehabilitation process.

Any injury that results in extreme pain or the possibility of a broken bone should be examined by a physician, who will likely order X-rays to determine whether there are any broken bones. The following treatment regimen should be followed for less severe injuries (first-degree strains and sprains, tendonitis, etc.).

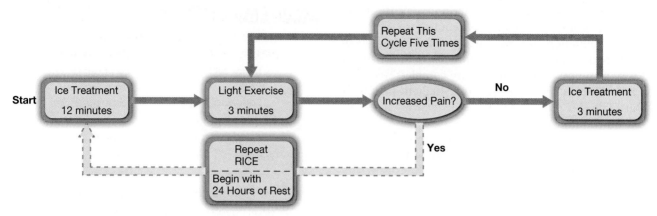

FIGURE 12.12 The steps of the cryokinetics procedure for rehabilitating injuries.

Initial Treatment of Exercise-Related Injuries

The objectives of the initial treatment of exercise-related injuries are to decrease pain, limit swelling, and prevent further injury (14). These objectives can be met by a combination of **R**est, **I**ce, **C**ompression, and **E**levation (**RICE**). Rest will help prevent further injury. Moving injured tissues will aggravate the injury and result in additional damage. Any movement that causes pain should be avoided.

Applying ice to an injury reduces swelling by reducing blood flow to the cooled area. Minimizing swelling will reduce the pain and lead to more rapid healing. Place ice (or an ice pack) in a cloth wrap to guard against skin damage, and apply it for 30-minute periods, three to four times a day, for 2 days after the injury.

Compressing the injured area also reduces swelling. The amount of compression should be enough to reduce fluid collection around the damaged area, but not tight enough to severely inhibit blood flow. Snugly wrapping the injured area with an elastic bandage is sufficient to control swelling. Placing a bag of ice in the last two or three wraps of the elastic bandage applies pressure and cools at the same time.

Finally, elevating the injured area (above the level of the heart if possible) reduces blood pressure and may therefore reduce swelling. Approximately 3 days following the injury, start an exercise rehabilitation program. If you have any doubts about whether the injury is ready for rehabilitation, delay another 24 to 48 hours.

Rehabilitation

Rehabilitation of minor injuries occurs naturally. After an injury has healed and swelling has subsided, most people will begin to move the injured area according to how much pain is involved. As the pain subsides, more movement can occur, until a normal range of motion is restored. However, this rehabilitation regimen has several drawbacks. First, it is very slow. Depending on the injury, the natural rehabilitation process may take five to ten times as long as an aggressive rehabilitation program. Second, the damaged area may be reinjured, because many people attempt to return to full use of the injured area too quickly. This secondary injury results in much greater damage than the first injury and can even weaken the tissue and lead to recurring injuries throughout life. Third, for many types of injury, the lack of an aggressive rehabilitation program can prevent the return of full function because the scar tissue that develops limits the normal range of motion. Fortunately, these problems may be overcome by an active rehabilitation process.

A popular rehabilitation technique that is implemented after the procedures have been followed is called **cryokinetics** (16). Ice is applied for approximately 12 minutes, followed by 3 minutes of light exercise, followed by another 3 minutes of cold. The 3 minutes of exercise and 3 minutes of ice should be repeated for five cycles. Exercise of the injured limb during this treatment must be guided by the pain associated with its use. Start with an exercise intensity that provides little or no pain, increasing intensity gradually as long as no increase in pain occurs. If pain increases during the cryokinetic therapy, stop the treatment and resume the procedures until the pain subsides (**FIGURE 12.12**).

---

stress fractures Tiny cracks or breaks in the bone.

RICE Acronym for a treatment protocol for exercise-related injuries; stands for **r**est, **i**ce, **c**ompression, and **e**levation.

cryokinetics Rehabilitation technique that incorporates alternating periods of treatment using ice, exercise, and rest.

The initial management of an injury is critical and determines how much time is required to complete the rehabilitation process. For example, a regimen of cryokinetics initiated after a third-degree ankle sprain (2–3 days post injury) results in complete recovery within 2 weeks. In contrast, if the cryokinetic treatment starts late (5–7 days post injury), the recovery may take 4 to 5 weeks.

As pain subsides and the range of motion returns, you may accelerate full recovery by adding a program of weight-training and flexibility exercises. This is especially true for muscle injuries, because the healing process may cause the muscle to shorten and thereby limit flexibility. An injury that does not heal properly may cause recurring pain during activity and may persist for years. Therefore, for extensive or complex injuries, you should seek the advice of a trained professional (athletic trainer, physical therapist, or physician).

MAKE SURE YOU **KNOW...**

- For treating injuries, remember the protocol: rest, ice, compression, and elevation.
- Cryokinetics is a rehabilitation technique that involves alternating periods of applying ice and exercising the injured area.

MasteringHealth™

Unintentional Injuries

 LO 7 Differentiate between *unintentional injury* and *accident*. List common unintentional injuries and describe how you can reduce your risk for each.

In addition to the exercise-related injuries that result from overstressing bones, muscles, ligaments, and tendons during physical activity, many Americans suffer from other **unintentional injuries** every year.

Unintentional injuries are the number-one killer of people between the ages of 1 and 44 in the United States (see **TABLE 12.2** for specific causes). Each year, unintentional injuries claim the lives of more than 5,100 children, or about 14 per day (17). In addition, for children under age 14, unintentional injuries result in about 6.2 million emergency room visits each year (17).

Although most unintentional injuries may seem to result from chance or "accidents," this is not the case. In fact, public health officials prefer using the term *unintentional injury* instead of **accident**, because the latter implies random events, bad luck, and an inability to change the outcome by modifying events or behavior (2). Keep in mind that *accident* refers to the sequence of events that lead up to the injury, whereas the injury is the

TABLE 12.2 ■ Five Leading Causes of Death among Young Adults		
Rank	Ages 15–24	Ages 25–34
1	Unintentional injury:	Unintentional Injury:
	Motor vehicle crash: 69.6%	Motor vehicle crash: 52.4%
	Poisoning: 14.6%	Poisoning: 27.9%
	Drowning: 3.7%	Drowning: 3.0%
	Other: 12.1%	Other: 16.7%
2	Suicide	Suicide
3	Homicide	Homicide
4	Malignant neoplasms	Malignant neoplasms
5	Heart disease	Heart disease

Source: National Center for Injury Prevention and Control. *CDC Injury Fact Book.* Atlanta: Centers for Disease Control and Prevention, 2013; National Center for Health Statistics. *Health, United States, 2013 with Chartbook.* Hyattsville, MD: National Center for Health Statistics, 2013.

health consequence of the accident. You can modify your behavior to control many risk factors.

Risk Factors for Unintentional Injury

One of the most significant risk factors is an unsafe attitude, which promotes risk-taking behaviors. For example, people who are overly confident in their driving skills may speed on a winding or wet road and thereby increase their risk of being in a crash. Similarly, people who are overconfident in their job skills may take unnecessary risks at work.

Some people crave excitement or the sensation of danger. Such a thrill-seeking attitude increases the risk of accidents. Such people often engage in high-risk activities such as skydiving, auto racing, or rock climbing, which increase their risk of injury due to accidents.

Stress increases your risk. During periods of emotional or physical stress, people tend to be less careful. If you find yourself having a series of small mishaps or "near misses" when performing routine activities such as yardwork, house cleaning, or sports activities, this may be an indication that you should reduce your stress level by resting and using stress management techniques.

Alcohol and other drugs also increase your risk of accidents. Drug use alters your judgment and decreases both reaction speed and motor coordination. Alcohol use is involved in about 25%–50% of deaths among

---

unintentional injury Injury resulting from unplanned actions; preferred term for accidental injury.

accident Event that results in unintended injury, death, or property damage; refers to the event itself, not to its consequences.

consider this! ////////////////////

Every 33 minutes in the United States, someone dies in an alcohol-related motor vehicle crash; every 2 minutes someone is injured.

adolescents and adults due to water recreation accidents; among adolescent men, alcohol is a contributing factor in 50% of drowning deaths (18). Sun exposure and heat increase the effects of alcohol on balance, coordination, and judgment. Similarly, cocaine and marijuana use are associated with a wide range of accidents, including falls, drownings, fires, and automobile accidents.

A number of environmental factors can increase your risk of accident. For example, storing combustible materials close to a heater and failing to have properly operating smoke detectors increase your risk of injury due to fire. Other factors, such as failing to properly maintain ladders or steps, increase the risk of falls or other accidental injury.

You can take steps to reduce your risk of injury. The key is to increase your awareness of the risk factors in your life. See the Steps for Behavior Change box on page 338. Use the tips there and in **FIGURE 12.13** to reduce your risk of injury from various causes.

Choking

Choking occurs when something (usually food) becomes stuck in the trachea (windpipe), blocking the airway. To assist a choking victim, you have to dislodge the trapped object, usually by performing the Heimlich maneuver. This first-aid protocol consists of a series of under-the-diaphragm thrusts. The rescuer stands behind the victim and circles his arms around the victim's waist. The rescuer then clasps his hands together and administers quick thrusts to the victim's abdomen. The thrusts lift the diaphragm and force enough air from the lungs to create an artificial cough, which usually expels the foreign body. The Heimlich maneuver is recommended for use on conscious adults and children over the age of 1. Other techniques are used for choking in infants under age 1 (see Weblinks).

Poisoning

Poisoning can occur when children accidentally ingest medications, cleaning products, or other household items. However, adults can also inadvertently be exposed to toxic or corrosive chemicals.

Bicycle or Motorcycle Accidents
• Always wear a helmet and use reflectors and protective clothing when riding.
• Ride with the traffic, or use bike paths when available.

Falls
• Maintain ladders and steps in good working condition.
• Use skidproof backing on rugs.
• Use handrails or nonslip mats in the bathtub and shower.

Drowning
• Never allow children to swim unsupervised.
• Learn to swim, and learn proper water safety procedures.
• Do not swim alone or in the dark.
• Dive only in designated areas.
• Do not swim immediately after eating, when tired, or when using drugs of any kind.
• Do not swim when using drugs of any kind.
• Avoid swimming in dangerous waters, such as rivers with strong currents.
• Learn cardiopulmonary resuscitation.
• Make sure residential pools are fenced.

Poisoning
• Properly label all drugs.
• Never take more of any drug than is recommended.
• Keep all drugs out of the reach of children.
• Store all drugs and chemicals in their proper containers.
• Use only nontoxic cleaning materials.
• Discard old or expired prescriptions.
• Do not combine drugs.
• Keep the poison control center's telephone number near your phone.

Fire
• Store combustible materials in a safe place.
• Maintain smoke detectors, fire extinguishers, and sprinkler systems in proper working condition.
• Know how to use a fire extinguisher.
• Practice safe evacuation procedures from your home and workplace.
• Never leave portable heaters unattended.
• Do not overload electrical outlets.

Motor Vehicle Crashes
• Do not drive when you are overly tired or sleepy.
• Maintain your motor vehicle in good mechanical condition.
• If you need assistance, in an accident, stay in your car and wait for help.

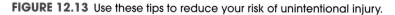

FIGURE 12.13 Use these tips to reduce your risk of unintentional injury.

steps ▶ FOR BEHAVIOR CHANGE

Does your behavior increase your likelihood of an unintentional injury?

Are you taking unnecessary risks that put you in danger of injury? Take this quiz to find out.

Y	N	
☐	☐	I often engage in thrill-seeking activities, such as bungee jumping, sky diving, and snowboarding.
☐	☐	I am a very confident driver and sometimes speed, or drive fast under subprime conditions, because I know I can handle it.
☐	☐	I have driven a car after consuming alcohol.
☐	☐	I quicken my pace when going up or down stairs or navigating a hill or other uncertain terrain.
☐	☐	I don't read package labels or directions when using a new cleaning product, gadget, or appliance.

If you answered yes to more than one of the above, you're probably on the road to some sort of unintentional injury.

Tips to Reduce Your Risk

Tomorrow, you will:

☑ Obey the rules of the road and drive defensively. Always wear your seat belt and drive within the legal speed limit. Do not drive when emotionally upset, and do not respond to aggressive drivers. Never drive while or after using drugs or alcohol.

☑ Use handrails when going up and down stairs, and never run up or down stairs. Additionally, do not attempt to climb ladders or stairs when you are ill or physically impaired because of alcohol or drug use.

☑ Read the label carefully when using a new medication to find out whether you need to avoid certain foods or substances. Don't use multiple medications without the express advice of your health-care provider.

☑ Read the directions when using a new gadget or appliance (particularly electrical ones) for the first time—don't assume you know how it works.

Within the next 2 weeks, you will:

☑ Adopt a realistic attitude toward sports and extracurricular activities. If you engage in a high-risk activity, such as sky diving, make sure you thoroughly understand the risks and take the proper precautions to avoid injury.

By the end of the semester, you will:

☑ Undergo adequate training by a qualified individual prior to trying a new activity that entails greater-than-normal risk of injury.

For poisoning accidents, always check the product label for first-aid information, and contact your poison control center. You may also need to contact 911 or a medical professional. For nonemergency situations, the following strategies may be useful:

■ **Poisons in the eye.** Flood the eye with lukewarm (never hot) water poured from a large glass 2 or 3 inches from the eye. Continue for 15 minutes. Blink the eye as much as possible during the flooding. Do not force the eyelid open, and do not allow the eyes to be rubbed. If lukewarm water is not available, rinse the eye quickly using a gentle stream from a hose for at least 15 minutes.

■ **Poisons on the skin.** Any poisons that come in contact with the skin must be removed as quickly as possible. Remove contaminated clothing, and flood the skin area with water for 10 minutes. Then gently wash the area with soap and water and rinse. Later, destroy contaminated clothing. For a chemical burn, remove clothing, rinse the affected area with lots of water and cover with a soft, clean cloth. Do not apply grease or ointments.

■ **Inhaled poisons.** Inhaled poisons are very serious because of the damage they can cause to the lungs and other tissues. Minimize your own risk of exposure, and immediately get the victim to fresh air. Send someone or call for help as quickly as possible. Loosen any restrictive clothing around the neck and chest. If the victim is not breathing, start CPR, and continue it until the victim is breathing or help arrives. Open the doors and windows so that no one else will be poisoned by the fumes.

■ **Swallowed poisons.** If you suspect that someone has swallowed a poisonous substance, first look into the victim's mouth and remove all tablets, powder, or any material that may be present. Examine the mouth for cuts, burns, swelling, unusual coloring, or odor. Rinse and wipe out the mouth with a cloth. If the person is awake and able to swallow, give one-half glassful of water.

Keep in mind that antidotes recommended on many product labels may be outdated or incorrect, so you should not rely on them. In addition, salt water, mustard water, and many other home remedies are ineffective and may be dangerous. Do not use them. In the past, ipecac syrup was sometimes used as a home remedy to induce vomiting, but experts disagree as to whether this is a safe and effective strategy. As of 2003, the American Academy of Pediatrics advises parents against keeping ipecac syrup in the home (19).

Bleeding

Although everyone occasionally experiences minor cuts and scrapes, massive blood loss is an extremely serious condition that can quickly lead to unconsciousness and even death. If you or someone near you experiences a wound that bleeds heavily, immediate attention is necessary. For serious wounds, call 911 and follow these steps until medical help arrives (20):

1. **Have the injured person lie down.** If possible, position the person's head slightly lower than the trunk, or elevate the legs. This position reduces the risk of fainting by increasing blood flow to the brain. If possible, elevate the site of bleeding.

2. **While wearing gloves, remove any obvious dirt or debris from the wound.** Don't remove any large or more deeply embedded objects. Don't probe the wound or attempt to clean it at this point. Your principal concern is to stop the bleeding.

3. **Apply pressure directly on the wound.** Use a sterile bandage, clean cloth, or even a piece of clothing. If nothing else is available, use your hand.

4. **Maintain pressure until the bleeding stops.** Hold continuous pressure for at least 20 minutes without looking to see whether the bleeding stopped. You can maintain pressure by binding the wound tightly with a bandage (or a piece of clean clothing) and adhesive tape.

5. **Don't remove the gauze or bandage.** If the bleeding continues and seeps through the gauze or other material you are holding on the wound, don't remove it. Instead, add more absorbent material on top of it.

6. **Immobilize the injured body part once the bleeding has stopped.** Leave the bandages in place, and get the injured person to the emergency room as soon as possible.

Stopped Breathing or Heartbeat

Cardiopulmonary resuscitation (CPR) may be necessary when an accident victim has stopped breathing or the heart has stopped. You need to take a course in CPR to be fully qualified to treat such victims. In short, here is what the rescuer should do:

1. First, check the victim for responsiveness. If there is no response, call 911 and return to the victim. In most locations, the emergency dispatcher can assist you with CPR instructions.

2. The following is what you will likely be instructed to do. Begin chest compressions immediately—hard and fast! Push down on the chest between the nipples (compress the chest about 2 inches), 30 times. Pump at the rate of 100 compressions per minute, faster than once per second. If a dispatcher is not available, keep compressions going. If a dispatcher is available, you may be instructed to perform step 3 below.

3. Tilt the head back, and listen for breathing. If the victim is not breathing normally, pinch the nose, cover the mouth with yours, and blow until you see the chest rise. Give two breaths. Each breath should take 1 second.

4. Continue with 30 pumps and two breaths until help arrives.

MAKE SURE YOU **KNOW...**

- Behavior and attitude can have a major impact on your likelihood of sustaining an unintentional injury. Motor vehicle accidents, falls, drowning,

and poisoning are the most common types of unintentional injuries.

- Avoiding or minimizing alcohol intake can reduce your risk of unintentional injury.

- There are a few key first-aid procedures that you should know, including the Heimlich maneuver and what to do in the case of poisoning or severe bleeding. You should take a course in first aid and CPR to be qualified to administer these procedures.

MasteringHealth™

study plan

Customize your study plan—and master your health!— in the Study Area of **MasteringHealth.**

summary

hear it! STUDY REVIEW

To hear an MP3 Chapter Summary, scan here or visit the Study Area in MasteringHealth™.

LO 1
- Evaporation is the most important means of heat loss during exercise in a hot environment. Wearing appropriate clothing maximizes the body surface area exposed to air and helps to ensure adequate release of body heat through evaporation.

- The body becomes acclimatized to heat after several days of exposure to a hot environment. Acclimatization increases the body's ability to lose heat and reduces the likelihood of heat injury. When exercising in hot environments, it is important to drink plenty of fluids to avoid dehydration.

- Although long-term exercise in a cold environment can result in hypothermia, short-term exercise in a cold environment does not generally pose a serious threat to heat balance. The key to avoiding hypothermia is to dress in layers of clothing.

LO 2
- Exercise at high altitude reduces the amount of oxygen in the blood, which reduces oxygen transport to the working muscles and lowers both $\dot{V}O_2$ max and exercise tolerance.

- At high altitudes, it is necessary to reduce the exercise intensity and ensure that you stay within your target heart rate range.

LO 3
- Ozone is produced by a chemical reaction between sunlight and vehicle exhaust, and carbon

monoxide is produced by the burning of fossil fuels. Both types of air pollution can impair exercise tolerance. It is advisable to avoid exercising outdoors when ozone or carbon monoxide levels are highest.

LO 4
- Overtraining poses the greatest risk for developing an exercise-related injury. Injuries associated with running occur primarily in the foot and knee because of the excessive stress placed on the legs and feet.

- Exercise-related injuries occur most often due to improper training techniques, inadequate shoes, and alignment problems in the legs and feet.

LO 5
- Exercise can help in preventing back pain and rehabilitating some back problems. Exercises to increase flexibility and strength, reduce body fat, improve muscle balance between the abdominal and back muscles, and prevent osteoporosis can decrease your risk of back problems.

- Acute muscle soreness may occur during or immediately after an exercise session. It may occur due to muscle damage, accumulation of fluid within the muscle, or chemical imbalances within the muscle.

- Delayed-onset muscle soreness (DOMS) usually occurs 24 to 48 hours after an exercise session. Eccentric exercise is a common cause of DOMS.

- When a muscle is forced to contract against excessive resistance, fibers are damaged. This injury is called a strain and can range from a minor separation of fibers to a complete tear.

- Tendonitis (inflammation of a tendon) is one of the most common overuse problems associated with physical activity.

- A sprain is caused by damage to a ligament, which is connective tissue that supports joints. Torn cartilage refers to damage to the tough, connective tissue that serves as a cushioning pad between the ends of bones.

- With patellofemoral pain syndrome (PFPS), the articular cartilage on the back of the kneecap (patella) may be damaged by chronic use during exercise. Shin splints describe injuries to the front of the lower leg, and stress fractures are microscopic breaks in the bone.

LO ■ For treating injuries, remember the protocol: rest, ice, compression, and elevation. Cryokinetics treatment calls for alternating periods of cold applications and exercise.

LO 7 ■ The three most common types of unintentional injuries are motor vehicle accidents, poisoning and drowning. Risk factors for accidents and injuries include an unsafe attitude, stress, and alcohol and drug use.

- Basic first aid involves knowing how to do the Heimlich maneuver and how to treat bleeding and poisoning. You should not perform CPR unless you have been trained and certified through the American Red Cross or other accredited program.

study questions

review it! QUIZZES

Find more review questions online MasteringHealth™.

LO 1. Which of the following is a major mechanism of heat loss during exercise?
   a. conduction
   b. radiation
   c. evaporation
   d. diffusion

2. During exercise, body temperature would rise to the highest level in which of the following environmental conditions?
   a. high temperature and low humidity
   b. high temperature and high humidity
   c. low temperature and high humidity
   d. low temperature and low humidity

3. The best strategy for dressing to exercise in the cold is to wear
   a. the thickest garment available.
   b. light-colored clothes.
   c. clothing that prevents moisture penetration.
   d. layers of clothing.

4. The greatest danger of exercising in the cold is
   a. reduced oxygen intake.
   b. increased likelihood of hypothermia.
   c. sweating too little.
   d. increased risk of lung damage.

5. List guidelines for fluid intake during and after exercise in hot environments.

6. Describe the appropriate clothing for exercising in hot and cold environments.

LO 7. Which of the following occurs to help the body cope with the stress of altitude?
   a. decrease in heart rate
   b. increase in breathing
   c. decrease in breathing
   d. increase in water content

8. Why does exercise at high altitude increase heart rate and breathing rate more than the same exercise performed at sea level?

LO 3 9. List the effects of air pollution on exercise tolerance.

LO 4 10. Define *overtraining*.

11. What are the primary causes of exercise-related injuries?

LO 5 12. Which of the following plays a major role in preventing back pain?
   a. exercise
   b. increasing body fat
   c. reducing hip flexibility
   d. all of the above

13. Pain developing immediately after an exercise session that has been too long or intense is referred to as
   a. delayed onset muscle soreness.
   b. acute muscle soreness.
   c. overtraining syndrome.
   d. lactate threshold.

14. Which of the following can help prevent shin splints?
   a. run on a soft surface
   b. wear well-padded shoes
   c. slowly increase exercise intensity
   d. all of the above

15. The primary means of preventing ligament sprains is to
    a. wear a joint brace.
    b. consume large amounts of protein.
    c. avoid intense exercise.
    d. refrain from activities that place a high force on joints.

16. Differentiate between a strain, a sprain, and a stress fracture.

17. Define *tendonitis,* and describe the best methods of prevention and treatment.

18. What is the cause of PFPS, and how should it be treated?

LO 6 19. Define the protocol, and describe its proper use in treating injuries.

LO 7 20. Describe the proper first aid response for each of the following:
    a. choking
    b. puncture wound with profuse bleeding
    c. swallowing of poison
    d. drowning victim who has stopped breathing

suggested reading

American College of Sports Medicine. Position stand: Exercise and fluid replacement. *Medicine and Science in Sports and Exercise* 39(2):377–390, 2007.

American College of Sports Medicine. Position stand: Prevention of cold injuries during exercise. *Medicine and Science in Sports and Exercise* 38(11):2012–2029, 2006.

Bärtsch, P., and B. Saltin. General introduction to altitude adaptation and mountain sickness. *Scandinavian Journal of Medicine and Science in Sports* 18(Suppl 1):1–10, 2008.

Bergeron, M. Heat stress and thermal strain challenges in running. *Journal of Orthopaedic and Sports Physical Therapy*. 44(10):831–838, 2014.

Burdon, C. A., H. T. O'Connor, J. A. Gifford, and S. M. Shirreffs. Influence of beverage temperature on exercise performance in the heat: A systematic review. *International Journal of Sport Nutrition and Exercise Metabolism* 20(2):166–174, 2010.

Corbett J., R. Neal, H. Lunt, and M. Tipton. Adaptation to heat and exercise performance under cooler conditions: A new hot topic. *Sports Medicine*. 44(10):1323–1331, 2014.

Fields, K. B. Running injuries: Changing trends and demographics. *Current Sports Medicine Reports* 10(5): 299–303, 2011.

Garrick, J., J. T. Bell, and P. Radetsky. *Anybody's Sports Medicine Book: The Complete Guide to Quick Recovery from Injuries,* 2nd ed. Tampa, FL: IFPA, 2009.

Herbert, R. D., M. de Noronha, and S. J. Kamper. Stretching to prevent or reduce muscle soreness after exercise. *Cochrane Database of Systematic Reviews* 6(7):CD004577, 2011.

Hill J, G. Howatson, K. van Someren, J. Leeder, and C. Pedlar. Compression garments and recovery from exercise-induced muscle damage: A meta-analysis. *British Journal of Sports Medicine*. 48(18):1340–1346, 2014.

Mazzeo, R. Physiological responses to exercise at altitude: An update. *Sports Medicine* 38(1):1–8, 2008.

Rundell, K. W. Effect of air pollution on athlete health and performance. *British Journal of Sports Medicine* 46(6): 407–412, 2012.

helpful weblinks

do it! WEBLINKS

For links to the organizations and websites listed, visit MasteringHealth™.

American College of Sports Medicine

Information on exercise in environmental extremes and pollution and how to deal with exercise-related injuries. **www.acsm.org**

American Lung Association

Information on air pollution and exercise, including how it affects your body and ways to minimize risk. **www.lung.org**

American Red Cross

Information on CPR and other first-aid techniques for use on adults, children, and infants. **www.redcross.org**

Mayo Clinic

Health information and research, including guidance on first aid for choking infants. **www.mayoclinic.org**

The Running Page

Information about racing, running clubs, places to run, products, magazines, and treating injuries. **www.runningpage.com**

WebMD

Information about preventing and treating exercise-related injuries. **www.webmd.com**

laboratory 12.1

do it! LABS
Complete Lab 12.1 online in the
study area of **MasteringHealth.com**

Name _____ Date _____

Exercising in Harsh Environments

Answer the following true-or-false questions related to exercise and the environment. If a statement is false, change it to make it true. You can check your answers against those provided below.

TRUE OR FALSE

1. Evaporation is the primary means of heat loss during exercise in a hot environment.

   T F _____

2. When exercising in a hot, humid environment, you should wear loose, dark-colored clothing.

   T F _____

3. Exercise at high altitude increases the amount of oxygen in the blood.

   T F _____

4. At high altitude, it is necessary to reduce the intensity of exercise to stay within your target heart rate range.

   T F _____

5. Ozone levels are highest during cool winter days.

   T F _____

6. Humans regulate their body temperature around the set point of 98.6°F.

   T F _____

7. Low-intensity exercise using small-muscle groups produces more body heat than high-intensity exercise incorporating large-muscle groups.

   T F _____

8. An increase in body temperature during exercise in a hot environment will result in larger increases in heart rate than will exercise in a cool environment.

   T F _____

9. The strategy for exercising in the cold is to wear enough clothing to trap just enough heat to maintain body temperature, but not to overheat.

   T F _____

10. Heat injuries are nonfatal conditions that result in cramps and fatigue.

    T F _____

ANSWERS

1. True: Of the ways you can lose heat during exercise, evaporation is the primary one because the process of evaporation takes heat away with the water vapor that is formed. The other methods do not use this principle of physics and are not as efficient in removing heat.

2. False: When exercising in a hot, humid environment, you should wear loose, light-colored clothing.

3. False: Exercise at high altitude reduces the amount of oxygen in the blood.

4. True: The low oxygen available to the blood causes the heart to work faster as it tries to transport more to the muscles. Thus, some of the increase in heart rate during exercise is due to low oxygen.

5. False: Ozone levels are highest during hot summer days.

6. True: Humans are homeotherms (meaning "to maintain the same temperature"). Thus, temperature changes due to environmental or exercise stress must be counteracted by the physiological systems in the body to maintain body temperature around "normal."

7. False: High-intensity exercise using large-muscle groups produces more body heat than low-intensity exercise incorporating small-muscle groups.

8. True: An increase in heart rate during exercise is due to the body trying to transport oxygen and nutrients to the muscles. If exercise is done in a hot environment, the body must pump blood faster in an attempt to cool the body as well.

9. True: Insulation is the key to comfortable exercise in the cold. If there is not enough trapped heat, the body will cool too much and injury or death could occur. If too much heat is trapped, you will start sweating. If you get wet with sweat, heat transfer away from the body could be dramatic and even life-threatening.

10. False: Heat injuries are serious and can result in damage to the nervous system and, in extreme cases, death.

Answer the three questions below to help you increase your awareness of safety issues in harsh environments.

1. If a friend planned to exercise in a warm, high-humidity environment, what safety advice would you give to him or her?

   _____

2. What advice would you give to a friend exercising in a cold climate?

   _____

3. What can you do to minimize the amount of air pollution in your immediate environment?

   _____

laboratory 12.2

do it! LABS
Complete Lab 12.2 online in the
study area of **MasteringHealth.com**

Name _____   Date _____

Assessing Flexibility and Back Pain Risk

Back pain is a multifactoral problem that is preventable in most cases. There are many sources of back pain, including improper lifting techniques, weak muscles, poor posture, inflexibility, and bone disorders. The following tests will assess the flexibility of your lower back, hamstrings, and hip flexors. Find a partner to assist you and use extreme caution in applying force.

Stretches and exercises to alleviate back pain or prevent future back injury are suggested in the Interpretation sections below.

TEST 1: BACK TO WALL

Stand with your back against a wall so that your head, shoulders, calves, and heels are all touching the wall. Try to flatten your neck and the hollow of your back by pressing your buttocks down. Your partner should be able to place just a hand between the wall and the small of your back.

        Pass _____   Fail _____

Interpretation

If this space is greater than the thickness of a flattened hand, you may have lumbar lordosis (increased curvature in the lower back with a forward pelvic tilt) with shortened lumbar and hip flexor muscles. To correct or prevent lumbar lordosis, flexibility exercises to lengthen the hip flexor muscles, as well as strength and endurance exercises for the abdominal muscles, are generally recommended. See the descriptions and videos for Hip Flexor Stretch, Abdominal Curl, and Abdominal Curl (stability ball).

TEST 2: STRAIGHT LEG LIFT

Lie on your back with your hands behind your neck. Your partner will kneel at your left side and stabilize your right leg by placing her right hand on your knee. With the left hand, your partner should grasp your left ankle and raise your left leg as near to a right angle (90 degrees) as possible. In this position, your lower back should be in contact with the floor, and your right leg should remain straight and on the floor. Repeat this test on the opposite side.

        Left side: Pass _____   Fail _____

        Right side: Pass _____   Fail _____

Interpretation

If your left leg bends at the knee, your hamstring muscles are short. If your back arches and/or your right leg does not remain on the floor, short lumbar muscles, short hip flexors, or both are implicated. To correct this condition, perform exercises to stretch your hamstrings; lower back stretches can be used to lengthen the lumbar muscles. See the descriptions and videos for Hamstrings Stretch (seated), Modified Hurdler Stretch, Low Back Knee-to-Chest Stretch, Torso Twist and Hip Stretch, Back Bridge, and Cat Stretch.

TEST 3: KNEE TO CHEST

(No partner is needed.) Lie on your back on a table or bench, with your right leg extended beyond the edge of the table (about one-third of your thigh is off the table). Bring your left knee to your chest, and grasp the back of your thigh, pulling down tightly toward your chest. Your right thigh should remain in contact with the table. Repeat this test on the opposite leg.

        Left side: Pass _____   Fail _____

        Right side: Pass _____   Fail _____

Interpretation

If your right thigh lifts off the table while you hug your knee to your chest, you have a tight right hip flexor muscle; if your left thigh lifts, then you have a tight left hip flexor. To stretch the right hip flexor, place the left knee directly above the left ankle, and stretch the right leg backward so that the right knee touches the floor. Press your pelvis forward and downward. Do not bend your front knee more than 90 degrees. Repeat on the opposite side to stretch the left hip flexor. See the description and video for Hip Flexor Stretch (thigh stretch).

SUMMARY

Awareness of flexibility problems may help you alleviate back pain or prevent future back discomfort. Remember that exercises designed to increase flexibility and strength, reduce body fat, improve muscle balance between the trunk flexors and extensors, and prevent osteoporosis can decrease your risk of developing back problems.

laboratory 12.3

do it! LABS
Complete Lab 12.3 online online in the
study area of **MasteringHealth.com**

Name _____   Date _____

Preventing Injuries during Exercise

This lab will help you identify and eliminate ways in which your exercise program may cause injuries. The following measures are associated with preventing exercise-related injury. Check those you have incorporated into your exercise program (or into your life in general). For any measure you check "No," write in the space provided exactly what changes you plan to implement to reduce or eliminate the risks associated with that measure.

1. I always wear the proper shoes for the activity.   Yes _____   No _____

   Changes to implement: _____

2. I always perform a proper warm-up before the exercise activity.   Yes _____   No _____

   Changes to implement: _____

3. I always stretch the muscles that will be involved in the activity.   Yes _____   No _____

   Changes to implement: _____

4. All muscle groups involved in the activity are strengthened and   Yes _____   No _____
   balanced.

   Changes to implement: _____

5. I avoid overstretching my neck and back.   Yes _____   No _____

   Changes to implement: _____

6. I avoid extending and rotating my spine.   Yes _____   No _____

   Changes to implement: _____

7. I avoid lifting heavy objects.   Yes _____   No _____

   Changes to implement: _____

8. I avoid quick, jerking movements.   Yes _____   No _____

   Changes to implement: _____

9. My training program has been properly designed.   Yes _____   No _____

   Changes to implement: _____

10. I use the appropriate frequency of exercise.   Yes _____   No _____

    Changes to implement: _____

11. I use the appropriate intensity of exercise.   Yes _____   No _____

    Changes to implement: _____

12. I use the appropriate duration of exercise.   Yes _____   No _____

    Changes to implement: _____

13. I use proper exercise techniques.   Yes _____   No _____

    Changes to implement: _____

14. I run only on a firm, level surface.   Yes _____   No _____

    Changes to implement: _____

15. I include a proper cool-down after exercising.   Yes _____   No _____

    Changes to implement: _____

347

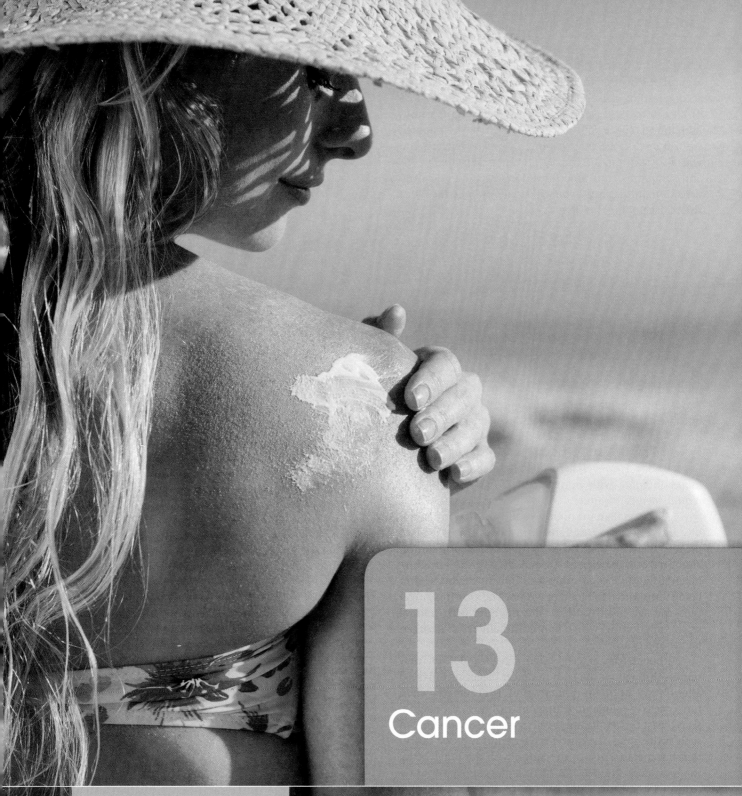

13
Cancer

LEARNING OUTCOMES

1 Define *cancer*.

2 Explain the process by which normal cells become cancerous.

3 List the most common types of cancer and rank them based on their mortality rates in men and women.

4 Describe the known risk factors for cancer and differentiate between controllable and uncontrollable factors.

CANCER REMAINS A major public health problem around the world. In the United States, cancer is the second leading cause of death, accounting for almost 25% of all deaths (1, 2). Therefore, understanding its causes and how to reduce your risk is critical (3). In this chapter, we will discuss the most common types of cancers. You will also learn about the significant risk factors, signs and symptoms, and procedures for screening and early detection. Importantly, you will learn how to reduce your risk of developing this disease.

What Is Cancer?

LO **1** Define *cancer*.

Cancer is actually a group of diseases characterized by the growth and spread of abnormal cells. It can occur in almost every tissue and organ in the body, and if the spread of cancer cells is not controlled, it can result in death (4, 5). Cancer cells form masses known as **tumors**. **Benign tumors** do not contain cancerous cells, but **malignant tumors** are cancerous. Generally, benign tumors are not serious health threats because the cells grow and divide less quickly and do not spread throughout the body. However, depending on their location, they might interfere with normal body functions and may require medical treatment.

Cells of malignant tumors tend to divide more rapidly and can spread throughout the body. This spreading process is called **metastasis**. With a malignant tumor, abnormal cells increase in size and often spread, invading neighboring tissues or other locations in the body after being transported in blood or lymph. The growing cancer cells damage healthy tissue and interfere with normal organ functioning, which may eventually result in organ failure and death.

Although cancer cells often spread and form new tumors throughout the body, a cancer diagnosis is named after the site of origin (primary site). For example, when cancer cells develop into a tumor in the breast, the diagnosis is breast cancer. If cancer cells spread to another organ such as the lungs, the cancer is referred to as breast cancer that has metastasized to the lungs, with the lungs being the secondary site (**FIGURE 13.1**). Metastasis significantly reduces a cancer patient's chances of survival because it is more difficult to treat tumors in multiple locations.

When a tumor or other abnormal tissue is detected, a sample is removed during a surgical procedure called a **biopsy**. The tissue sample is analyzed to determine if the cells are benign (noncancerous) or malignant (cancerous). If a tumor is malignant, its size is determined and various types of imaging procedures are used to determine if the cancer has spread to any other body regions. Physicians use this information to classify the "stage" of the cancer, which describes its extent or severity at the

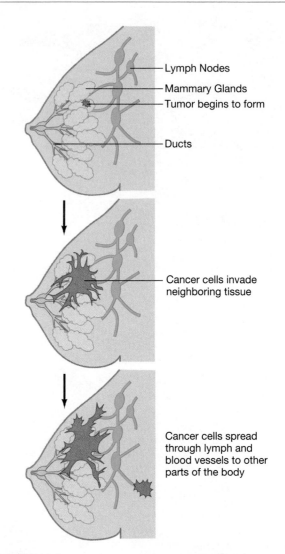

Lymph Nodes
Mammary Glands
Tumor begins to form

Ducts

Cancer cells invade neighboring tissue

Cancer cells spread through lymph and blood vessels to other parts of the body

FIGURE 13.1 Growth and metastasis of a malignant breast tumor.

time of diagnosis (1). A staging system used to describe many types of cancer is based on five numerical designations that range from Stage 0 (confined to the site of origin) to Stage IV (the most advanced stage in which the cancer has spread to distant organs in the body).

MAKE SURE YOU KNOW...

- Cancer is a group of diseases characterized by the growth and spread of abnormal cells. It can occur in almost every tissue and organ in the body.

- Cancer cells can spread through the bloodstream and lymphatic system in a process called metastasis. Uncontrolled spread of cancer cells can result in death.

- Cancer staging is used to describe the extent or severity of the disease at the time of diagnosis.

MasteringHealth™

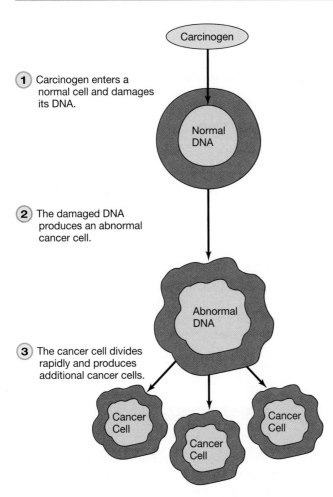

1. Carcinogen enters a normal cell and damages its DNA.

2. The damaged DNA produces an abnormal cancer cell.

3. The cancer cell divides rapidly and produces additional cancer cells.

FIGURE 13.2 The transformation of a normal cell into a cancer cell.

How Do Normal Cells Become Cancerous?

LO **2** Explain the process by which normal cells become cancerous.

Cancer can be caused by environmental factors such as tobacco use, ultraviolet radiation, infectious organisms, and an unhealthy diet. It can also be caused by inherited genetic mutations, hormonal dysfunction, and impaired immune function. So how do these various factors contribute to the development and growth of cancer cells?

Every cell contains deoxyribonucleic acid (DNA), the material that makes up the 25,000 genes contained in each cell. Cell growth and division is controlled by DNA, and when DNA functions normally, it regulates cell growth and division in an orderly manner. But when DNA is damaged, cell division can escalate out of control. Any substance or agent that can cause cancer is a **carcinogen**. Numerous environmental agents such

as radiation, chemicals, and drugs can lead to the DNA damage that causes a normal cell to become an abnormal cancer cell (**FIGURE 13.2**).

Although cancer cells grow rapidly, tumors take time to develop. A pea-sized tumor contains about a billion cells, so it may take years for a tumor to become large enough to be detected. Screening tests are used to detect early-stage cancer. Tumors in superficial tissues such as the breasts or testes can be felt as lumps during self-exams or clinical exams. However, tumors of deeper tissues or organs are not as easily detected and can develop into much larger masses before symptoms occur. This is why knowing the *seven warning signs* (**FIGURE 13.3** on page 352) is important for early detection and timely and appropriate medical treatment. Getting regular screenings at the recommended intervals is a key factor in early detection.

MAKE SURE YOU **KNOW...**

- Cell growth and division are regulated by DNA, and the uncontrolled growth of cancer cells is caused by damaged DNA.

- DNA can be damaged by various cancer-causing substances called carcinogens.

- Tumors in superficial tissue can be detected by self-exams and clinical exams; tumors in deeper tissues can only be detected via imaging or other screening procedures.

—————MasteringHealth™

cancer Disease that involves the uncontrolled growth and spread of abnormal cells; there are more than 100 types that can affect almost every body tissue.

tumor Abnormal growth of tissue; neoplasm.

benign tumor Tumor made up of noncancerous cells.

malignant tumor Tumor made up of cancerous cells.

metastasis Spread of cancer cells throughout the body.

biopsy Surgical removal of a tissue sample for laboratory analysis.

carcinogen Cancer-causing agent; includes radiation, chemicals, drugs, and other toxic substances.

Seven Warning Signs of Cancer

Change in bowel or bladder habits
Area or sore that does not heal or that heals slowly
Unusual bleeding or discharge from the bowel, nipples, or vagina,
   or unexplained blood in the urine
Thickening or lump in the breast or elsewhere
Indigestion, difficulty swallowing, or loss of appetite that persists
Obvious change in size or color of a wart or mole
Nagging or persistent cough or hoarseness

You should see your health care provider if you have any of
these symptoms.

FIGURE 13.3 Early detection is key to surviving cancer, and it is essential
to become familiar with these seven warning signs.

Common Types of Cancer

 List the most common types of cancer and rank them based on their mortality rates in men and women.

Cancer can develop in almost any organ (4, 5). The most common type is skin cancer, followed by prostate cancer in men and breast cancer in women. Other common cancer sites include the lungs, colon and rectum, uterus, kidneys, and liver (**TABLE 13.1**). Please note that skin cancer is not listed in Table 13.1 because the most common skin cancers (e.g., squamous cell and basal cell) constitute a small percentage of cancer deaths in the United States (1).

TABLE 13.1 ■ Leading sites of New Cancer and Deaths—2015 Estimates

Estimated New Cases*		Estimated Deaths	
Male	Female	Male	Female
Prostate	Breast	Lung & bronchus	Lung & bronchus
220,800 (26%)	231,840 (29%)	86,380 (28%)	71,660 (26%)
Lung & bronchus	Lung & bronchus	Prostate	Breast
115,610 (14%)	105,590 (13%)	27,540 (9%)	40,290 (15%)
Colon & rectum	Colon & rectum	Colon & rectum	Colon & rectum
69,090 (8%)	63,610 (8%)	26,100 (8%)	23,600 (9%)
Urinary bladder	Uterine corpus	Pancreas	Pancreas
56,320 (7%)	54,870 (7%)	20,710 (7%)	19,850 (7%)
Melanoma of the Skin	Thyroid	Liver & intrahepatic bile duct	Ovary
42,670 (5%)	47,230 (6%)	17,030 (5%)	14,180 (5%)
Non-Hodgkin lymphoma	Non-Hodgkin lymphoma	Leukemia	Leukemia
39,850 (5%)	32,000 (4%)	14,210 (5%)	10,240 (4%)
Kidney & renal pelvis	Melanoma of the skin	Esophagus	Uterine corpus
38,270 (5%)	31,200 (4%)	12,600 (4%)	10,170 (4%)
Oral cavity & pharynx	pancreas	Urinary bladder	Non-Hodgkin lymphoma
32,670 (40%)	24,120 (3%)	11,510 (4%)	8,310 (3%)
Leukemia	Leukemia	Non-Hodgkin lymphoma	Liver & intrahepatic bile duct
30,900 (4%)	23,370 (3%)	11,480 (4%)	7,520 (3%)
Liver & intrahepatic bile duct	Kidney & renal pelvis	Kidney & renal pelvis	Brain & other nervous system
25,510 (3%)	23,290 (3%)	9,070 (3%)	6,380 (2%)
All sites	All sites	All sites	All sites
848,200 (100%)	810,170 (100%)	312,150 (100%)	277,280 (100%)

*Excludes basal cell and squamous cell skin cancers and in situ carcinoma except urinary bladder.

Note that skin cancers are the leading site of new cases, but they are not included above because they constitute a very small percentage of annual cancer deaths in the United States (1).

Source: Data from the American Cancer Society.

Lung Cancer

In recent years, the number of new cases of lung cancer has decreased for men and has leveled off for women (1). However, lung cancer is still the leading cause of cancer deaths for both men and women. As you can see in **FIGURE 13.4** lung cancer has been the leading cause of cancer deaths in men since 1970 and is now the leading cause of cancer deaths in women, as well. The increase in lung cancer in women is likely due to the rise in the number of female smokers during the past several decades. Estimates indicate that over 159,000 men and women will die from lung cancer in 2015, and more than 341,000 new cases will be diagnosed (1). Although more cases of skin, prostate, and breast cancer are diagnosed each year, lung cancer results in more deaths than prostate, breast, and colon cancers combined (1).

Why does lung cancer contribute to so many more deaths than other cancers? One factor is the lack of screening tests for early detection (see Examining the Evidence for information on new screening tests). Lung cancer symptoms are often not present until the cancer has spread and become more advanced. Although new screening procedures are being studied, no effective screening methods have been developed to catch lung cancer in its early stages. Therefore, it is more difficult to treat lung cancer, and mortality rates are higher. The American Cancer Society reports 1-year survival rates have increased since the 1970s, but the 5-year survival rate across stages of lung cancer is approximately 17% (1).

Because early detection of lung cancer is difficult, knowing how to limit your risk factors, and how to spot the early signs and symptoms, is extremely important. The most significant thing you can do to reduce your risk of lung cancer is to not smoke. Smoking has long been linked to lung cancer, and the more and longer a person smokes, the greater the risk. However, the good news is that stopping smoking will lower the risk if cancer has not already developed. It is not just cigarette smoking that

consider this! ////////////////////////

Over 80% of lung cancers are linked to smoking, but risk is reduced 65% after 10 years of being smoke-free.

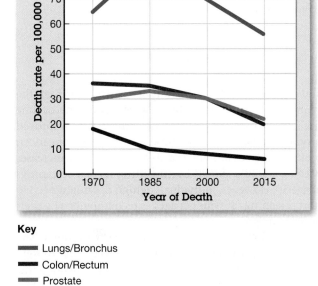

Trends in Cancer Death Rates Among Males

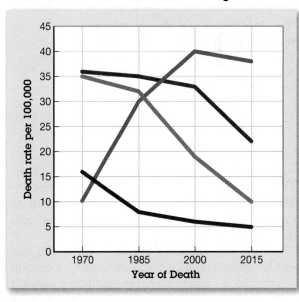

Trends in Cancer Death Rates Among Females

Key

■ Lungs/Bronchus
■ Colon/Rectum
■ Prostate
■ Stomach

Key

■ Lungs/Bronchus
■ Breast
■ Colon/Rectum
■ Uterus

FIGURE 13.4 Trends in death rates for the major cancers by gender from 1970–2015. Part (a) shows the rates for men and part (b) shows the rates for women. Note that the death rates for these cancers have declined during the past decades.

New Cancer Screening Tests on the Horizon

Numerous cancer screening tests exist, and more are currently under development. Effective screening tests

- detect cancer before symptoms appear,
- screen for cancers that are easier to treat and cure when detected early,
- test for cancer with a high level of accuracy (i.e., give few false-positive or false-negative results), and
- decrease the patient's chances of dying from cancer.

Currently, four major types of cancer screening are available:

1. A *medical history* is taken and a *physical exam* is performed by a physician to check for signs (such as a lump, growth, or unusual weight loss) that may indicate cancer.

2. *Laboratory tests* are conducted on various body tissues, blood, urine, or stool samples to detect abnormal (cancerous) cells.

3. *Imaging procedures* such as mammograms and CT scans are performed to allow the physician to look inside the body for evidence of tumors.

4. *Genetic tests* examine DNA from blood samples to determine if cancer-specific gene mutations exist.

Note that these screening tests do not lead to a definitive diagnosis of cancer. If an initial test result is considered abnormal, more tests are typically required. For example, a mammogram may reveal a lump in breast tissue. A lump can be benign or malignant, so

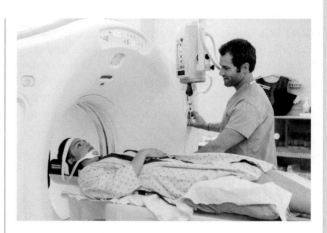

additional diagnostic tests may include a needle and/or tissue biopsy in which cells are removed and examined by a pathologist to determine if cancer is present.

Many cancers (such as pancreatic cancer) remain difficult to detect at an early stage, and some existing tests suffer from shortcomings. Therefore, ongoing research has focused on developing new and more sensitive cancer screening tests. A recently developed cancer screening test appears to be able to detect most major forms of cancer at early stages of development (8). This blood test is reported to be highly sensitive and capable of detecting both the presence and location of cancer (8). This is a highly promising development, and additional research will be conducted to confirm the attributes and accuracy of this new test.

increases the risk for lung cancer; smoking pipes, cigars, or marijuana also increases risk, as does exposure to secondhand smoke. Other risk factors include exposure to asbestos, radon, air pollution, and workplace carcinogens such as gasoline, diesel exhaust, and coal products.

Some research suggests that a diet rich in fruits and vegetables (and therefore rich in antioxidants) may help reduce the risk for lung cancer (6). Additional research is needed to confirm these findings. See **TABLE 13.2** for specific signs and symptoms that may be indicators of lung cancer.

Colon and Rectal Cancer

Colon and rectal cancer (sometimes called colorectal cancer) is the third leading cause of cancer deaths, contributing to 8–9% of cancer deaths among both men and women (1). But it is important to note that the number of deaths from these cancers is on the decline because of better screening procedures. These improved procedures can detect **polyps** and early stages of cancer, making early treatment possible. Because risk increases with age, adults should begin getting regular screenings at age 50. However, individuals at high risk might need to start screenings at younger ages as recommended by their health-care providers.

Several screening procedures can be performed. The American Cancer Society, along with other health organizations, recently updated screening recommendations. Tests of the stool are easier and less invasive, but they are not a sensitive test for detecting the presence of polyps. The more invasive tests that look directly into the colon using a scope or X-rays involve more complex preparation. However, these tests are preferred because

TABLE 13.2 ■ Signs and Symptoms of Specific Cancers	
Lung Cancer	■ A cough that does not go away ■ Chest pain, often aggravated by deep breathing, coughing, and even laughing ■ Hoarseness ■ Weight loss and loss of appetite ■ Bloody or rust-colored sputum (spit or phlegm) ■ Shortness of breath ■ Recurring infections such as bronchitis and pneumonia ■ New onset of wheezing
Colon and Rectal Cancer	■ Change in bowel habits, such as diarrhea, constipation, or narrowing of the stool, that lasts for more than a few days ■ A feeling that you need to have a bowel-movement that doesn't go away even after you do have a bowel movement ■ Bleeding from the rectum or blood in the stool ■ Cramping or gnawing stomach pain ■ Decreased appetite ■ Weakness and fatigue ■ Jaundice (yellow-green color of the skin and the white part of the eye)
Breast Cancer	■ A new lump or mass ■ Generalized swelling of part of a breast (even if no distinct lump is felt) ■ Skin irritation or dimpling ■ Nipple pain or retraction (turning inward) ■ Redness or scaliness of the nipple or breast skin ■ A discharge other than breast milk
Prostate Cancer	■ Blood in the urine (hematuria) ■ Difficulty getting an erection (impotence) ■ Pain in the hips, spine, ribs, or other areas if it spreads to the bones ■ Weakness or numbness in the legs or feet, or even loss of bladder or bowel control if it spreads to the spine and affects spinal nerves
Testicular Cancer	■ A slight enlargement of one of the testicles ■ A change in the consistency of a testicle ■ A dull ache in the lower abdomen or groin (may not occur in all cases of testicular cancer) ■ The sensation of dragging and heaviness in a testicle

they detect the presence of polyps or tumors. Fecal tests used for screening include the fecal occult blood test that is recommended annually, or a stool DNA test as recommended by the health-care provider. More invasive options include a flexible sigmoidoscopy, double contrast enema, or CT colonography every 5 years, or a colonoscopy every 10 years. Details of each procedure can be found on the American Cancer Society website.

Although early detection is relatively easy, prevention is still the key. Regular exercise and a high-fiber, low-fat diet are two behavioral factors that can reduce your risk for developing these two types of cancer. Engaging in the recommended 30 minutes of moderate activity at least 5 days a week is associated with a lower risk of colon cancer. Diets that are rich in a variety of fruits, vegetables, and whole grains will provide the fiber associated with lowering the risk for colon and rectal cancers. Other factors that might reduce your risk include consuming adequate calcium, vitamin D, and possibly a multivitamin that includes folic acid.

Risk factors for colon and rectal cancer include nonmodifiable factors such as heredity, and modifiable factors such as diet and exercise. Ashkenazi Jews of Eastern European descent have the highest rates in the world, and African Americans have the highest incidence and death rates from colon cancer in the United States (1). A family or personal history of colon and rectal cancer and a personal history of polyps and inflammatory bowel disease are also associated with increased risk. Certain inherited syndromes are also associated with the development of colon cancer. Modifiable risk factors include physical inactivity, poor diet, type 2 diabetes, heavy alcohol consumption, overweight, and smoking.

Breast Cancer

Breast cancer is the second most common type of cancer in women (after skin cancers) and is the second leading cause of cancer deaths in women. The American Cancer Society estimates that in one year (2015), more than 232,000 women will be diagnosed and approximately 40,000 will die from this disease (see Table 13.1). Fortunately, death rates from breast cancer are decreasing (1). Women today are more aware of the importance of regular screenings and of minimizing their risk. Hence this type of cancer is increasingly being detected in its earlier, more treatable stages. Although breast cancer occurs primarily in women, men can also develop breast cancer.

As with most cancers, breast cancer risk increases with age. Approximately two-thirds of the cases of invasive breast cancer occur in women 55 years of age and older. It is considered acceptable for women in their 20s not to perform self-exams, but starting at age 20, health-care providers should discuss the benefits and limitations of self-exams so women can make an informed decision. Younger women can also develop breast cancer, and getting to know their breasts through regular self-exams can assist in detecting a lump or growth if one

polyps Growths from mucous membranes; commonly found in the colon and rectum, where they can be indicators of colon cancer.

develops. Close to 70% of all breast cancers are discovered by women during routine self-exams. (See the Examining the Evidence box.)

Women in their 20s and 30s should get regular clinical exams at least every 3 years. Typically your health-care provider will perform a clinical breast exam when you have your annual Pap test. Beginning at age 50, women should have a **mammogram** done annually or at least every 2 years. Women at higher risk might need to start mammograms earlier as recommended by their health-care providers.

Knowing the signs and symptoms of breast cancer is very important for early detection. If you notice changes in your breasts or detect any of the signs during a self-exam,

you should see your health-care provider. Many of the lumps detected are not cancerous, but you cannot tell without a biopsy. If a lump is determined to be cancerous, there are multiple courses of treatment. Removal of the lump, and potentially the surrounding tissues and lymph nodes, is a typical first step. The specific surgical procedure will be determined by the stage and spread of the cancer and the woman's level of risk. Surgical procedures are typically followed by radiation and/or chemotherapy to kill any remaining cancer cells.

Many risk factors for breast cancer are nonmodifiable, such as age (over 50) and having a family history of breast cancer. There are also genetic factors involving specific cancer-susceptibility genes that increase the risk. According to the National Cancer Institute, race and ethnicity also play a role related to genetic risk. For example, Native Americans and Native Alaskans have the

see it!

ABC VIDEO

Watch the "How Effective is Breast Cancer Early Detection?" ABC News Video online at MasteringHealth™.

EXAMINING THE EVIDENCE | Breast Self-Examination

To do a self-exam, begin by standing in front of a mirror to inspect the breasts, looking for their usual symmetry. Some breasts are not symmetrical and, if this is not a change, it is okay. Raise and lower both arms while checking that the breasts move evenly and freely. Next, inspect the skin, looking for areas of redness, thickening, or dimpling, which might have the appearance of an orange peel. Look for any scaling on the nipple.

To feel for lumps, raise one arm above your head while either standing or lying. This will flatten out the breast, making it easier to feel the tissue. Using the index, middle, and fourth fingers of your opposite hand, gently push down on the breast tissue and move the fingers in small, circular motions, varying pressure from light to firm. Start at one edge of the breast and move upward and then downward, working your way across the breast

until all of the breast tissue has been covered. Often breast tissue will feel dense and irregular, and this is usually normal. It helps to do regular self-exams to become familiar with what your breast tissue feels like; then, if there is a change, you will notice. Cancers usually feel like a dense or firm little rock and are very different from the normal breast tissue.

Next, lower the arm and reach into the top of the underarm and pull downward with gentle pressure, feeling for any enlarged lymph nodes. To complete the exam, squeeze the tissue around the nipple. If you notice discharge from the nipple and you have not recently been breastfeeding, consult your doctor. Likewise, if you notice any asymmetry, skin changes, scaling on the nipple, or new lumps in the breast, you should see your health-care provider.

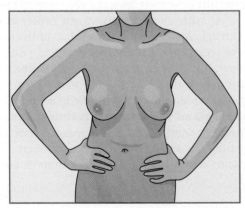

1 Face a mirror and check for changes in symmetry.

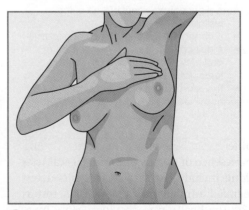

2 Either standing or lying down, use the pads of the three middle fingers to check for lumps. Follow an up and down pattern on the breast to ensure all tissue gets inspected.

lowest rates of breast cancer. Across the life span, white, non-Hispanic women have the highest overall incidence of breast cancer compared to other racial/ethnic groups. However, among women ages 40–50, African-American women have a higher incidence of breast cancer compared to white women.

Lifestyle and behavioral factors can also influence breast cancer risk. Having no children or having a first child after age 30 are associated with slightly elevated risk. By contrast, more than one pregnancy and pregnancy at a young age are associated with lower risk. The use of hormones, especially over a long period, such as taking oral contraceptives or hormone replacement therapy, has been linked to increased risk. However, risk associated with oral contraceptive use can decline to normal over time after discontinuation. Women who consume two to five alcoholic drinks per day have a risk one and a half times greater than women who do not consume alcohol (1). As with many types of cancer, obesity and a high-fat diet increase the risk. Performing regular bouts of moderate and vigorous aerobic exercise has been reported to reduce the risk of developing breast cancer in both pre- and post-menopausal women (7).

Prostate Cancer

The prostate is a small gland, about the size of a walnut, that produces seminal fluid in men. Cancer of the prostate is second only to skin cancer in the number of cases diagnosed per year in men, accounting for approximately 27% of all new cancers (see Table 13.1). After an increase in the death rate from prostate cancer from 1970 to 1985, mortality rates have leveled off and declined over the past 15 years thanks to improved early detection methods. Death rates from prostate cancer are second to lung cancer in men.

Prostate cancer is typically a slowly developing cancer. There are several signs and symptoms of advanced prostate cancer but typically no symptoms in the early stages. Two screening methods are available: the digital rectal exam and the prostate-specific antigen (PSA) blood test. During a digital rectal exam, a health-care provider inserts a gloved, lubricated finger into the rectum to feel for tumors. If a tumor is detected, then a biopsy will be performed to determine whether the mass is cancerous. The PSA test is a blood test in which levels of PSA are assessed. Higher-than-normal PSA is associated with prostate cancer.

Opinions differ regarding the value of PSA screening for prostate cancer. Therefore, men and their health-care providers should discuss the benefits and the risks associated with the tests and decide whether to have them done. Men at higher risk should begin testing at younger ages as recommended by their health-care providers.

Risk for prostate cancer increases with age, and most cases occur in men over 65 years of age. Race is a significant risk factor, with higher rates among African-American men

in the United States compared to other racial or ethnic groups. Asian men tend to have lower rates than white men. Rates are higher in North America and northwestern Europe than in Asia, Africa, and South and Central America. Family history is another nonmodifiable risk factor. Diet is a modifiable, behavioral risk factor. Diets high in red meat and high-fat dairy products are associated with increased risk.

Testicular Cancer

Although testicular cancer is not common overall, it is one of the most common cancers in younger men with 90% of cases in men 20 to 54 years of age (1). Testicular cancer is treatable and curable when detected early.

Lumps in the testes can be detected though routine self-exams (see the Examining the Evidence box on page 358). Men should also have a clinical examination of the testes performed during their regular physical exam. Risk factors for testicular cancer are primarily nonmodifiable. An undescended testicle (present at birth) is the most common risk factor. Other risk factors include race, previous testicular cancer, and family history. White men have higher rates than African-American, Asian, Hispanic, and Native-American men. Recent evidence suggests that HIV and AIDS increase the risk. Because the risk factors are not behavioral, there is little that can be done to prevent testicular cancer. Knowing your risk factors and participating in the recommended screenings are important for early detection and prompt treatment.

Skin Cancer

Skin cancer is the most common of all cancers, with more than 1 million cases diagnosed each year in the United States (1). There are three major types: basal cell carcinoma, squamous cell carcinoma, and **melanoma**. Basal cell carcinoma and squamous cell carcinoma (nonmelanoma skin cancers) occur most frequently. While both types are malignant cancers, they are unlikely to spread to other parts of the body and can be cured with early detection and treatment (5). Although malignant melanomas make up only a small fraction of skin cancers (~3%), these cancers are very aggressive and are often fatal even when detected early and treated (5).

Skin cancers begin as cells in which precancerous changes known as **dysplasia** have occurred. These cells

---

mammogram **X-ray image of the breast used for cancer screening.**

melanoma **Less common but more serious type of skin cancer; tends to spread aggressively.**

dysplasia **Abnormal development of cells or tissue.**

EXAMINING THE EVIDENCE

Testicular Self-Examination

Performing monthly testicular self-exams is often recommended to teen boys and young men as a means of detecting testicular cancer. These self-exams are important because most cases are discovered through self-exam, and there is currently no other screening test for the disease.

The testicular self-exam is best done after a hot shower, which will relax the scrotum and make the exam easier. Inspect the scrotum for any changes in color or in the size of each testicle. It is common for one testicle to be larger than the other and, if this is not a change, it is okay.

Hold a testicle using the three middle fingers of one hand. Using small circular motions and light pressure, move the index and middle fingers of the second hand over the testicle until the whole surface has been covered. Feel for changes in texture or small nodules that may feel like a pea or a grain of rice. Also note if there are areas where touch produces pain. Along the back of each testicle is the epididymis, which contains the spermatic cord and the blood vessels serving the

testicle. Feel this area with the index finger and the thumb, again looking for painful areas, changes in texture, or small lumps. Repeat the process for the second testicle. If you notice any of the above changes, see your health-care provider.

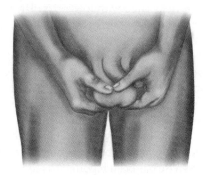

Source: Johnson, Michael, *Human Biology: Concepts and Current Issues with Interactive Physiology for Human Biology CD-ROM, 3rd Ed.,* © 2006. Reprinted and Electronically reproduced by permission of Pearson Education, Inc., Upper Saddle River, New Jersey.

pose a risk of developing into cancerous cells over time. Dysplastic changes that occur in the skin include the following:

- Actinic keratosis is an area of red or brown scaly, rough skin; this type of dysplasia can develop into squamous cell carcinoma.

- Moles are growths on the skin that rarely develop into cancer. Nonetheless, abnormal moles (dysplastic nevi) can develop, and they have the potential to develop into melanoma over time.

The most reliable way to catch skin cancer early is to perform routine self-exams (see Examining the Evidence). In addition to examining existing moles, you should examine blemishes and birthmarks for changes or new growth. Treatment for skin cancer varies depending on the type and severity and includes surgery, topical medications, chemotherapy, radiation, and other procedures to remove cancerous cells.

The keys to preventing both types of skin cancer are to avoid excessive exposure to ultraviolet (UV) light and, when you are exposed, to adequately protect your skin with sunscreen. In addition to wearing an adequate sunscreen (SPF 15 or higher; SPF stands for sun protection factor), avoid

sunlight at midday, and wear sunglasses and protective clothing as needed.

Although sunlight is the most common source of UV light, tanning beds also produce harmful UV rays that can damage your skin and increase cancer risk. Exposure to radiation and certain chemicals that might be present in the workplace are also associated with increased risk for skin cancer.

There are also nonmodifiable risk factors for both types of skin cancer. Women have higher rates than men at younger ages, but men have higher rates than women after age 40. People with fair skin, especially those who freckle or sunburn easily, have higher rates than people with darker skin. However, individuals with darker skin can develop skin cancer, so it is important for all people to use protective measures when exposed to UV light. Family history, personal history, and a weakened or suppressed immune system are risk factors for both types of skin cancer. Moles are an additional risk factor for melanoma. Risk for nonmelanoma is increased with smoking and certain skin conditions.

Uterine, Ovarian, and Cervical Cancers

Cancers of the female reproductive organs include uterine, ovarian, and cervical cancers. The most common type of uterine cancer is endometrial cancer, a cancer of the lining of the uterus. Many risk factors for endometrial

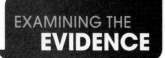

EXAMINING THE EVIDENCE

Early Detection of Skin Cancer

The key to early detection of skin cancer is self-examination. This exam should be performed monthly and should include the entire body, particularly those areas exposed to the sun. When examining your skin, begin by examining moles. Although moles are quite common and typically harmless, a change in a mole's appearance is a sign that you should see your health-care provider.

When examining moles, use the simple ABCD rule to remember the signs of melanoma and other skin cancers:

Asymmetry: Does one-half of a mole not match the other half?

Border: Is the border of the mole irregular, ragged, or notched?

Color: Is the color of the mole not the same all over? Does the mole have differing shades of black, brown, and/or patches of red or white?

Diameter: Is the diameter of the mole larger than 6 millimeters (about the size of a pencil eraser)? Does the mole appear to be growing in size?

Note that some skin cancers may not fit the ABCD rule, so it is particularly important for you to notice any changes in skin lesions or the appearance of a new lesion. Look for the following warning signs:

■ A sore that does not heal

■ A new growth of any kind

■ Spread of pigment from the border of a spot to the surrounding skin

■ Redness or a new swelling beyond the border of a mole

■ Change in sensation on the skin, such as itchiness, tenderness, or pain

■ Change in the surface of a mole, such as scaliness, oozing, bleeding, or the appearance of a bump

Schedule an appointment with your health-care provider as soon as possible if you observe any of these changes. Remember that many skin cancers can be successfully treated, but early detection is the key in the treatment of any cancer.

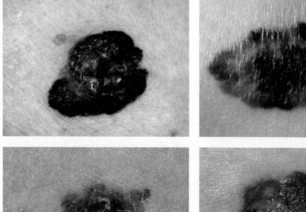

These four moles are examples of abnormalities that fit the ABCD rule for melanoma.

cancer are similar to those for breast cancer, but certain hormone therapies are associated with lower risk. Uterine cancer also includes cancer of the muscles and tissues of the uterus. These are less common than endometrial cancer, but risk factors are similar.

Ovarian cancer is the fifth leading cause of cancer deaths in women. Age, obesity, a longer menstrual history, family history, infertility, and breast cancer are all risk factors. The use of birth control pills, breastfeeding, one or more pregnancies, and a diet high in vegetables are associated with lower risk. During a routine pelvic exam, a health-care provider will check for lumps on the ovaries. Women at higher risk may have other clinical tests such as an ultrasound to screen for ovarian cancer.

Cervical cancer is most strongly linked to **human papillomavirus (HPV)**, a sexually transmitted virus that can cause genital warts. HPV can be spread though vaginal, anal, or oral sex. Additionally, it does not have to be spread through sex; it may spread as a result of any skin-to-skin contact with HPV. Vaccines for multiple types of HPV are now available for adolescents and young adults to prevent HPV prior to becoming sexually active. Smoking, long-term use of birth control pills, HIV infection, chlamydia, having many full-term pregnancies, a diet low in fruits and vegetables, low socioeconomic status, and family history are additional factors associated with increased risk for cervical cancer. In general, women should begin having Pap tests 3 years after they start having intercourse or at age 21, whichever is earlier, to screen for cervical cancer (9).

Oral and Pancreatic Cancers and Leukemia

Oral cancers include cancers of the lips, mouth, throat, and tongue. These cancers are strongly associated with tobacco use and alcohol consumption. Men are more likely to develop oral cancers than women. Exposure to UV light and HPV also increases risk. Early detection typically occurs through routine dental appointments and physical exams. Symptoms such as sores or a toothache may indicate oral cancer. Treatment depends on the location and stage of the cancer and can include surgery, radiation, chemotherapy, and medications.

Cancer of the pancreas is the fourth leading cause of cancer deaths for men and women. Increased risk is associated with age, family history, and race (African Americans have higher rates than whites). Behavioral risk factors include smoking, obesity, a sedentary lifestyle, exposure to pesticides and dyes, and diets high in fat, red meat, and pork. Early detection is difficult, but signs and symptoms include digestive problems, pain, jaundice, and weight loss. Treatment may include surgery, radiation, and chemotherapy.

Leukemia is cancer of the blood characterized by rapid abnormal cell growth but no tumor formation. Several types of leukemia can develop in children and adults. Because leukemia affects the blood and the production of blood cells, anemia and fatigue can be symptoms. Bruising easily, bleeding from the gums, and nosebleeds can be other indicators. White blood cells that fight infection are also affected, so leukemia impairs the body's ability to fight infection. The treatment will vary depending on the type of leukemia but can include bone marrow transplants, radiation, and chemotherapy.

What Are the Risk Factors for Cancer, and How Can You Reduce Your Risk?

LO Describe the known risk factors for cancer and differentiate between controllable and uncontrollable factors.

The cause of specific cancers is often unknown, but studies reveal that a variety of carcinogens can damage normal cells and start the cancer process. Several factors have been linked to an increased risk of cancer (1, 2). We have already mentioned risks for specific cancers; in this section we will further discuss risk factors commonly associated with multiple types of cancers, including family history/ heredity, race, nutrition/diet, exposure to toxins, viruses, tobacco and alcohol use, occupational carcinogens, and ultraviolet light. Risk factors include those that cannot be controlled and others that can be modified (**FIGURE 13.5**).

Factors You Cannot Control

Unfortunately, you cannot eliminate all of your risk for cancer. For instance, you cannot control your heredity or race; that is, you cannot modify your genetic makeup. But knowing your family history and whether you have nonmodifiable risk factors is important so you can discuss screening options with your health-care provider. Often screenings are recommended at earlier ages for individuals at high risk.

Heredity If a close relative, such as your father or mother, has had cancer, your chances of developing cancer are three times greater than average (10, 11). While the exact link between family history/heredity and cancer is often unclear, cancers of the breast, stomach, colon, prostate, uterus, ovaries, and lungs appear to run in families. Whether these patterns of increased risk are due to genetics or to the fact that people in the same family experience similar environmental risks remains unclear. It is important to learn as much about your family history as you can. For many types of cancer, different screening recommendations apply to individuals with a family history, and your health-care provider will help you determine the best plan for early detection.

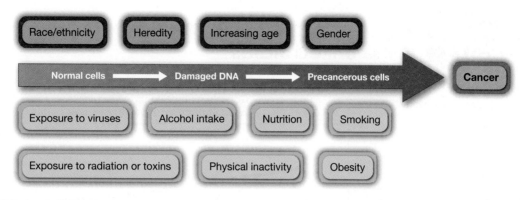

FIGURE 13.5 A summary of major cancer risk factors. Those risk factors that can be modified are shown in green, and those that cannot be modified are in red.

Race/Ethnicity Race and ethnic background also affect your risk of developing cancer. Overall incidence and death rates of cancer are higher among African Americans than whites (1). However, there are differences according to the specific sites (i.e., location) of cancer. Fortunately, there has been a decline in death rates among African-American adults, especially among men. One of the goals of the *Healthy People* objectives is to address health disparities, so increasing the awareness of cancer risk, preventive measures, and early detection procedures among African Americans is important in addressing the disproportionately high rates of cancer (see the Appreciating Diversity box on page 362).

Age Increasing age is a risk factor for most cancers (1). The influence of age on cancer risk is complex and may incorporate several factors including cumulative exposure to cancer-causing agents and less effective immune system function as a person ages.

Gender In the United States, the lifetime risk of developing cancer is higher in men (almost 1 in 2) than in women (slightly more than 1 in 3) (1). For some cancers, women are at greater risk; for example, women have a three times greater risk of developing lung cancer than men (1). The mechanisms responsible for gender differences are not known but may be linked to hormonal and lifestyle differences.

Factors You Can Control

Approximately 80% of all cancers are related to lifestyle, behavioral, and environmental factors that you can control (1). According to the National Cancer Institute, people who lead a healthy lifestyle have one-third to one-half the rate of cancer deaths compared with the

general population. The first step in reducing your risk is identifying the risk factors that apply to you (see Laboratory 13.1). The next step is to modify those aspects that increase your chances of developing cancer.

Nutrition/Diet Your diet is probably the most important behavioral factor in controlling your cancer risk (12). According to the National Academy of Sciences, diet is implicated in 60% of cancers in women and 40% of cancers in men. A high-fat diet has been linked to breast, colon, and prostate cancer. Further, a high-fat diet contributes to obesity, which is a risk factor for colon, breast, and uterine cancer. Additionally, salt-cured, smoked, and nitrite-cured foods have been linked to cancers of the esophagus and stomach.

Just as there are foods that increase cancer risk, there are foods and nutrients that seem to have a protective effect against cancer. For example, the antioxidant vitamins A, E, and C appear to protect cells against damage by free radicals (12). Free radicals, when produced in large quantities, promote the development of cancer by damaging DNA and producing abnormal cells that can become cancerous. (see Figure 13.2 on page 351). Antioxidants remove free radical cells, preventing DNA damage. Therefore, many cancer experts recommend a diet high in antioxidants.

A high-fiber diet lowers your risk of colon and rectal cancers by increasing the frequency of bowel movements, which decreases the time the colon and rectum are exposed to dietary carcinogens.

A high-fat diet has been hypothesized to be a risk factor for colon and rectal cancer, but recent studies suggest that fat itself is not a major risk factor in most cancers (13, 14). These studies indicate that consuming more than 4 ounces of red meat or more than 1 ounce

human papillomavirus (HPV) Sexually transmitted virus that can cause cervical cancer.

Race, Ethnicity, and Cancer Risk in the United States

More than 1.66 million Americans will be diagnosed with cancer this year, and more than 589,430 are expected to die from it (1). African Americans are more likely to die from cancer than individuals of any other racial or ethnic group. Data indicate that death rates in African Americans are 32% higher in men and 16% higher in women compared to white adults. New data also indicate that cancers are now the leading cause of death among Hispanic adults (24).

African Americans have the highest incidence of colon, rectum, and lung cancers, and black men are 50% more likely to develop prostate cancer than men of any other racial or ethnic group (24).

In most cases we do not have an explanation for the racial differences in the incidence and death rates. However, we do know that some risk factors for several types of cancers are higher in African Americans than in other groups. For example, the rates of physical inactivity and obesity are higher when compared to whites, especially in black women.

Also, disproportionate numbers of African Americans live in low socioeconomic status (SES) environments. Typically, people who have a low SES also have less access to quality health-care and are more likely to be uninsured. These conditions potentially decrease the likelihood of having routine screening procedures that would detect cancer early and increase survival rates. Additionally, behaviors such as smoking and eating a diet high in fat and low in fresh fruits and vegetables are more common among those in a low-SES environment. Increasing awareness about cancer risk, prevention, and screening are key in addressing the high rates of cancer among African Americans.

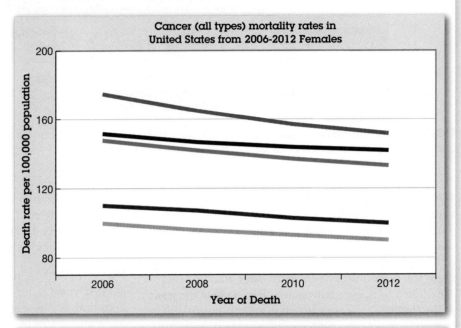

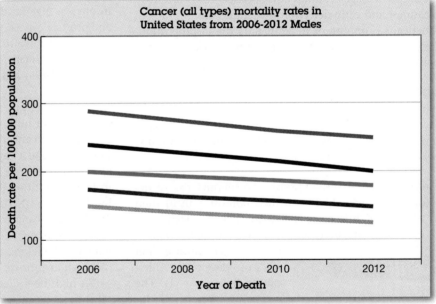

Key

━━ Asian/Pacific Islander ━━ American Indian/Alaska Na ━━ Black
━━ Hispanic ━━ White

*Age-adjusted to the 2000 U.S. standard population.
†Persons of Hispanic origin may be of any race.

Source: Data from the Division of Cancer Control and Population Sciences, National Cancer Institute. 2012. www.cancer.gov.

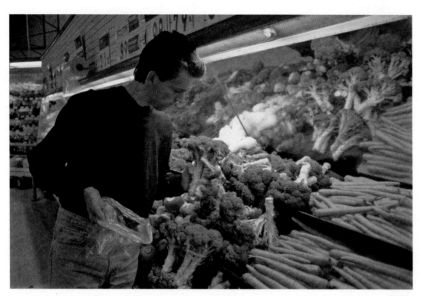

A diet rich in fruits and vegetables can provide antioxidants and other nutrients that help protect against cancer.

of processed meat per day increases your risk of colon and rectal cancers by 12%–49%. The link between cancer and the ingestion of red meat remains unclear and is the focus of intensive research.

Alcohol Use Heavy alcohol consumption increases the risk for oral, esophageal, liver, and breast cancer (15–17). Even moderate drinking is linked to a slightly increased risk of breast cancer in women. If you choose to drink alcohol, it is important to limit not just the quantity, but also the frequency of consumption. Having a drink one or two days a week is better than consuming alcohol on a daily basis. Also, consider other high-risk behaviors often associated with drinking. Many people combine drinking and smoking, creating an even greater cancer risk.

Tobacco Use Tobacco use is the single most significant cause of cancer deaths (approximately 25%) (1). Heavy smokers are 15 to 25 times more likely to die of cancer than are nonsmokers (1). Smoking also puts you at increased risk for oral cancers, as well as cancers of the pharynx, larynx, esophagus, pancreas, bladder, and colon (1). The average life expectancy for a chronic smoker is 7 years shorter than for a nonsmoker (18).

Cigarette smoking is responsible for 87% of all lung cancer cases (1). The risk of developing lung cancer and other smoking-related cancers is related to the total lifetime exposure to cigarette smoke (18–20). Lifetime exposure is measured in terms of the number of cigarettes smoked each day and the number of years a person has smoked. Risk of developing smoking-related cancer is greatest in heavy smokers with a long history of smoking. Secondhand tobacco smoke is also carcinogenic, so living with a smoker or working in an environment

where people smoke increases your risk for cancer as well.

Cigarettes do not pose the only risk from tobacco. Pipes, cigars, and smokeless tobacco also increase the risk for lung and oral cancers, and the use of chewing tobacco increases your risk of cancer of the mouth, larynx, throat, and esophagus (1). You can greatly reduce cancer risk by abstaining from all tobacco products. If you have never used any tobacco products, don't start. If you use tobacco, stopping can reverse your risk. Your risk of cancer decreases with each year you do not smoke. Even long-term smokers who quit after age 50 substantially reduce their risk of dying early from cancer (18, 19). It is never too late to quit!

Obesity The incidence of obesity has increased dramatically worldwide. Epidemiological evidence suggests that obesity is associated with an increased risk of several cancers (21). The underlying mechanisms linking obesity to cancer remain a topic of debate. Nonetheless, growing evidence suggests that obesity is associated with an increase in blood levels of several inflammatory factors that may directly or indirectly promote tumor growth (21). Therefore, maintaining a healthy body composition through diet and regular exercise can eliminate obesity as a risk factor.

Physical Inactivity A growing number of studies show that regular exercise may provide some protection against dying from cancer (**FIGURE 13.6** on page 364) (22, 23). The strongest evidence comes from studies demonstrating that regular exercise lowers the risk for colon cancer (23). Other studies show a relationship between exercise and the reduced risk for developing breast and uterine cancers in women (22).

How does exercise reduce cancer risk? One potential mechanism is an effect of exercise on the immune system. Tumors are formed in everyone from time to time, but the immune system typically destroys the abnormal cells before they increase in number. Thus, a strong immune system reduces the risk of cancer, while a weak immune system may increase your risk. Numerous studies suggest that physically active individuals have an increased resistance to infection and a decreased incidence of certain forms of cancer (22). It is also possible that regular exercise lowers chronic inflammation, known to be a cancer risk factor (22).

There are other potential explanations for the relationship between regular exercise and the reduced risk. Regular exercise helps you maintain a healthy body weight, and obesity is a risk factor for several types of cancer. Further, exercise is associated with increased bowel

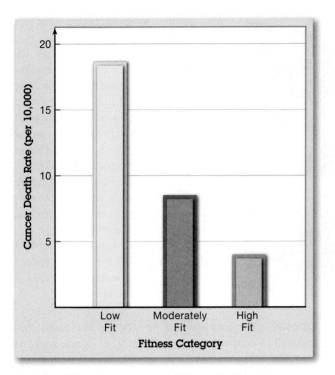

FIGURE 13.6 The declining risks of dying from cancer in men and women associated with increased exercise-related fitness.

Source: Data from Thune, I., and A. Furberg. Physical activity and cancer risk: Dose-response and cancer, all sites and site specific. *Medicine and Science in Sports and Exercise* 33:S530–S550, 2001. Also see Bauman, A. Updating the evidence that physical activity is good for health: An epidemiological review 2000–2003. *Journal of Science and Medicine in Sports* 7:6–19, 2004.

motility (22). Indeed, exercise has an effect similar to that of a high-fiber diet, increasing regularity and thereby reducing exposure to carcinogens in waste material. In summary, although the mechanism(s) to explain why regular exercise reduces the risk of some cancers remains unclear, abundant evidence indicates that exercise results in a reduced risk of cancer. Therefore, engaging in regular exercise and remaining active throughout life are important health behaviors that can lower your cancer risk.

Exposure to Ultraviolet Light Prolonged exposure to ultraviolet light from any source can damage your skin and increase your risk of cancer (1). Ultraviolet radiation from the sun and artificial tanning is responsible for most new cases of skin cancer each year (1). Tanning beds and sunlamps produce ultraviolet rays and present as much risk as the sun. Some tanning salons claim their equipment is less dangerous, but that is not true!

Limiting your sun exposure and avoiding tanning salons are the obvious ways to avoid the carcinogenic effect of ultraviolet light. However, we need some sun exposure to produce vitamin D, and few people want to completely avoid being in the sun. When you are exposed to the sun for more than 15 or 20 minutes (less if you have

fair skin), wear protective clothing and use sunscreen to block the effects of ultraviolet light.

All ultraviolet exposure to your skin can be damaging. While most people recognize the need to protect skin from the sun, they often think of it in terms of occasional extreme exposure (e.g., a day at the beach). However, long-term day-to-day sun exposure also increases your risk for skin cancer. Studies show that over the course of a lifetime, a person will receive tens of thousands of doses of damaging ultraviolet radiation (25). This cumulative exposure greatly increases your risk of developing skin cancer (25). Therefore, you need to protect yourself daily. Research shows that daily use of even low-level sunscreen (SPF 15) can reduce your lifetime ultraviolet exposure by 50% or more (25). See the Steps for Behavior Change box for ways to reduce your risk due to UV light.

Viruses Viruses can cause cancer by invading cells and damaging DNA. Research demonstrates that viruses play a role in several blood cancers (leukemia) as well as cancers of the lymphatic system (lymphomas). Evidence also suggests that viruses can cause liver, cervical, nose, and pharyngeal cancer (1). How can you control your exposure to viruses? In regard to the risk of cervical cancer, women do have some control. Cervical cancer is associated with HPV, a sexually transmitted virus. Abstaining, using condoms during intercourse, and limiting the number of sexual partners can reduce the risk of HPV. Vaccines are also available for adolescents and young adults that can prevent HPV infection.

Radiation Exposure Up to 5% of all cancers may be caused by radiation exposure due to medical X-rays, computer monitors, and environmental radiation (1). Further, many modern conveniences that emit electromagnetic fields may increase cancer risk by damaging cellular DNA. For example, electric blankets and low-frequency radio waves, such as those associated with cellular telephones, have been implicated in causing cancer. You can reduce your cancer risk by taking the recommended safety precautions if you work in an environment where you are exposed to radiation. Avoiding excessive use of items and devices that expose you to radiation can lower your risk.

Occupational Carcinogens Factory workers and people living near factories may have an increased risk of cancer due to exposure to chemical toxins used or produced in the factory. Industrial chemicals known to be carcinogenic include benzene, nickel, chromate, asbestos, and vinyl chloride (1). One of the most common occupational carcinogens is asbestos, which was formerly used in the construction, automobile, and shipbuilding industries. Being exposed to coal tars in mining or working near airborne carcinogens, such as in auto painting, is

steps ► FOR BEHAVIOR CHANGE

Do you protect your skin from ultraviolet light?

Taking the necessary precautions is very important to protect yourself against skin cancer. Answer the following questions to see how well you are doing in shielding your skin from ultraviolet light:

Y   N

☐ ☐   Do you wear sunscreen every time you know you will be exposed to the sun for more than 15 minutes?

☐ ☐   Do you avoid the use of tanning beds?

☐ ☐   Do you avoid being in the sun between 10:00 A.M. and 2:00 P.M.?

☐ ☐   Do you wear protective clothing when exposed to the sun?

If you answered yes to all of these questions, you are doing a good job of protecting your skin.

Tips to Protect Your Skin from UV Light

Tomorrow, you will:

☑ Use a sunscreen of at least SPF 15 on skin exposed to the sun, including when exercising outdoors. Reapply sunscreen during prolonged sun exposure. Make sure to apply to your face and lips.

Within the next 2 weeks, you will:

☑ If you must have a tan, use a sunless tanner instead of tanning in the sun or on a tanning bed.

☑ Wear sunglasses and a hat with a brim to protect your eyes and face.

By the end of the semester, you will:

☑ Regularly avoid sun exposure at midday when UV rays are the strongest.

☑ Perform regular exams to check for skin abnormalities or signs of skin cancer.

---

also dangerous. Many chemicals used to kill weeds (herbicides) and insects (pesticides) contain carcinogens and are found in excessive amounts in some water supplies.

Some professions require people to work around industrial pollutants, but being aware of the risk and following safety procedures can help lower risk. In particular, avoid exposure to industrial agents such as radon, dioxins, nickel, chromate, asbestos, and vinyl chloride. If you have questions concerning the risks of chemical exposure in your workplace, see the Environmental Protection Agency (EPA) website or contact the agency for a complete list of cancer-causing chemicals and help in identifying those used in your workplace.

MAKE SURE YOU **KNOW...**

- Even though the causes of specific cancers are often unknown, many cancer risk factors have been identified.

- Some risk factors, such as race/ethnicity, heredity, and age cannot be controlled.

- Several cancer risk factors can be controlled. Consuming a healthy diet, limiting alcohol intake, avoiding tobacco products and secondhand smoke, exercising regularly, and avoiding radiation and occupational carcinogens will reduce your risk for developing multiple types of cancers.

MasteringHealth™

study plan

Customize your study plan—and master your health!—in the Study Area of **MasteringHealth.**

summary

 hear it! STUDY REVIEW

To hear an MP3 Chapter Summary, scan here or visit the Study Area in MasteringHealth™.

LO **1** ■ Cancer is the uncontrolled growth and spread of abnormal cells. Groups of abnormal cells can form tumors, which can be classified as benign or malignant. Benign (noncancerous) tumors are generally not life-threatening; malignant tumors consist of cancerous cells that can spread to other tissues and disrupt organ function.

■ Currently, cancer is the number-two cause of death in the United States.

LO **2** ■ Carcinogens are cancer-causing agents. Normal cells become cancerous when DNA is damaged by carcinogens, resulting in uncontrolled cell division.

LO **3** ■ Common sites of cancer include the breasts, lungs, colon, and prostate gland.

■ Skin cancer is the most frequently diagnosed cancer, and lung cancer is the leading cause of cancer deaths.

■ Participating in cancer screenings is important for early detection. Recommendations for cancer screenings are based on age, gender, and the presence of risk factors.

LO **4** ■ Race/ethnicity, heredity, age, and gender are nonmodifiable risk factors for cancer. Modifiable risk factors include exposure to carcinogens such as radiation, viruses, tobacco, alcohol, occupational carcinogens, and ultraviolet light. Other behavioral factors that increase cancer risk include obesity, unhealthy diet, and lack of physical activity.

■ Approximately 80% of all cancers are related to lifestyle and environmental factors.

■ Diet may be the most important factor in reducing cancer risk. A diet rich in fruits and vegetables containing antioxidants and fiber will likely reduce your risk.

■ Exercise has been shown to reduce the risk of colon, uterine, and breast cancer.

study questions

review it! QUIZZES

Find more review questions online at MasteringHealth™.

LO **1** 1. _____ is the spread of cancerous cells throughout the body.

    a. Benign tumor   c. Carcinogen
    b. Malignant tumor   d. Metastasis

LO **2** 2. How do normal cells become cancerous?

3. Which of the following is not one of the seven warning signs of cancer?

    a. nagging cough or hoarseness
    b. a sore that does not heal
    c. unusual bleeding or discharge
    d. all are warning signs of cancer

LO **3** 4. What is the most common type of cancer?

    a. skin   c. lung
    b. leukemia   d. colon

5. Which type of cancer causes the most deaths in U.S. women?

    a. breast
    b. lung
    c. skin
    d. cervical

6. Describe the signs of skin cancer.

LO **4** 7. Which of the following is not a behavioral risk factor for developing cancer?

    a. unhealthy diet
    b. physical inactivity
    c. doing breast self-exams
    d. excessive alcohol consumption

8. Name and describe the cancer risk factors that can be controlled and those risk factors that cannot be modified.

9. Outline the dietary guidelines for reducing cancer risk.

suggested reading

American Cancer Society. *Cancer Facts and Figures 2015*. Atlanta: American Cancer Society, 2015. http://www.cancer.org.

National Cancer Institute. About Cancer. 2015. http://www.cancer.gov/

National Cancer Institute. NCI Fact Sheets. 2015. http://www.cancer.gov/publications/fact-sheets#risk

Parkin, M., et al. The fraction of cancer attributable to lifestyle and environmental factors in the UK in 2010. *British Journal of Cancer* 105 (Supp 2):S38–S41, 2011.

UK Cancer Research. Physical activity facts and evidence. 2015. http://www.cancerresearchuk.org/about-cancer/causes-of-cancer/physical-activity-and-cancer/physical-activity-facts-and-evidence

helpful weblinks

do it! WEBLINKS

For links to the organizations and websites listed, visit MasteringHealth™.

American Cancer Society

Includes up-to-date information, including cancer statistics, risk factors, and current treatments. **www.cancer.org**

National Breast Cancer Foundation, Inc.

Provides comprehensive information about breast cancer. **www.nationalbreastcancer.org**

National Cancer Institute

Presents up-to-date information about cancer for the general public, as well as clinicians and practitioners. **www.cancer.gov**

U.S. Environmental Protection Agency

Provides information about environmental and health concerns, including environmental factors associated with increased risk for cancers. **www.epa.gov**

WebMD

Contains information on a wide variety of diseases and medical problems, including cancer. **www.webmd.com/cancer/default.htm**

Name _____ Date _____

Determining Your Cancer Risk

The purpose of this laboratory is to increase your awareness of your risk of developing all forms of cancer. Answer the following questions by putting a check under either "Yes" or "No."

The more times you check "Yes," the more risk factors you have. If you check "Yes" even once, you should take steps to modify your lifestyle and reduce your risk.

	Yes	No
Do you have a family history of cancer?	_____	_____
Do you have a fair complexion?	_____	_____
Are you regularly exposed to occupational carcinogens or any type of radiation?	_____	_____
Is any part of your skin regularly exposed to excessive sunlight?	_____	_____
Do you consume more than 4 oz of red meat or 1 oz of processed meat per day?	_____	_____
Do you regularly eat smoked foods?	_____	_____
Is your diet low in fiber?	_____	_____
Are you obese?	_____	_____
Do you consume an excessive amount of alcohol?	_____	_____
Do you use tobacco products or breathe secondhand tobacco smoke?	_____	_____

1. How many "Yes" responses did you check?

   _____

2. Name any behaviors you can modify or change to reduce your risk for cancer.

   _____

   _____

3. Select one of your modifiable risk factors, and write out steps to change your behavior to reduce your risk. (Use the strategies for behavior change you learned in Chapter 1, if applicable.)

   _____

   _____

   _____

   _____

   _____

   _____

   _____

Name _____ Date _____

Early Detection

Early detection of cancer is very important in getting prompt and effective treatment. Several screening procedures outlined in this chapter are recommended for early detection. The purpose of this lab is to assess your behaviors related to early detection of cancer. Check the appropriate box to indicate your current level of participation for each screening.

	Never	Sometimes	As Recommended	N/A
Breast self-exam	_____	_____	_____	_____
Clinical breast exam	_____	_____	_____	_____
Mammogram (if over age 40 or 50)	_____	_____	_____	_____
Testicular self-exam	_____	_____	_____	_____
Clinical testicular exam	_____	_____	_____	_____
Colon cancer screening	_____	_____	_____	_____
PSA test (if over age 50)	_____	_____	_____	_____
Pap test	_____	_____	_____	_____
Skin exam	_____	_____	_____	_____

1. Do you meet the recommendations for cancer screenings based on your age, gender, and risk level?

_____

2. If not, which screenings do you need to start? Talk with your health-care provider to make a plan for scheduling any appropriate screenings.

_____

_____

_____

_____

_____

_____

_____

_____

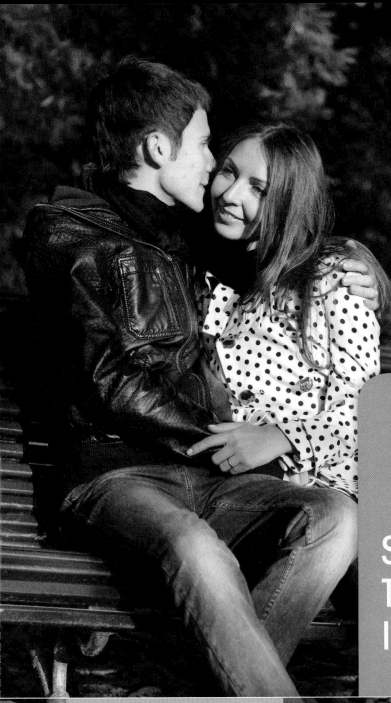

14

Sexually Transmitted Infections

HAVE YOU EVER asked a potential sexual partner about his or her sexual history? Were you surprised by his or her responses, and did you learn anything that caused you to reconsider entering into a sexual relationship? Such conversations may seem uncomfortable, but they are an essential component of practicing responsible sexual behavior. Asking questions, taking precautions, and educating yourself about the risks associated with sexual activities are the keys to protecting yourself from sexually transmitted infections. In this chapter, we will discuss the symptoms and transmission routes of some of the most common **sexually transmitted infections (STIs)**, also referred to as sexually transmitted diseases (STDs). We will also address strategies you can employ to ensure that any sexual activity you choose to engage in will not result in unpleasant, and sometimes deadly, sexually transmitted infections.

What Are Sexually Transmitted Infections?

 LO **1** Define *sexually transmitted infections* and list the microorganisms (i.e., bacteria, viruses, etc.) responsible for these infections.

STIs are infections that you can get and pass to others through vaginal, oral, or anal sex. STIs can be caused by more than 30 different viruses, bacteria, or parasites. Many STIs, such as those caused by bacteria or parasites, can be treated with antibiotics or other drugs, but STIs caused by viruses remain with the host for life.

STIs are more than just an embarrassing problem. In many cases, they can be life-altering and life-threatening. STIs can lead to infertility, complications during pregnancy, and cervical and other cancers. They can be passed on even when there are no symptoms present. These silent but sometimes deadly infections affect both men and women of all ages, races, and socioeconomic backgrounds.

STIs are often "silent" diseases, because early symptoms may be ignored and go untreated. Further, although STIs can be diagnosed through medical testing, routine screening programs are not widespread, and social stigmas about STIs often prevent infected individuals from visiting health-care professionals for testing (1). Thus, many cases of STIs go unreported, resulting in an underestimation of the total number of people infected with STIs.

STIs are a major public health challenge in the United States. The Centers for Disease Control and Prevention (CDC) estimates that 20 million new infections occur each year, almost half of them among young people between the ages of 15–24 (2). Because young people are among the groups most affected by STIs, there are several health objectives for *Healthy People 2020* that focus on preventing STIs and promoting responsible sexual behavior

among adolescents and young adults. The rate of STIs in the United States far exceeds those of every other industrialized nation (1–3). Lack of education and lack of public awareness of the dangers of STIs play a role in the high incidence of STIs in the United States. Statistics indicate that one in four Americans will contract at least one STI in their lifetime (1–3). STIs also pose a major health problem in many other countries (see the Appreciating Diversity box on page 376).

In addition to the health threat they pose, STIs pose an economic burden as well. Current estimates are that STIs add an estimated $16 billion to health-care costs in the United States each year (2). Some of the most common STIs include human immunodeficiency virus (HIV), trichomoniasis, chlamydia, hepatitis B, gonorrhea, human papillomavirus (HPV), genital herpes, and syphilis (3) (see **FIGURE 14.1**). Because of its important worldwide health ramifications, we begin our discussion of STIs with a detailed look at HIV.

MAKE SURE YOU **KNOW...**

- Every year millions of people in the United States are infected by one or more sexually transmitted infections (STIs).

- STIs can go undiagnosed for some time because of lack of symptoms and/or lack of screening, and they can be passed along even when no symptoms are present.

- The most common STIs in the United States include HIV, trichomoniasis, chlamydia, hepatitis B, gonorrhea, HPV, genital herpes, and syphilis.

— MasteringHealth™

HIV/AIDS

 LO **2** Define *HIV/AIDS* and describe the stages of HIV infection.

Acquired immunodeficiency syndrome (AIDS) is caused by a **virus**, called *human immunodeficiency virus (HIV)*. When HIV enters the bloodstream, immune cells rush to the virus in an attempt to destroy this invading agent. However, HIV enters the immune cells and uses them as hosts to replicate itself. The entry of HIV into immune cells eventually

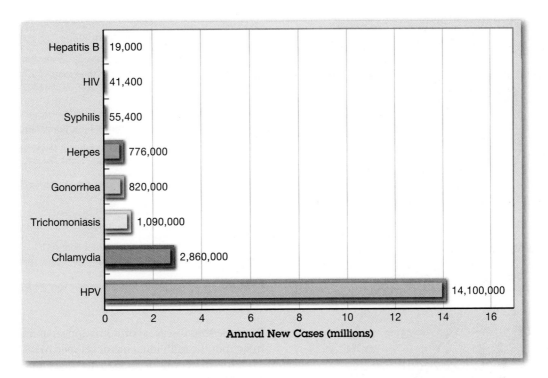

FIGURE 14.1 The most common STIs in the United States, as estimated by new cases of each type in 2013.

Source: Data are from the Centers for Disease Control and Prevention, 2015. www.cdc.gov/std/healthcomm/fact_sheets.htm.

disarms the immune cells and impairs the body's ability to fight infections. Over time, the level of HIV in the blood increases, and the immune system becomes weaker and weaker, resulting in immunodeficiency and the symptoms associated with AIDS.

Incidence of HIV/AIDS

The CDC estimates that over 900,000 people in the United States are living with HIV and that 20% of infected individuals are unaware they are infected. The total number of new AIDS diagnoses in the United States has declined during the past 20 years and plateaued with 41,400 new cases reported in 2013 (3). Importantly, the number of deaths from AIDS has decreased because of improved drug treatment (see Examining the Evidence on page 377).

In the beginning of the AIDS epidemic in the United States, the disease was predominantly one affecting homosexual men; however, the incidence of AIDS among heterosexual Americans is on the rise. Compared to whites, racial and ethnic minorities have been disproportionately infected with HIV. Moreover, the incidence of HIV infections is significantly higher in males compared to females. This gender difference is explained by the fact that about 63% of all new HIV infections occur through male-to-male sexual contact (4). See **FIGURE 14.2** on page 374 for the gender and race distributions of new HIV infections in the United States.

HIV/AIDS is a major health problem not just in the United States; the number of people infected with HIV is increasing all over the world. Current estimates are that over 35 million people worldwide are infected—more than 25 million in Africa alone. According to a 2013 UNAIDS/WHO report on the AIDS epidemic, there were 2.1 million new HIV infections in 2013, 1.5 million of which occurred in sub-Saharan Africa (5). Rates of HIV infection in many countries are declining as a result of improved awareness and prevention efforts. For example, the rates in 22 sub-Saharan African countries showed declines between 2001 and 2015. However, Africa remains the global epicenter of the AIDS **pandemic**. The majority of new cases are still found in these countries, and HIV prevention for women

sexually transmitted infections (STIs) **A group of more than 25 infections that are spread through sexual contact.**

acquired immunodeficiency syndrome (AIDS) **Fatal disease caused by the human immunodeficiency virus (HIV).**

virus **Infectious microorganism that cannot live independently and must invade a host cell to survive.**

pandemic **Illness or infection that occurs over a wide geographic area and affects a high proportion of the population.**

New HIV/AIDS Cases in 2013 by Gender

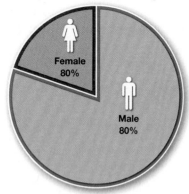

New HIV/AIDS Cases in 2013 by Race/Ethnicity

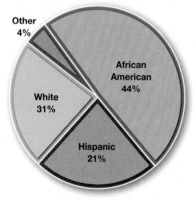

FIGURE 14.2 The pie charts above reveal that select groups of Americans are becoming infected with HIV disproportionately compared to other groups. For example, even though men make up about half of the population, approximately 80% of new HIV infections each year occur in men **(a)**. Although African Americans account for only 13% of the U.S. population, approximately 44% of the new HIV infections in 2013 occurred in that group **(b)**.

Source: From Centers for Disease Control and Prevention. HIV/AIDS in the United States, 2014. www.cdc.gov/hiv/resources/factsheets/PDF/us.pdf.

and girls is an area still in need of attention. Moreover, the infection rate for other STIs is also disproportionately high in these countries.

Stages of HIV Infection

Many people infected with HIV are unaware that they carry the virus because symptoms may not appear for months or even years after infection. Evidence suggests that in many cases, the virus remains dormant in the body for 5 to 10 years before creating health problems (6, 7). After this incubation period, the virus begins to multiply, damaging specific cells within the immune system. Because an impaired immune system is incapable of preventing infections, the body becomes vulnerable to a variety of diseases, from the common cold to cancer.

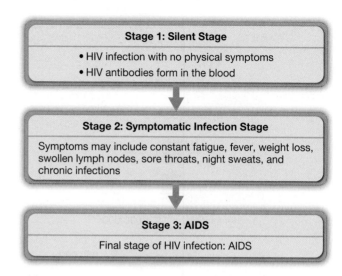

FIGURE 14.3 Stages in the development of AIDS.

When serious disease symptoms appear as a result of HIV infection, the individual has developed AIDS.

HIV infection progresses to AIDS in three stages (**FIGURE 14.3**). The first stage after HIV enters the body is the silent stage. During this stage, there are no physical symptoms, and the only evidence of HIV is the development of HIV antibodies in the blood. Typically, HIV antibodies are formed within 2 weeks after infection, but it can take up to 6 to 8 weeks before antibody levels are high enough to be detected by a blood test.

The second phase of HIV infection is called the symptomatic infection stage. This stage consists of several symptoms that may include constant fatigue, fever, weight loss, swollen lymph nodes, and sore throat. Symptoms that develop later in the second stage include night sweats, chronic infections, skin disorders, and ulcers of the membranes lining the nose, mouth, and other body cavities.

Unless medical research can develop a cure for HIV, all HIV-infected individuals will eventually progress to the third and final stage, AIDS. AIDS is characterized by all of the general symptoms associated with the second phase of HIV infection, plus one or more opportunistic diseases such as pneumonia or certain types of cancer such as Kaposi's sarcoma (see **TABLE 14.1**).

Although AIDS is a fatal disease, people now live with it for many years. This is possible because of improved medications, coupled with superior clinical management of the disease. In recent years, the National Institutes of Health has devoted millions of research dollars toward developing a cure. Because of this investment in AIDS research and the scientific progress that has been achieved, some researchers have concluded that eventually AIDS will be considered a chronic disease (like hypertension or diabetes) that can be controlled by appropriate medical treatment. For more about AIDS research, see Examining the Evidence on page 377.

TABLE 14.1 ■ Common Opportunistic Diseases Associated with the Development of AIDS	
Disease	**Symptoms**
Kaposi's sarcoma (type of cancer)	Brown or purple lesions on the skin that resemble bruises but do not heal.
Primary lymphoma of the brain (type of cancer)	Headache, loss of memory, personality changes, impaired vision
Tuberculosis (bacterial infection)	Fever, night sweats, fatigue, cough, weight loss
Pneumocystis pneumonia (rare form of pneumonia)	Chest pain, dry cough, difficulty breathing
Cytomegalovirus (viral infection that can occur in the lung, gastrointestinal tract, or central nervous system)	Symptoms vary depending on the location of the infection
Atypical mycobacterium (bacterial infection)	High fever, night sweats, fatigue, weakness

How HIV Is Transmitted

For HIV to replicate in the body, the virus must enter the bloodstream. Any exchange of body fluids such as blood, semen, or vaginal secretions is a possible mode for transmission. The three most common modes of transmission are

1. vaginal or anal intercourse without using a condom;

2. sharing needles contaminated with HIV-infected blood during injected drug use, tattooing, or body piercing; and

3. passage of the virus from mother to fetus in the uterus (20% to 50% chance) or in blood during delivery.

In addition to these common routes of transmission, the virus can also be spread from an HIV-infected mother to a baby by breastfeeding. It is also possible to transmit the virus by sharing sex toys if they are not properly disinfected and cleaned. Finally, HIV can be transmitted through accidental contamination when infected blood enters the body through the mucous membranes of the eyes or mouth or through breaks in the skin (i.e., cuts, abrasions, or punctures). Years ago, some individuals contracted the virus through a blood transfusion, but today's screening methods of all donated blood have minimized this risk.

Myths about HIV Transmission

Several myths about how HIV is transmitted create unnecessary fears in many people. This fear has caused some individuals to avoid any type of contact with infected individuals. It is critically important to understand both how HIV *can* be transmitted and how HIV *cannot* be transmitted. You cannot get HIV from any of the following:

■ *Casual contact with HIV-infected indivi-duals.* Normal household or social contact does not transmit HIV.

Shaking hands, hugging, or talking with someone with HIV are unlikely to transmit the virus.

■ *Contact with inanimate objects.* HIV cannot live outside the body. Therefore, HIV cannot survive on toilet seats, drinking fountains, countertops, doorknobs, or other areas. Alcohol, bleach, Lysol, or hydrogen peroxide can be used to disinfect a surface if it becomes contaminated with blood or semen containing HIV.

■ *Sports participation.* To date, there are no documented cases of HIV transmission through sports. Further, HIV is not found in the sweat of HIV-positive individuals, and HIV exists in only limited quantities in tears. Therefore, there is limited risk of contracting HIV during contact sports, even when bleeding occurs.

■ *Saliva.* Although HIV has been found in saliva and tears, there is no evidence that HIV has ever been transmitted from one person to another by kissing or by drinking from water fountains used by HIV-infected individuals.

■ *Swimming pools, hot tubs, or whirlpool baths.* HIV cannot live or replicate in water. Therefore, HIV cannot be transmitted by contact with water contained in hot tubs, whirlpools, or swimming pools.

■ *Contact with animals.* Household pets and farm animals cannot contract the HIV virus. Therefore, animals cannot spread HIV to humans.

■ *Insect bites.* Insects such as mosquitoes, biting flies, and bedbugs cannot transmit the HIV virus.

Diagnosis and Treatment

Diagnosis of HIV results from a blood test that detects the HIV virus in the blood and provides information about the status of the immune system. The treatment of HIV/AIDS has advanced markedly during the past decade and involves the use of numerous recently developed drugs.

MAKE SURE YOU **KNOW...**

■ AIDS is a fatal disease that develops from infection by the human immunodeficiency virus (HIV).

■ HIV is transmitted via infected body fluids, such as blood, semen, and vaginal secretions.

■ HIV cannot be transmitted through casual contact, kissing, water (such as in swimming pools or hot tubs), or dry surfaces.

■ Although no cure has yet been found for AIDS, many antiretroviral drugs are available to delay the onset of the disease and improve a patient's quality of life.

MasteringHealth™

Hepatitis B

 3 **Explain the health issues associated with hepatitis B infection.**

The CDC estimates that as of 2015, more than 420,000 people were infected with the **hepatitis B virus (HBV)**, a viral infection that causes liver disease (3). Although the mortality rate for hepatitis B is typically lower than for some other forms of hepatitis, it is estimated that more than 1,800 people die each year in the United States from this disease (3).

Hepatitis B virus can be transmitted by contact with infected blood, blood products, semen, vaginal secretions, and saliva. Consequently, people at risk for contracting hepatitis B include individuals having sex with an HBV-infected partner, sharing personal items such toothbrushes, sharing needles when injecting drugs, or working

APPRECIATING DIVERSITY
Sexually Transmitted Infections Are a Worldwide Problem

STIs are a major health problem in countries around the world. Nonetheless, the incidence of STIs varies widely. Some countries report a relatively low incidence, while other countries report a high prevalence of STIs (5). For example, the incidence tends to be lower in industrialized countries, but STIs constitute a large health risk in most developing countries. Each year there are an estimated 365 million new cases of curable STIs around the world, and more than 75% (274 million) of these cases occur in developing countries (5).

The reasons for the differences in the incidence of STIs between industrialized and developing countries are complex. Behavioral changes in young people, such as not having sex before age 15, increasing use of condoms, and having fewer sexual partners, offer possible explanations of why STI incidence is lower in industrialized countries (5). Social and cultural norms surrounding a woman's role in the family in some developing nations can contribute to her increased risk, because she has less control over her sexual activity and no control over her partner's promiscuity. Some people may also be at increased risk if they do not have access to condoms or decline to use them because it conflicts with their religious beliefs regarding birth control.

Lack of knowledge of safe sex and HIV remains high in many countries. A study by the World Health Organization reported that on a per-capita basis, sub-Saharan Africa has one of the highest incidences of STI infection in the world (see figure).

The good news is that government support for expanded access to treatment and new drug therapy programs are having a positive impact on reducing the number of STI deaths globally. Programs focused on educating people most at risk are demonstrating the most progress in preventing HIV and other STIs (5).

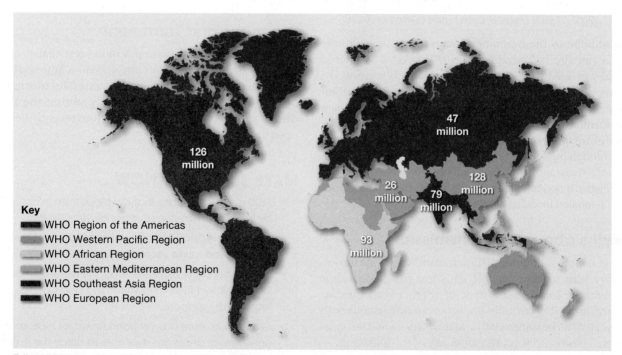

Key
- WHO Region of the Americas
- WHO Western Pacific Region
- WHO African Region
- WHO Eastern Mediterranean Region
- WHO Southeast Asia Region
- WHO European Region

Estimated new cases (each year) of STIs (AIDS, gonorrhea, chlamydia, syphilis, and trichomoniasis) around the world (5).

Source: Sexually transmitted infections (STIs), Fact sheet N°110, Updated November 2013, http://www.who.int/mediacentre/factsheets/fs110/en/. Courtesy World Health

The Search for a Cure for AIDS

Current estimates are that 35 million people worldwide are currently infected with HIV. In 2013, 1.5 million people died of AIDS-related illnesses (5). Without a cure for this disease, even more people will die, typically within 7–12 years after acquiring the virus.

A major problem confronting scientists in the treatment of HIV is that the virus is capable of mutating into many different strains. That is, the virus can change its characteristics, which makes developing a drug to kill all strains of the virus extremely difficult. Although no cure has yet been developed, advances in AIDS treatment (such as the use of several combinations of antiviral drugs) have lowered the mortality and morbidity rates of the disease. Indeed, many of the new antiviral drug treatments have resulted in a remission of AIDS for infected patients (9). Because of these recent advances in developing new treatments for AIDS, many scientists remain optimistic that a cure for the AIDS virus will be found (9).

---

in a job that involves handling human blood or other body fluids. Individuals at risk for contracting hepatitis B are often advised to be vaccinated against the disease.

Hepatitis promotes an inflammatory response in the liver that decreases normal liver function. The liver performs numerous functions, such as regulating blood glucose levels between meals, producing bile, and detoxifying the blood. Because many of the liver's functions are essential for life, severe liver dysfunction can be life-threatening. Therefore, hepatitis B is a very serious disease.

Symptoms

Approximately 30% of individuals infected with hepatitis B do not develop symptoms. In the remaining 70%, a variety of symptoms may be present. Common symptoms include jaundice (yellowing of skin and/or whites of the eyes), reduced appetite, nausea, joint pain, and chronic fatigue (8).

Diagnosis and Treatment

Hepatitis B is diagnosed by a blood test for antibodies that indicate infection with the hepatitis B virus. Unfortunately, there is currently no cure, so prevention of this disease is critical. Once hepatitis B is diagnosed, treatment consists of rest and consuming enough fluid to ensure adequate hydration. In people infected with the hepatitis B virus, the liver can become severely compromised. Two drugs (alpha interferon and lamivudine) are effective in reducing symptoms in patients with liver dysfunction.

Human Papillomavirus

LO **4** Explain the health issues associated with human papillomavirus infection.

Human papillomavirus (HPV) refers to a group of over 40 strains of a sexually transmitted virus; some of these strains cause genital warts. Most infected individuals do not realize they are infected because the virus lives in the skin or mucous membranes and usually causes no symptoms (8, 10). However, some people may get visible genital warts. Genital warts appear as soft pink or flesh-colored swellings that can be raised or flat. Infection generally occurs through sexual contact with an infected individual; after exposure, the virus penetrates the skin or mucous membranes of the genitals or anus, and warts may appear within weeks or even months after contact (10).

HPV is one of the most common causes of STIs in the world and the most frequent cause of STIs in the United States. Current estimates are that more than 79 million people in the United States are infected with HPV (10). Moreover, approximately 14 million Americans contract a new infection each year (10). The incidence of HPV varies across the population, with the highest rates in people between the ages of 19–30. In particular, studies suggest that the incidence of HPV in college students is extremely high.

Does HPV cause serious health problems? In some cases, HPV will clear on its own. However, when HPV does not disappear, it can cause problems such as genital warts and even lead to cancer. Untreated HPV is associated with cancer of the cervix, vulva, vagina, penis, anus, throat, tongue, and tonsils (10).

Symptoms

Many people infected with HPV are asymptomatic. In others, the infection results in genital warts or precancerous

see it!

ABC VIDEOS

Watch the "Oral HPV" ABC News Video online at MasteringHealth™.

---

hepatitis B virus (HBV) Viral infection that attacks the liver.

human papillomavirus (HPV) Group of sexually transmitted viruses that can cause genital warts and lead to cervical and other types of cancer.

changes in the cells of the cervix, vulva, anus, or penis. On dry areas of the external genitals (such as the penis and vulva), warts may develop as a series of small itchy bumps on the skin and may range in size from that of a pinhead to that of a pencil eraser. These warts can be detected by routine self-exams of the genital area to look for suspicious growths.

Diagnosis and Treatment

In women, a routine Pap test can reveal precancerous changes in cervical cells. To test for HPV, the Pap sample can be subjected to a DNA test to determine if the virus is present and, if so, the specific HPV type. At present, there is no diagnostic test for men. Genital warts are diagnosed based on visual inspection by a physician.

Genital warts can be treated with medications that cause the warts to dry up within a few days, or they can be removed by cryosurgery (freezing), laser surgery, or excision surgery. Removing the wart does not remove the virus from the body. Because the virus can remain dormant in cells, warts can reappear months or even years after treatment. The extent to which an individual can spread the virus after visible warts have been removed is unknown.

The greatest health risk associated with HPV infection affects women, since HPV infection increases the risk of uterine and cervical cancer. Indeed, within 5 years after infection, about 30% of all untreated HPV cases result in precancerous growths. Among precancerous growths that remain untreated, 70% will lead to cancer (10).

In 2006, the U.S. Food and Drug Administration (FDA) approved the first vaccine to help prevent cervical cancer caused by some types of HPV, and today two vaccines are available (3). The HPV vaccine is recommended for girls before the onset of sexual activity. The CDC recommends beginning the vaccination process when children are 11 to 12 years of age; uninfected adults up to age 26 can also receive the vaccine.

Genital Herpes

LO **5** Explain the health issues associated with herpes simplex viral infections.

Genital **herpes** infections are caused by two types of herpes simplex virus, HSV-1 and HSV-2 (11). HSV-1 infections commonly appear as sores on the lips or mouth (known as fever blisters or cold sores), and HSV-2 is the primary cause of genital herpes.

Genital herpes is highly contagious and can be transmitted through any form of sexual contact (such as hand-to-genital contact, oral sex, or intercourse). It is estimated that approximately 17% of people between the ages of 14–49 are infected with HSV-2, with rates being

higher among women and blacks (11). Data from the National Health and Nutrition Examination Survey III indicated that over 80% of those infected with the virus were unaware they had it. *Healthy People 2020* set a goal of reducing the number of young adults with genital herpes from 17% to fewer than 9% (12).

Symptoms

For most people infected with the herpes simplex virus, the initial infection is the most severe. The first symptoms generally appear within 2 weeks after exposure (11). Symptoms vary from sores (blisters) on the mouth, rectum, and genitals, to fever and swollen glands. Symptoms may disappear and then reappear without warning. Although symptoms may flare and subside, the virus remains in the body for life.

Treatment

At present, there is no cure for herpes, but newly developed drugs show promise to prevent or shorten outbreaks of symptoms (11). Although treatment with cold-sore medication reduces the pain and irritation of the sore, rubbing anything on the blister increases the chance of spreading herpes-laden fluids to other body parts or to other people.

MAKE SURE YOU **KNOW...**

- In addition to HIV/AIDS, several other STIs are caused by viruses, including hepatitis B, HPV, and genital herpes. Some viral STIs are treatable, but none are curable.

- Hepatitis B is a liver disease that can be transmitted by sexual activity. Symptoms include jaundice, reduced appetite, nausea, and vomiting.

- The human papillomavirus (HPV) is typically spread by sexual contact; it can result in genital warts that can be treated with medication and/or surgery. Untreated HPV in women increases the risk of uterine and cervical cancer. A vaccine against some types of HPV is available.

- Herpes is a viral STI that can be transmitted through any form of sexual contact; symptoms include sores on the mouth, rectum, and genitals.

————— MasteringHealth™

Chlamydia

LO **6** Describe the cause, symptoms, diagnosis, and treatment of chlamydia.

Chlamydia is an STI caused by **bacteria** known as *Chlamydia trachomatis*. It is common among heterosexual people worldwide (13). The bacteria cause infection

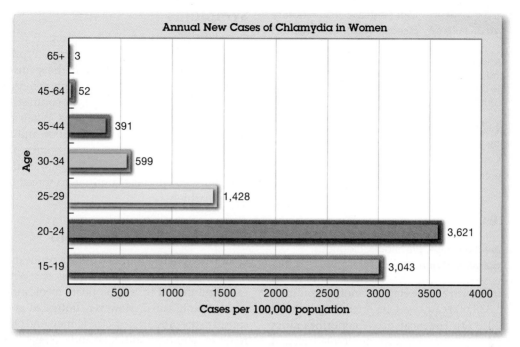

FIGURE 14.4 Females between the ages of 15 and 24 show the highest rates of chlamydia.

Source: Centers for Disease Control and Prevention. Trends in reportable sexually transmitted diseases in the United States, 2013. http://www.cdc.gov/std/stats10/trends.htm.

within the reproductive organs, and the infection is spread through vaginal, anal, and oral sex. The incidence of chlamydia infection in the United States has increased over the past 20 years, but increased screening rates contribute to the higher number of cases. A CDC report reveals that chlamydia is the most common bacterial STI in the United States, with 2.86 million new cases occurring each year (13). Equally alarming is the estimate that about 20% of all college students may have chlamydia and college-age women are the most susceptible. **FIGURE 14.4** shows the rates of chlamydia for females of all ages; high school and college-age females make up the bulk of the cases (3). The *Healthy People 2020* objective for chlamydia is to increase the number of women in high-risk groups who get screenings (12).

Symptoms

Symptoms often go unnoticed and may vary among individuals. In fact, over 75% of women and 50% of men infected do not develop symptoms and are unaware that they carry the bacteria. Early symptoms occur 7 to 21 days after infection. In women, early symptoms may include unusual vaginal discharge, burning sensation when urinating, and bleeding between menstrual periods. Later symptoms (months after initial infection) may include low back pain, abdominal pain, pain during intercourse, and low-grade fever.

Many men infected with chlamydia do not develop symptoms when first infected. However, several months later, infected men may experience an unusual discharge from the penis, burning sensation when urinating, pain in the testicles, and low-grade fever.

Diagnosis and Treatment

Chlamydia can be diagnosed based on swab or urine tests. In women, a cervical, vaginal, or urine sample can be analyzed to detect the bacteria. In men, a penile swab or urine test can be used. All sexually active women should be screened yearly, and all pregnant women should have a screening test. Early diagnosis and treatment is important to prevent potentially serious long-term health consequences.

Fortunately, chlamydia can be cured with antibiotics. If untreated, chlamydia can result in infertility in both men and women. Untreated chlamydia in women can

---

herpes General term used to describe infections caused by various types of herpes virus.

chlamydia The most common sexually transmitted infection among heterosexuals in the United States; caused by a bacterial infection within the reproductive organs.

bacteria Microorganisms that can cause infectious diseases. STIs caused by bacteria can be cured with antibiotics.

lead to **pelvic inflammatory disease (PID)**, an infection of the lining of the abdominal and pelvic cavity. Common symptoms of PID include pain in the lower abdominal cavity, fever, and menstrual irregularities. PID can lead to internal abscesses and long-lasting, chronic pain, and it can damage the fallopian tubes enough to cause infertility or increase the risk of ectopic pregnancy (3).

Gonorrhea

LO **7** Describe the cause, symptoms, diagnosis, and treatment of gonorrhea.

Gonorrhea (also known as "the clap") is another common STI. More than 333,000 cases were reported in the United States during 2013 (3). The incidence of gonorrhea ranks it as the second most common communicable bacterial infection. Only chlamydia is more prevalent. Fortunately, the rate of gonorrhea infection in the United States has declined over the past 40 years (**FIGURE 14.5**). The decline in gonorrhea may be due to improved testing and more frequent use of condoms. The *Healthy People 2020* goal for gonorrhea is to achieve a 10% reduction in the number of new cases (12).

The bacterium that causes gonorrhea is called *Neisseria gonorrhoeae;* it grows well within mucous membranes in the body. This bacterium cannot grow outside the body because it requires a warm and moist environment (8). Therefore, gonorrhea cannot be spread by contact with toilet seats, doorknobs, or other inanimate objects. However, it can be transmitted through vaginal, anal, or oral sex.

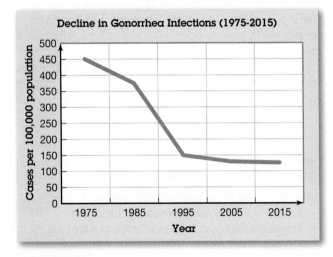

FIGURE 14.5 Reported rates of gonorrhea in the United States from 1975 to 2015.

Source: Centers for Disease Control and Prevention. Trends in reportable sexually transmitted diseases in the United States, 2015. http://www.cdc.gov/std/stats10/trends.htm.

Symptoms

Over 80% of men develop symptoms 2 to 10 days after sexual contact with an infected person. Typical symptoms include a milky discharge from the penis and painful urination (8). In some men, lymph glands in the groin become inflamed and swollen. In contrast, only 20% of infected women develop symptoms. When symptoms are present, they include painful urination and an occasional fever (8). The lack of symptoms in women poses a serious problem because women may be unaware that they have been infected and may continue to spread the disease to sexual partners.

Diagnosis and Treatment

Gonorrhea can be diagnosed using a penile or vaginal swab or a urine test. It is curable with antibiotics. When diagnosed early and treated with appropriate medication, gonorrhea can be easily cured. However, untreated gonorrhea may spread to the prostate, testicles, kidney, and bladder and can result in sterility in both men and women (3, 8). Like chlamydia, gonorrhea is a common cause of PID in women. As with all other STIs, early detection and treatment are essential to prevent serious negative health consequences.

Syphilis

LO **8** Describe the cause, symptoms, diagnosis, and treatment of syphilis and explain the stages of the disease.

Each year more than 15,000 new cases of **syphilis** are reported in the United States (3). Like chlamydia and gonorrhea, syphilis is caused by a bacterial infection. The spiral-shaped bacterium responsible for syphilis is *Treponema pallidum*. This bacterium requires a warm and moist environment, such as the genitals or the mucous membranes of the mouth, to survive.

Symptoms

The symptoms of untreated syphilis vary because the disease progresses through four stages: primary, secondary, latent, and tertiary. The early symptoms of primary syphilis include a dime-sized, painless sore called a **chancre**, located at the initial site of infection such as the penis, vaginal walls, or mouth. In both men and women, this chancre will disappear in 3–6 weeks. Secondary-stage symptoms may include a skin rash, hair loss, swollen lymph glands, and sores around the mouth or genitals. Later stages are often without symptoms. If untreated, the infected individual may spend several years in the latent stage during which the infection

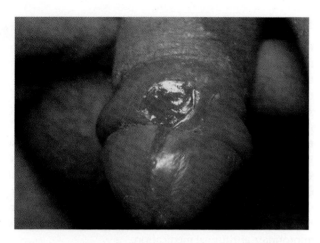

A chancre on the site of the initial infection is a symptom of primary syphilis.

slowly spreads to organs throughout the body. The final (tertiary) stage of untreated syphilis can result in heart damage, blindness, deafness, paralysis, and mental disorders.

Diagnosis and Treatment

Syphilis can be diagnosed with a blood test and can be cured by antibiotics. However, because of the progressive nature of this infection, early treatment is important to prevent serious, long-term health problems.

MAKE SURE YOU **KNOW...**

- Commons STIs caused by bacterial infections include chlamydia, gonorrhea, and syphilis. Bacterial STIs can be treated and cured with antibiotics.

- Chlamydia is the most common STI among heterosexuals. Symptoms vary among individuals; more than 75% of infected women and 50% of infected men do not develop symptoms and are unaware that they are infected.

- More than 80% of men infected with gonorrhea develop symptoms 2–10 days after sexual contact with an infected person; typical symptoms include a milky discharge from the penis and painful urination. Only 20% of infected women develop symptoms. If present, symptoms include painful urination and occasional fever.

- Syphilis infections progress through four stages, and symptoms vary depending on the stage of the infection. A chancre (painless sore) may develop during the primary stage, followed by hair loss, swollen lymph glands, and infectious sores around the mouth or genitals during the secondary stage. During the third (latent) stage, there may be no symptoms, but the infection spreads throughout the body. Tertiary (final stage) symptoms include heart and nervous system damage.

MasteringHealth™

Other Sexually Transmitted Infections

 LO **9** **Describe the cause, symptoms, diagnosis, and treatment for each of the following STIs: trichomoniasis, pubic lice, scabies, and candidiasis.**

In addition to the previously discussed STIs, numerous others occur. In this section, we present a brief discussion of four common STIs caused by organisms other than viruses or bacteria. See the Examining the Evidence box on page 384 for answers to frequently asked questions about STIs.

Trichomoniasis

Trichomonas vaginalis is a one-celled organism (protozoan) that infects the vaginal or urinary mucosa, causing a vaginal infection called **trichomoniasis**. Trichomoniasis is a common infection that affects approximately 3.7 million people in the United States (3, 15). The most common mode of transmission is by vaginal intercourse or other sexual contact with an infected person. Women can acquire the disease from infected men or women, whereas men usually acquire the disease from infected women (3). Trichomoniasis can also be contracted by prolonged exposure to moist material that harbors the protozoan (e.g., exposure to wet bathing suits or towels).

Most men and women experience symptoms of infection within days after contact with *Trichomonas vaginalis*. For women, common symptoms include a greenish-yellow vaginal discharge with a strong odor, itching of the genital area, and painful intercourse. Men may experience a discharge from the penis, burning sensation during urination, and irritation inside the penis. Trichomoniasis can be diagnosed by a simple laboratory test of vaginal or urethral fluid and treated with an oral dose of the prescription drug metronidazole (14). Although trichomoniasis is not considered a life-threatening infection, untreated trichomoniasis is associated with an increased risk of cancer.

---

pelvic inflammatory disease (PID) Inflammatory infection of the lining of the abdominal and pelvic cavity in women.

gonorrhea Sexually transmitted infection caused by the *Neisseria gonorrhoeae* bacterium; curable with antibiotics.

syphilis STI caused by the *Treponema pallidum* bacterium; curable with antibiotics.

chancre A sore that appears at the site of infection in primary-stage syphilis.

trichomoniasis STI caused by a single-celled protozoan parasite.

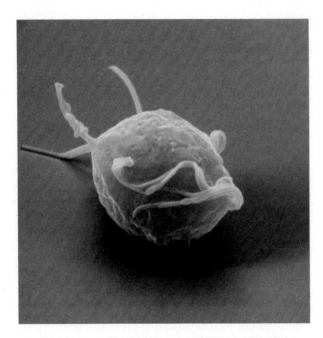

Trichomoniasis is one of the few STIs that can sometimes be transmitted without direct sexual contact. The protozoan that causes this infection can live on wet towels, bathing suits, and bedding, so sharing these items is not advised.

Pubic Lice

Pubic lice, commonly called "crabs," are usually transmitted via sexual contact but can also be spread through infected bed linen, clothes, or even toilet seats. These organisms grip pubic hair and feed on blood from tiny blood vessels in the surrounding skin. Once an infection occurs, the lice reproduce. When large numbers of lice are present, they can be seen as brown spots on pubic hairs and surrounding skin. As lice feed on blood vessels in the pubic area, they irritate the skin, causing itching and sometimes swelling. Fortunately, both over-the-counter and prescription topical medications are available that kill pubic lice. An infected individual also needs to wash all clothing and bed linen to avoid reinfection.

Scabies

Scabies is caused by a tiny mite that infects the skin between the fingers, on the wrists, under the breasts, and in the pubic area. Once an infection occurs, the female mite burrows under the skin, causing irritation and itching. Skin-to-skin contact (including sexual contact) with an infected individual can spread these parasites. Unlike pubic lice, scabies is rarely contracted from clothing, bedding, or toilet seats. A physician can diagnose scabies by scraping the infected area and performing a microscopic test to determine whether mites are present. Once diagnosed, scabies can be treated with several topical medications (2).

Candidiasis

Candidiasis is a common form of vaginitis (inflammation of the vagina) caused by the fungus *Candida albicans*. Although this fungus is normally found in small quantities in the vagina, its rapid growth can result in a "yeast infection" characterized by itching, discomfort, and a thick vaginal discharge. This fungus can be spread by sexual contact and can also manifest in the mouth and throat. Candidiasis requires different treatments depending on the location of the infection, but it is curable with the appropriate antifungal medication.

MAKE SURE YOU **KNOW...**

- Trichomoniasis is a common STI caused by a protozoan, *Trichomonas vaginalis*.

- Symptoms of trichomoniasis include a greenish-yellow vaginal discharge in women and a discharge from the penis in men. It is treatable with medication.

- Pubic lice, or "crabs," are parasites that infect the pubic area.

- Scabies is caused by a tiny mite that can infect the skin between the fingers, under the breasts, and in the pubic area.

- Candidiasis (yeast infection) is a common form of vaginitis that can also manifest in the mouth and throat.

MasteringHealth™

Reducing Your Risk for Sexually Transmitted Infections

LO **10** Outline several important actions you can take to reduce your risk for contracting STIs.

There is no cure for viral infections such as HIV, HPV, or genital herpes, and although many STIs can be treated, prevention is the best approach. The keys to preventing STIs are education and responsible action. You can assess your risk for contracting STIs with the Steps for Behavior Change box on page 385 and Laboratory 14.1. These questionnaires will help make you aware of the attitudes and behaviors that increase the risk of infection via sexual activity. The following sections highlight several steps you can take to avoid STIs.

Abstinence

Because all forms of sexual activity, including anal and oral sex, carry some risk of transmitting STIs, the only 100% effective means of prevention is abstinence.

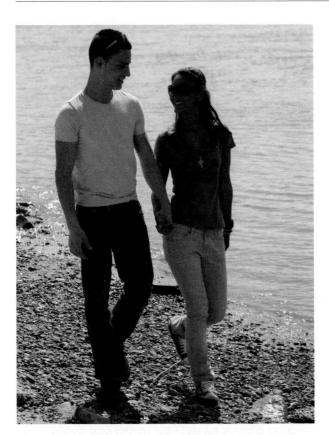

Maintaining a monogamous relationship with an STI-free partner is a strategy to prevent contracting an STI.

If abstinence is not an option, there are several strategies that can help minimize the risk of infection.

Limiting the Number of Sexual Partners

Maintaining a monogamous relationship with a sexual partner who is not infected with an STI is one way to avoid STIs. The keys to success with this strategy are that both partners be free of STIs and that the relationship remains monogamous. Failure of one member of the relationship to maintain monogamy will increase the risk of contracting an STI for *both* partners.

Limiting your number of sexual partners also decreases your risk of contracting an STI. The rationale is simple: The more sexual partners you have, the greater your odds of being exposed to an STI. Therefore, limiting the number will reduce your risk.

Using Male Latex Condoms

The pores of latex condoms are too small for most microorganisms to pass through; they therefore limit the

transmission of many STIs. Consistent and proper use of a latex condom during all sexual activity (including oral, anal, and vaginal sex) will reduce the risk of contracting and spreading an STI.

How effective are latex condoms in preventing the transmission of STIs? Studies show that use of latex condoms during sexual activities is effective against the transmission of HIV and gonorrhea in both men and women (16). Further, it appears that the use of male condoms will also reduce the risk of other STIs, including syphilis and chlamydia (3). Latex condoms will not prevent the transmission of parasites such as scabies or pubic lice, and HPV and genital herpes infections can occur in areas not covered by condoms. Therefore, although using condoms will reduce your risk for many STIs, it will not provide absolute protection against all STIs (3, 16).

Using Female Condoms

The CDC reports that female condoms are effective mechanical barriers against viruses, including HIV (17), so when used consistently and correctly, female condoms may reduce the risk of STIs including HIV (17). However, large clinical studies proving that female condoms prevent the spread of STIs have not been performed. Nonetheless, the CDC recommends that when male condoms cannot be used, sexual partners should consider the use of female condoms to reduce the risk of STIs (17).

Discussing Sexually Transmitted Infections with Sexual Partners

Prior to engaging in sexual activity with a new partner, you should talk about your concerns regarding STIs. Ask whether the person has been recently screened for STIs or has engaged in high-risk behaviors (such as having multiple sexual partners) that would increase the risk of being infected. This kind of conversation can lead to a mutual concern for preventing STIs and, in some cases, can result in the decision to refrain from sexual activity until medical screening has been completed.

Avoiding Drugs and Alcohol

The use of psychoactive drugs and alcohol prior to engaging in sexual activity can impair your judgment and increase your risk of engaging in risky sexual activity and/or failing to use condoms during sex. Because drugs

pubic lice STI caused by a parasitic insect that grips the hair in the pubic area; also called "crabs."

scabies Infection caused by a parasitic mite that can burrow under the skin between the fingers, on the wrists, under the breasts, and in the pubic area.

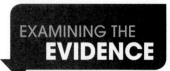

Frequently Asked Questions About STIs

What Percent of College Students Are Sexually Active?

Although the majority of students report being sexually active at some point in college, not all students are. Data from the National Center for Health Statistics indicate that the number of young adults who report being sexually active is between 53% and 76%.

What Is the Incidence, Prevalence, and Cost of STIs in the United States?

The annual incidence (number of new infections) of all STIs in the United States is approximately 20 million new cases (3). The prevalence (number of total infections) is estimated to be approximately 110 million (3). The estimated annual medical costs to treat these infections is about $16 billion (3). These large numbers serve as a reminder that STIs remain a major health and financial burden.

Who Should Get Tested for STIs?

Anyone who is at risk for STIs should get tested. You are at risk if you have had unprotected sex with anyone who has not been involved in a long-term, mutually monogamous relationship with you; either you or your partner has had unprotected sex with other people during the past several years; you have shared needles or syringes with anyone for injecting drugs; or you received a blood transfusion before 1985.

Getting tested for STIs if you are at risk is important because many people carrying HIV don't know they are infected, and because early treatment can improve the outcome of the infection. Blood tests are available from several sources, including any physician, your student health clinic, Planned Parenthood, and your local public health department.

Home testing kits exist for certain STIs, including HIV, chlamydia, and gonorrhea. For home testing, you collect a urine sample or an oral or genital swab and send it to a laboratory for analysis. The benefit of home testing is that samples are collected in the privacy of your home without requiring a doctor visit. When choosing a home testing kit, select only those clearly marked as FDA-approved.

Note that home-test samples may have a higher rate of false-positive results, indicating the presence of an STI that you really don't have. If you test positive using a home kit, visit your doctor or a public health clinic to confirm the results. If home-test results are negative, but you are experiencing symptoms, you should see a health-care provider to confirm your status.

and alcohol weaken your ability to reason, you should refrain from abusing these substances to reduce your risk of contracting STIs.

Other Protective Measures

There are several other steps that you can take to reduce your risk:

- Inspect yourself and your partner for signs of STIs.
- Do not share needles, scissors, or razors.
- Wash your genitals before and after sex.
- Do not handle towels, wet bedding, or underclothing that has been in contact with an individual who may be infected with an STI.

Note that vaginal spermicides containing nonoxynol 9 are not effective in preventing most STIs, including gonorrhea, HIV, and chlamydia. In fact, evidence indicates that nonoxynol 9 can increase the risk of contracting STIs by irritating the vaginal or anal lining and increasing the ease of entry of infectious agents into the body. Therefore, the CDC recommends avoiding condoms containing nonoxynol 9.

If you suspect that you have been exposed to an STI, you should contact your physician immediately for medical screening. Never try to diagnose an STI yourself, and do not delay seeking medical attention if you develop symptoms of any STI. Early diagnosis and treatment are essential to ensure that an STI does not lead to long-term health problems. If you learn that you are infected, you should immediately inform all of your sexual partners, past and present. Failing to tell a partner about an infection increases the risk of the spread of STIs to others.

live it!

ASSESS YOURSELF

Assess your relationship with the *How Healthy Is Your Relationship?* Take Charge of Your Health! Worksheet online at MasteringHealth™.

live it!

ASSESS YOURSELF

Assess your contraceptive choices with the *Choosing a Contraceptive* Take Charge of Your Health! Worksheet online at MasteringHealth™.

steps ➤ FOR BEHAVIOR CHANGE

Are you at increased risk for a sexually transmitted infection?

Answer the following questions to assess whether any of your behaviors put you at increased risk for an STI.

Y	N	
☐	☐	I sometimes end up having sex with someone without intending to, on the spur of the moment.
☐	☐	I am an intravenous drug user, and I have shared used needles with other drug users.
☐	☐	I am too uncomfortable to discuss STIs and sexual history with new sexual partners, so I do not address the topic.
☐	☐	I don't worry about using condoms during sexual intercourse.
☐	☐	I haven't been tested for STIs because I know there's no chance I have one, even though I am or have been sexually active.

If you answered yes to any of the above, then you could do more to protect yourself from an STI.

Tips to Lessen Your Risk of Contracting STIs

Tomorrow, you will:

☑ Have a candid talk with a sexual partner or potential sexual partner about your sexual histories.

☑ Purchase condoms if you are sexually active and not already using them regularly.

Within the next 2 weeks, you will:

☑ Get tested if there's even a slight chance of your having an STI. If you are sexually active, have periodic medical examinations that include blood, urine, and/or pelvic exams.

☑ Always use a condom.

By the end of the semester, you will:

☑ Ask yourself whether or not you are willing to engage in sex and under what circumstances it would be acceptable before entering a situation where spontaneous sex may occur. If you do decide to have sex, make sure you are protected.

☑ Always discuss your sexual histories with a new sexual partner. Remember that you're having sex not just with that person; you're having sex with everyone he or she has had sex with.

MAKE SURE YOU **KNOW...**

▪ Avoiding sexual activity (abstinence) is the only absolute means of preventing STIs. If abstinence is not an option, then monogamy or limiting your sexual partners is the next best strategy. Be sure to discuss STIs and sexual history with all sexual partners.

▪ Using latex condoms will reduce the risk of contracting an STI.

▪ Avoid using drugs or alcohol prior to engaging in sexual activities.

MasteringHealth™

study plan
Customize your study plan—and master your health!—
in the Study Area of **MasteringHealth.**

summary

hear it! STUDY REVIEW

To hear an MP3 Chapter Summary, scan here or visit
the Study Area in MasteringHealth™.

LO **1** ■ Every year, millions of U.S. residents are
infected by one or more sexually transmitted
infections (STIs).

■ Some of the most common sexually transmitted
infections include HIV/AIDS, hepatitis B, human
papillomavirus, genital herpes, chlamydia,
gonorrhea, syphilis, trichomoniasis, pubic lice,
and scabies.

LO **2** ■ Infection with the human immunodeficiency
virus (HIV) is the cause of AIDS, a fatal disease
for which there is presently no cure.

■ HIV is transmitted via infected body fluids.

LO **3** ■ STIs caused by viruses are not curable and remain
in the body for life.

■ Hepatitis B is a liver disease caused by a viral
infection that can be transmitted via sexual
activity.

LO **4** ■ Some strains of human papillomavirus (HPV)
cause genital warts. Untreated HPV is a primary
cause of cervical cancer.

LO **5** ■ Herpes is caused by a virus that can be transmitted
sexually; HSV-1 produces mouth sores, and HSV-2
can produce genital sores.

LO **6** ■ Chlamydia is a bacterial STI that is the most common among heterosexual adults in the United
States; often, it does not produce symptoms.

LO **7** ■ Gonorrhea (the "clap") is the second most common sexually transmitted bacterial infection.

LO **8** ■ Syphilis is a bacterial STI that progresses in four
stages; untreated, it can result in damage to the
heart and nervous system.

LO **9** ■ Trichomoniasis, pubic lice, scabies, and candidiasis (yeast infection) are STIs that can be spread
through vaginal, oral, and anal contact.

LO **10** ■ Most STIs can be avoided by abstaining from sex
or following safe-sex guidelines, including limiting
your number of sexual partners, using condoms,
and avoiding high-risk behaviors such as drug
or alcohol abuse.

study questions

review it! QUIZZES

Find more review questions online at MasteringHealth™.

LO **1** 1. Name the five most common STIs in the
United States. Which of these are currently
incurable?

LO **2** 2. Explain how HIV is transmitted.

3. Describe the three stages of AIDS, beginning
with infection with HIV and leading to the
final stage.

LO **3** 4. List the common symptoms of hepatitis B. Are
symptoms similar in men and women?

5. What is the treatment for a hepatitis B infection?

LO **4** 6. Genital warts are caused by
a. human papillomavirus (HPV).
b. hepatitis B.

c. herpes virus.
d. a single-celled protozoan parasite.

7. List the common symptoms of HPV. Are symptoms
similar in men and women?

8. What is the treatment for HPV infection?

9. Explain the relationship between HPV and uterine
and cervical cancer.

LO **5** 10. List the common symptoms of oral and genital herpes. Are symptoms similar in men and
women?

11. What is the treatment for a herpes simplex virus
infection?

LO **6** 12. List the common symptoms of chlamydia.
Are symptoms similar in men and women?

13. What is the treatment for chlamydia?

LO **7** 14. List the common symptoms of gonorrhea.
Are symptoms similar in men and women?

15. What is the treatment for gonorrhea?

LO ⑧ 16. Which of the following STIs is not caused by a virus?
    a. HPV
    b. hepatitis B
    c. genital herpes
    d. syphilis

17. Which stage of syphilis is characterized by a skin lesion called a chancre?
    a. stage 1—primary stage
    b. stage 2—secondary stage
    c. stage 3—latent stage
    d. stage 4—tertiary stage

18. List the symptoms associated with each stage of syphilis. Are symptoms similar in men and women?

19. What is the treatment for syphilis?

LO ⑨ 20. What is the common characteristic of trichomoniasis, scabies, and pubic lice?
    a. These STIs can be prevented by using a condom during sexual activity.
    b. These STIs are caused by parasites.
    c. These STIs are found in men only.
    d. Once you have had one of these STIs, you can never get it again.

21. List the symptoms associated with trichomoniasis, scabies, pubic lice, and candidiasis. Are symptoms similar in men and women?

22. How are trichomoniasis, scabies, pubic lice, and candidiasis treated?

LO ⑩ 23. Outline ways to reduce your risk of contracting STIs, and explain which population groups should get tested.

suggested reading

Centers for Disease Control and Prevention. Sexually transmitted diseases. Information from the CDC. 2015. www.cdc.gov/std

Donatelle, R. and P. Ketcham. *Access to Health*, 14th ed. San Francisco: Pearson/Benjamin Cummings, 2015.

Greenberg, J. S., C. E. Bruess, and S. Oswalt. *Exploring the Dimensions of Human Sexuality*, 5th ed. Burlington, MA: Jones and Bartlett, 2013.

McAnulty, R. (Ed.). *Sex in College*. Santa Barbara, CA: Praeger, 2012.

helpful weblinks

do it! WEBLINKS

For links to the organizations and websites listed, visit MasteringHealth™.

American Medical Association

Contains information about a wide variety of medical problems, including STIs. **www.ama-assn.org**

American Social Health Organization

Provides information, resources, and referrals in regard to STIs. **www.ashastd.org**

Centers for Disease Control and Prevention

Offers comprehensive information about STIs and prevention. **www.cdc.gov/std**

UNAIDS United Nations Program on HIV/AIDS

Information about HIV/AIDS worldwide. **www.unaids.org/en**

WebMD

Contains information about a wide variety of medical problems, including STIs. **www.webmd.com**

laboratory 14.1

do it! LABS
Complete Lab 14.1 online in the
study area of **MasteringHealth.com**

Name _____ Date _____

Inventory of Attitudes and Behaviors toward Sexually Transmitted Infections

This laboratory is designed to help you identify attitudes and behaviors that increase your risk of contracting an STI.

Read the following statements and determine whether each statement is true or false for you. Then score your answers and compute your level of risk.

	True	False
1. I maintain a monogamous sexual relationship with a trusted partner or I am not currently in a sexual relationship.	_____	_____
2. I never engage in sexual activities without using a condom.	_____	_____
3. I never use alcohol or drugs prior to sexual activities.	_____	_____
4. I am knowledgeable about the health risks associated with STIs.	_____	_____
5. I have a thorough knowledge of how all STIs are transmitted.	_____	_____
6. I do not share needles or syringes to inject drugs.	_____	_____
7. I am concerned about the risk of contracting an STI.	_____	_____
8. I always discuss STIs and safe sex with new partners prior to having sexual relations.	_____	_____
9. I always avoid sexual contact if I believe there is any risk of contracting an STI.	_____	_____
10. I believe that responsible safe sex is one of the best ways to reduce the chances of getting an STI.	_____	_____

SCORING AND INTERPRETATION

Count the number of "False" answers, and calculate your risk level as follows:

0 "False" answers = low risk for STI
1–3 "False" answers = high risk for STI
4 or more "False" answers = very high risk for STI

After calculating your risk, review the statements that you answered "False," and take action to correct this attitude or behavior. Answer the following questions to help you evaluate your sexual practices and think about STI prevention.

1. List three ways to bring up the subject of STIs with a new partner. How would you ask whether he or she has been exposed to any STIs or engaged in any risky behaviors?

_____

_____

_____

2. List three ways to bring up the subject of condom use with your partner. How might you convince someone to use a condom who does not want to?

_____

_____

_____

3. If you had an STI in the past that you can potentially pass on (e.g., herpes), how would you tell your partner(s), and what precautions would you take during each sexual encounter?

_____

_____

_____

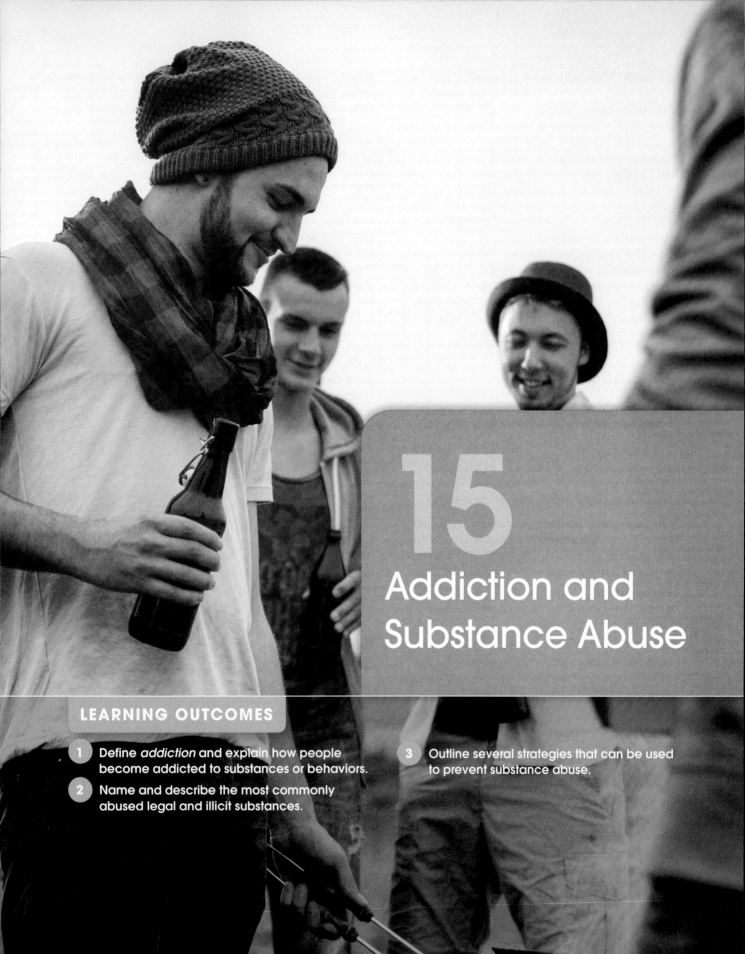

15

Addiction and Substance Abuse

1 Define *addiction* and explain how people become addicted to substances or behaviors.

2 Name and describe the most commonly abused legal and illicit substances.

3 Outline several strategies that can be used to prevent substance abuse.

THE MISUSE AND ABUSE of prescription and over-the-counter drugs in the United States remains an ongoing public health problem, and the abuse of both legal and illegal substances is common in our country and worldwide. Substance abuse can lead to addiction and negative consequences for individuals and societies. Estimates of the overall costs of substance abuse in the United States, including lost productivity, impaired health, and crime-related costs, exceeds $600 billion annually (1). Therefore, preventing substance abuse is an important goal for the nation.

Successful prevention involves public education about the negative consequences of specific drugs and the implementation of strategies to eliminate risk factors for abuse. In this chapter, we will discuss the nature of substance abuse and addiction, commonly used drugs, and strategies for prevention.

What Is Addiction?

 LO **1** Define *addiction* and explain how people become addicted to substances or behaviors.

The term **addiction** refers to a chronic psychological and physical dependence on a substance or practice that is beyond voluntary control (1). Specific addictive behaviors are often associated with the following traits (2):

- **Reinforcement leading to craving.** Repeated behaviors produce pleasurable emotional states that reinforce the behavior. This repeated reinforcement leads to a craving to engage in a particular behavior.

- **Loss of control.** Addictive behaviors lead to a loss of self-control, and the individual loses the ability to resist engaging in the activity.

- **Escalation.** Many addictive behaviors are associated with an increased need for the behavior. As addictive behavior is repeated, higher levels of the substance or activity are required to provide the same level of satisfaction.

- **Negative outcomes.** In all cases, addictive, unhealthy behaviors are associated with negative consequences, such as impairment in physical or mental health.

Because **denial** is often a characteristic of addiction, many people won't see their behaviors as destructive or seek treatment on their own. Family members, friends, or coworkers may need to persuade the user to undergo screening for addiction. In all cases, preventing an addiction is much easier than treating it.

Addiction Can Involve a Substance or Behavior

Almost anything can be addicting. In addition to substances such as drugs, alcohol, and tobacco, people can become addicted to behaviors such as gambling, Internet usage, pornography, sex, online/video gaming, eating, texting, and exercising (see Examining the Evidence on page 392).

Addiction occurs when a person loses the ability to control his or her behavior. For example, gambling addicts are unable to cut back on or stop gambling. They become preoccupied and experience frequent thoughts about their gambling experiences. An estimated 3 million American adults are compulsive gamblers. Compulsive gambling is classified as an impulse-control disorder (3), but it is similar to gaming and other addictive behaviors because the individual cannot resist the temptation to gamble. In men, compulsive gambling typically starts in adolescence, while women tend to start gambling later in life (3).

Compulsive shoppers and spenders share the same characteristics as compulsive gamblers. They shop to feel better, but the compulsive spending ultimately makes them feel worse. People with this disorder often have clothing and possessions that they have never used, with the price tags still attached. They are often in denial about the problem, and if family or friends complain, they hide their purchases and evidence of their spending such as credit card and bank records.

Another potentially addictive behavior is playing video games. Time spent playing video games does not necessarily qualify as an addiction, but an individual who cannot control the impulse to game has become addicted. Gaming becomes an escape from real-life problems, and the individual withdraws from other activities and social networks. The isolation that the person experiences can jeopardize jobs and relationships as he or she spends more and more time gaming.

Addiction Can Be Physical and/or Psychological

Addictions to drugs or alcohol often begin when an individual experiences a problem, discomfort, or some form of emotional or physical pain and looks for something to make him or her feel better. For example, you may miss friends and family when you move away from home to attend college. Establishing new friendships takes time and may involve an occasional rejection. Someone who feels like an outsider in a new environment or has been rejected by a person or group may turn to drugs or alcohol to ease the loneliness or the sting of rejection. At first, the drugs or alcohol seem to work because they dull the pain. As the person continues taking the substance, it may start to feel like the solution to their discomfort. Soon, **dependence** on the substance becomes the coping strategy for other painful or uncomfortable situations.

When drugs or alcohol are used on a regular basis, the body builds up a **tolerance** to them and larger amounts of

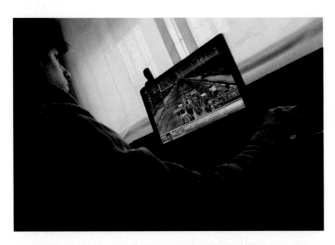

Not being able to control the amount of time spent playing video games or surfing the Internet can indicate an addiction to these behaviors.

the substance are required to achieve the same effects. Eventually, addiction results as the body cannot feel "normal" (physically and/or psychologically) without the substance. Because addiction can be a chronic relapsing disorder—meaning you tend to fall back into old addictive behaviors even after treatment—it is important to seek help and break the cycle as soon as possible.

The most serious forms of addiction involve **chemical dependence** on drugs or alcohol. This type of dependence means the body will experience physical **withdrawal symptoms** when the substance is no longer consumed. By the time a user develops a physical dependence, his or her body craves the substance and needs it to maintain equilibrium. Withdrawal symptoms may include restlessness, bone and muscle pain, vomiting, and diarrhea. Such symptoms usually peak between 24 and 48 hours after stopping intake and may last a week to several months. The severity of withdrawal symptoms depends on the level of addiction and the substance(s) involved. Drugs known to cause a high degree of physical dependence include nicotine, cocaine, and alcohol.

Causes of Addiction

Addictions can arise from numerous causes. Drugs vary in their potential to cause dependence, and some drugs such as alcohol, heroin, and cocaine can result in addiction more quickly than others. Similarly, using tobacco products poses a great risk for dependence, because nicotine is a highly addictive drug. By contrast, drugs such as marijuana and codeine are relatively less addictive (7). In some cases, addictive behaviors trigger the release of chemicals (neurotransmitters such as dopamine) in the brain, leading to a psychological "rush," or the sensation of pleasure (8).

In addition to the type of drug used, genetics, psychological makeup, and social factors also influence the risk of developing drug dependence. Research indicates that differences in brain chemistry and metabolism make some individuals more vulnerable to drug dependence (8). At present, the precise differences in brain chemistry and metabolism that contribute to increased risk of dependence remain unclear, and this topic remains an active area of research.

Personal characteristics such as poor coping skills, social environment (spending time with people who use drugs), and heredity can also play a role in the development of an addiction. Psychological risk factors for drug dependence include an inability to cope with stress or rejection, a strong need for excitement, and a tendency toward impulsive behavior. People may turn to drugs to avoid coping with stress, rejection, or depression. Social risk factors such as easy access to drugs, strong peer pressure, drug use in the family, and a low education level increase the risk of developing a dependence on drugs.

Drug use and abuse occurs in people of all ages, education and income levels, and ethnic groups. However, research shows that some people are more likely to try illegal drugs and are consequently at greater risk for abuse. For example, adolescents with risk-taking personalities are at high risk for experimenting with drugs (9). In contrast, drug use is less common in individuals who are independent thinkers and are not easily influenced by their peers. Children and teens who attend school regularly and earn good grades are less likely to try illegal drugs.

Although brain chemistry, personality traits, and social factors play a role in the development of some addictions, people are ultimately responsible for their own behavior and must take ownership of any addictive behaviors. Making a personal decision to not experiment with potentially addictive substances or behaviors is the key to prevention. In addition, having the ability to recognize the difference between a healthy habit and an addictive, unhealthy behavior is crucial.

see it!

ABC VIDEOS

Watch the "Woman's Shopping Addiction Revealed" ABC News Video online at MasteringHealth™.

---

addiction Habitual psychological and physical dependence on a substance or behavior.

denial Unconscious defense mechanism used to avoid facing painful or difficult circumstances or problems.

dependence A compulsive or chronic need for a substance or behavior.

tolerance Situation in which a drug/alcohol user requires increasingly larger amounts of the substance to experience the effects.

chemical dependence Physical and psychological habituation to a substance, such as alcohol or drugs.

withdrawal symptoms Symptoms that occur after stopping or reducing the intake of an addictive substance.

EXAMINING THE EVIDENCE

Behavior Addictions

Sex, work, and exercise are three behaviors that are a normal part of life. However, there are situations when participation in these activities becomes unhealthy. Abuse of or addiction to these behaviors can be associated with an impulse control problem. Such addictions are similar to substance addictions. Individuals need the behavior to feel "normal," and a tolerance develops. There can be negative effects on relationships, school, employment, finances, and self-esteem. Treatment involving psychological counseling and support groups is typically needed to address these problems.

Sex

Sexual addiction can have a significant impact on the lives of the individuals involved. Risk-seeking is associated with sexual addiction, and individuals are likely to participate in risky and potentially illegal behaviors, such as exhibitionism or prostitution. Risky sexual behavior does not mean one will become a sex offender, but individuals involved in risky behavior are not likely to have healthy monogamous sexual relationships because they seek the immediate gratification of sexual activity. Getting past denial is the first step toward treatment. Unfortunately, acknowledgment of the problem often does not occur until there are significant consequences such as the loss of a marriage or relationship. Addressing the addiction involves helping the individual develop a healthy perspective on sexual behavior. Treatment can include individual counseling, support groups, and family counseling. Medication might be needed to help reduce compulsive behaviors. Warning signs include a pattern of one-night stands, persistent use of pornography, compulsive masturbation, multiple affairs, and participation in phone or cybersex.

Work

Work addiction syndrome (WAS) is the term used to describe excessive and compulsive work habits. The term "workaholic" is often applied to this behavior. WAS is different from the positive behavior of being highly motivated and working hard to achieve goals. The true "workaholic" is a person who is compulsive in regard to his or her work habits. He or she may have low self-esteem, continually seek approval, and be overly submissive to those in authority. Perfectionism is also common. Such individuals may feel out of control in other areas of life, so they pour themselves into work to have control over one aspect. Those with WAS hide the truth about work habits and may even embellish their work successes. Work is also used as a means of escape from real-world issues such as family problems. Relationships are neglected and therefore suffer. Health also suffers due to stress, lack of sleep, and often the use of substances to increase energy level. Treatment can include individual and family counseling, support groups, and behavior change strategies to develop better work-life balance.

Exercise

While regular exercise is essential for health, too much exercise can be harmful. Exercise addiction describes exercise participation that is compulsive and excessive and has a negative impact on the individual's life. These habits might be driven by sport performance, weight loss, or body image. Exercise addicts experience stress, anxiety, and depressive symptoms when they are unable to exercise. They might also have an unrealistic perception of gaining weight or losing muscle mass when an exercise session is missed. This addiction may coexist with an eating disorder, but this is not always the case. Exercise addicts are at increased risk for overuse injuries and will exercise even when sick or injured. There is the potential for the use of steroids or other ergogenic aids to improve performance or body image. Exercise is often prioritized above family, friends, work, or school. Learning to develop healthy exercise habits and realistic expectations about exercise results are important in preventing exercise addiction. Engaging in group exercise is also a good strategy, as it provides accountability. Treatment involves counseling, which could also address any other issues such as substance abuse or an eating disorder.

Substance Use versus Substance Abuse

An individual can abuse a substance even if there is no full-blown addiction. There are many substances that are misused and abused without necessarily leading to addiction. In fact, you can think of the levels of drug use as a continuum, with complete abstinence at one end, progressing to occasional use, then to abuse, leading eventually to addiction. **Substance abuse** occurs when use of a drug interferes with other areas of one's life (academics, work, personal relationships) which can lead to legal or financial issues.

The American Psychiatric Association defines substance abuse as one or more of the following traits:

- Recurrent drug use, resulting in failure to perform major responsibilities at work, home, or school

- Continued drug use despite social or personal problems caused by the effects of the drug

- Recurrent drug use in situations where the drug poses a physical danger to the individual (e.g., using before driving)

- Recurrent legal problems associated with drug use

Many people who engage in intermittent drug use may not exhibit any of these traits on a regular basis. However, intermittent drug use has been shown to lead to drug abuse and is a warning sign to stop the behavior before the problem escalates.

MAKE SURE YOU **KNOW**...

- Addiction is a compulsive psychological and/or physical need for a drug or a particular behavior.

- In addition to drugs, alcohol, and tobacco, people can become addicted to video games, gambling, sex, shopping, using the Internet, and other behaviors.

- Drugs vary in their potential to cause dependence. Highly addictive drugs include nicotine, cocaine, and heroin.

- Addictions are often the result of several causes, including poor coping skills, environment, and heredity. Factors that determine risk for addiction are the type of drug used, genetics, psychological makeup, and social factors.

- Recognizing the difference between a healthy habit and an addictive, unhealthy behavior is important in preventing addiction.

—————————— MasteringHealth™

What Substances Are Commonly Abused?

LO **2** **Name and describe the most commonly abused legal and illicit substances.**

Millions of Americans abuse alcohol and misuse or abuse drugs, including marijuana, cocaine, heroin, hallucinogens, inhalants, prescription pain relievers, tranquilizers, stimulants, and sedatives (10). **Illicit drugs** are either illegal drugs or legal substances that are sold illegally. In addition to psychological and/or physical dependence,

live it!

ASSESS YOURSELF

Assess your drug I.Q. with the *Test Your Drug I.Q.* Take Charge of Your Health! Worksheet online at MasteringHealth™.

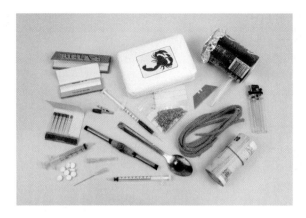

Psychoactive drugs can be ingested, smoked, injected, or inhaled. Drugs that are injected or inhaled enter the blood more quickly than drugs that are ingested, so their effects are felt more quickly.

abuse of alcohol or recreational drugs increases your risk of accidents and may damage your health.

Psychoactive Drugs

Any drug that produces an altered state of consciousness—feeling "high"—is a **psychoactive drug**. Soon after ingestion, injection, or inhalation, psychoactive drugs cross the blood-brain barrier. Users typically report feeling a surge of a pleasurable sensation (a "rush"). The intensity of the rush depends on how much of the drug is taken and how rapidly the drug enters the brain. Drugs that enter the brain rapidly, such as opiates (including heroin and morphine), are particularly potent. Alcohol, nicotine, opiates, marijuana, hallucinogens, and numerous other drugs are psychoactive drugs (see **TABLE 15.1** on page 394).

Examples of Psychoactive Drugs The most commonly abused drugs in the United States among individuals between the ages of 18–25 are marijuana, prescription medications, cocaine, Ecstasy, alcohol, and tobacco (10). **Marijuana** is the most commonly used illicit drug in the United States (1). It consists of dried leaves, flowers, stems, and seeds from the *Cannabis* (hemp) plant and contains the psychoactive chemical delta-9-tetrahydrocannabinol

---

substance abuse Use of illegal drugs, the inappropriate use of legal drugs, and/or the repeated use of drugs to produce pleasure, to alleviate stress, or to alter or avoid reality.

illicit drugs Illegal drugs or legal substances that are sold illegally.

psychoactive drugs Pharmacological agents that alter mood, behavior, and/or cognitive processes.

marijuana Psychoactive plant mixture (stems, leaves, or seeds) from *Cannabis sativa* or *Cannabis indica*.

TABLE 15.1 ■ Commonly Abused Drugs and Their Effects

Drug Classification and Names	How Administered	Intoxication Effects	Health Effects
Opiates			
Heroin	Injected, smoked, snorted	Pain relief, euphoria, drowsiness, staggering gait	Nausea, constipation, confusion, sedation, respiratory depression and arrest, tolerance, addiction, unconsciousness, coma, death
Opium	Swallowed, smoked	Same as for heroin	Same as for heroin
Stimulants			
Cocaine	Injected, smoked, snorted	Increased heart rate, blood pressure, metabolism; feelings of exhilaration, energy; increased mental alertness; increased temperature	Rapid or irregular heartbeat, reduced appetite, weight loss, heart failure, nervousness, insomnia
Methamphetamine	Injected, swallowed, smoked, snorted	Same as for cocaine, plus aggression, violence, psychotic behavior	Same as for cocaine, plus memory loss, cardiac and neurological damage; impaired memory and learning; tolerance, addiction
Nicotine	Smoked, snorted, taken in snuff and spit tobacco	Same as for cocaine	Same as for cocaine, plus adverse pregnancy outcomes, chronic lung disease, cardiovascular disease, stroke, cancer, tolerance, addiction
Ecstasy, also known as MDMA (methylene dioxymethamphetamine)	Taken orally in tablet form	Feelings of well-being, mental stimulation; distortion in time and other sensory perceptions	Increase in body temperature, leading to kidney failure; increase in heart rate and blood pressure; heart wall stress
Cannabinoid			
Marijuana	Swallowed or smoked	Euphoria, slowed thinking and reaction time, confusion, impaired balance and coordination	Cough, frequent respiratory infections, impaired memory and learning, increased heart rate, anxiety, panic attacks, tolerance, addiction
Hallucinogen			
Lysergic acid diethylamide, also known as LSD	Swallowed, absorbed through mouth tissues	Altered state of perception and feeling	Persisting perception disorder (flashbacks); increased body temperature, heart rate, and blood pressure; loss of appetite; sleeplessness; numbness, weakness, tremors
Narcotic			
Dextromethorphan, also known as DXM	Swallowed (found in some cough and cold medications)	Distorted visual perceptions to complete dissociative effects	At high doses, memory loss, numbness, nausea/vomiting
Hormones			
Anabolic steroids	Injected, swallowed, applied to the skin	No intoxication	Hypertension, blood clotting, and cholesterol changes; liver cysts and cancer; kidney cancer; hostility and aggression; acne; in adolescents: premature stoppage of growth; in men: prostate cancer, reduced sperm production, shrunken testicles, breast enlargement; in women: menstrual irregularities, development of beard and other masculine characteristics
Inhalants			
Laughing gas, whippets	Inhaled through nose or mouth	Stimulation, loss of inhibition; headache, nausea/vomiting, slurred speech, loss of motor coordination	Unconsciousness, cramps, weight loss, muscle weakness, depression, memory impairment, damage to cardiovascular and nervous systems, sudden death

Source: Based on National Institute on Drug Abuse. Commonly abused drugs. www.drugabuse.gov/drugs-abuse/commonly-abused-drugs/commonly-abused-drugs-chart.

EXAMINING THE EVIDENCE   Is Marijuana Medicine?

The marijuana plant contains chemicals that may prove useful in treating the symptoms of several illnesses (1, 15), and proponents are fighting for legalization of marijuana for medical purposes to treat pain and nausea caused by HIV/AIDS, cancer, and other conditions. As of early 2015, 23 states and the District of Columbia have legalized marijuana use for certain medical conditions.

The term "medical marijuana" is used to refer to the whole unprocessed plant or crude extracts. However, the FDA has not approved marijuana as a medication for two reasons:

■ There is not enough research demonstrating that the benefits of marijuana outweigh the safety concerns (1, 15). The known safety concerns of marijuana include impairment of short-term memory, altered decision making, and psychological effects that include severe anxiety (paranoia) and psychosis.

■ For FDA approval, a drug must have well-defined ingredients that are consistent from one dose to the next. The marijuana plant contains hundreds of chemical compounds that vary in concentration from plant-to-plant, so marijuana does not meet this requirement.

Scientists have investigated the active chemicals in marijuana (cannabinoids) believed to have medical applications. This research led to the development of two FDA-approved drugs designed to harness the therapeutic effects of cannabinoids while eliminating the potentially harmful side effects associated with smoking marijuana (1). Two cannabinoids that are of interest therapeutically are 9-tetrahydrocannabinol (THC) and cannabidiol (CBD) (1). THC is a psychoactive drug that stimulates appetite and reduces nausea. It may also reduce pain and inflammation; for these reasons, the THC-based medication dronabinol (brand name Marinol®) was approved by the FDA for treatment of nausea caused by chemotherapy and muscle wasting caused by AIDS (1). Nabilone (brand name Cesamet®) is also FDA-approved; it contains a synthetic cannabinoid similar to THC and is also used for nausea caused by cancer drug treatment (1).

CBD is a nonpsychoactive cannabinoid that reduces pain and inflammation and may have other therapeutic applications (1). Research funded by the National Institutes of Health is investigating the therapeutic uses of THC, CBD, and other cannabinoids to treat autoimmune disease, cancer, inflammation, pain, seizures, substance use disorders, and other mental disorders (1, 15).

(THC). The higher the THC concentration, the greater the psychoactive effect. THC content varies between 0.5% and 3%, with the average percentage of THC in marijuana sold in the United States being about 1% (11). Marijuana is smoked in pipes or in hand-rolled cigarettes (joints) or cigars (blunts). It can also be mixed in food or brewed as tea. Effects are generally felt within 15 to 30 minutes and disappear within 2 to 3 hours.

Marijuana is classified as a stimulant, and its immediate effects are increased heart rate and blood pressure, bloodshot eyes, and dry mouth and throat. Evidence suggests that short-term use increases the risk of stroke in male adolescent users (12). Use of marijuana also impairs motor coordination and may increase your risk of accidents. Further, marijuana use alters the normal function of memory centers in the brain. This memory loss resembles that observed as the brain ages. It is not yet clear if these changes in function put long-term marijuana users at risk for early mental disorders. On the other hand, marijuana is increasingly being used medically to treat the side effects of several diseases (see Examining the Evidence).

The use of **cocaine** ("coke") in the United States increased dramatically during the 1980s, and today more than 5 million Americans use the drug. Between 1990 and 2000, Americans spent $35 billion to $70 billion yearly on cocaine (13). In recent years, this number has dropped significantly to $28 billion per year. One survey suggests that as many as 6% of college students have experimented with cocaine, which makes cocaine the third most widely used drug among college students (13).

Cocaine is a powerful stimulant derived from the leaves of the coca plant, which grows primarily in the Andes Mountains in South America. Cocaine is extracted from the coca leaves, producing a white powder. Varying the extraction process can produce several different forms of cocaine, such as crack cocaine, rock cocaine, or freebase cocaine.

Common methods of taking cocaine include snorting, smoking, and intravenous injection. All routes of administration result in a rapid and short-lived high that lasts from 5 to 20 minutes. Cocaine is a highly addictive drug; when

---

cocaine Powerful stimulant derived from the leaves of the South American coca plant.

the initial high disappears, the user wants more. Spending over $1,500 per day for cocaine is not uncommon for an addict; job loss and financial ruin often result.

Cocaine is both an anesthetic and a central nervous system stimulant that increases heart rate and blood pressure. Other effects include a feeling of euphoria, heightened self-confidence, and increased alertness (14). In large doses, cocaine is extremely dangerous, and many people have died as a result of an overdose.

"Club drugs" are a group of popular psychoactive drugs. These include Ecstasy, gamma-hydroxybutyrate (GHB), ketamine, Rohypnol, methamphetamine, and LSD. The use of these drugs can cause serious health problems and in some cases can be fatal. When club drugs are taken in combination with alcohol, the dangers are multiplied.

Methamphetamine (meth) is a very addictive stimulant; it is chemically related to amphetamines, but is longer lasting, more potent, and more harmful to the central nervous system (CNS) (9). Methamphetamine is legally available only through a prescription that cannot be refilled. Illegal meth is manufactured in small, crude laboratories, where its production endangers not only those who "cook" it, but also neighbors and the environment. Short-term effects of methamphetamine use include increased wakefulness, increased physical activity, decreased appetite, increased respiration, rapid heartbeat, increased blood pressure, and hyperthermia. Cardiovascular collapse and death can occur from a single dose.

In addition to the street drugs that we often associate with drug abuse, there are numerous prescription medications that can also be highly addictive. One example is the prescription painkiller OxyContin. The illegal use of this habit-forming drug, which was developed to ease the suffering of patients with diseases such as cancer, has grown markedly across the United States. Its addictive qualities have led to abuse among some recreational users; many have overdosed, and others have turned to crime to feed their expensive habit.

Some people also misuse over-the-counter drugs to get a cheap high. Substances such as cough suppressants and expectorants (that can contain as much as 40% alcohol) are sometimes ingested to achieve the same effects as those derived from drinking alcohol. Cough and cold medications often contain dextromethorphan (DXM), a synthetic drug that is chemically similar to morphine. These medications are used to treat cold symptoms and do not lead to addiction, but they can be misused. Chronic misuse can lead to dependence and have long-term adverse health effects.

Recovery from addiction to any psychoactive drug often requires professional help. For information on drug treatment programs, consult the National Institute on Drug Abuse (see the web link at the end of this chapter).

Health Effects of Psychoactive Drug Use Long-term marijuana use can result in psychological dependence, and regular smoking causes lung damage similar to that caused by smoking tobacco (15). In fact, marijuana users usually inhale more deeply and hold their breath longer than tobacco smokers do, thereby increasing the lungs' exposure to carcinogenic smoke. The effect of long-term use on the heart is not well known; however, many investigators believe that marijuana increases the workload on the heart, which may eventually result in damage.

Some of the long-term complications from cocaine use are cardiovascular effects, including disturbances in heart rhythm and heart attacks; respiratory effects, such as chest pain and respiratory failure; neurological effects, including strokes, seizures, and headaches; and gastrointestinal complications, including abdominal pain and nausea. Long-term use of methamphetamines can result in paranoia, aggressiveness, extreme anorexia, memory loss, visual and auditory hallucinations, delusions, and severe dental problems.

Drug use by pregnant women can have serious health effects on the developing fetus. Prenatal exposure to marijuana results in the baby having weak responses to visual stimuli, increased tremulousness, and a high-pitched cry, which may indicate problems with neurological development. Many scientific studies have documented that babies born to mothers who abuse cocaine during pregnancy ("crack babies") are often delivered prematurely, have low birth weight, have smaller head circumference, and are shorter in length. Crack babies were once believed to suffer from severe, irreversible damage, such as reduced intelligence and social skills. Later research found that to be an exaggeration; however, these infants do exhibit subtle yet significant deficits in cognitive performance, attention to tasks, and information processing. Babies born to women who used heroin and were treated with methadone while pregnant require treatment for withdrawal symptoms after birth.

Alcohol

Alcohol (ethyl alcohol) is the most widely used recreational drug in the United States and the most popular drug on college campuses. The Centers for Disease Control and Prevention (CDC) estimates that approximately 51% of Americans over the age of 18 use alcohol more than 12 times a year. Numerous studies have described the incidence of alcohol use among college students. It has been reported that 40%–65% of full-time college students are current drinkers, and 10%–16% are heavy drinkers; 10%–22% of students reported using some type of illicit drugs (16, 17). Full-time college students are more likely to use alcohol, binge drink, and drink heavily than are

see it!

ABC VIDEOS

Watch the "Surge in Heroin Deaths" ABC News Video online at MasteringHealth™.

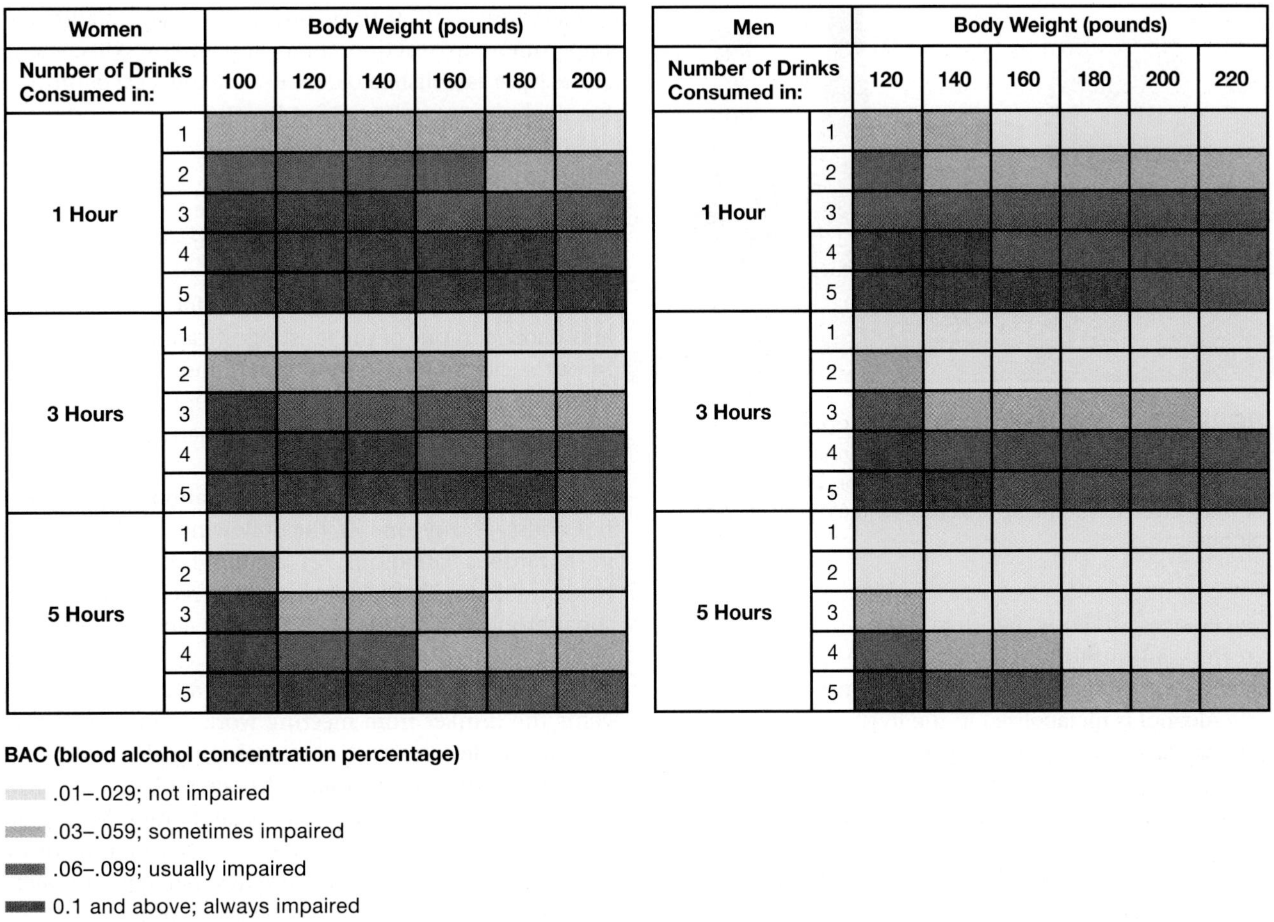

Women	Body Weight (pounds)					
Number of Drinks Consumed in:	100	120	140	160	180	200
1 Hour — 1						
2						
3						
4						
5						
3 Hours — 1						
2						
3						
4						
5						
5 Hours — 1						
2						
3						
4						
5						

Men	Body Weight (pounds)					
Number of Drinks Consumed in:	120	140	160	180	200	220
1 Hour — 1						
2						
3						
4						
5						
3 Hours — 1						
2						
3						
4						
5						
5 Hours — 1						
2						
3						
4						
5						

BAC (blood alcohol concentration percentage)

- .01–.029; not impaired
- .03–.059; sometimes impaired
- .06–.099; usually impaired
- 0.1 and above; always impaired

FIGURE 15.1 These charts approximate the blood alcohol concentration (BAC) for women and men, based on body weight and number of drinks consumed. The legal definition for alcohol intoxication is 0.08% BAC in many states.

part-time college students and people of the same age who do not attend college (16, 17). However, the number of college students who report binge drinking is on the decline among both full- and part-time college students (16, 17).

How much alcohol is contained in a drink? A drink is defined as 14 grams (0.6 ounces) of alcohol. This is the amount in one 12-ounce beer, 5 ounces of wine, or 1.5 ounces of hard liquor. The CDC defines "heavy drinking" as the consumption of 8 or more drinks per week for women and 15 or more drinks per week for men (16). Moderate drinking is defined as 1 drink per day for women and 2 drinks per day for men.

Although many people consume alcohol to "get high," alcohol is actually a central nervous system depressant that slows down the function of the brain. This depressive effect results in impaired vision, slowed reaction time, and impaired motor coordination (16, 17). Overconsumption of alcohol also impairs judgment. By decreasing the fear of danger, it can encourage risk-taking behaviors (such as driving too fast), which increases the likelihood of accidents (16, 17). Drinking too much can also increase the risk of poor judgment in social situations and in making decisions concerning sexual behavior.

The level of alcohol in the blood determines the magnitude of central nervous system depression. The **blood alcohol concentration (BAC)** is determined by the amount of alcohol consumed, body weight, and the rate of alcohol metabolism. For example, if two men of different weights (e.g., 200 pounds versus 150 pounds) consume the same amount of alcohol, the smaller individual will have the higher BAC (**FIGURE 15.1**). This difference in body size is also why many women feel the effects of alcohol sooner than men do. Women often have lower body weights and higher

see it!

ABC VIDEOS

Watch the "Sloppy Spring Breaker" ABC News Video online at MasteringHealth™.

blood alcohol concentration (BAC) The concentration of alcohol in the blood measured as a percentage by mass, by mass per volume, or a combination of both. A BAC of 0.20% can mean 2 grams of alcohol per 1000 grams of an individual's blood, or it can mean 0.2 gram of alcohol per 100 milliliters of blood.

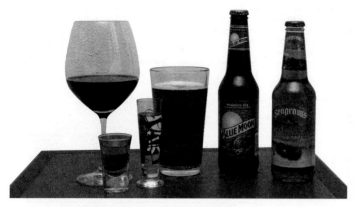

FIGURE 15.2 Ethyl alcohol is the psychoactive ingredient in all alcoholic beverages. A standard drink is defined as a 12-ounce beer, a 1.5-ounce cocktail, or a 5-ounce glass of wine. Each contains approximately 0.6 ounce of ethyl alcohol.

percentages of body fat than men, which results in greater concentrations of alcohol in the blood and consequently a greater central nervous system effect.

Alcohol is metabolized in the liver; and the body can remove 0.3 ounce of alcohol per hour. In practical terms, this rate of removal is approximately half of one drink (**FIGURE 15.2**) per hour. An individual who drinks slowly—that is, less than one drink per hour—can maintain a relatively low BAC. In contrast, someone who drinks rapidly, consuming more than two drinks per hour, will increase his or her BAC to higher levels, leading to intoxication.

Even low doses of alcohol can have significant behavioral and physical effects (see **TABLE 15.2**). Relatively small amounts of alcohol in your blood can decrease your level of alertness and increase your risk of injury (16). Higher doses can lead to impaired motor skills and slowed reaction times (16). These negative physical effects are the rationale behind state laws that specify the legal level of blood alcohol for driving.

Because 0.05–0.10% BAC results in significant impairment in reaction times and motor skills, many states have established 0.08% BAC as the legal definition for alcohol intoxication (13, 14).

Alcohol Abuse versus Alcohol Addiction Not everyone who uses alcohol will abuse it or become addicted. Many people drink moderate amounts of alcohol occasionally or on a regular basis without suffering any ill effects. However, because alcohol is widely available and affordable, it is one of the most significant drug problems in our society. Drinking too much and/or drinking too often are major contributors to alcohol abuse. Alcohol addiction is a very real problem for many people, and it can happen to anyone.

The American Psychiatric Association defines alcohol abuse as any one of the following: 1) alcohol use in hazardous situations; 2) alcohol-related school or work problems; 3) alcohol use causing recurrent interpersonal problems; and/or 4) alcohol use creating recurrent legal problems (2).

Alcohol abuse is particularly harmful when it prevents the drinker from meeting work, school, or family responsibilities. In addition, consuming alcohol during pregnancy has been linked to alcohol-related birth defects, including developmental disabilities. Moreover, alcohol abuse can also be deadly. The National Institute of Alcohol and Drug Abuse estimates that approximately 1,400 college students between the ages of 18 and 24 die each year as a result of alcohol abuse.

Alcoholism, also known as *alcohol dependence*, is a disease that involves craving alcohol and not being able to control the impulse to drink or limit the amount of drinking. Alcoholics develop a physical dependence on alcohol as their tolerance increases over time. Addiction to alcohol may have hereditary, psychological, and environmental components. Treatment for alcoholism involves medication and counseling to help a person

TABLE 15.2 ■ Behavioral and Physiological Effects of Alcohol		
Blood Alcohol Concentration (BAC)	Behavioral and Physiological Effects	Hours Required to Metabolize Alcohol
0.0%–0.05%	Increased relaxation, feeling of euphoria, and decreased alertness.	2–4
0.05%–0.10%	Reduced social inhibition and impairment in reaction time and motor skills. This level of alcohol may significantly impact driving skills. All states define legally drunk as a BAC of 0.08% or higher.	4–6
0.10%–0.15%	Increased impairment in reaction time and motor skills. Loss of peripheral vision.	6–10
0.15%–0.30%	Difficulty walking, slurred speech, impaired pain perception, and impairment in other sensory perceptions.	10–24
More than 0.30%	Can result in unconsciousness. Death possible at BAC levels of 0.35% or more. These levels of BAC are generally achieved by binge drinking.	More than 24

Source: Data from Ogden, E., and H. Moskowitz. Effects of alcohol and other drugs on driver performance. *Traffic Injury Prevention* 5(3):185–198, September 2004.

stop drinking. Several oral medications are currently FDA approved to treat alcohol dependence. These medications have been shown to help alcohol-dependent people reduce their drinking, avoid relapse, and remain sober. Nonetheless, these drugs are not a "magic bullet," because no single medication works in every case or for every person. There is no cure for alcoholism, and once a person has stopped drinking, he or she must avoid all alcohol for life or suffer the possibility of a relapse with the next drink.

Alcohol abuse and addiction are prevalent among college students. A survey of more than 14,000 students at 119 four-year colleges revealed that 31% of students met the criteria for a diagnosis of alcohol abuse, and 6% met the criteria for a diagnosis of alcohol dependence (16). For college students under age 24, nearly 10% of college men and 5% of college women met a 12-month diagnosis of alcohol dependence. Despite the prevalence of alcohol disorders on college campuses, few students reported having sought treatment for alcohol dependence.

Binge Drinking One common type of alcohol abuse among college students is binge drinking. The CDC defines **binge drinking** as 5 or more drinks for men and 4 or more drinks for women within a two-hour period. Binge drinking often begins in adolescence, as data indicate that approximately 25% of adolescents have reported binge drinking by the 12th grade. However, the habit seems to gradually decrease over time (17). In fact, the CDC estimates that 38 million Americans (1 in 6 people) engage in binge drinking (16, 17). The highest incidence occurs in those between the ages of 18-34, and the rate of binge drinking is twice as high in males as in females.

Bars and alcohol distributors in college towns often provide easy access to cheap alcohol, which promotes binge drinking. In one study, binge drinking among 18- to 22-year-old full-time college students was reported to be 42%, compared to 36% in people of the same age who were not enrolled full time in college (16). Students who live in fraternity or sorority houses tend to be the heaviest drinkers. Drinking games encourage consumption of excessive amounts of alcohol over a short time period.

Binge drinking is associated with a wide array of social, emotional, behavioral, and health problems. For example, alcohol poisoning, a potentially fatal physical reaction to an alcohol overdose, is the most serious consequence of binge drinking. The CDC estimates that approximately 88,000 deaths annually are due to alcohol-related health problems, including liver diseases and alcohol poisoning (16). A BAC of 0.35% or above can result in alcohol poisoning and death. Anyone who drinks to the point of unconsciousness may throw up and aspirate the vomit, leading to asphyxiation, or may

stop breathing. An unconscious individual whose breathing becomes too slow (fewer than 8 breaths per minute) or who cannot be awakened after drinking should be treated immediately by medical personnel because this is a life-threatening medical emergency.

consider this! ///////////////

In a national study, 91% of women and 78% of men who were frequent binge drinkers considered themselves to be moderate or light drinkers.

Most people who binge drink are not alcohol dependent; however, a consistent pattern of alcohol abuse can result in a need to drink more to feel the effects, which can lead to dependence.

Use the Steps for Behavior Change box on page 400 and Laboratory 15.1 to assess your drinking habits and determine whether you may be abusing alcohol. If you feel that you might be drinking too much, seek professional help from a health-care provider or an organization such as Alcoholics Anonymous or a rehab facility.

hear it!

CASE STUDY

How does Paulo know if he is a binge drinker? Listen to the online case study at MasteringHealth™.

Health Effects of Alcohol Abuse Chronic alcohol abuse over a period of years can result in liver disease (cirrhosis), nervous system damage, and an increased risk of certain cancers (16, 17). Liver disease due to years of drinking may eventually result in total liver failure and death. The damage to the nervous system

---

alcoholism Disease characterized by an addiction to alcohol and an inability to limit the amount of drinking despite adverse consequences.

binge drinking Drinking 5 or more drinks (for men) or 4 or more drinks (for women) within a 2-hour period.

steps > FOR BEHAVIOR CHANGE

Do you regularly abuse alcohol?

Take the following quiz to get a sense of your alcohol habits.

Y N

☐ ☐ Do you find it difficult to get through a week without drinking?

☐ ☐ Is going out with friends for the purpose of drinking a regular event?

☐ ☐ Do you and/or your friends engage in foolish or dangerous behavior while intoxicated?

☐ ☐ Would your grades or class attendance be better if you drank less alcohol?

☐ ☐ Do you regularly "black out" from drinking too much, to the extent that you don't remember periods of time?

If you answered yes to any of the above, you've engaged in at least one episode of alcohol abuse. While this doesn't necessarily mean you will become addicted to alcohol, it does mean you should take measures to modify your behavior.

Tips to Gain Control Over Your Drinking Habits

Tomorrow, you will:

☑ Write out a plan for alcohol consumption no more than 3 days per week (fewer is better).

☑ Set limits, and stay within them. If you are at a party and feel that you are drinking too much, learn to say no, dilute your drinks, or switch to a nonalcoholic beverage.

☑ Talk with a friend about the changes you want to make, and establish a support network when you attend parties and social events.

Within the next 2 weeks, you will:

☑ Stick to the rule of less than 0.3 ounce (one drink) of alcohol per hour. This will reduce the likelihood that you will become physically or mentally impaired by alcohol.

☑ Choose weaker drinks, such as wine, beer, and mixed drinks, instead of higher-alcohol beverages because they are less intoxicating than straight liquor.

☑ Eat before you plan to drink alcohol. Eating and drinking at the same time will slow the rate of alcohol absorption and reduce your chance of becoming impaired. Never drink on an empty stomach.

☑ Plan to have a designated driver or take extra money for a cab when you intend to drink alcohol while out.

By the end of the semester, you will:

☑ Drink alcohol no more than 2 days per week.

☑ Not drink alcohol every week.

---

from alcohol abuse is often localized to the left side of the brain, which is responsible for written and spoken language, logic, and mathematical skills. The degree of brain damage that occurs appears to be directly related to the amount of alcohol consumed (16, 17). Repeated irritation of the gastrointestinal system by alcohol has been linked to cancers of the esophagus, pancreas, stomach, mouth, tongue, and liver. Another, often overlooked problem linked to chronic alcohol consumption is **malnutrition**. Malnutrition occurs because the frequent presence of alcohol irritates the gastrointestinal system. An irritated gastric lining can result in impaired appetite, which in turn decreases food intake. A lowered food intake forces the body to function on a diet that is deficient in both calories and essential nutrients such as protein and vitamins. In extreme cases, loss of muscle mass and abnormal functioning of many organs can occur. The malnutrition accompanying chronic alcohol abuse can result in inadequate vitamin intake and numerous health problems. For example, a lack of vitamin A may contribute to liver disease and other alcohol-related health problems. Further, a lack of thiamin (vitamin B1) has been associated with a degenerative brain disorder called Wernicke-Korsakoff syndrome (17). Excessive alcohol intake, because of its high calorie content, can also contribute to overweight and obesity. Sweet mixed drinks can approach the calorie levels of many snacks and desserts.

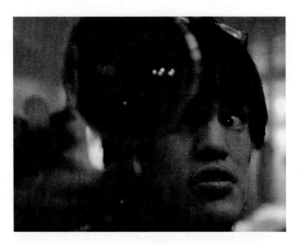

The effects of fetal alcohol syndrome last a lifetime. Justin is 20 years old, was born with FAS, and has the mental capabilities of a 6 year old. Typically, adults with FAS may exhibit autism, cerebral palsy, seizure disorder, gastrointestinal disorders, and developmental disabilities.

consider this! /////////////////////

An estimated 1,400 college students (age 18 to 24) die each year from alcohol-related injuries, including motor vehicle crashes.

Women who drink during pregnancy are subjecting the fetus to a wide range of preventable birth defects, including **fetal alcohol syndrome**. An estimated 1% of all live births show some alcohol-related prenatal damage, such as physical, behavioral, and learning problems. Babies born with fetal alcohol syndrome may have mild to severe learning disabilities and abnormal facial features (17). Any woman who is pregnant or thinks she may become pregnant should abstain from consuming alcohol.

Tobacco

Nicotine, contained in tobacco products, is the most heavily used addictive drug in the United States. The use of tobacco products in the United States has remained relatively constant from 2008 to 2015; approximately 25% of adults use tobacco (18). Cigarette smoking is the most common form, with about 42 million American smokers (18). Cigarette smoking remains more common among men than women. The good news is that smoking rates among young Americans have declined slightly. Nonetheless, a large number of Americans still use tobacco products and approximately 2 million start smoking each year (18). Cigarettes and all other forms of tobacco, such as snuff, chewing tobacco, and cigars, are associated with major health risks.

Cigarette smoking has been the most popular method of nicotine use since the early 20th century. Each cigarette contains 1.8 mg of nicotine, compared to 3.6 mg in snuff and 4.6 mg in chewing tobacco (18). A single cigar can contain anywhere from 1 to 20 grams (18, 19).

Nicotine Addiction Nicotine provides an almost immediate "psychological kick" to the body because it causes the release of epinephrine from the adrenal cortex

malnutrition Poor nutrition due to an insufficient or poorly balanced diet or to faulty digestion or utilization of foods.

fetal alcohol syndrome A cluster of birth defects that may include facial abnormalities and developmental disabilities caused by alcohol consumption during pregnancy.

nicotine Addictive and psychoactive substance in tobacco plants.

EXAMINING THE EVIDENCE

Are E-Cigarettes Safe?

Electronic cigarettes (e-cigarettes) are battery-operated devices designed to deliver nicotine and other chemicals in the form of vapor instead of smoke. More than 250 brands are currently on the market, and more than 40 million American adults, along with 1.8 million children, have tried them (5). Although e-cigarettes are promoted as safer alternatives to traditional cigarettes, little is known about potential long-term health risks.

Traditional cigarette smoking remains the leading preventable cause of disease and death in the United States. The worst health consequences—cancer and heart disease—are linked to the inhalation of tar and other chemicals. The pleasure and addictive properties of smoking are provided by nicotine.

E-cigarettes simulate the act of smoking by producing a flavored aerosol that delivers nicotine with fewer toxic chemicals than in tobacco smoke. Because they deliver nicotine without burning tobacco, it has been suggested that e-cigarettes are safer and less toxic than conventional cigarettes. Further, it has been proposed that e-cigarettes can help people quit smoking tobacco, but at present, it is unknown if they are effective as smoking cessation aids or if they actually contain fewer toxic chemicals than regular cigarettes (6).

While they do not produce tobacco smoke, e-cigarettes still contain nicotine and other potentially harmful chemicals. Nicotine is a highly addictive drug, and recent research reveals that nicotine exposure may prime the brain to become addicted to other drugs. A legitimate concern is the possibility that users may expose themselves to potentially toxic levels of nicotine.

Testing reveals that e-cigarette vapor contains carcinogens and other toxic chemicals (4). Studies also indicate that the inhaled vapor contains potentially harmful small particles (nanoparticles) from the vaporizing mechanism (4). The long-term health consequences of these harmful chemicals and nanoparticles remain unclear (6).

In summary, e-cigarettes have not been thoroughly evaluated, and limited research exists regarding the safety and health impact of using these products. It's important to note that because e-cigarettes are not marketed as a tobacco product or as a therapeutic device, they are not regulated by the FDA. This means there is no way to confirm the quality or safety of their contents. Therefore, consumers should be wary of e-cigarette use until more information becomes available.

(the outer portion of the adrenal glands). This stimulates the central nervous system and increases both heart rate and blood pressure. This stimulation is lost rapidly, which leads to depression and fatigue and causes the user to seek more nicotine.

Nicotine is absorbed readily from tobacco smoke in the lungs (19). Nicotine is also absorbed in the mouth when tobacco is chewed. With regular use, nicotine can accumulate in the body and remain for several hours (19).

Clove cigarettes have been used as an alternative to tobacco products; however, clove cigarettes contain about 60%–70% tobacco and amounts of nicotine equal to cigarettes (20). Exposure to tar, nicotine, and carbon monoxide is higher for smokers of clove cigarettes than for smokers of tobacco cigarettes.

Nicotine addiction results in withdrawal symptoms when a person tries to stop smoking. For example, studies indicate that when chronic smokers were deprived of cigarettes for 24 hours, they showed more anger, hostility, and aggression and less social cooperation (19). People suffering from nicotine withdrawal take longer to regain emotional equilibrium following exposure to stress. Moreover, during periods of abstinence, smokers show a wide range of physical and mental impairments, such as impaired psychomotor skills (movement coordination) and impaired cognitive function (19).

Studies have shown that some of the most successful long-term smoking cessation programs involve not only behavioral treatment but also pharmacological treatment (19). Most pharmacological treatments involve nicotine gum or transdermal patches (on the skin) to deliver nicotine during the initial stages of smoking cessation. It has been suggested that electronic cigarettes may assist in smoking cessation (see Examining the Evidence). The success of smoking cessation treatment varies widely. Generally, the rates of relapse are highest in the first few weeks after cessation and diminish greatly after about 3 months (19). If you smoke, it is possible to stop.

Secondhand Smoke   Secondhand smoke (also known as *sidestream smoke*) is a mixture of gases and particles from burning tobacco and smoke exhaled by smokers (also known as *mainstream smoke*). Secondhand smoke lingers in the air for hours after cigarettes have been extinguished; it contains toxic chemicals, more than 50 of which are

see it!

ABC VIDEOS

Watch the "GMA Investigates Liquid Nicotine" ABC News Video online at MasteringHealth™.

known to cause cancer. In addition to the absorption of nicotine, breathing secondhand smoke has immediate harmful effects on the cardiovascular system, increases the risk of lung cancer, and can cause respiratory disorders including bronchitis (21, 22). From 1965 to 2014, approximately 2.5 million people died from diseases related to secondhand smoke (19).

New legislation is being passed in almost every community in the United States to curb exposure to secondhand smoke. Smoking is banned in almost all government buildings, and many cities and states have passed legislation banning smoking in restaurants and bars. Because of these new laws, exposure rates have declined.

Health Effects of Tobacco Use Tobacco smoke contains over 7,000 chemicals that can affect every organ system (18). Smoking is the leading preventable cause of death in the United States, accounting for approximately one in every five deaths each year (23). Cigarette smoking can promote coronary heart disease, the leading cause of death in the United States, and doubles a person's chance for stroke (23). Regular tobacco use increases the risk of several forms of cancer, including cancers of the lung, larynx, esophagus, pancreas, bladder, and kidney (23). Compared to nonsmokers, men who smoke are 23 times more likely to develop lung cancer, and women who smoke are 13 times more likely (23). In the United States, it is estimated that tobacco use and secondhand smoke resulted in 21 million deaths and a total cost (medical costs and lost productivity) of $289 billion over the past 50 years (18).

Pregnant women who smoke are more likely to lose the baby during pregnancy or to deliver the baby prematurely, before the lungs are fully developed. Children born to women who smoke are lower in birth weight and tend to develop more illnesses. Nicotine and other harmful chemicals are absorbed in the mother's bloodstream and pass through the placenta to the fetus (18). Several of these chemicals may interfere with the developing baby's ability to get enough oxygen and nutrients, contributing to the low birth weight.

Caffeine

Caffeine is a bitter substance found in coffee, tea, soft drinks, chocolate, and certain over-the-counter drugs. Caffeine enters the bloodstream through the stomach and small intestine and can stimulate the central nervous system within 15 minutes after it is consumed (see Examining the Evidence on page 405). For most people, the amount of caffeine in two to four cups of coffee a day is not harmful. When consumed in moderate doses, caffeine can increase mental alertness; however, too much can make you restless and irritable. Caffeine has also been associated with insomnia, headaches, and abnormal heart rhythms. It is eliminated slowly and can remain in the body for up to 20 hours. If you have trouble sleeping at night, avoid ingesting caffeine products after 2:00 P.M.

Many investigations have studied the impact of moderate caffeine use on human health. In general, there is no evidence that caffeine is harmful (25). However, some studies suggest that caffeine causes psychological dependence (24), but there is no agreement on how much caffeine would have to be consumed daily to develop a dependence (24). Even if you consume caffeine in moderate doses, you could experience withdrawal symptoms when you stop using it. Typical withdrawal symptoms include headache and fatigue (24). Some people may find that they are more sensitive to the effects of caffeine than others and should limit intake or avoid it altogether. Certain drugs and supplements may interact with caffeine. If you have questions about whether caffeine is safe for you, talk with your health-care provider.

Anabolic Steroids

Anabolic steroids are synthetic substances related to male sex hormones (e.g., testosterone). Steroids are a class of drugs that are legally available only by prescription and are used primarily to treat conditions that occur when the body does not produce enough testosterone, such as in delayed puberty and some types of impotence. Anabolic steroids can be taken orally, injected into muscle, or applied topically.

More than 50 years ago, scientists discovered that anabolic steroids facilitated the growth of skeletal muscle in laboratory animals by mimicking the effect of naturally produced testosterone. This discovery led to abuse of these compounds, first by bodybuilders and weight

secondhand smoke Smoke from the burning end of a cigarette, cigar, or pipe and smoke exhaled by a smoker.

caffeine Stimulant found in coffee, tea, chocolate, and other foods and beverages.

anabolic steroids Synthetic hormones related to the male sex hormone testosterone.

lifters and then by athletes in other sports. Doses taken for sports-related purposes can typically be 100 times more than the dosage used for treating legitimate medical conditions.

Long-term steroid use can have serious psychological side effects. Users become aggressive, developing extreme, uncontrolled bouts of anger known as "roid rage." Depression often results when the drugs are stopped, which may contribute to dependence in an effort to avoid depression.

Anabolic steroids can cause potentially fatal liver cysts and liver cancer, increased blood cholesterol levels, increased blood clotting, and increased hypertension, which can promote heart attack and stroke in both men and women. In boys and men, anabolic steroid abuse can reduce sperm production, shrink the testicles, lead to impotence, and cause baldness and irreversible breast enlargement (gynecomastia) (26). In girls and women, anabolic steroid abuse causes the development of masculine characteristics such as decreased body fat and breast size, deepened voice, excessive body hair growth, acne, male pattern baldness, changes in the menstrual cycle, and enlargement of the clitoris (26).

The scope of steroid abuse in the United States is difficult to estimate because many users hide their habit. The National Institute of Drug Abuse estimates that more than 500,000 teens and more than 1 million adults abuse these drugs. Teenage boys are likely to use steroids to build muscle to improve their athletic performance. Teenage girls are likely to use steroids as body-shaping drugs to increase their lean body mass (27). Regardless of the motive, these drugs are illegal and can do permanent damage to a person's health and reproductive system.

hear it!

CASE STUDY

Should Evan, a bodybuilder, stop taking anabolic steroids? Listen to the online case study at MasteringHealth™.

MAKE SURE YOU **KNOW...**

- Psychoactive drugs alter brain function. Effects range from feelings of euphoria to increased heart rate, shallow breathing, a change in body temperature, and hallucinations.

- Commonly used psychoactive drugs include marijuana, cocaine, club drugs, alcohol, and tobacco. Common club drugs include Ecstasy, GHB, Rohypnol, ketamine, methamphetamine, and LSD.

- Alcohol is the most common recreational drug in the United States; it is estimated that 51% of adults drink. Relatively low levels of blood alcohol (0.05% to 0.10%) can impair both reaction time and motor skills, resulting in a diminished ability to drive.

- Nicotine is one of the most addictive drugs. Prolonged use of tobacco products can lead to

numerous health problems, including an increased risk of heart disease and cancer.

- Anabolic steroids are a class of synthetic substances related to the male sex hormone testosterone. Abusing steroids for bodybuilding or to enhance athletic performance can lead to harmful health effects, including psychological problems and physical side effects (e.g., changes in sexual characteristics and an impaired reproductive system).

————————— MasteringHealth™

Strategies to Prevent Drug Abuse

LO **3** Outline several strategies that can be used to prevent substance abuse.

Avoiding drug use requires self discipline and control. Several steps can help protect you from the temptation to use drugs (28):

1. **Increase your self-esteem.** Take pride in yourself and your achievements. This will boost your confidence and improve your ability to say "No."

2. **Learn how to cope with stress.** Master one or more stress management techniques (see Chapter 11).

3. **Develop varied interests.** Take the time to discover new hobbies or sports that you enjoy.

4. **Practice assertiveness.** Knowing how to stand up for yourself is key in resisting drug use.

5. **Seek professional help if you feel depressed.** Depression is a common cause of drug abuse. If you suspect that you are developing depression, seek medical help and/or counseling to avoid the risk of drug abuse.

6. **Focus on things in your life that make you happy.** Many people who develop drug addictions are unhappy. But instead of making an effort to change their circumstances, they seek drugs as a means of escape from their problems.

7. **Keep loving connections in your life.** Studies suggest that people who maintain positive, loving relationships with family and friends are less likely to abuse drugs. Pet owners are also less likely to abuse drugs versus those without pets. Having a person or animal to love is important, but be responsible—don't take on a pet unless your living situation and finances will allow you to provide proper care.

live it!

ASSESS YOURSELF

Assess your frequency of substance use and abuse with the *Substance Abuse Log* Take Charge of Your Health! Worksheet online at MasteringHealth™.

EXAMINING THE EVIDENCE — The Effects of Caffeine

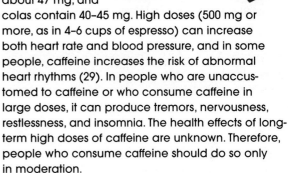

Caffeine is a stimulant found in a variety of foods and beverages, including chocolate, coffee, tea, soda, and energy drinks. It is one of the most frequently ingested psychoactive drugs in the world (25). Caffeine affects the central nervous system by stimulating a variety of brain centers, increasing alertness and decreasing drowsiness (29). In fact, caffeine has been shown to reduce fatigue and improve performance during prolonged endurance exercise (e.g., running a marathon) (30, 31). Evidence that caffeine may improve endurance exercise performance has prompted numerous organizations to consider banning high blood levels of caffeine during athletic competition.

As with other habit-forming drugs, chronic caffeine use can lead to withdrawal-related problems (25, 29). Abrupt discontinuation can result in severe headache, fatigue, irritability, and gastrointestinal distress, but, quitting caffeine use has been shown to be considerably easier than cessation of other stimulants, such as nicotine (25).

There is limited evidence that long-term caffeine use poses a significant health risk. Most experts conclude that moderate daily intake (less than 400 mg/day) is not associated with adverse health effects (25).

An 8-ounce cup of coffee contains about 85 mg of caffeine. A cup of tea contains about 47 mg, and colas contain 40–45 mg. High doses (500 mg or more, as in 4–6 cups of espresso) can increase both heart rate and blood pressure, and in some people, caffeine increases the risk of abnormal heart rhythms (29). In people who are unaccustomed to caffeine or who consume caffeine in large doses, it can produce tremors, nervousness, restlessness, and insomnia. The health effects of long-term high doses of caffeine are unknown. Therefore, people who consume caffeine should do so only in moderation.

Caffeine may have health effects during pregnancy. Some studies suggest that intake at or above three or more 8-ounce cups of coffee per day may increase the risk of miscarriage and of low birth weight (25). However, small amounts (one to two 8-ounce cups of coffee per day) appear to be safe during pregnancy.

study plan

Customize your study plan—and master your health!— in the Study Area of **MasteringHealth**.

summary

hear it! STUDY REVIEW

To hear an MP3 Chapter Summary, scan here or visit the Study Area in MasteringHealth™.

LO **1** ■ Addiction is a compulsive physical or psychological dependence on a substance or behavior.

LO **2** ■ Alcohol, nicotine (tobacco products), marijuana, and cocaine are the most widely used and abused drugs in the United States. Alcohol is the most common recreational drug.

■ Use of alcohol, marijuana, and cocaine increases your risk of accidents, and prolonged use may result in psychological dependence, physical addiction, and damaged health.

■ Chronic alcohol abuse can result in liver disease, nervous system damage, increased risk of certain cancers, and malnutrition.

■ Blood alcohol concentrations of 0.05%–0.10% can significantly reduce reaction time and impair motor skills.

■ Cocaine is a highly addictive drug that, when taken in large doses, can be lethal.

■ Use of tobacco products can lead to a nicotine addiction, and prolonged use can lead to numerous health problems, including increased risk of heart attack, stroke, and cancer.

- Caffeine is a central nervous system stimulant found in numerous foods and beverages.

- Regular consumption of small amounts of caffeine does not appear to have negative health consequences. It is not clear if chronic consumption of high amounts poses a significant health risk.

- Long-term use of anabolic steroids can cause psychological side effects, such as aggression and uncontrolled anger. In men, steroid use leads to

shrunken testicles, reduced sperm count, breast development, infertility, and increased risk of prostate cancer. In women, steroid use can cause growth of facial hair, male pattern baldness, menstrual cycle changes, enlargement of the clitoris, and a deepened voice.

LO   ■ You can decrease your risk of using drugs by increasing your self-esteem, managing stress, seeking help for depression, practicing assertiveness, developing varied interests, and focusing on positive activities and connections in your life.

study questions

review it! QUIZZES

Find more review questions online at MasteringHealth™.

LO 1. *Addiction* is defined as
   a. chronic psychological and/or physical dependence on a substance or behavior that is beyond voluntary control.
   b. dependence on a substance or behavior that is due to psychological factors only.
   c. dependence on a substance or behavior that is due to physical factors only.
   d. none of the above are correct.

2. Factors that determine risk for drug addiction include
   a. the type of drug used.
   b. genetics.
   c. psychological makeup.
   d. all of the above.

3. Differentiate between *substance use* and *substance abuse*.

LO 4. Which of the following drugs have been shown to have a high potential for physical dependence?
   a. LSD
   b. Marijuana
   c. Nicotine
   d. Mescaline

5. Psychoactive drugs are those that
   a. increase appetite.
   b. alter brain function and can cause a state of intoxication.
   c. increase metabolic rate.
   d. cause depression upon withdrawal.

6. The most common recreational drug in the United States is
   a. alcohol.
   b. marijuana.
   c. cocaine.
   d. LSD.

7. Blood alcohol levels of _____ have been shown to produce impaired motor functions.
   a. 0.01
   b. 0.03
   c. 0.04
   d. 0.08

8. Binge drinking is defined as
   a. 3 or more drinks for men and 2 or more drinks for women within a 2-hour period.
   b. 4 or more drinks for men and 2 or more drinks for women within a 2-hour period.
   c. 4 or more drinks for men and 4 or more drinks for women within a 2-hour period.
   d. 5 or more drinks for men and 4 or more drinks for women within a 2-hour period.

9. Describe the health effects of marijuana use.

10. Describe the health effects of alcohol use.

11. What changes in behavior and physical function occur as blood alcohol level increases?

12. Describe the health effects of using anabolic steroids.

13. Describe the health consequences of long-term smoking or breathing secondhand smoke.

LO 14. List several strategies that can help you avoid the temptation to use drugs.

suggested reading

Donatelle, R. *Access to Health*, 14th ed. San Francisco: Benjamin Cummings, 2015.

Donatelle, R. *Health: The Basics*, 11th ed. San Francisco: Benjamin Cummings, 2014.

Fields, R. *Drugs in Perspective*, 8th ed. St. Louis: McGraw-Hill, 2012.

Maguire, M., and C. Garoupa. *Annual Editions: Drugs, Society, and Behavior*, 30th ed. St. Louis: McGraw-Hill, 2015.

helpful weblinks

do it! WEBLINKS

For links to the organizations and websites listed, visit MasteringHealth™.

American Medical Association

Information about a wide variety of medical problems, including substance abuse. **www.ama-assn.org**

Higher Education Center for Alcohol and Other Drug Abuse Prevention

Information about alcohol and drug abuse on college campuses and links to related organizations. **www.higheredcenter.org**

National Institute on Drug Abuse

Information about commonly abused drugs, the incidence of drug abuse in the United States, and where to find help. **www.nida.nih.gov**

WebMD

Information about a wide variety of medical problems, including substance abuse. **www.webmd.com**

do it! LABS

Complete Lab 15.1 online in the
study area of **MasteringHealth.com**.

Name _____   Date _____

Alcohol Abuse Inventory

This laboratory is designed to increase your awareness of your drinking habits. To provide a valid assessment, you must answer each question honestly. Check Yes or No for each question below.

	Yes	No
1. Do you often drink alone?	_____	_____
2. When drinking, do you worry about running out of alcoholic beverages?	_____	_____
3. Do you drink alcohol daily?	_____	_____
4. Do you drink alcohol to reduce your stress?	_____	_____
5. Do you crave alcohol during all parts of the day?	_____	_____
6. Do you have trouble not drinking alcohol at a party?	_____	_____
7. After a night of drinking, do you sometimes have trouble remembering what you did?	_____	_____
8. Does your drinking impair your school or job performance?	_____	_____
9. Does your drinking impair your ability to use good judgment or cause you to have accidents?	_____	_____
10. Do you ever lie to friends or family about how much you drink?	_____	_____

Answering Yes to only one of the questions above suggests that you may be drinking too much. Answering Yes to two questions is a warning sign that you may have or are in the process of developing an alcohol abuse problem. Answering Yes to three or more questions indicates that you have a serious problem and that you should seek professional help.

Answer the following questions to help identify ways you can curb your alcohol consumption:

1. If you answered Yes to questions 1 and/or 2, you should reduce your access to alcohol. Identify two ways you can limit your access to alcohol in your home or environment.

    1. _____

    2. _____

2. If you answered Yes to questions 3 and/or 4, identify one healthy behavior you can substitute for the drinking behavior. Identify two stress management techniques you can try instead of drinking alcohol.

    Healthy behavior: _____

    Stress management technique: _____

    Stress management technique: _____

3. If you answered Yes to questions 5, 6, 7, 8, 9, and/or 10, recognize that alcohol is interfering with your life. Identify two campus resources and two community resources that you could use to get help with your alcohol-related behaviors.

    1. _____

    2. _____

laboratory 15.2

do it! LABS
Complete Lab 15.2 online in the
study area of **MasteringHealth.com**.

Name _____ Date _____

Tobacco Usage Inventory

This laboratory is designed to increase your awareness of your tobacco habits. Habits are sometimes difficult to break because they become unconscious acts. Unrecognized triggers may cause the desire to smoke or use the product. Breaking a habit may be as easy as identifying the trigger and substituting a healthy behavior instead.

Over the next 24 hours, take an inventory of the tobacco products you use. Identify the number of tobacco products you use each hour, where you use the product (such as a certain room or in the car), when you use it (such as after a meal), and any other factors, such as being alone or with friends or family, and so on. You must answer each question honestly to provide a valid assessment.

Time of Day	Number of Tobacco Products Used	Location	What Were You Doing Before and During Usage?	Other Factors
12:00 A.M.				
1:00				
2:00				
3:00				
4:00				
5:00				
6:00				
7:00				
8:00				
9:00				
10:00				
11:00				
12:00 P.M.				
1:00				
2:00				
3:00				
4:00				
5:00				
6:00				
7:00				
8:00				
9:00				
10:00				
11:00				

Analyze the above chart, noting any patterns to your tobacco use. Answer the following questions:

1. Do you smoke or use more than one cigarette or tobacco product in any given hour of the day? When?

    _____

    _____

2. Is there a particular location where you prefer to smoke? Where?

    _____

    _____

    _____

3. Do you use tobacco products more often at certain times, such as around meal time, when talking on the phone, or while driving?

    _____

    _____

    _____

4. Is someone else present or do you smoke alone?

    _____

    _____

    _____

Now that you have identified a potential pattern to your tobacco usage, consider ways that you can change that pattern. For example:

- Identify the number of cigarettes that you use during the day, and try cutting the number by half over the next 2 weeks. Every 2 weeks, cut your usage in half again.
- Identify one location that you will make off limits to any tobacco product over the next 2 weeks. Every 2 weeks, add another location to make off limits.
- Identify when you use a tobacco product and recognize the triggering situation or event. For example, you may find that eating, studying, or talking on the phone triggers your need to smoke. Try substituting a healthy behavior, such as taking a walk, eating a healthy snack, or drinking a glass of water.
- Examine other factors that may influence your tobacco usage. You may find that you smoke only when you are alone or when you are with a particular individual or group of people. Identify a way in which you can continue to socialize with your friends without tobacco. For example, you could meet friends in a smoke-free restaurant, bar, or building. If you smoke when alone, try performing other tasks that will keep your hands occupied.

Note that these steps may help you cut down on smoking, but by themselves they may not be enough to kick the habit. Nicotine is a highly addictive substance and you may require counseling and/or medical intervention to help you quit.

appendix A

Answers to Study Questions

Chapter 1

1. a. Although exercise is not a component of wellness, it can help you achieve physical health, which is one of the components of total wellness.

3. d. *Healthy People 2020* is the current health goals for the nation. The objectives address a broad range of health behaviors and outcomes needed to improve the health of the nation. See www.healthypeople.gov for a comprehensive list of the *Healthy People 2020* objectives.

4. c. Physical activity is any type of occupational, leisure, or lifestyle-related physical movement. Exercise is one example of leisure physical activity.

5. d. Reduced risk for osteoporosis and heart disease, as well as improved mental health, are all benefits of regular physical activity.

6. c. Agility may be important for sport performance, but it is not linked to improved overall health and therefore is not considered a major component of health-related physical fitness.

9. b. An individual in the action stage of change has been participating in a new health behavior for 6 months or less, but once this individual has moved beyond 6 months, she will be in the maintenance stage of change.

10. d. Assessing your current behavior—including number and effort of behaviors you want to change, your motive for behavior change, and current behaviors patterns—is an important step to take when planning a change.

12. c. For goals to be successful, it is important that they be specific and that the outcome can be measured to determine whether the goal was reached. It is also important to have a plan of action for meeting the goal. Goals should be challenging but realistic. Setting a time frame to achieve the goal provides direction and helps you maintain focus.

Chapter 2

1. d. Supercompensation is not one of the five key principles of exercise training.

9. c. Current guidelines indicate that a minimum of 30 minutes of moderate exercise each day can produce numerous health benefits.

Chapter 3

1. c. Aerobic exercises include activities that promote cardiorespiratory fitness, such as jogging, swimming, and cycling.

2. a. Arteries are the blood vessels that move oxygen-rich blood away from your heart. Veins return oxygen-depleted blood back to the heart.

7. a. Activities that promote muscle strength and endurance, such as wrestling, utilize the anaerobic energy pathway to create ATP and provide energy to muscles.

8. b. As an individual's cardiorespiratory fitness level increases, resting heart rate will decrease because the heart becomes more efficient at pumping blood throughout the body. This allows the heart to beat fewer times per minute to pump the same amount of blood.

9. d. Increases in heart rate, cardiac output, and breathing are normal physical changes you will experience during cardiorespiratory exercise.

11. b. A field test (e.g., 1.5 mile run) can provide an estimate of VO$_2$max.

12. c. You should exercise at a level of at least 50% of your heart rate reserve in order to improve health-related physical fitness and cardiorespiratory endurance.

Chapter 4

1. b. Maximal strength is determined by the cross-sectional area of the muscle and number of motor units activated, as well as the biomechanical aspects of the muscle/joint in question.

2. a. Strength training is specific to the muscle being used during the training. Lower back pains are often associated with weak and shortened back muscles. After strength training the back muscles, the incidence of lower back pain may be reduced.

4. b. Eccentric contractions are an important aspect of the adaptation to training. The eccentric contraction phase is responsible for muscle damage with overload/overtraining (DOMS).

5. a. The slow-twitch fiber is recruited first during low-intensity activities. Slow fibers are also the most fatigue resistant.

19. d. Muscle overload (high resistance) is necessary to see strength gains. With high resistance, the number of repetitions due to the overload is limited. Therefore, high resistance lifting necessitates low repetitions.

Chapter 5

1. d. The shape of the bones and tight skin and tendons can all affect one's flexibility at a joint. Bone length is typically not a factor.

5. d. The two types of proprioceptors are Golgi organs and muscle spindles; they are found in tendons and muscles, respectively. Motor units are not a type of proprioceptor.

7. d. An imbalance in muscle strength caused by weak hamstrings or abdominal muscles (or a combination of the two) can result in a forward curve (or hyperextension) of the lower back, resulting in back pain. Stretching and strengthening these muscles are important for avoiding LBP.

11. b. False. Most people, including athletes and non-athletes, would benefit from the improved flexibility that results from regular static stretching.

12. b. A few minutes of light exercise before stretching will minimize your risk of injury. Where and when you stretch is not likely to affect your risk. Stretching to the point of pain is more likely to result in injury than stretching to the point of mild discomfort.

Chapter 6

1. b. Several methods (e.g., skin fold measurements) exist to estimate the percent of fat in the body.

2. b. Essential fat, necessary fat the body requires to maintain certain functions, should be at least 3% of total body weight in men and 12% in women.

3. True. Excess fat stored in the abdomen or waist increases the risk of heart disease and diabetes.

4. d. Anemia is not a health consequence of overweight or obesity.

5. d. Type I diabetes does not result from being underweight or from most eating disorders.

8. a. While air displacement, underwater weighing, and bioelectrical impendence analysis are reliable methods for assessing body composition, the waist-to-hip ratio is the technique used to determine disease risk associated with body fat distribution.

9. c. A BMI of 30 kg/m^2 or greater is considered obese. A healthy BMI is less than 25 for men and less than 27 for women.

10. b. A skinfold test is an easy measure to obtain and can provide good estimates when done properly.

11. a. True. Your BMI is a good estimate of your weight status; however, BMI does not give you a direct measure of percent fat. The method can over- or underestimate body fatness.

13. c. Research suggests that a range between 8–19% body fat is an optimal health and fitness goal for men aged 20–39 years.

14. c. Experts agree that losing body weight as fast as possible is an unwise approach to weight loss. Further, when attempting to lose body fat, it is unwise to lose lean tissue because lean tissues comprise the vital organs of the body.

Chapter 7

1. c. Establishing goals is the first and most important step in establishing a successful personal fitness plan.

2. c. Most cardiorespiratory health benefits occur with 120–150 minutes per week of moderate-intensity aerobic exercise.

3. a. Exercise training to improve muscular strength should be performed 2–3 times per week.

8. b. Stretching should be performed at least 2 times per week.

11. b. Pregnant women should avoid exercises that require them to lie on their backs for 5 minutes or more. For this reason, pregnant women should avoid floor based abdominal toning exercises.

13. d. As you age, your maximal heart rate, cardiorespiratory fitness, and muscle mass all decrease.

16. d. Too rigid a schedule makes it much more difficult to stay on track with your plan. Being flexible with your scheduling can ease the implementation of your plan.

17. b. Understanding your health insurance coverage is important in knowing how best to manage your health in case of injury/sickness.

Chapter 8

2. b. Carbohydrates provide the main source of fuel for your brain and are the main source of energy during exercise.

3. c. Protein is used by the body to build muscle, skin, connective tissues, and other structural body tissues.

4. c. While water doesn't provide energy or build bone or protein, it is involved in numerous metabolic and other body processes, including blood formation.

5. d. A well-balanced diet consists of 58% carbohydrates, 30% fats, and 12% protein.

11. a. Calcium, iron, and vitamin C are classified as micronutrients. Protein is classified as a macronutrient.

16. c. Vitamin B12 is mostly available in animal sources and is absent in almost all vegetables. Therefore, Vegans are often encouraged to take a vitamin B12 supplement.

20. c. The most common cause of foodborne illness comes from food products that contain disease causing bacteria.

Chapter 9

1. b. Optimal body fat percentages for health and fitness in men range from 8% to 19%, and from 21% to 32% in women.

3. d. Energy balance occurs when the amount of calories you consume is equal to the amount of calories you burn, and therefore your weight will not change. If you consume more calories than you burn, you will gain weight. If you consume fewer calories than you burn, you will lose weight.

6. f. Leptin and ghrelin are hormones that play a role in appetite. Leptin depresses appetite, while ghrelin contributes to appetite.

7. c. Compared to strength training and cardiorespiratory endurance training, engaging in Pilates, yoga, or table tennis results in limited energy expenditure.

8. d. Research reveals that the energy deficit required to lose 1 pound per week is approximately 3,500 kilocalories.

Chapter 10

1. c. Cardiovascular disease is the leading cause of death in the United States for all ages.

3. d. Normal blood pressure is 120/80 mm/Hg, so a blood pressure reading of 140/90 would be considered high blood pressure, or hypertension.

4. d. Smoking, hypertension, and high blood cholesterol are major risk factors for cardiovascular disease. Resting pulse rate is not a risk factor.

5. b. Obesity, hypertension, and stress can all be modified by healthy lifestyle changes; however, heredity—the genes you are born with—cannot be changed.

Chapter 11

2. d. There are a variety of physical symptoms associated with stress, including headaches, anxiety, and muscle tension.

3. c. Eustress is positive stress that motivates and energizes us. Distress is the type of stress that can have a negative impact on our mental and physical health.

4. a. Epinephrine, cortisol, and norepinephrine are hormones released into the bloodstream during the stress response. Dopamine does not play a role in the body's response to stress.

6. d. Everyday life situations can contribute to our stress levels. These situations can include financial responsibilities, interpersonal relationship problems, and academic pressures.

10. b. Alcohol is not an effective way to cope with stress. Using alcohol to cope may eventually increase your stress level by affecting your ability to sleep and be productive, and may even lead to alcohol abuse.

Chapter 12

1. c. Evaporation is the body's major mechanism of heat loss during exercise. It is the only method that can dissipate enough heat during exercise to maintain a core temperature close to normal.

2. b. High humidity inhibits sweat evaporation. So, along with high heat, high humidity can cause a rapid rise in body temperature.

3. d. Layering clothing is the best method to insulate your body. Air is an excellent insulator, and layering clothing traps air between layers to insulate the body.

4. b. In cold weather the body's core temperature can decrease to dangerous levels, causing hypothermia.

7. b. At high altitudes, there is less oxygen available in the air, and thus there is a reduced level of oxygen in the blood. In order to compensate, breathing increases to maximize the available oxygen.

12. a. Because back pain is often associated with muscle weakness, exercise plays a role in prevention. In particular, core strength training, including your abdominal muscles, can readily prevent such damage.

13. b. Acute muscle soreness immediately after exercise is usually due to overuse or injury.

14. d. Because shin splints are typically caused by stress on the soft tissues, each of the listed precautions can reduce the stress on the tissues and reduce the risk of injury.

15. d. Ligaments cannot withstand much movement with- out injury. Thus, refraining from exercises that place a strain on joints is the best way to prevent damage.

20. a. The Heimlich maneuver is a procedure designed to produce a diaphragm thrust and artificial cough which would dislodge the foreign body blocking the airway.

Chapter 13

1. d. When a malignant tumor (one that is cancerous) metastasizes, this means that the cancer cells have spread to other parts of the body. A benign tumor is not cancer.

3. d. A nagging cough or hoarseness, a sore that does not heal, and unusual bleeding or discharge are three of the seven warning signs of cancer. If you have any one of these, make an appointment to see your doctor right away.

4. a. Skin cancer is the most common type of cancer, but is highly treatable if detected early. Among people under the age of 30, melanoma is the most common type of skin cancer.

5. b. Lung cancer is the leading cause of cancer deaths among women in United States. While more women are diagnosed with breast cancer per year than lung cancer, breast cancer is typically detected earlier and is more treatable than lung cancer.

7. c. Performing regular breast self-exams is one thing you can do to reduce your cancer risk. However, behaviors such as poor diet, physical inactivity, and excessive alcohol consumption can increase your risk.

Chapter 14

6. a. There are over 30 strains of human papillomavirus (HPV), and while many infected individuals do not experience noticeable symptoms, some strains of HPV are responsible for genital warts.

16. d. Syphilis is a bacterial infection. If it is treated early, it can be cured with antibiotics.

17. a. Stage 1, primary syphilis, generally includes a dime-sized, painless sore, called a chancre, located at the initial site of infection.

20. b. These infections are all caused by parasites.

Chapter 15

1. a. Addiction is defined as a chronic psychological and/or physical dependence on a substance or behavior that is beyond voluntary control.

2. d. The factors that determine the risk for addiction include the drug used, genetic makeup of the individual, and the psychological makeup of the individual.

4. c. LSD and mescaline are not physically addictive and the potential for physical addiction for marijuana remains unknown. In contrast, nicotine is known to be highly physically addictive.

5. b. Psychoactive drugs alter brain function and can cause a state of intoxication.

6. a. Alcohol remains the most widely used recreational drug in the United States.

7. d. Blood alcohol concentrations $\geq 0.05\%$ have been shown to impair motor functions.

8. d. Binge drinking is defined as 5 or more drinks for men and 4 or more drinks for women within a 2-hour period.

appendix B

Nutritive Value of Selected Foods and Fast Foods

The following table of nutrient values presents nutritional information about a wide array of foods, including many fast foods. Values are given for calories, protein, carbohydrates, fiber, fat, saturated fat, and cholesterol for common foods and serving sizes. Use this information to assess your diet and make improvements. This is only a selection of common foods. See the MyDietAnalysis database for an extensive list of foods. When using the software, the foods identified here can be quickly found by entering the MyDietAnalysis code in the search field.

Values are obtained from the USDA Nutrient Database for Standard Reference, Release 21.

A "0" displayed in any given field indicates that nutrient value is determined to be zero; a blank space indicates that nutrient information is not available.

Ener = energy (kilocalories); *Prot* = protein; *Carb* = carbohydrate; *Fiber* = dietary fiber; *Fat* = total fat; *Sat* = saturated fat; *Chol* = cholesterol.

Index:

MDA Code	Food Name	Amt	Wt (g)	Ener (kcal)	Prot (g)	Carb (g)	Fiber (g)	Fat (g)	Sat (g)	Chol (mg)
	BEVERAGES									
	Alcoholic									
22831	Beer	12 fl-oz	360	157	1	13		0	0	0
34067	Beer, dark	12 fl-oz	355.5	150	1	13		0	0	0
34053	Beer, light	12 fl-oz	352.9	105	1	5	0	0	0	0
22849	Beer, pale ale	12 fl-oz	360.2	179	2	17		0	0	0
22545	Daiquiri, frozen, from concentrate mix	1 ea	36	101	0	26	0	0	0	0
22514	Gin, 80 proof	1 fl-oz	27.8	64	0	0	0	0	0	0
22544	Liqueur, coffee, 63 proof	1 fl-oz	34.8	107	0	11	0	0	0	0
34085	Martini, prepared from recipe	1 fl-oz	28.2	69	0	1	0	0	0	0
22593	Rum, 80 proof	1 fl-oz	27.8	64	0	0	0	0	0	0
22515	Tequila, 80 proof	1 fl-oz	27.8	64	0	0	0	0	0	0
22594	Vodka, 80 proof	1 fl-oz	27.8	64	0	0	0	0	0	0
22670	Whiskey, 80 proof	1 fl-oz	27.8	64	0	0	0	0	0	0
22884	Wine, red	1 fl-oz	29	24	0	1		0	0	
22861	Wine, white	1 fl-oz	29.3	24	0	1		0	0	
	Coffee									
20012	Coffee, brewed w/tap water	1 cup	237	2	0	0	0	0	0	0
20686	Coffee, decaffeinated, brewed w/tap water	1 cup	236.8	0	0	0	0	0	0	0
20439	Coffee, espresso, restaurant prepared	1 cup	237	5	0	0	0	0	0.2	0
20023	Coffee, instant, prepared w/water	1 cup	238.4	5	0	1	0	0	0	0
21210	Coffee, instant, vanilla, sugar free, cafe style	1 Tbs	6	30	0	2	0	2	2	0
	Dairy Mixed Drinks and Mixes									
85	Chocolate milk, prepared w/syrup, whole milk	1 cup	282	254	9	36	1	8	4.7	25
46	Hot cocoa, sugar free, w/aspartame, prepared w/water	1 cup	256	74	3	14	2	1	0.4	0
21	Hot cocoa, prepared from recipe, w/milk	1 cup	250	192	9	27	2	6	3.6	20
48	Hot cocoa, prepared from dry mix	1 cup	274.7	151	3	32	1	2	0.9	0
166	Hot cocoa, w/marshmallows, dry packet	1 ea	28	112	1	21	1	4	4.2	0
29	Malted milk, natural, w/o add nutrients, prepared from powder w/milk	1 cup	265	233	10	27	0	10	5.4	32
41	Drink, strawberry, prepared from dry mix w/whole milk	1 cup	266	234	8	33	0	8	5.1	32
	Fruit and Vegetable Beverages and Juices									
20965	Apple cider, flavored, low calorie, w/vitamin C, prepared from instant	8 fl-oz	240	2	0	1	0	0	0	0
71080	Apple juice, unsweetened	1 ea	262	121	0	30	1	0	0.1	0
3015	Apricot nectar, canned	1 cup	251	141	1	36	2	0	0	0
72092	Blackberry juice, canned	0.5 cup	120	46	0	9	0	1	0	0
5226	Carrot juice, canned	1 cup	236	94	2	22	2	0	0.1	0
20042	Clam and tomato juice, canned	1 ea	166.1	80	1	18	1	0		0
3042	Cranberry juice cocktail, bottled	1 cup	252.8	137	0	34	0	0	0	0
20115	Cranberry juice cocktail, from frozen concentrate	1 cup	249.6	117	0	29	0	0	0	0
3275	Cranberry-grape juice	1 cup	244.8	137	0	34	0	0	0.1	0
20024	Fruit punch, w/added nutrients, canned	1 cup	248	117	0	30	0	0	0	0
20035	Fruit punch, from frozen concentrate	1 cup	247.2	114	0	29	0	0	0	0
20101	Grape drink, canned	1 cup	250.4	153	0	39	0	0	0	0
3052	Grapefruit juice, unsweetened, canned	1 cup	247	94	1	22	0	0	0	0
3053	Grapefruit juice, unsweetened, from frozen concentrate	1 cup	247	101	1	24	0	0	0	0
3068	Lemon juice, fresh	1 Tbs	15.2	4	0	1	0	0	0	0
20045	Lemonade, prepared from powder	1 cup	266	69	0	18	0	0	0	0
20047	Lemonade, low-calorie, w/aspartame, prepared from powder	1 cup	236.8	7	0	2	0	0	0	0

MDA Code	Food Name	Amt	Wt (g)	Ener (kcal)	Prot (g)	Carb (g)	Fiber (g)	Fat (g)	Sat (g)	Chol (mg)
20117	Lemonade, pink, from frozen concentrate	1 cup	247.2	99	0	26	0	0	0	0
3072	Lime juice, fresh	1 Tbs	15.4	4	0	1	0	0	0	0
20002	Limeade, from frozen concentrate	1 cup	247.2	129	0	34	0	0	0	0
20070	Orange drink, w/added vitamin C, canned	1 cup	248	122	0	31	0	0	0	0
20004	Orange breakfast drink, from powder	1 cup	248	122	0	31	0	0	0	0
71108	Orange juice, unsweetened, box	1 ea	263	124	2	29	1	0	0	0
3090	Orange juice, fresh	1 cup	248	112	2	26	0	0	0.1	0
3091	Orange juice, unsweetened, from frozen concentrate	1 cup	249	112	2	27	0	0	0	0
3170	Orange-grapefruit juice, unsweetened, canned	1 cup	247	106	1	25	0	0	0	0
3101	Peach nectar, canned	1 cup	249	134	1	35	1	0	0	0
20059	Pineapple-grapefruit juice, canned	1 cup	250.4	118	1	29	0	0	0	0
20025	Pineapple-orange juice, canned	1 cup	250.4	125	3	30	0	0	0	0
3120	Pineapple juice, unsweetened, canned	1 cup	250	132	1	32	1	0	0	0
3128	Prune juice, canned	1 cup	256	182	2	45	3	0	0	0
3985	Punch, fruit	1 cup	247.2	128	0	31	0	0	0	0
20106	Punch, fruit, prepared from frozen concentrate, w/water	8 fl-oz	234.4	98	0	24	0	0	0	0
14594	Punch, tropical, w/artificial sweetener, from dry packet	1 indv pkt	8	30	0	7	0	0	0	0
3140	Tangerine juice, sweetened, canned	1 cup	249	124	1	30	0	0	0	0
5397	Tomato juice, unsalted, canned	1 cup	243	41	2	10	1	0	0	0
20849	Vegetable-fruit juice, mixed	4 oz	113.4	33	0	8	0	0		0
20080	Vegetable juice, mixed, canned	1 cup	242	46	2	11	2	0	0	0
	Soft Drinks									
20006	Club soda	1 cup	236.8	0	0	0	0	0	0	0
20685	Low-calorie caffeine-free cola, w/aspartame	12 fl-oz	355.2	4	0	1	0	0	0	0
20843	Cola, w/higher caffeine	12 fl-oz	370	152	0	39	0	0	0	0
20028	Cream soda	1 cup	247.2	126	0	33	0	0	0	0
20008	Ginger ale	1 cup	244	83	0	21	0	0	0	0
20031	Grape soda	1 cup	248	107	0	28	0	0	0	0
20032	Lemon-lime soft drink	1 cup	245.6	98	0	25	0	0		0
20027	Pepper-type soft drink	1 cup	245.6	101	0	26	0	0	0.2	0
20009	Root beer	1 cup	246.4	101	0	26	0	0	0	0
	Teas									
20436	Iced tea, lemon flavor	1 cup	240	86	0	22	0	0	0	
20040	Instant tea powdered mix, lemon flavor, w/saccharin	1 cup	236.8	5	0	1	0	0	0	0
20014	Tea, brewed	1 cup	236.8	2	0	1	0	0	0	0
444	Tea, decaffeinated, brewed	1 cup	236.8	2	0	1	0	0	0	0
20118	Tea, herbal, chamomile, brewed	1 cup	236.8	2	0	0	0	0	0	0
20036	Tea, herbal (not chamomile), brewed	1 cup	236.8	2	0	0	0	0	0	0
	Other Drinks									
22606	Beer, nonalcoholic	12 fl-oz	352.9	73	1	14	0	0	0	0
17	Eggnog	1 cup	254	343	10	34	0	19	11.3	150
8889	Rice milk, enriched, original	8 fl-oz	248	120	1	25	0	2	0	0
20033	Soy milk	1 cup	245	132	8	15	1	4	0.5	0
21070	Soy milk, plain, "lite"	1 cup	245	90	4	15	2	2	0	0
21064	Soy milk, vanilla	1 cup	245	190	11	25	5	5	0.5	0
20041	Water, tap, (municipal)	1 cup	236.6	0	0	0	0	0	0	0
	Breakfast Cereals									
61211	Bran, w/malted flour	0.33 cup	29	83	4	23	8	1	0.1	0
40095	All-Bran/Kelloggs	0.5 cup	30	78	4	22	9	1	0.2	0
40295	Apple Cinnamon Cheerios/General Mills	0.75 cup	30	120	2	25	1	2	0	0

MDA Code	Food Name	Amt	Wt (g)	Ener (kcal)	Prot (g)	Carb (g)	Fiber (g)	Fat (g)	Sat (g)	Chol (mg)
40098	Apple Jacks/Kelloggs	1 cup	30	117	1	27	0	0	0.1	0
40394	Basic 4/General Mills	1 cup	55	210	4	44	3	3	0.5	0
40259	Bran Flakes/Post	0.75 cup	30	96	3	24	5	1	0.1	0
40032	Capn' Crunch/Quaker Oats	0.75 cup	27	109	1	23	1	2	1.1	0
40297	Cheerios/General Mills	1 cup	30	110	3	22	3	2	0.3	0
40414	Cinnamon Grahams/General Mills	0.75 cup	30	113	2	26	1	1	0.2	0
60924	Chex, multi-bran/General Mills	0.75 cup	47	154	3	40	6	1	0.2	0
40126	Cinnamon Toast Crunch/General Mills	0.75 cup	30	130	2	24	1	3	0.4	0
40102	Cocoa Krispies/Kelloggs	0.75 cup	31	118	2	27	1	1	0.6	0
40425	Cocoa Puffs/General Mills	1 cup	30	120	1	26	2	2	0	0
40325	Corn Chex/General Mills	1 cup	30	110	2	26	1	1	0.1	0
40195	Corn Flakes/Kelloggs	1 cup	28	101	2	24	1	0	0.1	0
40089	Corn Grits, instant, plain, prepared/Quaker Oats	1 ea	137	93	2	21	1	0	0	0
40206	Corn Pops/Kelloggs	1 cup	31	117	1	28	0	0	0.1	0
40205	Cracklin' Oat Bran/Kelloggs	0.75 cup	55	221	4	39	7	8	3.4	0
40179	Rice cereal, hot, prepared with salt	1 cup	244	127	2	28	0	0	0	0
40182	Farina, hot, instant, prepared with salt	1 cup	241	149	4	32	1	1	0.1	0
40104	Crispix/Kelloggs	1 cup	29	109	2	25	0	0	0.1	0
40130	Fiber One/General Mills	0.5 cup	30	60	2	25	14	1	0.1	0
40218	Froot Loops/Kelloggs	1 cup	30	118	1	26	1	1	0.6	0
40217	Frosted Flakes/ Kelloggs	0.75 cup	31	114	1	28	1	0	0	0
11916	Frosted Mini Wheats, bite-size/Kelloggs	1 cup	55	189	6	45	6	1	0.2	0
40197	Granola, lowfat w/raisins/Kelloggs	0.66 cup	55	211	4	45	4	3	0.8	0
40265	Grape Nuts Flakes	0.75 cup	29	106	3	24	3	1	0.2	0
61155	Honey Bunches Of Oats	0.75 cup	30	118	2	25	1	1	0.1	0
40378	Honey Nut Clusters	1 cup	57	218	4	48	3	3	0	0
40010	Kix/General Mills	1.33 cup	30	110	2	25	3	1	0.2	0
40011	Life, plain/Quaker Oats	0.75 cup	32	119	3	25	2	1	0.3	0
40300	Lucky Charms/General Mills	1 cup	30	122	2	25	1	1	0.2	0
40186	Wheat cereal, hot, prepared w/salt	1 cup	249	189	6	39	2	1	0.2	0
40434	Oat Bran/Quaker Oats	1.25 cup	57	212	7	43	6	3	0.5	0
61223	Oat, corn & wheat squares, maple flavor, w/add sugar	1 cup	30	129	2	24	1	3	0.4	0
40358	Oatmeal Squares, cinnamon	1 cup	60	227	6	48	5	3	0.5	0
40430	Oatmeal Squares/Quaker Oats	1 cup	56	212	6	44	4	2	0.5	0
40073	Oatmeal, hot, apple-cinnamon, instant Quaker Oats	1 ea	149	130	3	26	3	1	0.2	0
40343	Peanut Butter Puffs (Reeses)/General Mills	0.75 cup	30	130	2	23	1	4	0.5	0
40018	Puffed Rice/Quaker Oats	1 cup	14	54	1	12	0	0	0	0
40242	Puffed Wheat, fortified	1 cup	12	44	2	10	1	0	0	0
40209	Raisin Bran/Kelloggs	1 cup	61	196	5	47	7	1	0.2	0
40117	Raisin Squares, mini wheats	0.75 cup	55	188	5	44	5	1	0.2	0
40333	Rice Chex/General Mills	1.25 cup	31	118	2	26	0	0	0.1	0
40210	Rice Krispies/Kelloggs	1.25 cup	33	128	2	28	0	0	0.1	0
60887	Shredded Wheat, no added sugar or salt, round biscuits	2 ea	37.8	127	4	30	5	1	0.2	0
40288	Shredded Wheat 'N Bran	1 cup	237	792	30	189	32	3	0.5	0
60879	Smart Start/Kelloggs	1 cup	50	182	4	43	3	1	0.1	0
40211	Special K/Kelloggs	1 cup	31	117	7	22	1	0	0.1	0
40413	Toasty Os/Malt-O-Meal	1 cup	30	121	4	22	3	2	0.4	0
40382	Total Raisin Bran/General Mills	1 cup	55	170	3	42	5	1	0.2	0
40021	Total Wheat/General Mills	0.75 cup	30	100	2	23	3	1	0.1	0
40306	Trix/General Mills	1 cup	30	120	1	26	1	2	0.2	0

MDA Code	Food Name	Amt	Wt (g)	Ener (kcal)	Prot (g)	Carb (g)	Fiber (g)	Fat (g)	Sat (g)	Chol (mg)
40202	Wheat Bran Flakes, complete	0.75 cup	29	92	3	23	5	1	0.1	0
40335	Wheat Chex/General Mills	1 cup	30	108	3	24	3	1	0.1	0
61208	Wheat & malt barley flakes	0.75 cup	29	106	3	24	3	1	0.2	0
40307	Wheaties/General Mills	1 cup	30	110	3	24	3	1	0.1	0
	Dairy									
7	Buttermilk, lowfat, cultured	1 cup	245	98	8	12	0	2	1.3	10
500	Cream, half & half	2 Tbs	30	39	1	1	0	3	2.1	11
218	Milk, 2% w/added vitamins A & D	1 cup	245	130	8	13	0	5	3	20
21109	Milk, chocolate, reduced fat w/added calcium	1 cup	250	195	7	30	2	5	2.9	20
19	Milk, chocolate, reduced fat	1 cup	250	158	8	26	1	2	1.5	8
11	Milk, condensed, sweetened	2 Tbs	38.2	123	3	21	0	3	2.1	13
134	Milk, evaporated, whole, w/added vitamin A	2 Tbs	31.5	42	2	3	0	2	1.4	9
68	Milk, nonfat/skim, w/added vitamin D, dry	0.5 cup	60	217	22	31	0	0	0.3	12
6	Milk, nonfat/skim, w/added vitamin A	1 cup	245	83	8	12	0	0	0.1	5
1	Milk, whole, 3.25%	1 cup	244	146	8	11	0	8	4.6	24
20	Milk, whole, chocolate	1 cup	250	208	8	26	2	8	5.3	30
2834	Yogurt, blueberry, fruit on the bottom	1 ea	227	220	9	41	1	2	1	10
2315	Yogurt, blueberry, lowfat	1 ea	113	110	3	23	0	1	0.5	10
72636	Yogurt, blueberry, nonfat	1 ea	227	120	7	21	0	0	0	5
72639	Yogurt, creamy vanilla, nonfat	1 ea	227	120	7	21	0	0	0	5
2001	Yogurt, fruit, lowfat	1 cup	245	250	11	47	0	3	1.7	10
15408	Yogurt, fruit, nonfat	1 cup	245	233	11	47	0	0	0.3	5
2450	Yogurt, lemon, nonfat	1 cup	227	130	8	24	0	0	0	5
	Cheese									
1287	American, nonfat, slice/Kraft	1 pce	21.3	32	5	2	0	0	0.1	3
47855	Blue, 1" cube	1 ea	17.3	61	4	0	0	5	3.2	13
47859	Brie, 1" cube	1 ea	17	57	4	0	0	5	3	17
48333	Cheddar, 1" cube, processed, pasterized, fat-free	1 ea	16	24	4	2	0	0	0.1	2
1440	Cheese, fondue	2 Tbs	26.9	62	4	1	0	4	2.3	12
48313	Cheese spread, cream cheese base	1 Tbs	15	44	1	1	0	4	2.7	14
13349	Cheese sauce, pasturized, processed/Kraft	2 Tbs	33	91	4	3	0	7	4.3	25
1014	Cottage cheese, 2% fat	0.5 cup	113	97	13	4	0	3	1.1	11
47867	Cottage cheese, fat-free, small curd, dry	0.5 cup	113	81	12	8	0	0	0.2	8
1015	Cream cheese	2 Tbs	29	99	2	1	0	10	5.6	32
1452	Cream cheese, fat-free	2 Tbs	29	30	5	2	0	0	0.2	3
1016	Feta, crumbled	0.25 cup	37.5	99	5	2	0	8	5.6	33
1054	Gouda	1 oz	28.4	101	7	1	0	8	5	32
1442	Mexican, queso anejo, crumbled	0.25 cup	33	123	7	2	0	10	6.3	35
47885	Monterey jack, slice	1 ea	28.4	106	7	0	0	9	5.4	25
47887	Mozzarella, whole milk, slice	1 ea	34	102	8	1	0	8	4.5	27
1075	Parmesan, grated	1 Tbs	5	22	2	0	0	1	0.9	4
47900	Provolone, slice	1 ea	28.4	100	7	1	0	8	4.9	20
1064	Ricotta, whole milk	0.25 cup	62	108	7	2	0	8	5.1	32
	Eggs and Egg Substitutes									
19510	Egg, hard boiled, large	1 ea	50	78	6	1	0	5	1.6	212
19517	Egg, poached, large	1 ea	50	71	6	0	0	5	1.5	211
19525	Egg substitute, liquid	0.25 cup	62.8	53	8	0	0	2	0.4	1
19506	Egg whites, raw, large	1 ea	33.4	16	4	0	0	0		0
19509	Egg, whole, large, fried	1 ea	46	90	6	0	0	7	2	210
19516	Egg, scrambled	1 ea	61	102	7	1	0	7	2.2	215
19508	Egg yolk, raw, large	1 ea	16.6	53	3	1	0	4	1.6	205

MDA Code	Food Name	Amt	Wt (g)	Ener (kcal)	Prot (g)	Carb (g)	Fiber (g)	Fat (g)	Sat (g)	Chol (mg)
	Fruit									
71079	Apples, fresh, chopped w/peel	1 cup	125	65	0	17	3	0	0	0
3004	Apples, fresh, peeled, slices	1 cup	110	53	0	14	1	0	0	0
3001	Apple, fresh, w/peel, medium, 3"	1 ea	182	95	0	25	4	0	0.1	0
3330	Applesauce, unsweetened, w/vitamin C, canned	1 cup	244	102	0	27	3	0	0	0
72101	Apricots, w/heavy syrup, canned, drained	1 cup	182	151	1	39	5	0	0	0
3657	Apricots, raw, sliced	1 cup	165	79	2	18	3	1	0	0
3210	Avocado, California, raw	1 ea	173	289	3	15	12	27	3.7	0
3024	Blackberries, fresh	1 cup	144	62	2	14	7	1	0	0
3032	Boysenberries, w/heavy syrup, canned	0.5 cup	128	113	1	29	3	0	0	0
3026	Boysenberries, fresh	0.5 cup	72	31	1	7	4	0	0	0
71082	Banana, fresh, extra small, 6" or shorter	1 ea	81	72	1	19	2	0	0.1	0
3642	Cantaloupe, fresh, wedge, 1/8 of a medium melon	1 pce	69	23	1	6	1	0	0	0
72094	Cherries, maraschino, canned, drained	1 ea	4	7	0	2	0	0	0	0
3336	Cherries, sweetened, canned, w/juice	0.5 cup	125	68	1	17	2	0	0	0
3045	Fruit cocktail, canned, w/heavy syrup	0.5 cup	124	91	0	23	1	0	0	0
3164	Fruit cocktail, canned, w/juice	0.5 cup	118.5	55	1	14	1	0	0	0
3414	Fruit salad, canned, w/heavy syrup	0.5 cup	127.5	93	0	24	1	0	0	0
44023	Fuit salad, canned, w/juice	0.5 cup	124.5	62	1	16	1	0	0	0
72093	Cranberries, dried, sweetened	0.25 cup	30.3	93	0	25	2	0	0	0
3673	Cranberries, fresh, chopped	0.5 cup	55	25	0	7	3	0	0	0
3192	Currants, zante, dried	0.25 cup	36	102	1	27	2	0	0	0
72111	Dates, medjool, w/o pit	1 ea	40	111	1	30	3	0		
3677	Figs, fresh, small, 1-1/2"	1 ea	40	30	0	8	1	0	0	0
71976	Grapefruit, fresh, medium	0.5 ea	154	60	1	16	6	0	0	0
3634	Guava, fresh	0.5 cup	82.5	56	2	12	4	1	0.2	0
3055	Grapes, Thompson seedless, fresh	0.5 cup	80	55	1	14	1	0	0	0
3342	Grapefruit, canned, w/juice, sections	0.5 cup	124.5	46	1	11	0	0	0	0
3644	Honeydew, fresh, 6"-7"	1 ea	1280	461	7	116	10	2	0.5	0
71979	Lemon, fresh, medium	1 ea	58	15	0	5	1	0	0	0
3071	Lime, fresh, peeled, 2"	1 ea	67	20	0	7	2	0	0	0
71743	Lychee (Litchi), dried, shelled	1 ea	2.5	7	0	2	0	0	0	0
71990	Mandarin orange, fresh, medium	1 ea	109	50	1	15	3	0	0	0
71927	Mango, dried	0.33 cup	40	140	0	34	1	0	0	0
3221	Mango, fresh, whole	1 ea	207	135	1	35	4	1	0.1	0
3644	Melon, honeydew, fresh, 6"-7"	1 ea	1280	461	7	116	10	2	0.5	0
3085	Orange, all types, fresh, large, 3-1/16"	1 ea	184	86	2	22	4	0	0	0
71990	Orange, mandarin, fresh, medium	1 ea	109	50	1	15	3	0	0	0
3228	Orange, navel, fresh, 2-7/8"	1 ea	140	69	1	18	3	0	0	12
3098	Peaches, canned, w/heavy syrup	1 cup	262	194	1	52	3	0	0	0
3194	Persimmon, native, fresh	1 ea	25	32	0	8	0	0		0
3168	Mixed fruit, prunes apricots & pears, dried	1 ea	293	712	7	188	23	1	0.1	0
3216	Nectarines, fresh, slices	0.5 cup	71.5	31	1	8	1	0	0	0
3721	Papaya, fresh, small, 4 1/2" × 2 3/4"	1 ea	152	59	1	15	3	0	0.1	0
3726	Peaches, fresh, small, w/o skin, 2.5"	1 cup	130	51	1	12	2	0	0	0
3106	Pear, fresh, large	1 ea	209	121	1	32	6	0	0	0
72113	Pineapple, fresh, slice	1 pce	84	38	0	10		0		
3748	Plantain, cooked, mashed	1 cup	200	232	2	62	5	0	0.1	0
3121	Plum, fresh	1 ea	66	30	0	8	1	0	0	0
3197	Pomegranate, fresh	1 ea	154	128	3	29	6	2	0.2	0

MDA Code	Food Name	Amt	Wt (g)	Ener (kcal)	Prot (g)	Carb (g)	Fiber (g)	Fat (g)	Sat (g)	Chol (mg)
3766	Raisins, seedless	50 ea	26	78	1	21	1	0	0	0
9758	Raisins, golden, seedless	0.25 cup	40	130	1	31	2	0	0	0
71987	Raspberries, fresh	1 cup	125	50	1	17	8	0	0	0
3354	Strawberries, frozen, sweetened, thawed, whole	0.5 cup	127.5	99	1	27	2	0	0	0
3135	Strawberries, fresh, slices	1 cup	166	53	1	13	3	0	0	0
3717	Tangerine, fresh, large	1 ea	98	52	1	13	2	0	0	0
3143	Watermelon, fresh, 1/16 melon	1 pce	286	86	2	22	1	0	0	0

GRAIN AND FLOUR PRODUCTS

Breads, Rolls, Bread Crumbs, and Croutons

MDA Code	Food Name	Amt	Wt (g)	Ener (kcal)	Prot (g)	Carb (g)	Fiber (g)	Fat (g)	Sat (g)	Chol (mg)
62740	Bagel, blueberry	1 ea	85	190	7	40	5	2	0	0
71170	Bagel, cinnamon raisin, mini, 2-1/2"	1 ea	26	71	3	14	1	0	0.1	0
71167	Bagel, egg, mini, 2-1/2"	1 ea	26	72	3	14	1	1	0.1	6
71152	Bagel, sesame, mini, enriched, w/calcium propionate, 2-1/2"	1 ea	26	67	3	13	1	0	0.1	0
42039	Banana bread, homemade w/margarine, slice	1 pce	60	196	3	33	1	6	1.3	26
42433	Biscuit	1 ea	82	273	5	28	1	16	3.9	1
47709	Biscuit, buttermilk, refrigerated dough/Pillsbury	1 ea	64	150	4	29	1	2	0.3	0
71192	Biscuit, plain, lowfat, refrigerated dough	1 ea	21	63	2	12	0	1	0.3	0
42004	Bread crumbs, dry	1 Tbs	6.8	27	1	5	0	0	0.1	0
49144	Bread, garlic, Italian, crusty	1 pce	50	186	4	21		10	2.4	6
42090	Bread, egg, slice	1 pce	40	113	4	19	1	2	0.6	20
42069	Bread, oat bran, slice	1 pce	30	71	3	12	1	1	0.2	0
42076	Bread, oat bran, reduced calorie, slice	1 pce	23	46	2	9	3	1	0.1	0
42136	Bread, wheat bran, slice	1 pce	36	89	3	17	1	1	0.3	0
42095	Bread, whole wheat, reduced calorie, slice	1 pce	23	46	2	10	3	1	0.1	0
71247	Bread, white, soft, w/o crust, thin slice	1 pce	9	24	1	5	0	0	0.1	0
42084	Bread, white, reduced calorie, slice	1 pce	23	48	2	10	2	1	0.1	0
71259	Breadsticks, plain, small, 4-1/4" Long	1 ea	5	21	1	3	0	0	0.1	0
26561	Buns, hamburger/Wonder	1 ea	43	117	3	22	1	2	0.4	
42021	Buns, hot dog/frankfurter	1 ea	43	120	4	21	1	2	0.5	0
71364	Buns, whole wheat, hot dog/frankfurter	1 ea	43	114	4	22	3	2	0.4	0
42115	Cornbread, prepared from dry mix	1 pce	60	188	4	29	1	6	1.6	37
42016	Croutons, plain, dry	0.25 cup	7.5	31	1	6	0	0	0.1	0
71227	Pita bread, white, enriched, small, 4"	1 ea	28	77	3	16	1	0	0	0
71228	Pita bread, whole wheat, small, 4"	1 ea	28	74	3	15	2	1	0.1	0
42159	Roll, dinner, egg, 2-1/2"	1 ea	35	107	3	18	1	2	0.6	18
42161	Roll, dinner, french	1 ea	38	105	3	19	1	2	0.4	0
71056	Roll, Kaiser	1 ea	57	167	6	30	1	2	0.3	0
42297	Tortilla, corn, unsalted, medium, 6"	1 ea	26	58	1	12	1	1	0.1	0
90645	Taco shells, baked, medium, 6"	1 ea	10	46	0	6	0	2	0.4	0

Crackers

MDA Code	Food Name	Amt	Wt (g)	Ener (kcal)	Prot (g)	Carb (g)	Fiber (g)	Fat (g)	Sat (g)	Chol (mg)
71277	Cheese crackers, bite size	1 cup	62	312	6	36	1	16	5.8	8
71451	Goldfish cheese crackers, low sodium	55 pce	33	166	3	19	1	8	3.2	4
43532	Rye crispbread crackers	1 ea	10	37	1	8	2	0	0	0
71284	Melba toast crackers, plain, peices	1 cup	30	117	4	23	2	1	0.1	0
43507	Oyster crackers	1 cup	45	189	4	33	1	4	0.9	0
70963	Butter crackers, original/Kraft	5 ea	16	79	1	10	0	4	0.9	
43587	Saltine crackers, original/Kraft	5 ea	14	56	1	10	0	1	0	0
43664	Saltine crackers, fat free, low sodium	6 ea	30	118	3	25	1	0	0.1	0
43659	Oyster crackers, low sodium	1 cup	45	189	4	33	1	4	0.9	0
43545	Crackers w/cheese filling	4 ea	28	134	3	17	1	6	1.7	1

MDA Code	Food Name	Amt	Wt (g)	Ener (kcal)	Prot (g)	Carb (g)	Fiber (g)	Fat (g)	Sat (g)	Chol (mg)
43501	Crackers, cheese, w/peanut butter filling	4 ea	28	139	3	16	1	7	1.2	0
43546	Crackers w/peanut butter filling	4 ea	28	138	3	16	1	7	1.4	0
43581	Crackers, wheat, original/Kraft	16 ea	29	140	3	20	1	6	0.9	0
12683	Crackers, Wheat Thins/Kraft	5 ea	16	80	1	10	0	4	1	0
43508	Crackers, whole wheat	4 ea	32	142	3	22	3	6	1.1	0
	Muffins									
42723	English muffin, plain/Thomas'	1 ea	57	132	5	26		1	0.2	
42153	English muffin, wheat	1 ea	57	127	5	26	3	1	0.2	0
62916	Muffin, blueberry, mini, 1-1/4"	1 ea	11	43	1	5	0	2	0.4	4
44521	Muffin, corn, 2-1/4" × 2-1/2"	1 ea	57	174	3	29	2	5	0.8	15
44514	Muffin, oat bran, 2-1/4" × 2-1/2"	1 ea	57	154	4	28	3	4	0.6	0
44518	Toaster muffin, blueberry	1 ea	33	103	2	18	1	3	0.5	2
44522	Toaster muffin, cornmeal	1 ea	33	114	2	19	1	4	0.6	4
	Noodles and Pasta									
66103	Angel hair pasta, semolina, dry	2 oz	56	201	7	41	2	1	0.3	0
91313	Bow tie pasta, enriched, dry	1.5 cup	56	204	8	42	2	1	0.2	0
38048	Chow mein noodles, dry	1 cup	45	237	4	26	2	14	2	0
38047	Egg pasta, enriched, cooked	0.5 cup	80	110	4	20	1	2	0.3	23
91316	Elbow pasta, enriched, dry	0.5 cup	56	204	8	42	2	1	0.2	0
38356	Fettuccine pasta, frozen/Kraft	70 g	70	200	8	38	2	2	0	0
91293	Fettuccine pasta, spinach, enriched, dry	1.33 cup	56	202	8	40	2	1	0.3	1
38102	Macaroni pasta, enriched, cooked	1 cup	140	221	8	43	3	1	0.2	0
66121	Pasta shells, low protein, wheat free, dry, small	2 oz	56.7	194	0	48	0	0	0	0
92830	Penne pasta, dry	2 oz	57	210	7	41	1	1		0
38067	Ramen noodles, cooked	0.5 cup	113.5	77	2	10	1	3	0.8	0
38551	Rice pasta, cooked	0.5 cup	88	96	1	22	1	0	0	0
38094	Soba noodles, cooked	1 cup	114	113	6	24		0	0	0
38118	Spaghetti, enriched, cooked	0.5 cup	70	111	4	22	1	1	0.1	0
38066	Spaghetti, spinach, cooked	1 cup	140	182	6	37	5	1	0.1	0
38060	Spaghetti, whole wheat, cooked	1 cup	140	174	7	37	6	1	0.1	0
	Grains									
38003	Barley, pearled, cooked	0.5 cup	78.5	97	2	22	3	0	0.1	0
38028	Bulgur, wheat, cooked	1 cup	182	151	6	34	8	0	0.1	0
38279	Cornmeal, yellow, dry	0.25 cup	41.5	151	4	31	3	2	0.3	0
38076	Couscous, cooked	0.5 cup	78.5	88	3	18	1	0	0	0
5470	Hominy, yellow, canned	0.5 cup	80	58	1	11	2	1	0.1	0
38078	Oat bran, cooked	0.5 cup	109.5	44	4	13	3	1	0.2	0
38080	Oats, whole grain, unprocessed	0.25 cup	39	152	7	26	4	3	0.5	0
38010	Rice, brown, long grain, cooked	1 cup	195	216	5	45	4	2	0.4	0
38082	Rice, brown, medium grain, cooked	0.5 cup	97.5	109	2	23	2	1	0.2	0
38256	Rice, white, enriched, long grain, cooked w/salt	1 cup	158	205	4	45	1	0	0.1	0
38019	Rice, white, enriched, long grain, instant, cooked	1 cup	165	193	4	41	1	1	0	0
38097	Rice, white, medium grain, cooked	0.5 cup	93	121	2	27	0	0	0.1	0
38034	Tapioca, pearl, dry	0.25 cup	38	136	0	34	0	0	0	0
38025	Wheat, germ, crude, raw	0.25 cup	28.8	104	7	15	4	3	0.5	0
	Pancakes, French Toast, and Waffles									
42155	French toast, frozen	1 pce	59	126	4	19	1	4	0.9	48
42156	French toast, homemade w/2% milk	1 pce	65	149	5	16		7	1.8	75
45192	Pancakes, buttermilk, frozen/Eggo	1 ea	42.5	99	3	16	0	3	0.6	5
45118	Pancakes, blueberry, homemade, 6"	1 ea	77	171	5	22	1	7	1.5	43

MDA Code	Food Name	Amt	Wt (g)	Ener (kcal)	Prot (g)	Carb (g)	Fiber (g)	Fat (g)	Sat (g)	Chol (mg)
45117	Pancakes, plain, homemade, 6"	1 ea	77	175	5	22	1	7	1.6	45
45193	Waffles, homestyle, low fat, frozen/Eggo	1 ea	35	83	2	15	0	1	0.3	9
45003	Waffles, homemade, 7"	1 ea	75	218	6	25	1	11	2.1	52
	MEAT AND MEAT SUBSTITUTES									
	Beef									
10093	Beef, average of all cuts, cooked, 1/4" trim	3 oz	85.1	260	22	0	0	18	7.3	75
10705	Beef, average of all cuts, lean, cooked, 1/4" trim	3 oz	85.1	184	25	0	0	8	3.2	73
10108	Beef, brisket, whole, braised, 1/4" trim	3 oz	85.1	328	20	0	0	27	10.5	80
10035	Beef, breakfast strips, cured, cooked	3 ea	34	153	11	0	0	12	4.9	40
58099	Beef, chuck tender steak, broiled, 0" trim	3 oz	85.1	136	22	0	0	5	1.6	54
10264	Beef, cured, thin sliced	5 pce	21	37	6	1	0	1	0.3	9
10624	Beef, short ribs, braised, choice	3 oz	85.1	401	18	0	0	36	15.1	80
10133	Beef, whole rib, roasted, 1/4" trim	3 oz	85.1	305	19	0	0	25	10	71
10008	Corned beef, cured, slices, canned	3 oz	85.1	213	23	0	0	13	5.3	73
58129	Ground beef, hamburger, pan browned, 25% fat	3 oz	85.1	236	22	0	0	15	6	76
58114	Ground beef, hamburger, pan browned, 10% fat	3 oz	85.1	196	24	0	0	10	4	76
58109	Ground beef, hamburger, pan browned, 5% fat	3 oz	85.1	164	25	0	0	6	2.9	76
10791	Porterhouse steak, broiled, 1/4" trim	3 oz	85.1	280	19	0	0	22	8.7	61
58257	Rib eye steak, broiled, 0" trim	3 oz	85.1	210	23	0	0	13	4.9	94
58094	Skirt steak, broiled, 0" trim	3 oz	85.1	187	22	0	0	10	4	51
58328	Strip steak, top loin, lean, broiled, choice, 1/8" trim	3 oz	85.1	171	25	0	0	7	2.7	67
10805	T-bone steak, broiled, 1/4" trim	3 oz	85.1	260	20	0	0	19	7.6	55
58299	Top round steak, lean, broiled, select, 1/8" trim	3 oz	85.1	151	27	0	0	4	1.4	52
58098	Tri-tip steak, loin, broiled, 0" trim	3 oz	85.1	226	26	0	0	13	4.9	58
11531	Veal, average of all cuts, cooked	3 oz	85.1	197	26	0	0	10	3.6	97
	Chicken									
81185	Chicken, breast, mesquite flavor, fat free, sliced	2 pce	42	34	7	1	0	0	0.1	15
81186	Chicken, breast, oven roasted, fat free, sliced	2 pce	42	33	7	1	0	0	0.1	15
15013	Chicken breast, w/skin, batter fried	3 oz	85.1	221	21	8	0	11	3	72
15057	Chicken breast, w/o skin, fried	3 oz	85.1	159	28	0	0	4	1.1	77
15113	Chicken, dark meat, w/skin, batter fried	3 oz	85.1	254	19	8		16	4.2	76
15080	Chicken, dark meat, w/skin, roasted	3 oz	85.1	215	22	0	0	13	3.7	77
15030	Chicken drumstick, w/skin, batter fried	3 oz	85.1	228	19	7	0	13	3.5	73
15042	Chicken drumstick, w/o skin, fried	3 oz	85.1	166	24	0	0	7	1.8	80
15111	Chicken, light meat, w/skin, batter fried	3 oz	85.1	236	20	8	0	13	3.5	71
15077	Chicken, light meat, w/skin, roasted	3 oz	85.1	189	25	0	0	9	2.6	71
15072	Chicken, whole, w/skin, batter fried	3 oz	85.1	246	19	8		15	3.9	74
15000	Chicken, whole, w/o skin, roasted	3 oz	85.1	162	25	0	0	6	1.7	76
15036	Chicken thigh, w/skin, batter fried	3 oz	85.1	236	18	8	0	14	3.8	79
15011	Chicken thigh, w/o skin, fried	3 oz	85.1	186	24	1	0	9	2.4	87
15034	Chicken wing, w/skin, batter fried	3 oz	85.1	276	17	9	0	19	5	67
15048	Chicken wing, w/o skin, fried	3 oz	85.1	180	26	0	0	8	2.1	71
15059	Chicken wing, w/o skin, roasted	3 oz	85.1	173	26	0	0	7	1.9	72
	Turkey									
51151	Turkey bacon, cooked	1 oz	28.4	108	8	1	0	8	2.4	28
51098	Turkey, thick slice, breaded & batter fried, 3" × 2" × 3/8"	1 ea	42	119	6	7	0	8	2	32
16308	Turkey, roast, light & dark meat, from frozen	1 cup	135	209	29	4	0	8	2.6	72
16110	Turkey breast, w/skin, roasted	3 oz	85.1	130	25	0	0	3	0.7	77
16038	Turkey breast, w/o skin, roasted	3 oz	85.1	115	26	0	0	1	0.2	71

MDA Code	Food Name	Amt	Wt (g)	Ener (kcal)	Prot (g)	Carb (g)	Fiber (g)	Fat (g)	Sat (g)	Chol (mg)
16101	Turkey, dark meat, w/skin, roasted	3 oz	85.1	155	24	0	0	6	1.8	100
16099	Turkey, light meat, w/skin, roasted	3 oz	85.1	140	24	0	0	4	1.1	81
16003	Turkey, ground patty, 13% fat, raw	1 ea	113.4	193	22	0	0	11	2.8	84
Lamb										
13604	Lamb, average of all cuts, cooked, choice, 1/4" trim	3 oz	85.1	250	21	0	0	18	7.5	83
13616	Lamb, average of all cuts, cooked, choice, lean 1/4" trim	3 oz	85.1	175	24	0	0	8	2.9	78
13522	Lamb, kabob meat, lean, broiled, 1/4" trim	3 oz	85.1	158	24	0	0	6	2.2	77
13524	Lamb, ground, broiled, 20% Fat	3 oz	85	241	21	0	0	17	6.9	82
Pork										
12000	Bacon, medium slice, cooked	3 pce	19	103	7	0	0	8	2.6	21
28143	Bacon, Canadian/Hormel	1 ea	56	68	9	1		3	1	27
12212	Ham, extra lean, 5% fat, roasted	1 cup	140	203	29	2	0	8	2.5	74
12211	Ham, 11% fat, roasted	1 cup	140	249	32	0	0	13	4.4	83
12309	Pork, loin & spareribs, average of retail cuts, cooked	3 oz	85.1	232	23	0	0	15	5.3	77
12097	Pork, backribs, roasted	3 oz	85.1	315	21	0	0	25	9.4	100
12099	Pork, ground, cooked	3 oz	85.1	253	22	0	0	18	6.6	80
Lunch Meats										
13103	Beef, chopped, smoked, cured, 1oz slice	1 pce	28.4	38	6	1	0	1	0.5	13
13335	Beef, smoked, sliced, package/Carl Buddig	1 pce	71	99	14	0	0	5	1.8	48
13000	Beef, thin slice	1 oz	28.4	33	5	1	0	1	0.3	14
58275	Bologna, beef & pork, lowfat, 1" cube	1 ea	14	32	2	0	0	3	1	5
58280	Bologna, beef, lowfat, medium slice	1 ea	28	57	3	1	0	4	1.5	12
58212	Bologna, beef, reduced sodium, thin slice	1 pce	14	44	2	0	0	4	1.6	8
13176	Bologna, beef, light	1 pce	28	56	3	2	0	4	1.6	12
13152	Chicken, oven roasted, breast (white) meat, serving	1 oz	28	36	5	1	0	2	0.4	17
13306	Corned beef, chopped, cooked, serving, packaged/Carl Buddig	1 ea	71	101	14	1	0	5	2	46
13263	Ham, 11% fat	1 oz	28	46	5	1	0	2	0.8	16
13264	Ham, slices, regular, 11% fat	1 cup	135	220	22	5	2	12	4	77
13049	Olive loaf, w/pork, 4" × 4" × 3/32" slice	1 pce	28.4	67	3	3	0	5	1.7	11
13337	Pastrami, beef, smoked, chopped, package/Carl Buddig	1 oz	28.4	40	6	0	0	2	0.9	18
13101	Pastrami, beef, cured, 1 oz slice	1 oz	28.4	41	6	0	0	2	0.8	19
13020	Pastrami, turkey, slices	2 pce	56.7	75	9	1	0	4	1	39
11913	Pork & ham, canned/Spam	2 oz	56.7	176	8	2	0	15	5.6	40
13123	Bologna, turkey/Louis Rich	1 oz	28.4	52	3	1	0	4	1.1	19
16160	Turkey, breast, 3-1/2" slice	1 pce	21	22	4	1	0	0	0.1	9
58279	Turkey ham, extra lean, package	1 cup	138	171	27	4	0	5	1.5	92
13014	Turkey ham, thigh, cured	1 oz	28	35	5	1	0	1	0.4	20
Sausage & Wursts										
58009	Bacon & beef stick	2 oz	56.7	293	16	0	0	25	9.1	58
58230	Beef sausage, cooked from fresh	2 oz	56.7	188	10	0	0	16	6.2	46
58228	Beef sausage, precooked	2 oz	56.7	230	9	0	0	21	8.6	47
13035	Beerwurst, salami, pork & beef	2 oz	56.7	157	8	2	1	13	4.8	35
13077	Blood sausage, 5" × 4-5/8" × 1/16" slice	1 pce	25	95	4	0	0	9	3.3	30
13079	Bratwurst, pork, cooked	1 ea	85	283	12	2	0	25	8.5	63
58012	Bratwurst, pork, beef & turkey, light, smoked	3 oz	85.1	158	12	1	0	12		48
13070	Chorizo, pork & beef sausage, 4" link	1 ea	60	273	14	1	0	23	8.6	53
13190	Frankfurter, beef, bun length/Kraft	1 ea	57	185	6	2	0	17	7.1	34
13191	Hot dog, beef/Kraft	1 ea	45	147	5	1	0	14	5.6	25

MDA Code	Food Name	Amt	Wt (g)	Ener (kcal)	Prot (g)	Carb (g)	Fiber (g)	Fat (g)	Sat (g)	Chol (mg)
13129	Frankfurter, turkey & chicken/Kraft	1 ea	45	85	5	2	0	6	1.7	41
57877	Frankfurter, beef, 5″ × 3/4″	1 ea	45	148	5	2	0	13	5.3	24
57966	Frankfurter, beef, 97% fat free	1 ea	49	45	6	3	0	2	1	15
13260	Frankfurter, chicken	1 ea	45	100	7	1	0	7	1.7	43
13012	Frankfurter, turkey	1 ea	45	100	6	2	0	8	1.8	35
57890	Pork sausage, Italian, link, cooked, 1/4 lb (before cooking)	1 ea	83	286	16	4	0	23	7.9	47
13043	Kielbasa beef & pork sausage, link	1 pce	26	80	3	1	0	7	2.4	17
58020	Kielbasa turkey & beef sausage, smoked	3 oz	85.1	192	11	3	0	15	5.3	60
13044	Knockwurst beef & pork sausage, link	1 ea	68	209	8	2	0	19	6.9	41
13019	Liverwurst pork sausage, 2.5″ × 1/4″ slice	1 pce	18	59	3	0	0	5	1.9	28
13021	Pepperoni, beef & pork, slice	1 pce	5.5	27	1	0	0	2	0.8	6
13022	Polish sausage, pork, 10″ × 1.25″	1 ea	227	740	32	4	0	65	23.4	159
58227	Pork sausage, precooked	3 oz	85	321	12	0	0	30	9.9	63
13184	Smokie sausage links/Oscar Mayer	1 ea	43	130	5	1	0	12	4	27
13200	Summer sausage, slice/Kraft	2 ea	46	140	7	0	0	12	4.9	39
13066	Sausage, liver, braunschweiger, slice, 2-1/2″ × 1/4″	1 pce	18	59	3	1	0	5	1.7	32
13025	Salami, turkey, cooked, serving	1 oz	28.4	48	5	0	0	3	0.8	22
13267	Sausage, pork, cooked	2 oz	56	190	11	0	0	16	5.1	47
17345	Salami, beef cotto	1 slc	23	47	3	0	0	4	1.6	19
58007	Turkey sausage, breakfast link, mild	2 ea	56	129	9	1	0	10	2.1	90
	Meat Substitutes									
27044	Bacon bits, meatless	1 Tbs	7	33	2	2	1	2	0.3	0
7509	Bacon strips, meatless	3 ea	15	46	2	1	0	4	0.7	0
7561	Beef substitute, patty	1 ea	56	110	12	4	3	5	0.8	0
62359	Breakfast sausage patty, meatless, frozen/Morningstar Farms	1 ea	38	80	10	3	2	3	0.4	1
91055	Burger, vegetarian, frozen, Grillers Vegan/Morningstar Farms	1 ea	85	112	14	8	4	3	0.4	0
91489	Burger, vegan, original	1 ea	71	70	13	6	4	1		0
7547	Chicken, vegetarian	1 cup	168	376	40	6	6	21	3.1	0
7722	Garden Veggie Patties, vegetarian, frozen/Morningstar Farms	1 ea	67	118	12	9	3	4	0.5	1
7674	Harvest Burger, vegetarian, original, frozen/Gardetto's	1 ea	90	138	18	7	6	4	1	0
90626	Sausage, vegetarian, slices	1 ea	28	72	5	3	1	5	0.8	0
7726	Spicy Black Bean Burger, vegetarian, frozen/Morningstar Farms	1 ea	78	133	13	15	5	4	0.6	1
7549	Vegetarian fish sticks	1 ea	28	81	6	3	2	5	0.8	0
	Nuts and Seeds									
63195	Cashews, raw	2 oz	56.7	314	10	17	2	25	4.4	0
4519	Cashews, whole dry roasted, salted	0.25 cup	34.2	196	5	11	1	16	3.1	0
4645	Chinese chestnuts, dried	1 oz	28.4	103	2	23		1	0.1	0
63081	Flaxseeds, whole	0.25 cup	42	224	8	12	11	18	1.5	0
4728	Macadamias, whole, dry roasted, unsalted	1 cup	134	962	10	18	11	102	16	0
4592	Mixed nuts, dry roasted, salted	0.25 cup	34.2	203	6	9	3	18	2.4	0
4626	Peanut butter, chunky	2 Tbs	32	188	8	7	3	16	2.6	0
4756	Peanuts, dry roasted, unsalted	30 ea	30	176	7	6	2	15	2.1	0
4696	Peanuts, raw	0.25 cup	36.5	207	9	6	3	18	2.5	0
4540	Pistachios, dry roasted, salted	0.25 cup	32	182	7	9	3	15	1.8	0
4523	Sesame seeds, whole, dried	0.25 cup	36	206	6	8	4	18	2.5	0
4551	Sunflower seeds, kernels dry roasted, unsalted	0.25 cup	32	186	6	8	4	16	1.7	0

MDA Code	Food Name	Amt	Wt (g)	Ener (kcal)	Prot (g)	Carb (g)	Fiber (g)	Fat (g)	Sat (g)	Chol (mg)
	Seafood									
19041	Abalone, fried, mixed species	3 oz	85.1	161	17	9	0	6	1.4	80
17029	Bass, freshwater, mixed species, fillet, baked/broiled	3 oz	85.1	124	21	0	0	4	0.9	74
17104	Bass, striped, fillet, baked/broiled	3 oz	85.1	106	19	0	0	3	0.6	88
17088	Catfish, channel, fillet, breaded, fried	3 oz	85.1	195	15	7	1	11	2.8	69
19002	Clams, mixed species, canned, drained	3 oz	85.1	126	22	4	0	2	0.2	57
71140	Clams, mixed species, raw	4 oz	113.4	84	14	3	0	1	0.1	39
17037	Cod, Atlantic, fillet, baked/broiled	3 oz	85.1	89	19	0	0	1	0.1	47
19036	Crab, Alaska king, leg, steamed	3 oz	85.1	83	16	0	0	1	0.1	45
19037	Crab, Alaska king, imitation	3 oz	85.1	81	6	13	0	0	0.1	17
17289	Eel, mixed species, fillet, w/o bone, baked/broiled, 1" cube	3 oz	85.1	201	20	0	0	13	2.6	137
17291	Halibut, Atlantic/Pacific, fillet, baked/broiled	3 oz	85.1	119	23	0	0	3	0.4	35
17049	Mackerel, Atlantic, fillet, baked/broiled	3 oz	85.1	223	20	0	0	15	3.6	64
17115	Mackerel, king, fillet, baked/broiled	3 oz	85.1	114	22	0	0	2	0.4	58
19044	Mussels, blue, steamed	3 oz	85.1	146	20	6	0	4	0.7	48
17093	Perch, ocean, Atlantic, fillet, baked/broiled	3 oz	85.1	103	20	0	0	2	0.3	46
19048	Octopus, steamed	3 oz	85.1	140	25	4	0	2	0.4	82
19089	Oysters, eastern, farmed, medium, raw	4 oz	113.4	67	6	6	0	2	0.5	28
17095	Pike, northern, fillet, baked/broiled	3 oz	85.1	96	21	0	0	1	0.1	43
17074	Rockfish, Pacific, mixed species, fillet, baked/broiled	3 oz	85.1	103	20	0	0	2	0.4	37
17121	Orange Roughy, orange fillet, baked/broiled	3 oz	85.1	89	19	0	0	1	0	68
17181	Salmon, Atlantic, farmed, fillet, baked/broiled	3 oz	85.1	175	19	0	0	11	2.1	54
17123	Salmon, Atlantic, fillet, baked/broiled, wild	3 oz	85.1	155	22	0	0	7	1.1	60
17099	Salmon, sockeye, fillet, baked/broiled	3 oz	85.1	184	23	0	0	9	1.6	74
17086	Sea bass, mixed species, fillet, baked/broiled	3 oz	85.1	106	20	0	0	2	0.6	45
17023	Sea trout, mixed species, fillet, baked/broiled	3 oz	85.1	113	18	0	0	4	1.1	90
17076	Shark, mixed species, Batter Fried	3 oz	85.1	194	16	5	0	12	2.7	50
17022	Snapper, mixed species, fillet, baked/broiled	3 oz	85.1	109	22	0	0	1	0.3	40
71707	Calamari, mixed species, fried	3 oz	85.1	149	15	7	0	6	1.6	221
71139	Sturgeon, mixed species, baked/broiled	3 oz	85.1	115	18	0	0	4	1	66
17066	Swordfish, fillet, baked/broiled	3 oz	85.1	132	22	0	0	4	1.2	43
17185	Trout, rainbow, farmed, fillet, baked/broiled	3 oz	85.1	144	21	0	0	6	1.8	58
17082	Trout, rainbow, wild, fillet, baked/broiled	3 oz	85.1	128	20	0	0	5	1.4	59
56007	Tuna salad spread	2 Tbs	25.6	48	4	2	0	2	0.4	3
17101	Tuna, bluefin, fillet, baked/broiled	3 oz	85.1	157	25	0	0	5	1.4	42
17151	Tuna, white, w/water, drained, canned	3 oz	85.1	109	20	0	0	3	0.7	36
17083	Tuna, white, w/oil, canned, drained	3 oz	85.1	158	23	0	0	7	1.1	26
17162	Whitefish, mixed species, fillet, baked/broiled	3 oz	85.1	146	21	0	0	6	1	66
17164	Yellowtail, mixed species, fillet, baked/broiled	3 oz	85.1	159	25	0	0	6		60
	VEGETABLES AND LEGUMES									
	Beans									
7038	Baked beans, plain/vegetarian, canned	1 cup	254	239	12	54	10	1	0.2	0
56101	Baked beans, w/frankfurters, canned	0.5 cup	129.5	184	9	20	9	9	3	8
5197	Bean sprouts, mung, mature, canned, drained	1 cup	125	15	2	3	1	0	0	0
7012	Black beans, mature, cooked	1 cup	172	227	15	41	15	1	0.2	0
92152	Chili beans, ranch style, bbq, cooked	1 cup	253	245	13	43	11	3	0.4	0
9574	Black eyed peas, immature, cooked w/salt, drained	1 cup	165	155	5	33	8	1	0.2	0
90018	Cowpeas, mature, cooked w/salt	1 cup	171	198	13	35	11	1	0.2	0
7913	Fava beans, immature, in pod	1 cup	126	111	10	22		1	0.1	0

MDA Code	Food Name	Amt	Wt (g)	Ener (kcal)	Prot (g)	Carb (g)	Fiber (g)	Fat (g)	Sat (g)	Chol (mg)
7081	Hummus (garbanzo or chickpea spread), homemade	1 Tbs	15.4	27	1	3	1	1	0.2	0
7087	Kidney beans, all types, mature, canned	1 cup	256	215	13	37	14	2	0.3	0
7006	Lentils, mature, cooked	1 cup	198	230	18	40	16	1	0.1	0
7011	Lima beans, large, mature, canned	1 cup	241	190	12	36	12	0	0.1	0
7022	Navy beans, mature, cooked	1 cup	182	255	15	47	19	1	0.2	0
7122	Navy beans, mature, canned	1 cup	262	296	20	54	13	1	0.3	0
7051	Pinto beans, mature, canned	1 cup	240	206	12	37	11	2	0.4	0
5854	Pinto beans, immature, cooked from frozen w/salt, drained	3 oz	85.1	138	8	26	7	0	0	0
5856	Snap beans, green, cooked w/salt, drained	1 cup	125	44	2	10	4	0	0.1	0
6748	Snap beans, green, fresh, 4" Long	10 ea	55	17	1	4	2	0	0	0
90026	Green peas, mature, split, cooked w/salt	0.5 cup	98	114	8	20	8	0	0.1	0
7053	White beans, mature, cooked	1 cup	179	249	17	45	11	1	0.2	0
7054	White beans, mature, canned	1 cup	262	299	19	56	13	1	0.2	0
	Vegetables									
9577	Artichoke, French, fresh, cooked w/salt, drained	1 ea	20	11	1	2	2	0	0	0
5723	Artichoke, globe, frozen	3 oz	85.1	32	2	7	3	0	0.1	0
6033	Arugula greens, fresh, chopped	1 cup	20	5	1	1	0	0	0	0
5841	Asparagus, cooked w/salt, drained	0.5 cup	90	20	2	4	2	0	0	0
6755	Beet slices, canned, drained	1 cup	170	53	2	12	3	0	0	0
5573	Beet slices, fresh	0.5 cup	68	29	1	7	2	0	0	0
5558	Broccoli, stalks, fresh	1 ea	114	32	3	6	3	0	0.1	0
6091	Broccoli, chopped, cooked w/salt, drained	0.5 cup	78	27	2	6	3	0	0.1	0
5870	Brussels sprouts, cooked w/salt, drained	0.5 cup	78	28	2	6	2	0	0.1	0
5036	Cabbage, fresh, shredded	1 cup	70	18	1	4	2	0	0	0
5042	Cabbage, red, fresh, shredded	0.5 cup	35	11	1	3	1	0	0	0
90605	Carrots, fresh, baby, large	1 ea	15	5	0	1	0	0	0	0
5281	Carrots, w/peas, in liquid, canned	0.5 cup	127.5	48	3	11	3	0	0.1	0
5887	Carrot slices, cooked w/salt, drained	0.5 cup	78	27	1	6	2	0	0	0
5199	Carrot slices, canned, drained	0.5 cup	73	18	0	4	1	0	0	0
5045	Carrots, fresh, whole, 7-1/2" long	1 ea	72	30	1	7	2	0	0	0
5049	Cauliflower, fresh	0.5 cup	50	12	1	3	1	0	0	0
5891	Cauliflower, cooked w/salt, drained, 1" pieces	0.5 cup	62	14	1	3	1	0	0	0
90436	Celery stalk, fresh, small, 5" long	1 ea	17	3	0	1	0	0	0	0
6093	Greens, collard, chopped, cooked w/salt, drained	1 cup	190	49	4	9	5	1	0.1	0
6801	Corn, sweet, yellow, fresh, small ear, 5.5" – 6.5" long	1 ea	73	63	2	14	2	1	0.1	0
7202	Corn, sweet, white, fresh, kernels from small ear	1 ea	73	63	2	14	2	1	0.1	0
5900	Corn, sweet, yellow, cooked w/salt, drained	0.5 cup	82	89	3	21	2	1	0.2	0
5908	Eggplant, cubes, cooked w/salt, drained	1 cup	99	33	1	8	2	0	0	0
5450	Fennel, bulb, fresh, slices	0.5 cup	43.5	13	1	3	1	0		0
9182	Jicama, fresh, slices	1 cup	120	46	1	11	6	0	0	0
5915	Kale, chopped, cooked w/salt, drained	0.5 cup	65	18	1	4	1	0	0	0
90445	Lettuce, butterhead, small leaf	1 pce	5	1	0	0	0	0	0	0
5089	Lettuce, romaine, fresh, inner leaf	2 pce	20	3	0	1	0	0	0	0
9545	Lettuce, red leaf, fresh, shredded	1 cup	28	4	0	1	0	0		
5926	Mushrooms, shiitake, cooked w/salt, pieces	1 cup	145	78	2	20	3	0	0.1	0
51069	Mushrooms, crimini, fresh	2 ea	28	8	1	1	0	0	0	0
90457	Mushrooms, canned, drained, caps	8 ea	47	12	1	2	1	0	0	0
51067	Mushrooms, portabella, fresh	1 oz	28	7	1	1	0	0	0	0
5927	Mustard greens, chopped, cooked w/salt, drained	0.5 cup	70	10	2	1	1	0	0	0
6971	Okra, pod, cooked w/salt, drained, sliced	0.5 cup	80	18	1	4	2	0	0	0

MDA Code	Food Name	Amt	Wt (g)	Ener (kcal)	Prot (g)	Carb (g)	Fiber (g)	Fat (g)	Sat (g)	Chol (mg)
6074	Onion, cooked w/salt, drained	0.5 cup	105	44	1	10	1	0	0	0
9548	Onion, sweet, fresh	1 oz	28	9	0	2	0	0		0
9547	Onion, green, fresh, stalk-top only	1 Tbs	6	2	0	0	0	0	0	0
7270	Palm hearts, canned	0.5 cup	73	20	2	3	2	0	0.1	0
5938	Peas, green, cooked w/salt, drained	0.5 cup	80	67	4	13	4	0	0	0
5116	Peas, green, fresh	1 cup	145	117	8	21	7	1	0.1	0
9611	Peppers, green chili, canned	0.5 cup	69.5	15	1	3	1	0	0	0
7932	Peppers, jalapeno, fresh, sliced	1 cup	90	27	1	5	2	1	0.1	0
9632	Peppers, serrano chili, fresh, chopped	1 cup	105	34	2	7	3	0	0.1	0
90493	Peppers, bell, green, sweet, fresh, strips	10 pce	27	5	0	1	0	0	0	0
9549	Peppers, bell, green, sweet, sauteed	1 oz	28	36	0	1	1	3	0.4	0
6990	Peppers, bell, red, sweet, fresh, ring, 3" × 1/4" thick	1 ea	10	3	0	1	0	0	0	0
9551	Peppers, bell, red, sweet, sauteed	1 oz	28	37	0	2	1	4	0.4	0
90589	Pickles, sweet, spears	1 ea	20	18	0	4	0	0	0	0
9251	Potatoes, red, baked, w/skin, small	1 ea	138	123	3	27	2	0	0	0
9245	Potatoes, russet, baked, w/skin, small	1 ea	138	134	4	30	3	0	0	0
90564	Potatoes, peeled, cooked w/salt, large, 3" to 4-1/4"	1 ea	299.6	258	5	60	6	0	0.1	0
5950	Potatoes, skin, baked w/salt	1 ea	58	115	2	27	5	0	0	0
5964	Pumpkin, canned, salted	0.5 cup	122.5	42	1	10	4	0	0.2	0
90505	Radishes, fresh, red, small	10 ea	20	3	0	1	0	0	0	0
90508	Sauerkraut, canned, drained	0.5 cup	71	13	1	3	2	0	0	0
5260	Seaweed, spirulina, dried	0.5 cup	59.5	173	34	14	2	5	1.6	0
5972	Spinach, cooked w/salt, drained	0.5 cup	90	21	3	3	2	0	0	0
5149	Spinach, canned, drained	0.5 cup	107	25	3	4	3	1	0.1	0
5146	Spinach, fresh, chopped	1 cup	30	7	1	1	1	0	0	0
5984	Squash, butternut, baked w/salt, cubes	0.5 cup	102.5	41	1	11	3	0	0	0
5975	Squash, summer, all types, cooked w/salt, drained	0.5 cup	90	18	1	4	1	0	0.1	0
5981	Squash, winter, all types, baked w/salt, cubes	0.5 cup	102.5	40	1	9	3	1	0.1	0
90525	Squash, zucchini, fresh, w/skin, small	1 ea	118	19	1	4	1	0	0	0
6921	Squash, zucchini, w/skin, cooked w/salt, drained, mashed	0.5 cup	120	19	1	5	2	0	0	0
5989	Succotash, cooked w/salt, drained	0.5 cup	96	107	5	23	5	1	0.1	0
6924	Sweet potato, dark orange, baked in skin, w/salt	0.5 cup	100	92	2	21	3	0	0.1	0
5555	Sweet potato, dark orange, w/syrup, canned, drained	1 cup	196	212	3	50	6	1	0.1	0
5445	Tomatillo, fresh, medium	1 ea	34	11	0	2	1	0	0	0
5476	Tomato puree, canned	0.5 cup	125	48	2	11	2	0	0	0
5180	Tomato sauce, canned	0.5 cup	122.5	29	2	7	2	0	0	0
6887	Tomatoes, red, whole, w/juice, 6.7 oz can	1 ea	190	32	1	8	2	0	0	0
90532	Tomatoes, red, fresh, year round average, small, thin slice	1 pce	15	3	0	1	0	0	0	0
5447	Tomatoes, sun dried	10 pce	20	52	3	11	2	1	0.1	0
6002	Turnips, cooked w/salt, drained, mashed	0.5 cup	115	25	1	6	2	0	0	0
7955	Wasabi root, fresh	1 ea	169	184	8	40	13	1		0
5388	Water chestnuts, Chinese, whole w/liquid, canned	4 ea	28	14	0	3	1	0	0	0
5223	Watercress greens, fresh, sprig	10 ea	25	3	1	0	0	0	0	0
6010	Yams, tropical, baked w/salt, drained, cubes	0.5 cup	68	78	1	18	3	0	0	0
	Soy Products									
7503	Miso	1 Tbs	17.2	34	2	5	1	1	0.2	0
7564	Tempeh	0.5 cup	83	160	15	8		9	1.8	0
7015	Soybeans, mature, cooked	1 cup	172	298	29	17	10	15	2.2	0
4707	Soybeans, mature, roasted, salted	0.25 cup	43	203	15	14	8	11	1.6	0
71584	Soy yogurt, peach/Silk	1 ea	170.1	160	4	32	1	2	0	0

MDA Code	Food Name	Amt	Wt (g)	Ener (kcal)	Prot (g)	Carb (g)	Fiber (g)	Fat (g)	Sat (g)	Chol (mg)
7542	Tofu, firm, silken, 1" slice/Mori-Nu	3 oz	85.1	53	6	2	0	2	0.3	0
7799	Tofu, firm, silken, light, 1" slice/Mori-Nu	3 oz	85.1	31	5	1	0	1	0.1	0
7541	Tofu, soft, silken, 1" slice/Mori-Nu	3 oz	85.1	47	4	2	0	2	0.3	0
7546	Tofu yogurt	1 cup	262	246	9	42	1	5	0.7	0
MEALS AND DISHES										
Homemade										
57482	Coleslaw, homemade	0.5 cup	60	47	1	7	1	2	0.2	5
56102	Falafel, patty, homemade, 2-1/4"	1 ea	17	57	2	5		3	0.4	0
53125	Mole poblana, sauce, homemade	2 Tbs	30.3	50	1	4	1	3		0
56005	Potato salad, homemade	0.5 cup	125	179	3	14	2	10	1.8	85
5786	Potatoes au gratin, w/butter, homemade	1 cup	245	323	12	28	4	19	11.6	56
92216	Tortellini pasta, cheese filled	1 cup	108	332	15	51	2	8	3.9	45
Packaged or Canned Meals or Dishes										
56634	Chimichanga, beef	1 ea	174	425	20	43		20	8.5	9
57705	Egg noodles, w/creamy alfredo sauce, dry mix/Lipton	1 ea	124	518	19	77		15	5.7	139
1753	Enchilada & tamale meal, beef	1 ea	311.9	450	10	56	9	20	8	30
90098	Beef ravioli, w/meat sauce, canned, serving/Chef Boyardee	1 ea	244	224	8	33	1	7	2.8	7
25279	Beefaroni, w/tomato sauce, canned, serving/Chef Boyardee	1 ea	212.6	196	7	29	1	6	2.5	6
82002	Burrito, mild, beef & bean	1 ea	142	294	9	43	5	10	3.5	7
70442	Chicken, orange glazed, low fat	1 serving	241	300	12	54	2	4	1	20
92265	Chicken & dumplings, canned	1 cup	247	230	11	24	2	10	4.5	35
57658	Chili con carne, w/beans, canned	1 cup	222	269	16	25	9	12	3.9	29
56001	Chili w/beans, canned	1 cup	256	287	15	30	11	14	6	44
57700	Chili w/o beans, canned/Hormel	1 cup	236	194	17	18	3	7	2.2	35
57701	Chili, turkey, w/beans, canned/Hormel	1 cup	247	203	19	26	6	3	0.7	35
57703	Chili, vegetarian, w/beans, canned/Hormel	1 cup	247	205	12	38	10	1	0.1	0
50317	Chili w/beans, canned/Chef-Mate	1 cup	253	420	18	34	8	24	10.1	40
90738	Cheeseburger macaroni pasta/Hamburger Helper	1.5 oz	42.5	168	5	27		4	1.2	4
57068	Macaroni & cheese, original, dry mix/Kraft	1 ea	70	259	11	48	1	3	1.3	10
57470	Meatloaf, w/gravy & mashed potatoes	1 ea	396.9	540	23	42	5	30	12	95
1751	Pasta, chicken alfredo	1 cup	194.4	270	11	28	3	12	7	40
83107	Pasta, chicken cacciatore	1.25 cup	295	330	23	44	3	6		40
57484	Potatoes, scalloped, from dry mix, w/milk & butter	1 ea	822	764	17	105	9	35	21.6	90
90103	Ravioli, beef, w/sauce, mini, canned, serving/Chef Boyardee	1 ea	252	232	8	31	3	8	3.5	8
47708	Spaghetti, w/meatballs canned/Chef Boyardee	1 ea	240	240	10	29	3	9	3.8	17
70959	Spinach au gratin, frozen	1 ea	155	222	7	11	2	17	7.6	42
70470	Stir fry, rice & vegetables	1 serving	226	350	7	45	3	16	4	15
42147	Stuffing, cornbread, from dry mix	0.5 cup	100	179	3	22	3	9	1.8	0
Frozen Meals or Dishes										
11112	Beef macaroni, serving	1 ea	226.8	200	13	32	4	2	0.6	14
70893	Beef pot pie	1 ea	198	436	14	44	2	23	8.2	42
83051	Beef pot roast, w/potatoes & gravy/Stouffers	1 ea	255	184	13	21	3	5	1.4	20
70950	Beef w/gravy & vegetables, sliced	1 ea	255	207	15	26	4	5	1.3	31
11047	Beef, oriental, w/vegetables & rice	1 serving	255	189	13	28	4	3	1.1	23
57474	Beef stroganoff, w/noodles & vegetables/Marie Callender's	1 ea	368	420	25	40	7	18	7.2	63
56915	Broccoli, w/cheese sauce/Gardettos	0.5 cup	84	56	2	7		2	0.4	
56738	Cabbage, stuffed, w/whipped potatoes/Lean Cuisine	1 ea	269	196	11	24	4	6	1.7	13

MDA Code	Food Name	Amt	Wt (g)	Ener (kcal)	Prot (g)	Carb (g)	Fiber (g)	Fat (g)	Sat (g)	Chol (mg)
4104	Chicken & noodles, escalloped	1 ea	227	330	14	28	2	18	4	35
16195	Chicken & vegetables w/vermicelli/Lean Cuisine	1 ea	297	232	20	26	4	5	1.9	30
16262	Chicken, mesquite BBQ	1 ea	298	277	17	42	7	4	1.2	33
16198	Chicken enchilada w/rice & cheese sauce/Stouffer's	1 ea	283	424	15	61	4	13	7.4	51
83028	Chicken fajita kit, serving/Tyson	1 ea	107	128	7	17	2	4	0.9	12
1746	Chicken, thigh, fried, w/mashed potatoes & corn/ Banquet	1 ea	228	388	22	30	4	20	4.4	68
70899	Chicken pot pie	1 ea	217	464	13	50	3	24	7.8	52
16266	Chicken teriaki/Healthy Choice	1 ea	312	250	16	36	9	5	1.6	22
70582	Chicken nuggets, w/macaroni & cheese	1 ea	257	457	19	51	7	20	5.6	57
70895	Egg, scrambled, & sausage, w/hash browns	1 ea	177	361	13	17	1	27	7.3	283
70917	Hot Pockets beef & cheddar pocket sandwich	1 ea	142	403	16	39		20	8.8	53
70918	Hot Pockets chicken broccoli cheddar pocket sandwich	1 ea	128	301	11	39	1	11	3.4	37
18119	Hot Pockets, chicken parmesan	1 ea	127	340	9	41	3	15	6	10
4096	Lasagna, w/Italian sausage	1 ea	308.4	410	18	41	4	19	9	50
56757	Lasagna w/meat sauce	1 ea	215	249	17	27	2	8	4.1	28
11029	Macaroni & beef, w/tomato sauce, serving/Lean Cuisine	1 ea	283	258	17	37	5	4	1.7	17
90491	Onion rings, cooked from frozen	1 cup	48	195	3	18	1	13	4.1	0
83156	Pasta, chicken, garlic, w/vegetables	1.67 cup	178	240	11	21	3	8	2	30
56762	Peppers, stuffed, w/beef & tomato sauce/Stouffers	0.5 ea	219.5	160	8	19	3	6	2.2	18
5587	Potatoes, mashed, granules w/milk, prepared w/water & margarine	0.5 cup	105	122	2	17	1	5	1.3	2
15972	Pot Pie, chicken	1 ea	283	733	20	64	4	44	17.8	62
70898	Pizza, pepperoni serving	1 ea	146	432	16	42	3	22	7.1	22
11034	Salisbury steak, w/potatoes & corn	1 ea	269	339	15	27	4	19	9.4	30
81146	Sausage w/biscuit sandwich/Jimmy Dean	1 ea	48	192	5	12	1	14	4.3	16
56703	Spaghetti w/meat sauce, serving/Lean Cuisine	1 ea	326	284	14	49	5	4	1.1	13
56760	Spaghetti, w/meatballs, 12.6 oz	1 serving	357.2	360	19	45	6	12	3.5	35
6246	Spinach, creamed, w/real cream sauce	0.5 cup	124	100	3	7	1	7	3	35
11099	Swedish meatballs & pasta, serving/Lean Cuisine	1 ea	258	273	22	31	3	7	2.8	49
4128	Turkey beast, w/potatoes & vegetables	1 serving	453.6	460	22	51	5	19	6	65
70892	Turkey pot pie	1 ea	397	699	26	70	4	35	11.4	64
16306	Turkey w/gravy, 5 oz pkg	1 ea	141.8	95	8	7	0	4	1.2	26
6999	Vegetables, cooked, from frozen, w/salt, drained, 10 oz pkg	1 ea	275	165	8	36	12	0	0.1	0
Snack Foods and Granola Bars										
3307	Banana chips	1 oz	28.4	147	1	17	2	10	8.2	0
10051	Beef jerky, large piece	1 ea	19.8	81	7	2	0	5	2.1	10
10052	Beef meat stick, smoked	1 ea	19.8	109	4	1		10	4.1	26
63331	Breakfast bar w/oats, raisins & coconut	1 ea	43	200	4	29	1	8	5.5	0
53227	Cereal bar, mixed berry/Kelloggs	1 ea	37	137	2	27	1	3	0.6	0
61251	Cheese puffs & twists, corn based, low fat	1 oz	28.4	123	2	21	3	3	0.6	0
44032	Chex snack mix, original	1 cup	42.5	180	4	32	2	4	0.6	
44034	Corn Nuts, BBQ	1 oz	28.4	124	3	20	2	4	0.7	0
44031	Corn Nuts, original	1 oz	28.4	127	2	20	2	4	0.7	0
11594	Fruit leather, bar	2 ea	28	104	0	24		1	0.3	
23404	Fruit leather, roll, large	1 ea	21	78	0	18	0	1	0.1	0
23103	Granola bar, peanut butter, hard	1 ea	23.6	114	2	15	1	6	0.8	0
23059	Granola bar, plain, hard	1 ea	24.5	115	2	16	1	5	0.6	0
23101	Granola bar, chocolate chip, hard	1 ea	23.6	103	2	17	1	4	2.7	0

MDA Code	Food Name	Amt	Wt (g)	Ener (kcal)	Prot (g)	Carb (g)	Fiber (g)	Fat (g)	Sat (g)	Chol (mg)
23096	Granola bar, chocolate chip, chocolate coated, soft	1 ea	35.4	165	2	23	1	9	5	2
23107	Granola bar, nut & raisin, soft	1 oz	28.4	129	2	18	2	6	2.7	0
72602	Nachos, cheese, serving	1 serving	57	120	4	5	0	9	4	10
44036	Oriental mix, rice based	1 oz	28.4	144	5	15	4	7	1.1	0
44012	Popcorn, air popped	1 cup	8	31	1	6	1	0	0	0
44014	Popcorn, caramel coated, w/o peanuts	1 oz	28.4	122	1	22	1	4	1	1
44038	Popcorn, cheese flavored	1 cup	11	58	1	6	1	4	0.7	1
44066	Popcorn, low fat, low sodium, microwaved	1 cup	8	34	1	6	1	1	0.1	0
44013	Popcorn, oil popped, microwaved	1 cup	11	64	1	5	1	5	0.8	0
61252	Popcorn, fat free, sugar syrup/caramel	1 cup	37.3	142	1	34	1	1	0.1	0
12080	Pork skins, plain	1 oz	28	153	17	0	0	9	3.2	27
44043	Potato chips, reduced fat	1 oz	28.4	134	2	19	2	6	1.2	0
44076	Potato chips, plain, unsalted	1 oz	28.4	152	2	15	1	10	3.1	0
5437	Potato chips, sour cream & onion	1 oz	28.4	151	2	15	1	10	2.5	2
61257	Potato chips, reduced fat, unsalted	1 oz	28.4	138	2	19	2	6	1.2	0
44015	Pretzels, hard	5 pce	30	113	3	24	1	1	0.1	0
44079	Pretzels, enriched, plain, hard, unsalted	10 ea	60	229	5	48	2	2	0.4	0
61182	Pretzels, soft, medium	1 ea	115	389	9	80	2	4	0.8	3
44021	Rice cake, brown rice, plain	1 ea	9	35	1	7	0	0	0.1	0
44020	Taro chips	1 oz	28.4	141	1	19	2	7	1.8	0
44058	Trail mix, regular	0.25 cup	37.5	173	5	17		11	2.1	0
44059	Trail mix, w/chocolate chips, salted nuts & seeds	0.25 cup	36.2	175	5	16		12	2.2	1
	Soups									
92160	Bean & ham, reduced sodium, canned, prepared w/water	0.5 cup	128	95	5	17	5	1	0.3	3
17776	Beef & barley	1 cup	242	140	9	18	2	4	1.5	15
92192	Beef mushroom, chunky, low sodium, canned	1 cup	251	173	11	24	1	6	4.1	15
50198	Beef mushroom, canned, prepared w/water	1 cup	244	73	6	6	0	3	1.5	7
57659	Beef stew, canned, serving	1 ea	232	220	11	16	3	12	5.2	37
50052	Chicken, chunky, ready to serve	1 cup	245	174	12	17	1	6	1.9	29
50077	Chicken gumbo, canned, prepared w/water	1 cup	244	56	3	8	2	1	0.3	5
50080	Chicken mushroom, canned, prepared w/water	1 cup	244	132	4	9	0	9	2.4	10
50081	Chicken noodle, chunky, canned, ready to serve	1 cup	240	89	8	10	1	2	1	12
50085	Chicken rice, chunky, canned, ready to serve	1 cup	240	127	12	13	1	3	1	12
50088	Chicken vegetable, chunky, canned, ready to serve	1 cup	240	166	12	19		5	1.4	17
40675	Cream of broccoli, microwave	1 serving	305	143	3	17	7	7	2	6
50049	Cream of mushroom, canned, prepared w/water	1 cup	244	102	2	8	0	7	1.6	0
50197	Cream of potato, canned, prepared w/water	1 cup	244	73	2	11	0	2	1.2	5
50050	Green pea, canned, prepared w/water	1 cup	250	152	8	25	5	3	1.3	0
50021	Clam chowder, Manhattan, canned, prepared w/water	1 cup	244	73	2	12	1	2	0.4	2
50009	Minestrone, canned, prepared w/water	1 cup	241	82	4	11	1	3	0.6	2
92163	Ramen noodle soup, any flavor, from dry packet	0.5 cup	38	172	4	25	1	6	2.9	0
28172	Ramen noodle soup, chicken flavor, from dry packet	1 serving	43	188	5	27	1	7	3.1	
50025	Split pea & ham, canned, prepared w/water	1 cup	253	190	10	28	2	4	1.8	8
50028	Tomato, canned, prepared w/water	1 cup	244	85	2	16	1	1	0.2	0
15774	Tomato & vegetable, from dry, prepared w/water	1 cup	245	54	2	10	1	1	0.4	0
50014	Vegetable beef, canned, prepared w/water	1 cup	244	76	5	10	2	2	0.8	5
92189	Vegetable chicken, low sodium	1 cup	241	166	12	21	1	5	1.4	17
7559	Vegetarian stew	1 cup	247	304	42	17	3	7	1.2	0

MDA Code	Food Name	Amt	Wt (g)	Ener (kcal)	Prot (g)	Carb (g)	Fiber (g)	Fat (g)	Sat (g)	Chol (mg)
	DESSERTS, CANDIES, AND PASTRIES									
	Brownies and Fudge									
62904	Brownie, square, large, 2-3/4" × 7/8"	1 ea	56	227	3	36	1	9	2.4	10
47019	Brownie, homemade, 2" square	1 ea	24	112	1	12		7	1.8	18
23127	Fudge, chocolate marshmallow, w/nuts, homemade	1 pce	22	104	1	15	0	5	2.3	5
23025	Fudge, chocolate, homemade	1 pce	17	70	0	13	0	2	1.1	2
	Cakes, Pies, and Donuts									
46062	Cake, chocolate, homemade, w/o frosting, 9"	1 pce	95	352	5	51	2	14	5.2	55
12722	Cake, chocolate, w/cream, snack size	3 ea	85	280	3	54	0	6	2	75
46000	Cake, gingerbread, homemade, 8"	1 pce	74	263	3	36		12	3.1	24
46092	Coffee cake, w/cheese, 16 oz	1 pce	76	258	5	34	1	12	4.1	65
46003	Cake, white, w/coconut frosting, homemade, 9"	1 pce	112	399	5	71	1	12	4.4	1
46085	Cake, white, homemade, w/o frosting, 9"	1 pce	74	264	4	42	1	9	2.4	1
46091	Cake, yellow, homemade, w/o icing, 8"	1 pce	68	245	4	36	0	10	2.7	37
49001	Cheesecake, from dry mix, 9"	1 pce	99	271	5	35	2	13	6.6	29
46426	Cupcake, low fat, chocolate, w/frosting	1 ea	43	131	2	29	2	2	0.5	0
46011	Cupcake, snack, chocolate, w/frosting & cream filling	1 ea	50	200	2	30	2	8	2.4	0
71338	Doughnut, cake, chocolate, glazed, 3-3/4"	1 ea	60	250	3	34	1	12	3.1	34
71337	Doughnut, cake, w/chocolate icing, large, 3-1/2"	1 ea	57	258	3	29	1	14	7.7	11
45525	Doughnut, cake, glazed/sugared, medium, 3"	1 ea	45	192	2	23	1	10	2.7	14
71335	Doughnut holes	1 ea	14	59	1	6	0	3	1	1
45527	Doughnut, French cruller, glazed, 3"	1 ea	41	169	1	24	0	8	1.9	5
45563	Doughnut, creme filled, 3-1/2" oval	1 ea	85	307	5	26	1	21	4.6	20
48044	Pie filling, pumpkin, canned	0.5 cup	135	140	1	36	11	0	0.1	0
46001	Sponge cake, 1/12 of 16 oz	1 pce	38	110	2	23	0	1	0.3	39
	Candy									
51150	Candied fruit	1 oz	28.4	91	0	23	0	0	0	0
4148	Candy, Bit O Honey/Nestle	6 pce	40	150	1	32	0	3	2.2	0
23115	Candy, butterscotch	5 pce	30	117	0	27	0	1	0.6	3
23015	Candy, caramel	1 pce	10.1	39	0	8	0	1	0.3	1
92202	Candy, caramel, w/nuts, chocolate covered	1 ea	14	66	1	8	1	3	0.7	0
90671	Candy, jellybeans, large	10 ea	28.4	106	0	27	0	0		0
23480	Candy, milk chocolate, package, 1.69 oz	1 pkg	48	236	2	34	1	10	6.3	7
92212	Candy, milk chocolate covered coffee beans	1 oz	28.4	156	2	16	2	9	5.2	6
23022	Candy, milk chocolate covered raisins	1.5 oz	42.5	166	2	29	1	6	4.4	1
23047	Candy, milk chocolate w/peanuts	0.25 cup	42.5	219	4	26	2	11	4.3	3
23021	Candy, milk chocolate w/coated peanuts	10 ea	40	208	5	20	2	13	5.8	4
92201	Candy, nougat w/almonds	1 ea	14	56	0	13	0	0	0.2	0
23081	Candy, peanut brittle, homemade	1.5 oz	42.5	207	3	30	1	8	1.8	5
23152	Candy, Peppermint Patty/York 1-1/2 oz	1 ea	43	165	1	35	1	3	1.9	0
90698	Candy, Rolo, caramels in milk chocolate, 1.74 oz roll	1 ea	49.3	234	3	33	0	10	7.2	6
23142	Candy, sesame crunch	20 pce	35	181	4	18	3	12	1.6	0
23144	Candy, Starburst, original	8 ea	40	163	0	33	0	3	3.1	0
92198	Candy, strawberry, pkg, 8 oz	4 pce	45	158	1	36	0	1	0	0
90682	Candy bar, milk chocolate w/almonds 1.55 oz	1 ea	43.9	231	4	23	3	15	7.8	8
91509	Candy, milk chocolate, w/almonds, bites/Hershey's Bites	17 pce	39	214	4	20	1	14	6.8	7
90681	Candy bar, milk chocolate, mini	1 ea	7	37	1	4	0	2	1.3	2
90685	Candy bar, milk chocolate, w/crisped rice, mini	1 ea	10	51	1	6	0	3	1.6	2
23145	Candy bar, sweet chocolate, 1.45 oz	1 ea	41.1	208	2	24	2	14	8.3	0
23405	Candy bar, Almond Joy, fun size, 7 oz	1 ea	19.8	95	1	12	1	5	3.5	1

MDA Code	Food Name	Amt	Wt (g)	Ener (kcal)	Prot (g)	Carb (g)	Fiber (g)	Fat (g)	Sat (g)	Chol (mg)
23110	Candy bar, Baby Ruth, 2.1 oz	1 ea	60	275	3	39	1	13	7.3	0
23066	Candy bar, Butterfinger, 2.16 oz	1 ea	60	275	3	44	1	11	5.7	0
23116	Candy bar, Caramello, 1.6 oz	1 ea	45.4	210	3	29	1	10	5.8	12
23060	Candy bar, Kit Kat, 1.5 oz	1 ea	42.5	220	3	27	0	11	7.6	5
23061	Candy bar, Krackle, 1.45 oz	1 ea	42.5	218	3	27	1	11	6.8	5
23037	Candy bar, Mars, almonds, 1.76 oz	1 ea	50	234	4	31	1	12	3.6	8
90688	Candy bar, Milky Way, 2.05 oz	1 ea	58	262	2	41	1	10	7	5
23062	Candy bar, Mr. Goodbar, 1.75 oz	1 ea	49.6	267	5	27	2	16	7	5
23135	Candy bar, Oh Henry!, 2 oz	1 ea	56.7	262	4	37	1	13	5.4	4
23036	Candy bar, Skor, toffee, 1.4 oz	1 ea	39.7	212	1	25	1	13	7.5	21
23057	Candy bar, Special Dark, sweet chocolate, 1.45 oz	1 ea	41.1	229	2	25	3	13		2
23076	Candy bar, 3 Musketeers, fun size	2 ea	28	120	1	22	0	4	2.4	1
23149	Candy bar, Twix, caramel cookie, 2.06 oz pkg	1 ea	56.7	285	3	37	1	14	10.8	4
90712	Chewing gum, Chiclets	10 pce	16	40	0	11	0	0	0	0
	Cookies									
47026	Animal crackers	10 ea	12.5	56	1	9	0	2	0.4	0
90636	Chocolate chip cookie, enriched, higher fat, large, 3.5" to 4"	1 ea	40	190	2	26	1	9	4	0
47037	Chocolate chip cookie, homemade w/butter, 2-1/4"	2 ea	32	156	2	19		9	4.5	22
47032	Chocolate chip cookie, lower fat	3 ea	30	136	2	22	1	5	1.1	0
47001	Chocolate chip cookie, soft	2 ea	30	136	1	20	1	6	3	
45787	Chocolate peanut butter wafer, Nutty Bar	1 ea	57	312	5	31		19	3.6	
47006	Chocolate sandwich cookie, crème filled	3 ea	30	141	2	21	1	6	1.9	0
71272	Graham crackers, cinnamon, small rectangular peices	4 ea	14	59	1	11	0	1	0.2	0
47380	Graham crackers, chocolate, individual package	1 ea	31	144	2	22		5	1	
47526	Coconut macaroon cookie, home style	1 ea	22	101	1	13	1	5	4.4	0
62905	Fig bar, 2 oz pkg	1 ea	56.7	197	2	40	3	4	0.6	0
47043	Fortune cookie	3 ea	24	91	1	20	0	1	0.2	0
90638	Gingersnap, large, 3-1/2" to 4"	1 ea	32	133	2	25	1	3	0.8	0
90639	Molasses, cookie, large, 3-1/2" to 4"	1 ea	32	138	2	24	0	4	1	0
90640	Oatmeal cookie, big, 3-1/2" to 4"	1 ea	25	112	2	17	1	5	1.1	0
47003	Oatmeal raisin cookie, homemade, 2-5/8"	1 ea	15	65	1	10		2	0.5	5
47010	Peanut butter cookie, homemade, 3"	1 ea	20	95	2	12		5	0.9	6
47056	Peanut butter cookie, soft type	1 ea	15	69	1	9	0	4	0.9	0
47059	Peanut butter sandwich cookie	2 ea	28	134	2	18	1	6	1.4	0
47007	Shortbread cookie, plain, 1-5/8" square	4 ea	32	161	2	21	1	8	2	6
47559	Sugar cookie, home style/Archway	1 ea	24	99	1	17	0	3	0.7	4
62907	Sugar cookie, from refrigerated dough, pre-sliced	1 ea	23	111	1	15	0	5	1.4	7
90642	Sugar wafer cookie, crème filled, small	1 ea	3.5	18	0	2	0	1	0.1	0
90643	Vanilla sandwich cookie, crème filled, oval	2 ea	30	145	1	22	0	6	0.9	0
49065	Vanilla wafer cookie, golden, artificial flavor	1 ea	31	147	2	22		6	1.1	
	Custards, Gelatin, and Puddings									
2622	Custard, egg, from dry mix, w/2% milk	0.5 cup	133	148	5	23	0	4	1.8	64
57896	Custard, flan, dry mix, serving	1 ea	21	73	0	19	0	0	0	0
14734	Gelatin, strawberry, sugar free, from dry, serving	1 ea	2.9	10	2	1		0	0	
57894	Pudding, chocolate, ready to eat, 4 oz can	1 ea	113.4	161	2	26	0	5	1.4	1
2612	Pudding, vanilla, ready to eat, 4 oz can	1 ea	113.4	147	2	26	0	4	1.2	1
2651	Pudding, rice, ready to eat, 4 oz can	1 ea	141.8	167	5	28	1	4	2.5	26
57902	Pudding, tapioca, ready to eat, 3.5 oz can	1 ea	113.4	147	2	25	0	4	1.1	1
57989	Pudding, banana, snack cup	1 serving	98.9	130	1	21	0	5	2	
57995	Pudding, vanilla, fat free, snack cup	1 ea	113.4	80	1	18	0	0	0	0

MDA Code	Food Name	Amt	Wt (g)	Ener (kcal)	Prot (g)	Carb (g)	Fiber (g)	Fat (g)	Sat (g)	Chol (mg)
	Ice Cream and Frozen Desserts									
71819	Frozen yogurt, chocolate, nonfat, w/artificial sweetener	1 cup	186	199	8	37	2	1	0.9	7
72124	Frozen yogurt, all flavors not chocolate	1 cup	174	221	5	38	0	6	4	23
70640	Ice cream bar, vanilla & dark chocolate	1 ea	85	300	4	23	1	21	13	70
49111	Ice cream cone, wafer/cake type, large	1 ea	29	121	2	23	1	2	0.4	0
49014	Ice cream cone, sugar, rolled type	1 ea	10	40	1	8	0	0	0.1	0
2010	Ice cream, vanilla, light, soft serve	0.5 cup	88	111	4	19	0	2	1.4	11
90723	Popsicle, 2 fl-oz bar	1 ea	59	47	0	11	0	0	0	0
	Pastries									
45788	Apple turnover, frozen/Pepperidge Farm	1 ea	89	284	4	31	2	16	4	
42264	Cinnamon rolls, w/icing, refrigerated dough/Pillsbury	1 ea	44	145	2	23	0	5	1.5	0
45675	Éclair shell, homemade, 5″ × ; 2″ × 1-3/4″	1 ea	48	174	4	11	0	12	2.7	94
71299	Croissant, butter, large	1 ea	67	272	5	31	2	14	7.8	45
71301	Croissant, cheese, large	1 ea	67	277	6	31	2	14	7.1	38
45572	Danish, cheese	1 ea	71	266	6	26	1	16	4.8	11
71330	Danish, cinnamon nut, 15 oz ring	1 pce	53.2	229	4	24	1	13	3.1	24
70913	Pie crust, Nilla, ready to use/Nabisco	1 ea	28	144	1	18	0	8	1.4	3
49015	Strudel, apple	1 pce	71	195	2	29	2	8	1.5	4
42164	Sweet roll, cheese	1 ea	66	238	5	29	1	12	4	50
71348	Sweet roll, honey bun, enriched, 5″ × 13-1/2″	1 ea	85	339	5	43	2	16	4.6	26
42166	Sweet roll, cinnamon, frosted, from refrigerated dough	1 ea	30	109	2	17		4	1	0
71367	Sweet roll, cinnamon raisin, large	1 ea	83	309	5	42	2	14	2.6	55
45683	Toaster pastry, brown sugar & cinnamon	1 ea	50	206	3	34	0	7	1.8	0
45593	Toaster pastry, Pop Tarts, apple cinnamon	1 ea	52	205	2	37	1	5	0.9	0
45768	Toaster pastry, Pop Tarts, chocolate fudge, frosted, lowfat	1 ea	52	190	3	40	1	3	0.5	0
45601	Toaster pastry, Pop Tarts, chocolate fudge, frosted	1 ea	52	201	3	37	1	5	1	0
	Toppings and Frostings									
23000	Apple butter	1 Tbs	18	31	0	8	0	0	0	0
23070	Caramel topping	2 Tbs	41	103	1	27	0	0	0	0
23014	Chocolate fudge topping, hot	2 Tbs	38	133	2	24	1	3	1.5	0
46039	Cream cheese frosting, creamy	1 oz	28.4	118	0	19	0	5	1.3	0
54334	Hazelnut spread, chocolate flavored	1 oz	28	151	2	17	2	8	8	0
23164	Strawberry topping	2 Tbs	42.5	108	0	28	0	0	0	0
510	Whipped cream topping, pressurized	2 Tbs	7.5	19	0	1	0	2	1	6
514	Dessert topping, pressurized	2 Tbs	8.8	23	0	1	0	2	1.7	0
508	Dessert topping, semi-solid, frozen	2 Tbs	9.4	30	0	2	0	2	2	0
54387	Whipped topping, low fat, frozen	2 Tbs	9.4	21	0	2	0	1	1.1	0
	FATS AND OILS									
44469	Butter, light, salted	1 Tbs	13	66	0	0	0	7	4.5	14
44470	Butter, light, unsalted	1 Tbs	13	65	0	0	0	7	4.5	14
44952	Butter, organic, salted	1 Tbs	14	100	0	0	0	11	7	30
90210	Butter, unsalted, stick	1 Tbs	14	100	0	0	0	11	7.2	30
90209	Butter, salted, whipped, stick	1 Tbs	9.4	67	0	0	0	8	4.7	21
8003	Fat, bacon grease	1 tsp	4.3	39	0	0	0	4	1.7	4
8005	Fat, chicken	1 Tbs	12.8	115	0	0	0	13	3.8	11
8107	Fat, Lard	1 Tbs	12.8	115	0	0	0	13	5	12
8135	Margarine & butter, blend, w/soybean oil	1 Tbs	14.2	101	0	0	0	11	2	2
44476	Margarine, 80% fat, tub	1 Tbs	14.2	101	0	0	0	11	2	0
8067	Oil, fish, cod liver	1 Tbs	13.6	123	0	0	0	14	3.1	78
8084	Oil, canola	1 Tbs	14	124	0	0	0	14	1	0

MDA Code	Food Name	Amt	Wt (g)	Ener (kcal)	Prot (g)	Carb (g)	Fiber (g)	Fat (g)	Sat (g)	Chol (mg)
8008	Oil, olive, salad/cooking	1 Tbs	13.5	119	0	0	0	14	1.9	0
8111	Oil, safflower, salad/cooking, more than 70% Oleic	1 Tbs	13.6	120	0	0	0	14	0.8	0
8027	Oil, sesame, salad/cooking	1 Tbs	13.6	120	0	0	0	14	1.9	0
44483	Shortening, vegetable, household	1 Tbs	12.8	113	0	0	0	13	3.2	0
8007	Shortening, household, hydrogenated soybean & cottonseed oil	1 Tbs	12.8	113	0	0	0	13	3.2	0
	CONDIMENTS, SAUCES, AND SYRUPS									
9713	Barbecue sauce, hickory smoked flavor	2 Tbs								
4936	Barbecue sauce, original flavor	2 Tbs	40	50	1	11	0	0	0	0
27001	Catsup, packet	1 ea	6	6	0	2	0	0	0	0
53523	Cheese sauce, ready to serve	0.25 cup	63	110	4	4	0	8	3.8	18
13095	Chicken spread, canned	1 oz	28.4	45	5	1	0	5	0.9	16
27019	Cranberry orange relish, canned	0.25 cup	68.8	122	0	32	0	0	0	0
54388	Cream substitute, light, powder	1 Tbs	5.9	25	0	4	0	1	0.2	0
9054	Enchilada sauce	0.25 cup	61	20	0	3	0	1	0	0
53474	Fish sauce	2 Tbs	36	13	2	1	0	0	0	0
53036	Gravy, brown, from dry mix	1 Tbs	6	22	1	4	0	1	0.2	0
53472	Hoisin sauce	2 Tbs	32	70	1	14	1	1	0.2	1
9533	Hollandaise sauce, w/butter fat, from dehydrated w/water, packet	1 ea	204	188	4	11	1	16	9.1	41
27004	Horseradish	1 tsp	5	2	0	1	0	0	0	0
92174	Hot sauce, chili, from immature green peppers	1 Tbs	15	3	0	1	0	0	0	0
92173	Hot sauce, chili, from mature red peppers	1 Tbs	15	3	0	1	0	0	0	0
23003	Jelly	1 Tbs	19	51	0	13	0	0	0	0
25002	Maple syrup	1 Tbs	20	52	0	13	0	0	0	0
23005	Marmalade, orange	1 Tbs	20	49	0	13	0	0	0	0
44697	Mayonnaise, light	1 Tbs	15	49	0	1	0	5	0.8	5
8145	Mayonnaise, w/safflower & soy oil	1 Tbs	13.8	99	0	0	0	11	1.2	8
8502	Miracle Whip, light/Kraft	1 Tbs	16	37	0	2	0	3	0.5	4
435	Mustard, yellow	1 tsp	5	3	0	0	0	0	0	0
27011	Olives, black, small, canned	1 ea	3.2	4	0	0	0	0	0	0
53473	Oyster sauce	2 Tbs	8	4	0	1	0	0	0	0
23042	Pancake syrup	1 Tbs	20	47	0	12	0	0	0	0
23172	Pancake syrup, reduced calorie	1 Tbs	15	25	0	7	0	0	0	0
53524	Pasta sauce, spaghetti/marinara, ready to serve	0.5 cup	125	109	2	17	3	3	0.9	2
53344	Pasta sauce, traditional	0.5 cup	130	81	2	13	3	3	1	0
53470	Pepper/hot sauce	1 tsp	4.7	1	0	0	0	0	0	0
93303	Pickles, bread & butter, slices	1 ea	7.5	7	0	2	0	0	0	0
53461	Plum sauce	2 Tbs	38.1	70	0	16	0	0	0.1	0
92229	Preserves	1 Tbs	20	56	0	14	0	0	0	0
27019	Relish, cranberry orange, canned	0.25 cup	68.8	122	0	32	0	0	0	0
90594	Relish, sweet pickle, packet	1 ea	10	13	0	4	0	0	0	0
90280	Salsa, ready to serve, packet	1 ea	8.9	2	0	1	0	0	0	0
92614	Salsa, chipotle, chunky	2 Tbs	32	8	0	2	1	0	0	0
91457	Salsa, green chili & tomato, chunky	2 Tbs	31	7	0	3	0	0	0	0
91458	Salsa, picante, chunky	2 Tbs	31	7	0	1		0	0	0
26014	Salt, table	0.25 tsp	1.5	0	0	0	0	0	0	0
504	Sour cream, cultured	2 Tbs	28.8	56	1	1	0	6	3.3	15
54383	Sour cream, fat free	1 oz	28	21	1	4	0	0	0	3

MDA Code	Food Name	Amt	Wt (g)	Ener (kcal)	Prot (g)	Carb (g)	Fiber (g)	Fat (g)	Sat (g)	Chol (mg)
54381	Sour cream, light	1 oz	28	38	1	2	0	3	1.8	10
515	Sour cream, cultured, reduced fat	2 Tbs	30	40	1	1	0	4	2.2	12
516	Sour dressing, non butterfat, cultured, filled cream type	1 Tbs	14.7	26	0	1	0	2	2	1
53063	Soy sauce, tamari	1 Tbs	18	11	2	1	0	0	0	0
90035	Soy sauce, low sodium, from wheat & soy	1 Tbs	18	10	1	2	0	0	0	0
53264	Sweet & sour sauce	1 Tbs	33	56	0	14	0	0	0	0
14867	Taco sauce, green	2 Tbs	16	4	0	1		0	0	0
14869	Taco sauce, red	1 Tbs	16	8	0	2	0	0	0	0
4655	Tahini sauce, from roasted & toasted kernels	1 Tbs	15	89	3	3	1	8	1.1	0
53004	Teriyaki sauce	1 Tbs	18	16	1	3	0	0		0
53468	White sauce, medium, homemade	1 cup	250	368	10	23	1	27	7.1	18
53099	Worcestershire sauce	1 Tbs	17	13	0	3	0	0	0	0
	Salad Dressing									
44497	Thousand island, fat free	1 Tbs	16	21	0	5	1	0	0	1
8024	Thousand island	1 Tbs	15.6	58	0	2	0	5	0.8	4
8013	Blue cheese	2 Tbs	30.6	146	0	1	0	16	2.5	9
92511	Caesar	2 Tbs	30	150	1	1	0	16	3	5
44467	French, fat free	1 Tbs	16	21	0	5	0	0	0	0
8255	French, reduced fat, unsalted	1 Tbs	16.3	38	0	5	0	2	0.2	0
90232	French, packet	1 ea	12.3	56	0	2	0	6	0.7	0
92510	Italian	2 Tbs	30	140	0	2	0	15	2.5	0
44498	Italian, fat free	1 Tbs	14	7	0	1	0	0	0	0
44720	Italian, reduced calorie	1 Tbs	14	28	0	1	0	3	0.4	0
44499	Ranch, fat free	1 oz	28.4	34	0	8	0	1		2
44696	Ranch, reduced fat	1 Tbs	15	29	0	3	0	2	0.2	2
8022	Russian	1 Tbs	15.3	54	0	5	0	4	0.4	0
8144	Sesame seed	2 Tbs	30.6	136	1	3	0	14	1.9	0
8035	Vinegar & oil, homemade	2 Tbs	31.2	140	0	1	0	16	2.8	0
	FAST FOOD									
	Generic Fast Food									
6178	Baked potato w/cheese sauce & bacon	1 ea	299	451	18	44		26	10.1	30
6177	Baked potato w/cheese sauce	1 ea	296	474	15	47		29	10.6	18
6181	Baked potato w/sour cream & chives	1 ea	302	393	7	50		22	10	24
66025	Burrito, bean	1 ea	108.5	224	7	36		7	3.4	2
56629	Burrito, bean & cheese	1 ea	93	189	8	27		6	3.4	14
66023	Burrito, beef, bean & cheese	1 ea	101.5	165	7	20		7	3.6	62
66024	Burrito, beef	1 ea	110	262	13	29		10	5.2	32
56600	Breakfast biscuit w/egg sandwich	1 ea	136	373	12	32	1	22	4.7	245
56601	Breakfast biscuit w/egg & bacon sandwich	1 ea	150	458	17	29	1	31	8	352
56602	Breakfast biscuit w/egg & ham sandwich	1 ea	192	442	20	31	1	27	5.9	300
66028	Breakfast biscuit w/egg & sausage sandwich	1 ea	180	562	20	38	0	37	11.6	290
66029	Breakfast biscuit w/egg, cheese & bacon sandwich	1 ea	144	433	17	35	0	25	8.1	239
56604	Biscuit w/ham sandwich	1 ea	113	386	13	44	1	18	11.4	25
66030	Biscuit w/sausage sandwich	1 ea	124	460	12	37	0	30	9.2	35
66013	Cheeseburger, double patty, w/condiments & vegetables	1 ea	166	417	21	35		21	8.7	60
66016	Cheeseburger, double patty, plain	1 ea	155	477	27	32	1	27	11	85
56651	Cheeseburger, w/bacon & condiments, large	1 ea	195	550	31	37	3	31	11.9	98
56649	Cheeseburger, w/condiments & vegetables, large	1 ea	219	451	25	37	3	23	8.5	74
15063	Chicken drumstick & thigh, dark meat, breaded & fried	3 oz	85.1	248	17	9		15	4.1	95
15064	Chicken breast & wing, white meat, breaded & fried	3 oz	85.1	258	19	10		15	4.1	77

MDA Code	Food Name	Amt	Wt (g)	Ener (kcal)	Prot (g)	Carb (g)	Fiber (g)	Fat (g)	Sat (g)	Chol (mg)
56656	Chicken fillet sandwich w/cheese	1 ea	228	632	29	42		39	12.4	78
56000	Chicken fillet sandwich, plain	1 ea	182	515	24	39		29	8.5	60
50312	Chili con carne	1 cup	253	256	25	22		8	3.4	134
56635	Chimichanga, beef & cheese	1 ea	183	443	20	39		23	11.2	51
19110	Clams, breaded & fried	3 oz	85.1	334	9	29		20	4.9	65
5461	Coleslaw	0.75 cup	99	147	1	13		11	1.6	5
6175	Corn cob w/butter	1 ea	146	155	4	32		3	1.6	6
56668	Corn dog	1 ea	175	460	17	56		19	5.2	79
56606	Croissant sandwich w/egg & cheese	1 ea	127	368	13	24		25	14.1	216
56607	Croissant sandwich w/egg, cheese & bacon	1 ea	129	413	16	24		28	15.4	215
56608	Croissant sandwich w/egg, cheese & ham	1 ea	152	474	19	24		34	17.5	213
45588	Cheese Danish, cheese	1 ea	91	353	6	29		25	5.1	20
45513	Danish, fruit	1 ea	94	335	5	45		16	3.3	19
66021	Enchilada, cheese	1 ea	163	319	10	29		19	10.6	44
66022	Enchilada, beef & cheese	1 ea	192	323	12	30		18	9	40
66020	Enchirito, beef, bean & cheese	1 ea	193	344	18	34		16	7.9	50
42064	English muffin w/butter	1 ea	63	189	5	30	2	6	2.4	13
66031	English muffin sandwich w/cheese & sausage	1 ea	115	389	15	29	1	24	9.4	49
66032	English muffin sandwich w/egg, cheese & Canadian bacon	1 ea	146	323	20	31	1	13	5.4	245
66010	Fish sandwich, w/tartar sauce	1 ea	158	431	17	41		23	5.2	55
66011	Fish sandwich w/tartar sauce & cheese	1 ea	183	523	21	48		29	8.1	68
90736	French fries, fried in vegetable oil, medium size	1 ea	134	427	5	50	5	23	5.3	0
90498	French fries, w/salt, from frozen, 9 oz pkg	1 pkg	198	265	5	55	6	10	2	0
42354	French toast sticks	5 pce	141	479	8	58	2	25	5.6	0
42353	French toast w/butter	2 pce	135	356	10	36		19	7.7	116
56638	Frijoles (refried beans) w/cheese	0.5 cup	83.5	113	6	14		4	2	18
42368	Garlic bread, from frozen, 2″	1 pce	50	170	5	21	1	8	2	6
56664	Ham & cheese sandwich	1 ea	146	352	21	33		15	6.4	58
56665	Ham, egg & cheese sandwich	1 ea	143	347	19	31		16	7.4	246
69150	Hamburger w/condiments, large	1 ea	171.5	439	27	38	2	20	8.2	69
56662	Hamburger, double patty, w/condiments & vegetables, large	1 ea	226	540	34	40		27	10.5	122
56661	Hamburger w/condiments & vegetables, large	1 ea	218	512	26	40		27	10.4	87
56659	Hamburger w/condiments & vegetables, medium	1 ea	110	279	13	27		13	4.1	26
66007	Hamburger, plain	1 ea	90	266	13	30	1	10	3.2	30
5463	Hash browns	0.5 cup	72	235	2	23	2	16	3.6	0
56667	Hot dog w/chili & bun	1 ea	114	296	14	31		13	4.9	51
66004	Hot dog, plain, w/bun	1 ea	98	242	10	18		15	5.1	44
2032	Hot fudge sundae	1 ea	158	284	6	48	0	9	5	21
56666	Hush puppies	5 pce	78	257	5	35		12	2.7	135
6185	Mashed potatoes	0.5 cup	121	100	3	20		1	0.6	2
90214	Mayonnaise, w/soybean oil, packet	1 ea	10	72	0	0	0	8	1.2	4
71129	Milk shake, chocolate, small, 12 fl-oz	1 ea	249.6	317	8	51	5	9	5.8	32
71132	Milk shake, vanilla, small, 12 fl-oz	1 ea	249.6	369	8	49	2	16	9.9	57
56639	Nachos, w/cheese	7 pce	113	346	9	36		19	7.8	18
56641	Nachos w/cheese, beans, beef & peppers	7 pce	225	502	17	49		27	11	18
6176	Onion rings, serving	8 pce	78.1	259	3	29		15	6.5	13
19109	Oysters, breaded & battered, fried	3 oz	85.1	226	8	24		11	2.8	66
45122	Pancakes, w/butter & syrup	1 ea	116	260	4	45		7	2.9	29
6173	Potato salad	0.333 cup	95	108	1	13		6	1	57

MDA Code	Food Name	Amt	Wt (g)	Ener (kcal)	Prot (g)	Carb (g)	Fiber (g)	Fat (g)	Sat (g)	Chol (mg)
56669	Roast beef sandwich, w/cheese	1 ea	176	473	32	45		18	9	77
66003	Roast beef sandwich, plain	1 ea	139	346	22	33		14	3.6	51
56643	Taco salad	1.5 cup	198	279	13	24		15	6.8	44
56644	Taco salad, w/chili con carne	1.5 cup	261	290	17	27		13	6	5
19115	Shrimp, breaded & fried	4 ea	93.7	260	11	23		14	3.1	114
56670	Steak sandwich	1 ea	204	459	30	52		14	3.8	73
56671	Submarine sandwich, w/cold cuts	1 ea	228	456	22	51		19	6.8	36
56673	Submarine sandwich, w/tuna salad	1 ea	256	584	30	55		28	5.3	49
57531	Taco, small	1 ea	171	371	21	27		21	11.4	56
66017	Tostada, bean & cheese	1 ea	144	223	10	27		10	5.4	30
56645	Tostada, beef & cheese	1 ea	163	315	19	23		16	10.4	41
	Arby's									
6429	Baked potato w/broccoli & cheese	1 ea	384	517	12	69	8	21	10.9	46
9011	Chicken tenders, 5 piece serving	1 ea	192	555	37	41	3	27	4.8	61
8987	French fries, curly, large	1 ea	198	631	8	73	7	37	6.8	0
9006	French fries, large	1 ea	212.6	565	6	82	6	37	6.7	0
9008	Cheese sticks, mozzarella, fried	1 ea	137	426	18	38	2	28	12.9	45
69055	Submarine sandwich, beef & swiss cheese	1 ea	311	678	35	47	4	36	10.9	91
9014	Breakfast biscuit, bacon, egg & cheese	1 ea	144	420	15	27	1	25	7.3	153
69043	Submarine sandwich, french dip, w/au jus	1 ea	285	453	29	49	3	18	7.2	59
8991	Submarine sandwich, hot, ham & swiss	1 ea	278	501	28	46	2	18	4.2	55
56336	Sandwich, roast beef	1 ea	157	326	20	35	1	14	5.5	45
81506	Sandwich, roast beef sourdough melt	1 ea	166	356	17	40	2	14	4.7	30
53256	Sauce, Arby's, packet	1 ea	14	15	0	4	0	0	0	0
9018	Sauce, barbecue, dipping, packet	1 serving	28.4	45	0	11	0	0	0	0
	Source: Arby's									
	Burger King									
56352	Cheeseburger	1 ea	133	380	19	32	4	20	9.1	60
56355	Cheeseburger, Whopper	1 ea	316	790	35	53	3	48	18.3	114
56357	Cheeseburger, Whopper, double	1 ea	399	1061	58	54	6	68	27.9	188
9087	Chicken tenders, 4 piece serving	1 ea	62	179	11	11	1	10	2.6	32
9065	French fries, large	1 ea	160	530	6	64	5	28	7	
56351	Hamburger	1 ea	121	333	17	33	2	15	6.1	42
56354	Hamburger, Whopper	1 ea	291	678	31	54	5	37	12.4	87
9071	Hash browns, round, medium	1 ea	128	472	4	44	4	31	7.6	0
2127	Milk shake, chocolate, medium 16 fl-oz	1 ea	397	440	13	80	4	8	5	35
2129	Milk shake, vanilla, medium, 16 fl-oz	1 ea	397	667	13	76	0	35	21.2	123
9041	Onion rings, large	1 ea	137	480	7	60	5	23	6	0
69071	Breakfast biscuit, bacon, egg & cheese	1 ea	189	692	27	51	1	61	18.6	253
56360	Sandwich, chicken	1 ea	224	660	25	53	3	39	8	70
57002	Sandwich, Chicken Broiler	1 ea	258	550	30	52	3	25	5	105
9084	Sandwich, croissant w/sausage & cheese	1 ea	107	402	15	25	1	27	9.2	46
	Source: Burger King Corporation									
	Chik-Fil-A									
69185	Chargrilled Chicken breast fillet, chargrilled	1 ea	79	100	20	1	0	2	0	60
15263	Chicken nuggets, 8 piece serving	1 ea	113	260	26	12	1	12	2.5	70
15262	Chicken strips, 4 piece serving	1 ea	108	250	25	12	0	11	2.5	70
52138	Cole slaw, small	1 ea	105	210	1	14	2	17	2.5	20
48214	Lemon pie, slice	1 pce	113	320	7	51	3	10	3.5	110
52134	Salad, garden, chargrilled chicken	1 ea	278	180	23	8	3	6	3	70

MDA Code	Food Name	Amt	Wt (g)	Ener (kcal)	Prot (g)	Carb (g)	Fiber (g)	Fat (g)	Sat (g)	Chol (mg)
52137	Salad, side	1 ea	164	80	5	6	2	5	2.5	15
69155	Sandwich, chicken salad, whole wheat	1 ea	153	350	20	32	5	15	3	65
69189	Sandwich, chicken, deluxe	1 ea	208	420	28	39	2	16	3.5	60
69176	Sauce, honey mustard, dipping, packet	1 ea	28	45	0	10	0	0	0	0
69182	Wrap, spicy chicken	1 ea	225	390	31	51	3	7	3.5	70
	Source: Chik-Fil-A									
	Dairy Queen									
56372	Cheeseburger, double, homestyle	1 ea	219	540	35	30	2	31	16	115
72142	Frozen dessert, banana split, large	1 ea	527	810	17	134	2	23	15	70
71693	Frozen dessert, Brownie Earthquake	1 ea	304	740	10	112	0	27	16	50
72139	Frozen dessert, chocolate cookie dough, large	1 ea	560	1320	21	193	0	52	26	90
72134	Frozen dessert, chocolate sundae, large	1 ea	333	580	11	100	1	15	10	45
72138	Frozen dessert, Oreo, large	1 ea	500	1010	19	148	2	37	18	70
72135	Frozen dessert, strawberry sundae, large	1 ea	333	500	10	83	1	15	9	45
72137	Frozen dessert, Triple Chocolate Utopia	1 ea	284	770	12	96	5	39	17	55
2222	Ice cream cone, chocolate, medium	1 ea	198	340	8	53	0	11	7	30
2136	Ice cream cone, dipped, medium	1 ea	220	490	8	59	1	24	13	30
2143	Ice cream cone, vanilla, medium	1 ea	213	355	9	57	0	10	6.5	32
2134	Ice cream sandwich	1 ea	85	200	4	31	1	6	3	10
72129	Milk shake, chocolate malt, large	1 ea	836	1320	29	222	2	35	22	110
	Source: International Dairy Queen, Inc.									
	Domino's Pizza									
91365	Breadsticks	1 ea	37.2	116	3	18	1	4	0.8	0
91369	Chicken, buffalo wings	1 ea	24.9	50	6	2	0	2	0.6	26
56386	Pizza, cheese, hand tossed, 12"	2 pce	159	375	15	55	3	11	4.8	23
91356	Pizza, Deluxe Feast, hand tossed, 12"	2 pce	200.8	465	19	57	3	18	7.7	40
91358	Pizza, MeatZZa Feast, hand tossed, 12"	2 pce	216.2	560	26	57	3	26	11.4	64
91361	Pizza, Pepperoni Feast, hand tossed, 12"	2 pce	196.1	534	24	56	3	25	10.9	57
91357	Pizza, Veggie Feast, hand tossed, 12"	2 pce	203.2	439	19	57	4	16	7.1	34
	Source: Domino's Pizza Incorporated									
	Hardee's									
9295	Apple turnover	1 ea	91	270	4	38		12	4	0
42330	Biscuit, cinnamon raisin	1 ea	75	250	2	42		8	2	0
15201	Chicken wing, serving	1 ea	66	200	10	23	0	8	2	30
9278	Hot dog sandwich w/chili	1 ea	160	451	15	24	2	32	12	55
9284	Chicken strips, 5 piece serving	1 ea	92	201	18	13	0	8	1.7	25
9277	Hamburger, Monster	1 ea	278	949	53	35	2	67	25	185
9275	Hamburger, Six Dollar	1 ea	353	911	41	50	2	61	27	137
2247	Ice cream cone, twist	1 ea	118	180	4	34		2	1	10
6147	French fries, large	1 ea	150	440	5	59	0	21	3	0
9281	Chicken sandwich, barbecue, grilled	1 ea	171	268	24	34	2	3	1	60
56423	Sandwich, fish, Fisherman's Fillet	1 ea	221	530	25	45		28	7	75
	Source: Hardee's Food Systems, Inc.									
	Jack in the Box									
56437	Cheeseburger, Jumbo Jack	1 ea	296	714	26	56	3	43	16.6	72
62547	Cheeseburger, Bacon Ultimate	1 ea	302	974	41	47	2	69	26.8	125
56445	Egg roll, 3 piece serving	1 ea	170	400	14	44	6	19	6	15
62558	French toast sticks, original, serving	1 ea	120	466	7	58	4	23	5	25
56433	Hamburger	1 ea	104	273	14	26	1	12	5.3	35
2964	Milk shake, Oreo cookie, medium	1 ea	419	941	15	112	1	46	25.8	157

MDA Code	Food Name	Amt	Wt (g)	Ener (kcal)	Prot (g)	Carb (g)	Fiber (g)	Fat (g)	Sat (g)	Chol (mg)
2165	Milk shake, vanilla, medium	1 ea	332	664	13	75	1	34	21	134
56446	Onion rings, serving	1 ea	120	504	6	51	3	30	6.1	0
6425	French fries, curly, medium	1 ea	125	404	6	44	4	23	4.4	0
6150	French fries, natural cut, small	1 ea	113	306	5	40	3	14	3.5	0
62551	Potato wedges, bacon & cheddar, serving	1 ea	268	692	21	53	6	44	14.8	49
56441	Sandwich, chicken fajita pita	1 ea	230	317	24	33	3	11	4.7	69
56431	Sandwich, breakfast, sausage croissant	1 ea	181	603	22	38	2	41	13.5	265
56377	Taco, beef, regular	1 ea	90	189	6	18	2	9	3.6	18
	Source: Jack in the Box									
	KFC									
42331	Biscuit, buttermilk	1 ea	57	203	4	24	1	10	2.4	1
15169	Chicken breast, extra crispy	1 ea	162	447	37	13	1	28	5.9	123
15185	Chicken breast , hot & spicy	1 ea	179	460	33	20	0	27	8	130
15163	Chicken breast, original recipe	1 ea	161	377	39	9	1	21	4.8	132
81292	Chicken breast, original recipe, w/o skin, breaded	1 ea	108	185	32	0	0	6	1.4	94
81293	Chicken, drumstick, original recipe	1 ea	59	145	13	3	0	9	2.1	69
15166	Chicken, thigh, original recipe	1 ea	126	335	24	9	1	23	5.4	125
416	Chicken, wing, honey barbecue, peices	6 ea	157	540	25	36	1	33	7	150
56451	Cole slaw, serving	1 ea	130	187	1	20	3	11	1.7	3
9535	Corn cob, small	1 ea	82	76	3	13	4	2	0.5	0
2897	Dessert, strawberry shortcake, LilBucket	1 ea	99	200	2	34	0	6	4	20
56681	Macaroni & cheese	1 ea	287	130	5	15	1	6	2	5
56453	Potatoes, mashed w/gravy, serving	1 ea	136	130	2	18	1	4	1	0
45166	Pie, pecan, slice	1 pce	95	370	4	55	2	15	2.5	40
81090	Pot pie, chicken, chunky	1 ea	423	770	29	70	5	40	15	115
56454	Potato salad, serving	1 ea	128	180	2	22	1	9	1.5	5
49148	Sandwich, chicken, honey bbq flavor, w/sauce	1 ea	147	300	21	41	4	6	1.5	50
81301	Sandwich, chicken, tender roasted, w/o sauce	1 ea	177	260	31	23	1	5	1.5	65
81093	Sandwich, chicken roasted, w/sauce	1 ea	196	390	31	24	1	19	4	70
81302	Sandwich, chicken, Twister	1 ea	252	670	27	55	3	38	7	60
	Source: Yum! Brands, Inc.									
	Long John Silver's									
91388	Cheese sticks, fried	3 ea	45	140	4	12	1	8	2	10
91390	Clam chowder, serving	1 ea	227	220	9	23	1	10	4	25
56477	Hush puppies, serving	1 ea	23	60	1	9	1	2	0.5	0
56461	Fish, batter dipped, regular	1 pce	92	230	11	16	0	13	4	30
92415	Cod, baked, serving	1 ea	100.7	120	21	0	0	5	1	90
91392	Sandwich, fish, batter dipped, Ultimate	1 ea	199	500	20	48	3	25	8	50
92290	Battered Shrimp, battered, 4 piece serving	1 ea	65.8	197	7	14	0	13	4.1	64
92292	Shrimp, breaded, fried, basket	1 ea	114	340	12	32	2	19	5	105
	Source: Yum! Brands, Inc.									
	McDonald's									
81465	Breakfast, big, w/eggs, sausage, hash browns & biscuit	1 ea	266	758	27	47	3	52	17	460
56675	Burrito, sausage, breakfast	1 ea	113	296	13	24	1	17	6.1	173
69010	Cheeseburger, Big Mac	1 ea	219	563	26	44	4	33	8.3	79
81458	Cheeseburger, double	1 ea	173	458	26	34	1	26	10.5	83
69012	Cheeseburger, Quarter Pounder	1 ea	199	513	29	40	3	28	11.2	94
49152	Chicken McNuggets, 6 piece serving	6 pce	100	291	15	17	1	18	3.1	44
42334	Croutons, serving	1 ea	12	50	1	9	1	1	0	0
42335	Danish, apple	1 ea	105	340	5	47	2	15	3	20

MDA Code	Food Name	Amt	Wt (g)	Ener (kcal)	Prot (g)	Carb (g)	Fiber (g)	Fat (g)	Sat (g)	Chol (mg)
72902	Dessert, apple dipper, w/low fat caramel sauce	1 ea	89	99	0	23		1	0.4	3
81440	French fries, large	1 ea	171	540	7	67	7	28	3.6	0
1747	Frozen dessert, Butterfinger	1 ea	348	620	16	90	1	22	14	70
2171	Frozen Dessert, hot fudge sundae	1 ea	179	333	7	54	1	11	6.4	23
69008	Hamburger	1 ea	105	265	13	32	1	10	3.1	28
69011	Hamburger, Quarter Pounder	1 ea	171	417	24	38	3	20	6.9	67
6155	Hash browns	1 ea	53	139	1	14	1	9	1.2	0
72913	Milk shake, chocolate, triple thick, large	1 ea	713	1162	26	199	1	32	16.4	100
81453	Pancakes, hotcake, w/2 pats margarine & syrup	1 ea	221	601	9	102	2	18	1.8	20
81154	Parfait, fruit n' yogurt, w/o granola	1 ea	142	128	4	25	1	2	0	7
48136	Pie, apple, snack	1 ea	77	249	2	34	2	12	3.1	
69218	Salad, bacon ranch, w/crispy chicken	1 ea	316	348	28	19	3	20	5.1	70
608	Salad, caesar, w/chicken, shaker	1 ea	163	100	17	3	2	2	1.5	40
61674	Salad, California cobb, w/grilled chicken	1 ea	325	273	34	11	3	11	4.8	143
57764	Salad, chef, Shaker	1 ea	206	150	17	5	2	8	3.5	95
61667	Salad, fruit & walnut	1 ea	264	312	5	44		13	1.8	5
81466	Sandwich, breakfast, McGriddle w/bacon, egg & cheese	1 ea	168	457	20	44	1	22	7.1	247
81532	Sandwich, chicken, grilled, classic	1 ea	229	419	32	51	3	10	2	78
69013	Sandwich, Filet O Fish, w/tartar sauce	1 ea	141	388	15	39	1	19	3.7	39
81456	Sandwich, Filet O Fish w/o tartar sauce	1 ea	123	299	15	38	1	9	2.2	31
53176	Sauce, barbecue, packet	1 ea	28	46	0	10	0	0	0	
53177	Sauce, sweet & sour, packet	1 ea	28	48	0	11	0	0	0	
12230	Sausage, pork, serving	1 ea	43	170	6	0	0	16	5	35
42747	Sweet roll, cinnamon	1 ea	105	418	8	56	2	19	4.7	61
	Source: McDonald's Nutrition Information Center									
	Pizza Hut									
92497	Breadsticks, cheese	1 ea	67	200	7	21	1	10	3.5	15
92526	Dessert pizza, cherry, slice	1 pce	102	240	4	47	1	4	0.5	0
92519	Pasta Bakes, primavera w/chicken, serving	1 ea	540	1050	52	97	6	50	12	75
57394	Pizza, beef, medium, 12", slice	1 pce	91	230	11	21	2	11	5	25
56489	Pizza, cheese, medium, 12", slice	1 pce	96	260	11	30	2	10	4.8	23
56481	Pizza, cheese, pan, medium, 12", slice	1 pce	100	280	12	30	2	13	5.2	21
57781	Pizza, chicken supreme, 12", medium, slice	1 pce	120	230	14	30	2	6	3	25
830	Pizza, super supreme, medium, 12"	1 pce	127	309	14	33	3	14	5.8	25
92483	Pizza, green pepper, onion & tomato, 12", medium, slice	1 pce	104	150	6	24	2	4	1.5	10
92482	Pizza, ham, pineapple & tomato, 12" medium, slice	1 pce	99	160	8	24	2	4	2	15
57810	Pizza, Meat Lovers, 12", medium, slice	1 pce	169	450	21	43	3	21	10	55
56486	Pizza, pepperoni, 12" medium, slice	1 pce	77	210	10	21	1	10	4.5	25
57811	Pizza, Veggie Lovers, 12", medium, slice	1 pce	172	360	16	45	3	14	7	35
	Source: Yum! Brands, Inc.									
	Subway									
47658	Cookie, chocolate chip, M & M's	1 ea	45	220	2	30	1	10	4	15
52119	Salad, chicken breast, roasted	1 ea	303	140	16	12	3	3	1	45
52115	Salad, club	1 ea	322	150	17	12	3	4	1.5	35
52118	Salad, tuna, w/light mayonnaise	1 ea	314	240	13	10	3	16	4	40
52113	Salad, veggie delite	1 ea	233	50	2	9	3	1	0	0
91761	Sandwich, chicken teriyaki, w/sweet onion, white bread, 6"	1 ea	269	380	26	59	4	5	1.5	50
69117	Sandwich, club, white bread, 6"	1 ea	255	320	24	46	4	6	2	35
69113	Sandwich, cold cut trio, white bread, 6"	1 ea	257	440	21	47	4	21	7	55
91763	Sandwich, ham, w/honey mustard, white bread, 6"	1 ea	232	310	18	52	4	5	1.5	25

MDA Code	Food Name	Amt	Wt (g)	Ener (kcal)	Prot (g)	Carb (g)	Fiber (g)	Fat (g)	Sat (g)	Chol (mg)
69139	Sandwich, Italian BMT, white bread, 6"	1 ea	248	480	23	46	4	24	9	55
69129	Sandwich, meatball, white bread, 6"	1 ea	287	530	24	53	6	26	10	55
69103	Sandwich, roast beef, deli style	1 ea	151	220	13	35	3	4	2	15
69143	Tuna Sandwich, tuna, w/Llight mayonnaise, white bread, 6"	1 ea	255	450	20	46	4	22	6	40
69101	Sandwich, turkey, deli style	1 ea	151	220	13	36	3	4	1.5	15
69109	Sandwich, veggie delight, white bread, 6"	1 ea	166	230	9	44	4	3	1	0
91778	Soup, roasted chicken noodle	1 cup	240	90	7	7	1	4	1	20
91791	Soup, cream of broccoli	1 cup	240	130	5	15	2	6	0	10
91783	Soup, minestrone	1 cup	240	70	3	11	2	1	0	10
91788	Soup, chicken w/ brown & wild rice	1 cup	240	190	6	17	2	11	4.5	20
	Source: Subway International									
	Taco Bell									
92107	Border Bowl, chicken, zesty, w/sauce	1 ea	417	730	23	65	12	42	9	45
56519	Burrito, bean	1 ea	198	404	16	55	8	14	4.8	18
56522	Burrito, beef, supreme	1 ea	248	469	20	52	8	20	7.6	40
57668	Burrito, chicken, fiesta	1 ea	184	370	18	48	3	12	3.5	30
56691	Burrito, seven layer	1 ea	283	530	18	67	10	22	8	25
92113	Burrito, steak, grilled, Stuft	1 ea	325	680	31	76	8	28	8	55
92118	Chalupa, beef, nacho cheese	1 ea	153	380	12	33	3	22	7	20
92120	Chalupa, chicken, Baja	1 ea	153	400	17	30	2	24	6	40
92122	Chalupa, steak, supreme	1 ea	153	370	15	29	2	22	8	35
45585	Cinnamon twists, serving	1 ea	35	160	1	28	0	5	1	0
57666	Gordita, beef, Baja	1 ea	153	350	14	31	4	19	5	30
57669	Gordita, chicken, Baja	1 ea	153	320	17	29	2	15	3.5	40
57662	Gordita, steak, Baja	1 ea	153	320	15	29	2	16	4	30
56530	Guacamole, serving	1 ea	21	35	0	2	1	3	0	0
38561	Mexican rice, serving	1 ea	131	210	6	23	3	10	4	15
56534	Nachos, Bell Grande, serving	1 ea	308	780	20	80	12	43	13	35
56536	Pintos & cheese, serving	1 ea	128	180	10	20	6	7	3.5	15
56531	Pizza, Mexican	1 ea	216	550	21	46	7	31	11	45
57689	Quesadilla, chicken	1 ea	184	540	28	40	3	30	13	80
92098	Salsa, fiesta	1 ea	21	5	0	1		0	0	0
53186	Sauce, hot, Border, packet	1 ea	11	4	0	0	0	0	0	0
92105	Steak bowl, southwest	1 ea	443	700	30	73	13	32	8	55
56524	Taco	1 ea	78	184	8	14	3	11	3.6	24
57671	Taco, double decker, supreme	1 ea	191	380	15	40	6	18	8	40
56693	Taco, soft shell	1 ea	127	286	15	22	2	15	4.3	39
56537	Taco salad, w/salsa & shell	1 ea	533	906	36	80	16	49	15.9	101
56528	Tostada	1 ea	170	250	11	29	7	10	4	15
	Source: Taco Bell/Yum! Brands, Inc.									
	Wendy's									
56579	Baked potato w/bacon & cheese	1 ea	380	580	18	79	7	22	6	40
56582	Baked potato, w/sour cream & chives	1 ea	312	370	7	73	7	6	4	15
81445	Cheeseburger, single, classic	1 ea	236	522	35	34	3	27	12.3	90
56571	Cheeseburger, bacon, junior	1 ea	165	380	20	34	2	19	7	55
15176	Chicken nuggets, 5 piece serving	1 ea	75	250	12	12	1	17	3.7	38
50311	Chili, small	1 ea	227	200	17	21	5	6	2.5	35
6169	French fries, large	1 ea	159	507	6	63	6	26	5.1	

MDA Code	Food Name	Amt	Wt (g)	Ener (kcal)	Prot (g)	Carb (g)	Fiber (g)	Fat (g)	Sat (g)	Chol (mg)
2177	Frozen dessert, dairy, medium	1 ea	298	393	10	70	10	8	4.9	48
56574	Hamburger, bacon big, classic	1 ea	282	570	34	46	3	29	12	100
56566	Hamburger, single, classic	1 ea	218	464	28	37	3	23	8	76
8457	Dressing, blue cheese, packet	1 ea	71	290	2	3	0	30	6	45
8461	Dressing, french, packet	1 ea	71	90	0	21	1	0	0	0
71595	Dressing, sesame, oriental, packet	1 ea	71	280	2	21	0	21	3	0
81444	Sandwich, Homestyle Chicken Fillet	1 ea	230	492	32	50	3	19	3.7	71
81443	Sandwich, Ultimate Grill Chicken	1 ea	225	403	33	42	2	11	2.3	90
52080	Salad, side, caesar, w/o dressing	1 ea	99	70	7	2	1	4	2	15
71592	Salad, chicken, mandarin, w/o dressing	1 ea	348	150	20	17	3	2	0	10
52083	Salad, side, garden, w/o dressing	1 ea	167	35	2	7	3	0	0	0
	Source: Wendy's Foods International									

references

Chapter 1

1. Margen, S., et al. (Eds.). *The Wellness Encyclopedia*. Boston: Houghton Mifflin, 1995.

2. National Institute of Mental Health. *The Numbers Count: Mental Disorders in America*. Fact Sheet. http://www.nimh.nih.gov/publicat/numbers.cfm#MajorDepressive.

3. Koeing, H. G. Religion, spirituality and medicine: Research findings and implications for clinical practice. *Southern Medical Journal* 97:1194–1200, 2004.

4. Katon, W., E. H. B. Lin, and K. Kroenke. The association of depression and anxiety with medical symptom burden in patients with chronic medical illness. *General Hospital Psychiatry* 29:147–155, 2007.

5. Weaver, A. J., and K. J. Flannelly. The role of religion/spirituality for cancer patients and their caregivers. *Southern Medical Journal* 97:1210–1214, 2004.

6. Caspersen, C. J., K. E. Powell, and G. M. Christenson. Physical activity and exercise: Definitions and distinctions for health related-fitness research. *Public Health Reports* 100:126–130, 1985.

7. Paffenbarger, R., J. Kampert, I. Lee, R. Hyde, R. Leung, and A. Wing. Changes in physical activity and other lifeway patterns influencing longevity. *Medicine and Science in Sports and Exercise* 26:857–865, 1994.

8. Powell, K.E., A. Paluch, and S.N. Blair. Physical activity for health: What kind? How much? How intense? On top of what? *Annual Review of Public Health*. 32:349–365, 2011.

9. Helmrich, S., D. Ragland, and R. Paffenbarger. Prevention of non-insulin-dependent diabetes mellitus with physical activity. *Medicine and Science in Sports and Exercise* 26:824–830, 1994.

10. Penedo, F. and J. Dahn. Exercise and well-being: a review of mental and physical health benefits associated with physical activity. *Current Opinion in Psychiatry*. 18:189–193, 2005.

11. Morris, J. Exercise in the prevention of coronary heart disease: Today's best buy in public health. *Medicine and Science in Sports and Exercise* 26:807–814, 1994.

12. Blair, S. N., M. LaMonte, and M. Nichaman. The evolution of physical activity recommendations: How much is enough? *American Journal of Clinical Nutrition* 79:913S–920S, 2004.

13. Thompson, P., et al. Exercise and physical activity in the prevention and treatment of atherosclerotic cardiovascular disease. *Circulation* 107:3109–3116, 2003.

14. Brooks, G. A., N. Butte, W. Rand, J. Flatt, and B. Caballero. Chronicle of the Institute of Medicine physical activity recommendation: How a physical activity recommendation came to be among dietary recommendations. *American Journal of Clinical Nutrition* 79:921S–930S, 2004.

15. Brown, D., D. Brown, G. Heath, L. Balluz, W. Giles, E. Ward, and A. Mokdad. Associations between physical activity dose and health-related quality of life. *Medicine and Science in Sports and Exercise* 36:890–896, 2004.

16. U.S. Department of Health and Human Services. *Physical Activity and Health: A Report of the Surgeon General*. Atlanta, GA: U.S. Department of Health and Human Services, Centers for Disease Control and Prevention, National Center for Chronic Disease Prevention and Health Promotion, 1996.

17. Rogers, V. L. et al. Heart disease and stroke statistics—2012 update. *Circulation* 125:e12–e230, 2012.

18. Opie, L.H. and A. J. Dalby. Cardiovascular prevention: lifestyle and statins—competitors or companions? *South African Medical Journal*. 104:168–173, 2014.

19. Williams, P. T. Relationship between distance run per week to coronary heart disease risk factors in 8283 male runners: The National Runners Health Study. *Archives of Internal Medicine* 157:191–198, 1997.

20. Fagard, R. Physical activity in the prevention and treatment of hypertension in the obese. *Medicine and Science in Sports and Exercise* 31:S624–S630, 1999.

21. Williams, P. Physical fitness and activity as separate heart disease risk factors: A meta-analysis. *Medicine and Science in Sports and Exercise* 33:754–761, 2001.

22. Borges J.P.,et al., Delta Opioid Receptors: The Link between Exercise and Cardioprotection. *PLoS ONE* 9(11): e113541. doi:10.1371/journal.pone.0113541, 2014.

23. Powers, S.K., A. J. Smuder, A.N. Kavazis, and J. C. Quindry. Mechanisms of exercise-induced cardioprotection. *Physiology*. 29:27–38, 2014.

24. Lee, Y., K. Min, E.E. Talbert, A.N. Kavazis, A.J. Smuder, W. T. Willis, and S.K. Powers. Exercise protects against cardiac mitochondria against ischemia-reperfusion injury. *Medicine and Science in Sports and Exercise*. 44:397–405, 2012.

25. Lee, I., and R. Paffenbarger. Associations of light, moderate, and vigorous intensity physical activity with longevity: The Harvard Alumni Health Study. *American Journal of Epidemiology* 151:293–299, 2000.

26. Powell, K., and S. Blair. The public health burdens of sedentary living habits: Theoretical but realistic estimates. *Medicine and Science in Sports and Exercise* 26:851–856, 1994.

27. Rodnick, K., J. Holloszy, C. Mondon, and D. James. Effects of exercise training on insulin-regulatable glucose-transporter protein levels in rat skeletal muscle. *Diabetes* 39:1425–1429, 1990.

28. Pan, X. R., et al. Effects of diet and exercise in preventing NIDDM in people with impaired glucose tolerance. *Diabetes Care* 20:537–544, 1997.

29. Rankin, J. Diet, exercise, and osteoporosis. *Certified News* (American College of Sports Medicine) 3:1–4, 1993.

30. Wheeler, D., J. Graves, G. Miller, R. Vander Griend, T. Wronski, S. K. Powers, and H. Park. Effects of running on the torsional strength, morphometry, and bone mass on the rat skeleton. *Medicine and Science in Sports and Exercise* 27:520–529, 1995.

31. Farr, J. N., D. R. Laddu, and S.B. Going. Exercise, hormones, and skeletal adaptations during childhood and adolescence. *Pediatric Exercise Science*. 26:384–391, 2014.

32. Jackson, A.S., X. Sui, J.R. Herbert, T.S. Church, and S.N. Blair. Role of lifestyle and aging on the longitudinal change in cardiorespiratory fitness. *Archives Internal Medicine*. 169:1781–1787, 2009.

33. Fleg, J., and E. Lakatta. Role of muscle loss in the age-associated reduction in VO2max. *Journal of Applied Physiology* 65:1147–1151, 1988.

34. Nakamura, E., T. Moritani, and A. Kanetaka. Effects of habitual physical exercise on physiological age in men and women aged 20–85 years as estimated using principal component analysis. *European Journal of Applied Physiology* 73:410–418, 1996.

35. Hammeren, J., S. Powers, J. Lawler, D. Criswell, D. Martin, D. Lowenthal, and M. Pollock. Exercise training–induced alterations in skeletal muscle oxidative and antioxidant enzyme activity in senescent rats. *International Journal of Sports Medicine* 13:412–416, 1992.

36. Dickinson, J. M., E. Volpi, and B.B. Rasmussen. Exercise and nutrition to target protein synthesis impairments in aging skeletal muscle. *Exercise and Sport Science Reviews.* 41:216–223, 2013.

37. Holloszy, J. Exercise increases average longevity of female rats despite increased food intake and no growth retardation. *Journal of Gerontology* 48:B97–B100, 1993.

38. Lee, I., R. Paffenbarger, and C. Hennekens. Physical activity, physical fitness, and longevity. *Aging* (Milano) 9:2–11, 1997.

39. Franklin, B. Improved fitness = increased longevity. *ACSM's Health and Fitness Journal* 5:32–33, 2001.

40. Blair, S. N., and M. Wei. Sedentary habits, health, and function in older men and women. *American Journal of Health Promotion* 15:1–8, 2000.

41. Blair, S. N., H. W. Kohl, R. Paffenbarger, D. Clark, K. Cooper, and L. Gibbons. Physical fitness and all-cause mortality: A prospective study of healthy men and women. *Journal of the American Medical Association* 262:2395–2401, 1989.

42. Penedo, F. J., and J. R. Dahn. Exercise and well-being: A review of mental and physical health benefits associated with physical activity. *Current Opinion in Psychiatry* 18:198–193, 2005.

43. Jones, M. A., G. Stratton, T. Reilly, and V. B. Unnithan. Biological risk indicators for recurrent non-specific low back pain in adolescents. *British Journal of Sports Medicine* 39:137–140, 2005.

44. Mikkelson, L. O., H. Nupponen, J. Kaprio, H. Kautiainen, and U. M. Kujala. Adolescent flexibility, endurance strength, and physical activity as predictors of adult tension neck, low back pain and knee injury: A 25 year follow up. *British Journal of Sports Medicine* 40:107–113, 2006.

45. Kruk, J. and U. Czerniak. Physical activity and its relation to cancer risk: Updating the evidence. *Asia Pacific Journal of Cancer Prevention.* 14:3993–4003, 2013.

46. Owen, N., P. Sparling, G. Healy, D. Durstan, and C. Mathews. Sedentary Behavior: Emerging Evidence for a New Health Risk. Mayo Clinic Proceedings. 85:1138–1141, 2010.

47. Durstan, D., B. Howard, G. Healy, and N. Owen. Too much sitting-a health hazard. Diabetes Research and Clinical Practice. 97:368–376, 2012.

Chapter 2

1. Howley, E., and D. Thompson. *Fitness Professional's Handbook.* Champaign, IL: Human Kinetics, 2012.

2. Powers, S., and E. Howley. *Exercise Physiology: Theory and Application to Fitness and Performance,* 8th ed. New York: McGraw-Hill, 2012.

3. Stone, M., S. Plisk, and D. Collins. Training principles: Evaluation of modes and methods of resistance training—A coaching perspective. *Sports Biomechanics* 1:79–103, 2002.

4. Abernethy, P., J. Jurimae, P. Logan, A. Taylor, and R. Thayer. Acute and chronic response of skeletal muscle to resistance exercise. *Sports Medicine* 17:22–28, 1994.

5. Powers, S., D. Criswell, J. Lawler, L. Ji, D. Martin, R. Herb, and G. Dudley. Influence of exercise and fiber type on antioxidant enzyme activity in rat skeletal muscle. *American Journal of Physiology* 266:R375–R380, 1994.

6. Coyle, E., W. Martin, D. Sinacore, M. Joyner, J. Hagberg, and J. Holloszy. Time course of loss of adaptations after stopping prolonged intense endurance training. *Journal of Applied Physiology* 57:1857–1864, 1984.

7. Costill, D., and A. Richardson. *Handbook of Sports Medicine: Swimming.* London: Blackwell Publishing, 1993.

8. Bushman, B. (Ed). *ACSM's Complete Guide to Fitness and Health.* Champaign, IL: Human Kinetics, 2011.

9. Wilmot, E.G., C. Edwardson, F. Achana et al. Sedentary time in adults and the association with diabetes, cardiovascular disease and death: systematic review and meta analysis. *Diabetologia.* 55:2895–2905, 2012.

10. Levine, J.A. Lethal sitting: homo sendentarius seeks answers. *Physiology.* 29: 300–301, 2014.

11. Solomon, T.P., and J.P. Thyfault. Type 2 diabetes sits in a chair. *Diabetes Obesity Metabolism.* 15:987–992, 2013.

12. Warburton, D., C. Nicol, and S. Bredin. Prescribing exercise as preventative therapy. *Canadian Medical Association Journal* 28:961–974, 2006.

13. Walsh, N., M. Gleeson, D. Pyne, D. Nieman, Dhabhar, R. Shephard, S. Oliver, S. Bermon, and A. Kajeniene. Position statement. Part two: Maintaining immune health. *Exercise Immunology Review.* 17:64–103, 2011.

14. Paffenbarger, R., J. Kampert, I. Lee, R. Hyde, R. Leung, and A. Wing. Changes in physical activity and other lifeway patterns influencing longevity. *Medicine and Science in Sports and Exercise* 26:857–865, 1994.

15. Fiuza-Luces, C., N. Garatachea, N.A. Berger, and A. Lucia. Exercise is the real polypill. *Physiology.* 28:330–358, 2013.

16. Garber, C. B. Blissmer, M. Deschenes, B. Franklin, M. Lamonte, I. Lee, D. Nieman, D. Swain. American College of Sports Medicine position stand. Quality and quantity of exercise for developing and maintaining cardiorespiratory, musculoskeletal, and neuromotor fitness in apparently healthy adults: Guidance for prescribing exercise. *Medicine and Science in Sports and Exercise.* 43:1334–1359, 2011.

17. Howley, E. T. You asked for it: Is rigorous exercise better than moderate activity in achieving health-related goals? *ACSM's Health and Fitness Journal* 4(2):6, 2000.

18. Thompson, P., et al. Exercise and physical activity in the prevention and treatment of atherosclerotic cardiovascular disease. *Circulation* 107:3109–3116, 2003.

19. Blair, S., M. LaMonte, and M. Nichman. The evolution of physical activity recommendations: How much exercise is enough? *American Journal of Clinical Nutrition* 79: 913S–920S, 2004.

20. Brooks, G., N. Butte, W. Rand, J. P. Flatt, and B. Caballero. Chronicle of the institute of medicine physical activity recommendation: How a physical activity recommendation came to be among dietary recommendations. *American Journal of Clinical Nutrition* 79:921S–930S, 2004.

21. Brown, D., D. Brown, G. Heath, L. Balluz, W. Giles, E. Ford, and A. Mokdad. Associations between physical activity dose and health-related quality of life. *Medicine and Science in Sports and Exercise* 36:890–896, 2004.

22. Swain, D. Moderate or vigorous intensity exercise: What should we prescribe? *ACSM's Health and Fitness Journal* 10:21–27, 2006.

23. Ishikawa-Takata, K., T. Ohta, and H. Tanaka. How much exercise is required to reduce blood pressure in essential hypertensive: A dose-response study. *American Journal of Hypertension* 16:629–633, 2003.

24. U.S. Department of Health and Human Services. *2008 Physical Activity Guidelines for Americans.* 2008. http://www .health.gov/paguidelines.

25. Blair, S. N. Physical inactivity: The biggest public health problem of the 21st century. *British Journal of Sports Medicine* 43:1–2, 2009.

26. Powell, K. A. Paluch, and S. Blair. Physical activity for health: What kind? How much? How intense? On top of what? *Annual Review of Public Health.* 32:349–395, 2011.

27. Lee, D., E. Artero, X. Sui, and S. Blair. Mortality trends in the general population: The importance of cardiorespiratory fitness. *Journal of Psychopharmacology.* 24:27–35, 2010.

28. Gleeson, M., N. Bishop, D. Stensel, M. Lindley, S. Mastana, and M. Nimmo. The anti-inflammatory effects of exercise: Mechanisms and implications for the prevention and treatment of disease. *Nature Review Immunology.* 11:607–615, 2011.

Chapter 3

1. Evert, A. and M. Riddell. Lifestyle intervention: Nutrition therapy and physical activity. *Medical Clinics of North America.* 99(1)69–85, 2015.

2. Foulds, H., S. Bredin, S. Charlesworth, A. Ivey and D. Warburton. Exercise volume and intensity: a dose-response relationship with health benefits. *European Journal of Applied Physiology.* 114(8):1563–1571, 2014.

3. Powers, S., and E. Howley. *Exercise Physiology: Theory and Application to Fitness and Performance,* 9th ed. New York: McGraw-Hill, 2015.

4. Kilpatrick, M., M. Jung and J. Little. High-intensity interval training: A review of physiological and psychological responses. *ACSM's Health & Fitness Journal* 18(5):11–16, 2014.

5. Myer, J., P. McAuley, C. Lavie, J-P. Despres, R. Arena, P. Kokkinos. Physical Activity and Cardiorespiratory Fitness as Major Markers of Cardiovascular Risk: Their Independent and Interwoven Importance to Health Status. *Progress in Cardiovascular Diseases.* (57)4:306–314, 2015.

6. Meeusen, R. Exercise, nutrition and the brain. *Sports Medicine.* (44)1: 47–56, 2014.

7. Erlachera, C., D. Erlachera, and, M. Schredlc. The effects of exercise on self-rated sleep among adults with chronic sleep complaints. *Journal of Sort and Health Science.* (3)1:1–10, 2014.

8. American College of Sports Medicine. *ACSM's Guidelines for Exercise Testing and Prescription,* 9th ed. Philadelphia: Lippincott Williams, & Wilkins, 2013.

9. Mays, R., F. Goss, E. Nagle, M. Gallagher, M. Schafer, K. Kim, and R. Robertson. Prediction of VO₂peak using OMNI ratings of perceived exertion from a submaximal cycle exercise test. *Perceptual and Motor Skills* 118(1): 863–881, 2014.

10. Paradisis, G., E. Zacharogiannis, & D. Mandila. Multi-Stage 20-m Shuttle Run Fitness Test, Maximal Oxygen Uptake and Velocity at Maximal Oxygen Uptake. *Journal of Human Kinetics* 41(1):81–87, 2014.

11. DiVencenzo, H., A. Morgan, C. Laurent & K. Keylock. Metabolic demands of law enforcement personal protective equipment during exercise tasks *Ergonomics* 57(11):306–314, 2014.

12. Kayihan, G., A. Özkan, Y. Köklü, E. Eyuboğlu, F. Akça, M. Koz, & G. Ersöz. Comparative analysis of the 1-mile run test evaluation formulae: Assessment of aerobic capacity in male law enforcement officers aged 20–23 years. *International Journal of Occupational Medicine and Environmental Health* 27(2):165–174, 2014.

13. Gault, M. and M. Willems. Walking and Aerobic Capacity in Old Adults after Concentric and Eccentric Endurance Exercise at Self-Selected Intensities. *Health* 6(8):1–10, 2014.

14. Trappe S., E Hayes, A. Galpin, L Kaminsky, & B. Jemiolo. Lifelong endurance athletes. New records in aerobic power among octogenarians. *Journal of Applied Physiology* 114:3–10, 2013.

15. Lox, C., K. Ginis and S. Petruzzello. *The Psychology of Exercise Integrating Theory and Practice,* 3rd ed. Scottsdale, AZ: Holcomb Hathaway Publishers, 2010.

16. Mullen, S., T. Wójcicki, E. Mailey, A. Szabo, N. Gothe, E. Olson, J. Fanning, A. Kramer, & E. McAuley. A Profile for Predicting Attrition from Exercise in Older Adults. *Prevention Science* 14(5):489–496, 2013.

17. Lepp, A., J. Barkley, G. Sander, M. Rebold1 & P. Gates. The relationship between cell phone use, physical and sedentary activity, and cardiorespiratory fitness in a sample of U.S. college students. *International Journal of Behavioral Nutrition and Physical Activity* (10)79:1–9, 2013.

18. Borg, G. *Borg's Perceived Exertion and Pain Scales.* Champaign, IL: Human Kinetics, 1998.

19. Kuzy, K. and J. Zielinski. Sprinters versus Long-distance Runners: How to Grow Old Healthy. *Exercise & Sport Sciences Reviews* 43(1):57–64, 2015.

20. Perry, C., G. Heigenhauser, A. Bonen, A., L. Spriet. High-intensity aerobic interval training increases fat and carbohydrate metabolic capacities in human skeletal muscle. *Applied Physiology, Nutrition, and Metabolism.* 33(6): 1112–1123, 2008.

21. Thompson, W. Worldwide survey of fitness trends for 2015: What's driving the market. *ACSM's Health & Fitness Journal.* 18(6), 8–17, 2014.

22. Smith, M., A. Sommer, B. Starkoff, S. Devor. Crossfit-Based High-Intensity Power Training Improves Maximal Aerobic Fitness and Body Composition. *Journal of Strength and Conditioning Research.* 27(11):3159–3172, 2013.

Chapter 4

1. Kell, R. T., and G. J. Asmundson. A comparison of two forms of periodized exercise rehabilitation programs in the management of chronic nonspecific low-back pain. *Journal of Strength and Condition- ing Research* 23(2):513–523, 2009.

2. Olson, T., C. Chebny, J. Willson, T. Kernozek, and J. Straker. Comparison of 2D and 3D kinematic changes during a single leg step down following neuromuscular training. *Physical Therapy and Sport* 12(2):93–99, 2010.

3. Gianoudis J., C. Bailey, P. Ebeling, C. Nowson, K. Sanders, K. Hill, R. Daly. Effects of a targeted multimodal exercise

program incorporating high-speed power training on falls and fracture risk factors in older adults: a community-based randomized controlled trial. *Journal of Bone Mineral Research.* 29(1):182–91, 2014.

4. Hopps, E., and G. Caimi. Exercise in obesity management. *Journal of Sports Medicine and Physical Fitness* 51(2):275–282, 2011.

5. Powers, S., and E. Howley. *Exercise Physiology: Theory and Application to Fitness and Performance,* 9th ed. New York: McGraw-Hill, 2015.

6. Oberbach A., Y. Bossenz, S. Lehmann, J. Niebauer, V. Adams, R. Paschke, M. R. Schön, M. Blüher, and K. Punkt. Altered fiber distribution and fiber-specific glycolytic and oxidative enzyme activity in skeletal muscle of patients with type 2 diabetes. *Diabetes Care* 29(4):895–900, 2006.

7. Karjalainen, J., H. Tikkanen, M. Hernelahti, and U. Kujala. Muscle fiber-type distribution predicts weight gain and unfavorable left ventricular geometry: A 19 year follow-up study. *BMC Cardiovascular Disorders* 10(6):1–8, 2006.

8. Ehrenborg, E., and A. Krook. Regulation of skeletal muscle physiology and metabolism by peroxisome proliferator-activated receptor delta. *Pharmacological Reviews* 61(3):373–393, 2009.

9. Brito, A., C. de Oliveira, M. Santos and A. Santos. High-intensity exercise promotes postexercise hypotension greater than moderate intensity in elderly hypertensive individuals. *Clinical Physiology and Functional Imaging.* 34(2): 126–132, 2014.

10. American College of Sports Medicine. American College of Sports Medicine position stand: Progression models in resistance training for healthy adults. *Medicine and Science in Sports and Exercise* 41(3):687–708, 2009.

11. Bodine, S. and K. Baar. Analysis of Skeletal Muscle Hypertrophy in Models of Increased Loading. *Myogenesis: Methods in Molecular Biology.* 798: 213–229, 2012.

12. Knuttgen, H. G. Strength training and aerobic exercise: Comparison and contrast. *Journal of Strength and Conditioning Research* 21(3):973–978, 2007.

13. American College of Sports Medicine. Quantity and quality of exercise for developing and maintaining cardiorespiratory, musculoskeletal, and neuromotor fitness in apparently healthy adults: Guidance for prescribing exercise. *Medicine and Science in Sports and Exercise* 43(7):1334–1359, 2011.

14. Fleck, S. and W. Kraemer. *Designing resistance training programs.* 4th Ed., Champaign, Il., Human Kinetics, 2014.

15. Tillin, N. A., M. T. G. Pain, and J. P. Folland. Short-term training for explosive strength causes neural and mechanical adaptations. *Experimental Physiology* 23(8):817–824, 2012.

16. Rønnestad, B. R., B. S. Nymark, and T. Raastad. Effects of in-season strength maintenance training frequency in professional soccer players. *Journal of Strength and Conditioning Research* 25(10): 2653–2660, 2011.

Chapter 5

1. Magee, D. Orthopedic Physical Assessment. 6th Ed., Philadelphia: Elsevier Publishing, 2014.

2. Esposito, F., E. Limonta, and E. E. Cè. Passive stretching effects on electromechanical delay and time course of recovery in human skeletal muscle: new insights from an electromyographic and mechanomyographic combined approach. *European Journal of Applied Physiology* 111(3):485–495, 2011.

3. Ryan, E. E., M. Rossi, and R. Lopez. The effects of the contract-relax-antagonist-contract form of proprioceptive neuromuscular facilitation stretching on postural stability. *Journal of Strength and Conditioning Research* 24(7):1888–1894, 2010.

4. American College of Sports Medicine position stand: Quantity and quality of exercise for developing and maintaining cardiorespiratory, musculoskeletal, and neuromotor fitness in apparently healthy adults: Guidance for prescribing exercise. *Medicine and Science in Sports and Exercise* 43(7):1334–1359, 2011.

5. Opar, D., M. Williams, and A. Shield. Hamstring Strain Injuries. *Sports Medicine.* 42(3): 209–226, 2012.

6. Manchikanti, L., Singh, V. Falco, F., Benyamin, R. and Hirsch, J. Epidemiology of low back pain in adults. *Neuromodulation.* 17(S2), 3–10, 2014.

7. Brackley, H. M., J. M. Stevenson, and J. C. Selinger. Effect of backpack load placement on posture and spinal curvature in prepubescent children. *Work* 32(3):351–360, 2009.

8. Tracy, BL and Hart, CEF. Bikram yoga training and physical fitness in healthy young adults. J Strength Cond Res 27(3): 822–830, 2013.

9. O'Hora, J., A. Cartwright, C. D. Wade, A. D. Hough, and G. L. K. Shum. Efficacy of static stretching and proprioceptive neuromuscular facilitation stretch on hamstrings length after a single session. *Journal of Strength and Conditioning Research* 25(6):1586–1591, 2011.

10. Fasen, J. M., A. M. O'Connor, S. L. Schwartz, J. O. Watson, C. T. Plastaras, C. W. Garvan, C. Bulcao, S. C. Johnson, and V. Akuthota. A randomized controlled trial of hamstring stretching: Comparison of four techniques. *Journal of Strength and Conditioning Research* 23(2):660–667, 2009.

Chapter 6

1. Swain, D.P. and C.A. Brawner. *ACSM'S Resource Manual for Guidelines for Exercise Testing and Prescription.* 7th Ed. Philadelphia: Lippincott, Williams and Wilkins, 2013.

2. Kumanyika, S., and R. Brownson (Ed.). *Handbook of Obesity Prevention: A Resource for Health Professionals.* New York: Springer, 2010.

3. Rosen, L., and E. Rossen. *Obesity 101.* New York: Springer, 2011.

4. Cook, C., and D. Schoeller. Physical activity and weight control. *Current Opinion in Clinical Nutrition and Metabolic Care* 14:419–424, 2011.

5. Flegal, K., B. Kit, H. Orpana, B. Graubard. Association of All-Cause Mortality With Overweight and Obesity Using Standard Body Mass Index Categories. JAMA. 309(1):71–82, 2013.

6. Dubnov-Raz, G., and E. Berry. The dietary treatment of obesity. *Medical Clinics of North America* 95:939–952, 2011.

7. Bouchard, C., S. Blair, and W. Haskell (Eds.). *Physical Activity and Health.* Champaign, IL: Human Kinetics, 2012.

8. Center for Disease Control. Statistics on obesity and overweight. 2014. http://www.cdc.gov/obesity/data/index.html.

9. Congressional Budget Office: Economic and Budget Issue Brief. How does Obesity in Adults Affect Spending on Health Care? *www.CBO.gov.* Sept., 2010.

10. Nguyen, D. and H. Serag. The Epidemiology of Obesity. *Gastroenterology Clinics of North America.* 39(1): 1–7, 2010.

11. Wright, S. and L. Aronne. Causes of obesity. *Abdominal Imaging.* http://link.springer.com/article/10.1007/s00261-012-9862-x#page-2, Mar., 2012.

12. Kohl, H., and T. Murray. *Foundations of Physical Activity and Public Health.* Champaign, IL: Human Kinetics, 2012.

13. U.S. Department of Health and Human Services: National Diabetes Information Clearinghouse. http://diabetes.niddk.nih.gov/dm/a-z.aspx. Oct., 2014.

14. American Psychological Association. Mind/body health: Obesity. http://www.apa.org/helpcenter/obesity.aspx. Jan., 2015.

15. U.S. Department of Health and Human Services: National Heart, Lung, and Blood Institute. What are the health risks of overweight and obesity? http://www.nhlbi.nih.gov/health/health-topics/topics/obe. July, 2012.

16. Howley E., and Thompson D. *Fitness Professional's handbook.* Champaign, IL: Human Kinetics, 2012.

17. Powers, S., and E. Howley. *Exercise Physiology: Theory and Application to Fitness and Performance,* 8th ed. New York: McGraw-Hill, 2012.

18. Lee, S., and D. Gallagher. Assessment methods in body composition. *Current Opinion in Clinical Nutrition and Metabolic Care* 11:566–572, 2008.

19. Dehghan, M., and A. Merchant. Is bioelectrical impedance accurate for use in large epidemiological studies? *Nutrition Journal* 7:26–35, 2008.

20. Rankinen, T., T. Rice, M. Teran-Garcia, D. Rao, and C. Brouchard. FTO genotype is associated with exercise training-induced changes in body composition. *Obesity* 18:322–326, 2010.

21. Pride, A., D. Hey, T. Hagobian, A. McDermott and L. Hall. Weight and Percent Body Fat Increased Significantly over Freshman Year in a Subset of the FLASH College Health Study. *The FASEB Journal.* 27:851.16, 2013.

Chapter 7

1. Byrd, N. What gets measured is more likely to get done. *ACSM's Health and Fitness Journal* 15:26–29, 2011.

2. Fieger, H. *Behavior Change.* New York: Morgan James, 2009.

3. Howley, E., and D. Thompson. *Fitness Professional's Handbook.* Champaign, IL: Human Kinetics, 2012.

4. Baechle, T., and R. Earle. *Essentials of Strength Training and Conditioning.* Champaign, IL: Human Kinetics, 2008.

5. Powers, S., and E. Howley. *Exercise Physiology: Theory and Application to Fitness and Performance,* 9th ed. New York: McGraw Hill, 2015.

6. Earle, R., and T. Baechle. *NSCA's Essentials of Personal Training 2nd Edition.* Champaign, IL: Human Kinetics, 2011.

7. Weiglein, L., Herrick, J., Kirk, S., Kirk, E.P. The 1-Mile Walk Test is a Valid Predictor of VO_2 max and is a Reliable Alternative Fitness Test to the 1.5-Mile Run in US Air Force Males. *Military Medicine,* 176: 669–673, 2011.

8. Plante, T., M. Madden, S. Mann, G. Lee, A. Hardesty, N. Gable, A. Terry, and G. Kaplow. Effects of perceived fitness level of exercise partner on intensity of exertion. *Journal of Social Science* 6: 50–54, 2010.

9. Volpe, S. L. Can dogs help with maintaining motivation? *ACSM's Health and Fitness Journal* 15:36–37, 2011.

10. Kushner, R., D. Blatner, D. Jewell, and K. Rudloff. The PPET Study: people and pets exercising together. *Obesity* 14: 1762–1770, 2006.

11. Pate, R. Overcoming barriers to physical activity: helping youth be more active. *ACSM's Health and Fitness Journal* 15:7–12, 2011.

12. Chaput, J., L. Klingenberg, and A. Sjodin. Do all sedentary activities lead to weight gain: sleep does not. *Current Opinion in Clinical Nutrition and Metabolic Care* 13:601–607, 2010.

13. Walsh, N., M.Gleeson, D. Pyne, D. Nieman, F. Dhabhar, R. Shephard, S. Oliver, S. Bermon, and A. Kajeniene. Position statement. Part 2: Maintaining immune health. *Exercise Immunology Review* 17:64–103, 2011.

14. Bonnet, M. H., and D. L. Arand. Clinical effects of sleep fragmentation versus sleep deprivation. *Sleep Medicine Reviews* 7:297–310, 2003.

15. National Center for Chronic Disease and Health Promotion, Division of Adult and Community Health. Insufficient sleep is a public health epidemic. Centers for Disease Control and Prevention (CDC): http://www.cdc.gov/features/dssleep/ Accessed March 30, 2015.

16. Sharma, S. and M. Kavuru. Sleep and metabolism: An — overview. *International Journal of Endocrinology* Volume 2010: 12 pages, 2010. http://www.hindawi.com/journals/ije/2010/270832/

17. Kokkinos, P. Physical activity, health benefits, and mortality risk. ISRN Cardiology, Volume 2012, Article ID 718789, 14 pages. http://www.ncbi.nlm.nih.gov/pmc/articles/PMC3501820/ Accessed March 20, 2015.

18. Warburton, D., C. Nicol, and S. Bredin. Health benefits of physical activity: The evidence. *Canadian Medical Association Journal* 174:801–809, 2006.

19. Kohl, H., C. Craig, E. Lambert, S. Inoue, J. Alkandari, G. Leetongin, & S. Kahlmeier. The pandemic of physical inactivity: global action for public health. The Lancet. 380 (9838): 294–30, 2012.

20. Evenson, K., D. Buchner, & K. Morland. Objective Measurement of Physical Activity and Sedentary Behavior Among US Adults Aged 60 Years or Older. *Preventing Chronic Disease.* Centers for Disease Control and Prevention. 9: E26, 2012.

21. Hallal, P., L. Andersen, F. Bull, R. Guthold, W. Haskell, U. Ekelund. Global physical activity levels: surveillance progress, pitfalls, and prospects. *The Lancet* 380(9838): 247–257, 2012.

22. Williamson, P. *Exercise for Special Populations.* Philadelphia: Lippincott Williams and Wilkins, 2011.

23. Bain, E., M. Crane, J. Tieu, S. Han, C. Crowther, P. Middleton. Diet and exercise interventions for preventing gestational diabetes mellitus. *The Cochrane Library.* Wiley & Sons, Issue 4, DOI: 10.1002/14651858.CD010443, 2015.

24. American College of Sports Medicine. *ACSM's Guidelines for Exercise Testing and Prescription,* 9th ed. Philadelphia: Lippincott Williams and Wilkins, 2013.

25. Hicks, A., K Ginis, C. Pelletier, D. Ditor, B. Foulon and D. Wolfe. The effects of exercise training on physical capacity, strength, body composition and functional performance among adults with spinal cord injury: a systematic review. *Spinal Cord.* 49:1103–1127, 2011.

26. Babson, K., A. Heinza, G. Ramirezb, M. Puckettb, J. Ironsc, M. Bonn-Millerd, and S. Woodward. The interactive role of

exercise and sleep on veteran recovery from symptoms of PTSD. *Mental Health and Physical Activity*. 8: 15–20, 2015.

27. Rando, T. and H. Chang. Aging, Rejuvenation, and Epigenetic Reprogramming: Resetting the Aging Clock. Cell 148(1–2): 46–57, 2012.

28. Louis, J., C. Hausswirth, C. Easthope, J. Brisswalter. Strength training improves cycling efficiency in master endurance athletes. *European Journal of Applied Physiology*. 112(2):631–640, 2012.

29. Mitchell, W., J.Williams, P. Atherton, M.Larvin, J. Lund, and M.Narici. Sarcopenia, Dynapenia, and the Impact of Advancing Age on Human Skeletal Muscle Size and Strength; a Quantitative Review. Frontiers in Physiology. 3: 260, 2012.

30. Saxon, S., M. Etten, and E. Perkins. Physical Change and Aging; A Guide for the Helping Professions. 6th Ed., New York, Springer Pub., 2012.

31. Chapman, S., S. Aslan, J. Spence, L. DeFina, M. Keebler, N. Didehbani, and H. Lu. Shorter term aerobic exercise improves brain, cognition, and cardiovascular fitness in aging. Frontiers in Aging Neuroscience. 5: 75, 2013.

32. Liberman, D., and A. Cheung. Practical Approach to Osteoporosis Management in the Geriatric Population. *Canadian Geriatric Journal*. 18(1): 29–34, 2015.

Chapter 8

1. Mokdad AH, Marks JS, Stroup DF, Gerberding JL: Actual causes of death in the United States, 2000. *JAMA* 2004, 291(10):1238–1245.

2. Olshansky SJ, Passaro DJ, Hershow RC, Layden J, Carnes BA, Brody J, Hayflick L, Butler RN, Allison DB, Ludwig DS: A potential decline in life expectancy in the United States in the 21st century. *N Engl J Med* 2005, 352(11):1138–1145.

3. Kushi LH, Meyer KA, Jacobs DR, Jr.: Cereals, legumes, and chronic disease risk reduction: evidence from epidemiologic studies. *Am J Clin Nutr* 1999, 70(3 Suppl):451S–458S.

4. Byrd-Bredbenner C, Moe G, Beshgetoor D, Berning J: Wardlaw's Perspectives in Nutrition. New York: McGraw; 2012.

5. Wardlaw G, Smith A: Contemporary Nutrition: A functional approach. New York: McGraw Hill; 2014.

6. Powers SK, Howley ET: Exercise Physiology. New York: McGraw-Hill; 2015.

7. Jeukendrup A: Carbohydrate supplementation during exercise: does it help? How much is too much? *Sports Science Exchange* 2007, 20(3):1–6.

8. Jeukendrup A, Gleeson M: Sport Nutrition. Champaign: Human Kinetics; 2009.

9. Maughan R, Burke L: Nutrition for athletes. In.: International Olympic Committee; 2012.

10. Kenney WL: Dietary water and sodium requirements for active adults. *Sports Science Exchange* 2004, 17(92):1–7.

11. Phillips SM: Protein consumption and reistance exercise: maximizing anabolic potential. *Sports Science Exchange* 2013, 26(107):1–5.

12. van Loon L: Protein ingestion prior to sleep: potential for optimizing post-exercise recovery. *Sports Science Exchange* 2013, 26(117):1–5.

13. van Loon L: Is there a need for protein ingestion during exercise? *Sports Science Exchange* 2013, 26(109):1–6.

14. Powers SK, DeRuisseau KC, Quindry J, Hamilton KL: Dietary antioxidants and exercise. *J Sports Sci* 2004, 22(1):81–94.

15. Powers SK, Sollanek KJ: Endurance exercise and antioxidant supplement: sense or nonsense? Part 1. *Sports Science Exchange* 2014, 27(137):1–4.

16. Powers SK, Sollanek KJ: Endurance exercise and antiodixant supplementation: sense or nonsense?-part 2. *Sports Science Exchange* 2014, 27(138):1–4.

17. Centers for Disease Control. Foodborne illness. http://www.cdc.gov/foodsafety/facts.html 2015.

Chapter 9

1. *Obesity and overweight*. Geneva (Switzerland): World Health Organization; 2014. Available: www.who.int/mediacentre/factsheets/fs311/en.

2. Hu, F. *Obesity Epidemiology*. New York: Oxford University Press, 2008.

3. American Society for Metabolic and Bariatric Surgery. News release: Bariatric Surgical Society Takes on New Name, New Mission and New Surgery. August 22, 2007. http://www.asbs.org/Newsite07/resources/press_release_8202007.pdf.

4. Swain, D.P. (Ed.). *ACSM'S Resource Manual for Guidelines for Exercise Testing and Prescription*. Philadelphia: Wolters Kluwer/Lippincott, Williams and Wilkins, 2013.

5. Poehlman, E. T. A review: exercise and its influence on resting energy metabolism in man. *Medicine and Science in Sports and Exercise* 21:515–525, 1989.

6. Power, M., and J. Schulkin. *The Evolution of Obesity*. Baltimore, MD: John Hopkins University Press. 2009.

7. Melanson, E., P. MacLean, and J. Hill. Exercise improves fat metabolism in muscle but does not increase 24-h fat oxidation. *Exercise and Sport Science Reviews* 37:93–101, 2009.

8. Powers, S., and E. Howley. *Exercise Physiology: Theory and Application to Fitness and Performance*, 9th ed. New York: McGraw-Hill, 2015.

9. van Vliet-Ostaptchouk, J., H. Snieder, and V. Vasiliki. Gene-lifestyle interactions in obesity. *Current Nutrition Reports*. 1: 184–196, 2012.

10. Bell, C., A. J. Walley, and P. Froguel. The genetics of human obesity. *Nature Reviews* 6:221–234, 2005.

11. Yeo, G. Are my genes to blame when my jeans don't fit. *Physiology News* 96: 12–13, 2014.

12. Ismail, L., S. Keating, M. Baker, and N. Johnson. A systematic review and meta-analysis of the effect of aerobic vs. resistance exercise training on visceral fat. *Obesity Reviews* 13:68–91, 2012.

13. Johnson, R., M. Segal, Y. Sautin, T. Nakagawa, D. Feig, D. Kang, M. Gersh, S. Benner, and L. Sanchez-Lozada. Potential role of sugar (fructose) in the epidemic of hypertension, obesity and the metabolic syndrome, diabetes, kidney disease, and cardiovascular disease. *American Journal of Clinical Nutrition* 86:899–906, 2007.

14. Samuel, V. Fructose induced lipogenesis: From sugar to fat to insulin resistance. *Trends in Endocrinology and Metabolism* 22:60–65, 2011.

15. Stanhope, K. Role of fructose-containing sugars in the epidemics of obesity and metabolic syndrome. *Annual Review of Medicine* 63:19.1–19.15, 2012.

16. Wolff, E., and M. Dansinger. Soft drinks and weight gain: How strong is the Link? *Medscape Journal of Medicine* 10:89–97, 2008.

17. Johnson, R. J., and R. Murray. Fructose, exercise, and health. *Current Sports Medicine Reports* 9:253–258, 2010.

18. Onakpoya, I., R. Perry, J. Zhang, and E. Ernst. Efficacy of calcium supplementation for management of overweight and obesity: Systematic review of randomized clinical trials. *Nutrition Reviews* 69:335–343, 2011.

19. Manore, M. Dietary supplements for improving body composition and reducing body weight: Where is the evidence? *International Journal of Sport Nutrition and Exercise Metabolism* 22:139–154, 2012.

20. Jeukendrup, A., and R. Randell. Fat burners: Nutrition supplements that increase fat metabolism. *Obesity Reviews* 12:841–851, 2011.

21. Dansinger, M., J. Gleason, and J. Griffith, H. Selker, and E. Schaefer. Comparison of the Atkins, Ornish, Weight Watchers, and Zone diets for weight loss and heart disease risk reduction. *Journal of American Medical Association* 293:43–53, 2005.

22. Gardner, C., A. Kizzand, S. Alhassan, S. Kim, R. Stafford, R. Balise, H. Kraemer, and A. King. Comparison of the Atkins, Zone, Ornish, and LEARN diets for change in weight and related risk factors among overweight premenopausal women. *Journal of American Medical Association* 297:969–977, 2007.

23. Shai, I., D. Schwarzfuchs, et al. Weight loss with a low carbohydrate, Mediterranean, or low-fat diet. *New England Journal of Medicine* 359:229–241, 2008.

24. Sachs, F., G. Bray, et al. Comparison of weight-loss diets with different compositions of fat, protein, and carbohydrates. *New England Journal of Medicine* 360:859–873, 2009.

25. Broom, D. R., R. Batterham, J. A. King, and D. Stensel. Influence of resistance and aerobic exercise on hunger, circulating levels of acylated ghrelin, and peperide YY in healthy male. *American Journal of Physiology*. 296: R29–R35, 2009.

26. Stensel, D. Exercise, appetite, and appetite-regulating hormones: Implications for food intake and weight control. Annuals Nutrition and Metabolism. 57: 36–42, 2010.

27. Romijn, J., E. Coyle, L. Sidossis, et al. Regulation of endogenous fat and carbohydrate metabolism in relation to exercise and duration. *American Journal of Physiology* 265:E380–E391, 1993.

28. De Feo, D. Is high-intensity exercise better than moderate intensity exercise for weight loss? *Nutrition, metabolism, and cardiovascular diseases* 23:1037–1042, 2013.

29. Forman, E. M., and M. L. Butryn. A new look at the science of weight control: How acceptance and commitment strategies can address the challenge of self-regulation. *Appetite* 84: 171–180, 2015.

30. Steelman, G. and E. Westman (Eds.). Obesity: Evaluation and treatment essentials. *Informa Healthcare*, 2010.

31. Yeomans, M. Alcohol, appetite, and energy balance: Is alcohol intake a risk for obesity? *Physiology of Behavior* 100:82–89, 2010.

32. Sharkey, B., and S. Gaskill. *Fitness and Health*. Champaign, IL: Human Kinetics, 2006.

33. Weight-Control Information Network. *Gastrointestinal Surgery for Severe Obesity*. NIH Publication No. 04-4006. December 2004. http://win.niddk.nih.gov/publications/gastric.htm.

34. Coelho, G., A. Gomes, B. Ribeiro, and E. Soares. Prevention of eating disorders in female athletes. *Open Access Journal of Sports Medicine* 5:105–113, 2014.

Chapter 10

1. American Heart Association. Heart disease and stroke statistics—2015 update. *Circulation* 131:e29–e322, 2015.

2. Trogdon, P., O. Khavjou, J. Butler, K. Dracup, M. Ezekowitz, et al. Forecasting the future of cardiovascular disease in the United States: A policy statement from the American Heart Association. *Circulation* 123:933–944, 2011.

3. Centers for Disease Control and Prevention. Heart Disease and Stroke Prevention: Heart Disease, 2015. http://www.cdc.gov/heartdisease/index.htm

4. Powers, S., and E. Howley. *Exercise Physiology: Theory and Application to Fitness and Performance*, 9th ed. New York: McGraw-Hill, 2015.

5. Mann, D., D. P. Zipes, P. Libby, and R. O. Bonow. Braunwalds's Heart Disease. Elsevier/Saunders, 2014.

6. Rigotti, N.A. and R. C. Pasternak. Cigarette smoking and coronary heart disease: risk and management. *Cardiology Clinical* 14: 51–68, 19996.

7. Tran, D.M. and L. M. Zimmerman. Cardiovascular risk factors in young adults: A literature review. *Journal of Cardiovascular Nuring* 2014.

8. Gordon, B. S. Chen, and J. L. Durstine. The effects of exercise training on the traditional lipid profile and beyond. *Current Sports Medicine Reports* 13:253–259, 2014.

9. Superko, H.R., L. Pendyala, P. Williams, K. Momary, S. B. King, and B.C. Garrett. High density lipoprotein subclasses and their relationship to cardiovascular disease. *Journal of Clinical Lipidology* 6: 496–523, 2012.

10. Pescatello, L.S. (Editor) ACSM's Guidelines for Exercise Testing and Prescription. 9th edition, Wolters Kluwer/ Lippincott Williams and Williams, 2013.

11. Zalesin, K., B. Franklin, W. Miller, E. Peterson, and P. McCullough. Impact of obesity on cardiovascular disease. *Medical Clinics of North America* 95:919–937, 2011.

12. Sattelmair, J., J. Pertman, E. L. Ding, H.W. Kohl, W. Haskell, and I. Lee. Dose-response between physical activity and risk of coronary heart disease. *Circulation* 124:789–795, 2011.

13. Paffenbarger, R. S., R. T. Hyde, A. L. Wing, and C. C. Hsieh. Physical activity, all-cause mortality of college alumni. *New England Journal of Medicine* 314:605 613, 1986.

14. Arts, J. M. L. Fernandez, and I. E. Lofgren. Coronary heart disease risk factors in college students. *Advances in Nutrition* 5:177–187, 2014.

15. Gotto, A. Statins: Powerful drugs for lowering cholesterol. *Circulation* 105:1514–1516, 2002.

16. Bybee, K., J. Lee, and J. O'Keefe. Cumulative clinical trial data on atorvastatin for reducing cardiovascular events: The clinical impact of atorvastatin. *Current Medical Research Opinion* 24:1217–1229, 2008.

17. Franklin, B. Aspirin for the primary prevention of cardiovascular events: Considerations regarding the risk/benefit. *Physician and Sports Medicine* 38:158–161, 2010.

18. Thompson, P. D., et al. Exercise and acute cardiovascular events placing the risks into perspective: A scientific statement from the American Heart Association Council on Nutrition, Physical Activity, and Metabolism and Council on Clinical Cardiology. *Circulation* 115:2358–2368. 2007.

Chapter 11

1. Canon, W. *The Wisdom of the Body*. New York: Norton Publishing, 1963.

2. Selye, H. *The Stress of Life*, rev. ed. New York: McGraw-Hill, 1978.

3. Friedman, M., and R. Rosenman. Type A behavior pattern: Its association with coronary heart disease. *Annals of Clinical Research* 3(6):300–312, 1971.

4. Knox, S., G. Wiedner, A. Adelman, S. Stoney, and R. Ellison. Hostility and physiological risk in the National Heart, Lung, and Blood Institute Family Heart Study. *Archives of Internal Medicine* 164(22): 2442–2448, 2004.

5. Sher, L. Type D personality: the heart, stress, and cortisol. *QJ Med* 98: 323–329, 2005.

6. Denollet, J. Type D Personality. *Encyclopedia of Behavioral Medicine*, 2014–2018, 2013.

7. Kessler, R., W. Chui, O. Demler, K. Merikangas, and E. Walters. Prevalence, severity, and comorbidity of 12-month DSM-IV disorders in the National Comorbidity Survey Replication Study. *Archives of General Psychiatry* 62:590–592, 2005.

8. American Psychological Association (2013). How Does Stress Affect Us? *Psych Central*. Retrieved on April 29, 2015, from http://psychcentral.com/lib/how-does-stress-affect-us/0001130

9. Baum, A. & R. Contrada. The Handbook of Stress Science: Biology, Psychology, and Health. New York: Springer Publishing Company, 2010.

10. Margen, S., et al. (Eds.). *The Wellness Encyclopedia*. Boston: Houghton Mifflin, 1992.

11. Carlson N. Physiology of behavior, 8th ed. New York: Allyn & Bacon, 2004.

12. McEwen, B. Allostasis and allostatic load: Implications for neuropsychopharmacology. *Neuropsychopharmacology* 22:108–124, 2000.

13. Abercrombie, H., et. al. Flattened cortisol rhythms in metastatic breast cancer patients. *Psychoneuroendocrinology* 29(8):1082–1092, 2004.

14. Holroyd, K., et al. Management of chronic tension-type headache with tricyclic antidepressant medication, stress management therapy, and their combination: A randomized trial. *Journal of the American Medical Association* 285(17):2208–2215, 2001.

15. Howley, E., and B. Franks. *The Fitness Professional's Handbook*, 5th ed. Champaign, IL: Human Kinetics, 2007.

16. Salmon, P. Effects of physical exercise on anxiety, depression, and sensitivity to stress: A unifying theory. *Clinical Psychology Review* 21 (1): 33–61, 2001.

17. Jahnke, R.,L Larkey,, C. Rogers,, J. Etiner,.& F. Lin. A comprehensive review of health benefits of Qigong and Tai Chi. *American Journal of Health Promotion* 24 (6): e1–e25, 2011.

18. Rocha, K., A. Ribeiro, K. Rocha, F. Albuquerque, S. Ribeiro, and R. H Silva. Improvement in physiological and psychological parameters after 6 months of yoga practice. *Consciousness and Cognition*. [Epub ahead of print] 2012. http://www.ncbi.nlm.nih.gov/pubmed/22342535.

19. Netz, Y., M. Wu, B. Becker & G. Tenenbaum. Physical activity and psychological well-being in advanced age: A meta-analysis of intervention studies. *Psychology and Aging* 20 (2): 272–284, (2005).

20. Blumenthal, J., A. Sherwood, M. Babyak, et al. Effects of exercise and stress management training on markers of cardiovascular risk in patients with ischemic heart disease. JAMA 293 (13): 1626-1634, 2005.

21. Dishman, R. P. O'Connor. Lessons in exercise neurobiology: the case of endorphins. *Mental Health and Physical Activity* 2:4–9, 2009.

Chapter 12

1. Radomski, M. Sports injuries. *Wellness Options* 6:52, 2003.

2. Centers for Disease Control, National Center for Injury Prevention and Control. WISQARS Leading Causes of Death Reports, National and Regional, 2013. http://www.cdc.gov/injury/.

3. Nelson, N. G., C. L. Collins, R. D. Comstock, and L. B. McKenzie. Exertional heat-related injuries treated in emergency departments in the U.S., 1997–2006. *American Journal of Preventive Medicine.* 40(1):54–60, 2011.

4. Nichols, A. Heat-related illness in sports and exercise. Current Reviews in Musculoskeletal Medicine. 7(4): 355–365, 2014.

5. McArdle, W. D., F. I. Katch, and V. L. Katch. *Exercise Physiology: Nutrition, Energy, and Human Performance*, 8th ed. Philadelphia: Lippincott Williams and Wilkins, 2014.

6. American College of Sports Medicine. Position stand: Exercise and fluid replacement. Medicine and Science in Sports and Exercise. 39(2):377–390, 2007.

7. American College of Sports Medicine. Position stand: Prevention of cold injuries during exercise. *Medicine and Science in Sports and Exercise* 38(11):2012–2029, 2006.

8. Giles L. and, M. Koehle. The health effects of exercising in air pollution. *Sports Medicine.* 44(2):223–49, 2014.

9. Tenforde, A. S., L. C. Sayres, M. L. McCurdy, H. Collado, K. L. Sainani, and M. Fredericson. Overuse injuries in high school runners: Lifetime prevalence and prevention strategies. *Physical Medicine and Rehabilitation* 3(2):125–131, 2011.

10. Steinberg, N., I. Siev-Ner, S. Peleg, G. Dar, Y. Masharawi, A. Zeev, and I. Hershkovitz. Extrinsic and intrinsic risk factors associated with injuries in young dancers aged 8–16 years. *Journal of Sports Sciences*. 30(5):485–495, 2012.

11. Dvorak, H., C. Kujat, and J. Brumitt. Effect of therapeutic exercise versus manual therapy on athletes with chronic low back pain. *Journal of Sport Rehabilitation* 20(4):494–504, 2011.

12. Powers, S., and E. Howley. *Exercise Physiology: Theory and Application to Fitness and Performance*, 9th ed. New York: McGraw-Hill, 2015.

13. Lewis, P. B., D. Ruby, and C. A. Bush-Joseph. Muscle soreness and delayed-onset muscle soreness. *Clinics in Sports Medicine.* 31(2):255–262, 2012.

14. Prentice, W. *Therapeutic Modalities: For Sports Medicine and Athletic Training*. New York: McGraw-Hill, 2009.

15. Harrast, M. A., and D. Colonno. Stress fractures in runners. *Clinics in Sports Medicine* 29(3):399–416, 2010.

16. Denegar, C. R., E. Saliba, and S. F. Saliba. *Therapeutic Modalities for Musculoskeletal Injuries*. Champaign, IL: Human Kinetics, 2009.

17. Safe Kids USA. *Report to the Nation: Trends in Unintentional Childhood Injury Mortality and Parental Views on Child Safety*. Washington, DC: Safe Kids Worldwide, 2008.

18. National Center for Injury Prevention and Control. *CDC Injury Fact Book*. Atlanta, GA: Centers for Disease Control and Prevention, 2009.

19. American Academy of Pediatrics. Syrup of Ipecac Is No Longer Recommended. http://www.healthychildren.org.

20. Mayo Clinic. Severe Bleeding: First Aid. http://www.mayoclinic.com/health/first-aid-severe-bleeding/FA00038.

Chapter 13

1. American Cancer Society. Cancer Facts and Figures 2015. Atlanta: American Cancer Society, 2015.

2. Siegel, R., J. Ma, Z. Zou, and A. Jemal. Cancer statistics, 2014. Cancer Journal for Clinicians 64:9–29, 2014.

3. American Institute for Cancer Research. *Diet and Cancer*. http://www.aicr.org/reduce-your-cancer-risk/diet.

4. Kumar, V., A. Abbas, and J. C. Aster. *Robbins and Cotran Pathologic Basis of Disease*. Philadelphia: Elsevier/Saunders, 2014.

5. Niederhuber, J. E., J. Armitage, J. Doroshow, M. Kastan, and J. Tepper. Abeloff's Clinical Oncology. 5th edition, Philadelphia: Elsevier/Saunders, 2013.

6. Neuhouser, M. L. Reivew: Dietary flavonoids and cancer risk: evidence from human population studies. *Nutrition and Cancer*. 50:1–7, 2004.

7. Howell, A., A. Anderson, R. Clarke, S. Duffy, D. Evans, M. Garcia-Closas, A. Gescher, T. Key. J. Saxton, and M. Harvie. Risk determination and prevention of breast cancer. *Breast Cancer Research*. 16:1–19, 2014.

8. Hanau, C., D. Morre, and D. Morre. Cancer prevention trial of a synergistic mixture of green teac concentrate plus capsicum in a random population of subjects 40–84. *Clinical Proteomics*. 11: 1–11, 2014.

9. Centers for Disease Control. Gynecologic Cancers: What should I know about screening? http://www.cdc.gov/cancer/cervical/basic_info/screening.htm

10. Shiovitz, S. and L. Korde. Genetics of breast cancer: a topic in evolution. *Annuals of Oncology*. 2015. Epub-ahead of publication.

11. Mocellin, S., D. Verdi, K. Pooley, and D. Nitti. Genetic variation and gastric cancer risk: a field synopsis and meta analysis. Gut. 2015 epubl ahead of print.

12. Bishop, K. and L. Ferguson. The interaction between epigenetics, nutrition, and the development of cancer. *Nutrients*. 7:922–947, 2015.

13. Sandu, M., I. White, and K. McPherson. Systematic review of prospective cohort studies on meat consumption and colorectal cancer risk: A meta-analytical approach. *Cancer, Epidemiology, Biomarkers and Prevention* 10:439–496, 2001.

14. Norat, T., and E. Roboli. Meat consumption and colorectal cancer: A review of epidemiological evidence. *Nutritional Reviews* 59:37–47, 2001.

15. Brown, L. M. Epidemiology of alcohol-associated cancers. *Alcohol* 35:161–168, 2005.

16. McPherson, K. Moderate alcohol consumption and cancer. *Annals of Epidemiology* 17:S46–S48, 2007.

17. Roswall, N. and E. Weiderpass. Alchohol as a risk factor for cancer: Existing evidence in a global perspective. *Journal of preventive medicine and public health*. 48:1–9, 2015.

18. Bernhard, D., C. Moser, A. Backovic, and G. Wick. Cigarette smoke—an aging accelerator? *Experimental Gerontology* 42:160–165, 2007.

19. Edwards, R. The problem of tobacco smoking. *British Medical Journal* 328:217–219, 2004.

20. Westmaas, J., and T. Brandon. Reducing risk in smokers. *Current Opinion in Pulmonary Medicine* 10:284–288, 2004.

21. Ungefroren, H., F. Gieseler, S. Fliedner, and H. Lehnert. Obesity and cancer. *Hormone molecular biology and clinical investigation*. 2015. Epub before print

22. Kruk, J. and U. Czerniak. Physical activity and its relation to cancer risk: updating the evidence. *Asian Pacific Journal of Cancer prevention*. 14:3993–4003, 2013.

23. Keimling, M. G. Behrens, D. Schmid, C. Jochem, and M. Leitzmann. The association between physical activity and bladder cancer: systematic review and meta-analysis. *British Cancer Journal* 110:1862–1870.

24. Siegel, R., and Naishadham, D. Cancer statistics for Hispanics/Latinos, *A Cancer Journal for Clinicians* 62(5): 279–348, 2012.

25. Nole, G., and A. Johnson. An analysis of cumulative lifetime solar ultraviolet radiation exposure and the benefits of daily sun protection. *Dermatology Therapy* 17:57–62, 2004.

Chapter 14

1. Center for HIV/AIDS, Viral Hepatitis, STD, and TB Prevention. Reported STDs in the United States. http://www.cdc.gov/nchhstp/newsroom/docs/std-trends-508.pdf December, 2014.

2. Centers for Disease Control and Prevention. Sexually transmitted disease Surveillance 2013. Atlanta: U.S. Department of Health and Human Services, 2014.

3. Centers for Disease Control and Prevention. CDC Fact Sheet. Incidence, prevalence, and cost of sexually transmitted infections in the United States. February 2013.

4. Kaiser Family Foundation. The HIV/AIDS Epidemic in the United States. 2014.

5. World Health Organization. HIV/AIDS Fact Sheet, November 2014.

6. UNAIDS. *UNAIDS 2010 Report on the Global AIDS Epidemic*. Geneva, Switzerland: UNAIDS, 2010.

7. Watanabe, M. AIDS: 20 years later. *The Scientist* 15:1, 2001.

8. V., A. Abbas, and J. C. Aster. *Robbins and Cotran Pathologic Basis of Disease*. Philadelphia: Elsevier/ Saunders, 2014.

9. Anderson, J., R. Fromentin, G. Corbelli, L. Ostergaard, and A. Ross. Progress toward an HIV Cure: Update from the 2014 International AIDS Society Symposium. Aids Research and Human Retroviruses. 31:36–44, 2015.

10. Centers for Disease Control and Prevention. Human papillomavirus. 2015, http://www.cdc.gov/hpv.

11. Centers for Disease Control and Prevention. Genital herpes fact sheet. Updated January 2012. http://www.cdc.gov/std/herpes/STDFact-Herpes.htm

12. Healthy People 2020. Sexually Transmitted Diseases. http://www.healthypeople.gov/2020/topicsobjectives2020/overview.aspx? topicid=37.

13. Centers for Disease Control and Prevention. Chlamydia fact sheet. 2015. http://www.cdc.gov/std/chlamydia/STDFact-Chlamydia.htm.

14. Centers for Disease Control and Prevention. Gonorrhea fact sheet. 2015. http://www.cdc.gov/std/gonorrhea/STDFact-gonorrhea.htm.

15. Centers for Disease Control and Prevention. Trichomoniasis fact sheet. 2015. http://www.cdc.gov/std/trichomonas/STDFact-Trichomoniasis.htm.

16. American Public Health Association. Condoms proved effective against HIV transmission. *The Nation's Health* 4, September 2001.

17. Centers for Disease Control and Prevention. Sexually transmitted diseases treatment guidelines. *Morbidity and Mortality Weekly Report* 51:1–80, 2002.

Chapter 15

1. National Institute on Drug Abuse. Drug facts: Understanding drug abuse and addiction. http://www.drugabuse.gov/publications/drugfacts/understanding-drug-abuse-addiction. 2015.

2. National Institute of Mental Health. *The Numbers Count: Mental Disorders in America.* Fact Sheet. http://www.nimh.nih.gov/publicat/numbers.cfm#MajorDepressive. 2015.

3. Subramaniam, M., Lerner, C., I. Sundar, R. Watson, A. Elder, R. Jones, D. Done, R. Kurtzman, D. Ossip, R. Robinson, S. McIntosh, and I. Rahman. Environmental health hazards of e-cigarettes and their components: oxidants and copper in e-cigarette aerosols. *Environmental Pollutants.* 198: 100–107, 2014.

4. Callahan-Lyon, P. Electronic cigarettes: human health effects. *Tobacco Control.* 23: ii36–ii40, 2014.

5. Wu, Q., D. Jiang, M. Minor, and H. Chu. Electronic cigarette liquid increases inflammation and virus infection in primary human airway epithelial cells. Plos One. 9:e108342, 2014.

6. Callahan-Lyon, P. Electronic cigarettes: human health effects. *Tobacco Control.* 23: ii36–ii40, 2014.

7. WebMD: Cocaine use and its effects. June 2012. http://www.webmd.com/mental-health/cocaine-use-and-its-effects.

8. Cannon, C., and M. Bseikri. Is dopamine required for natural reward? *Physiology of Behavior* 81:741–748, 2004.

9. National Institute on Drug Abuse. DrugFacts: Understanding drug abuse and addiction. Revised March 2011. http://www.drugabuse.gov/publications/drugfacts/understanding-drug-abuse-addiction.

10. Substance Abuse and Mental Health Services Administration. *Results from the 2010 National Survey on Drug Use and Health: Mental Health Findings.* NSDUH Series H-42, HHS Publication No. (SMA) 11–4667. Rockville, MD: Substance Abuse and Mental Health Services Administration, 2012.

11. Liska, K. *Drugs and the Human Body.* Englewood Cliffs, NJ: Prentice Hall, 2008.

12. Geller T., L. Loftis, and D. Brink. Cerebellar infarction in adolescent males associated with acute marijuana use. *Pediatrics* 113:e365–370, 2004.

13. Office of National Drug Control Policy. *National Drug Control Strategy Data Supplement 2014.* Washington, DC: Office of National Drug Control Policy, 2014.

14. White, S., and C. Lambe. The pathophysiology of cocaine abuse. *Journal of Clinical Forensic Medicine* 10:27–39, 2003.

15. Panlilo, L.V. and S. R. Goldberg. Cannainoid abuse and addiction:Clinical and preclinical findings. *Clinical Pharmacology and Therapeutics.* doi: 10.1002/cpt.118,. 2015.

16. Alcohol-related impact. Atlanta, GA. Centers for Disease Control. 2015.

17. Vital and Health Statistics. Series 10, number 260. Atlanta, GA. Centers for Disease Control. 2014.

18. The Health Consequences of Smoking-50 years of progress. Office of Surgeon General. US Department of Health and Human Services. Centers for Disease Control, Atlanta, GA. 2014.

19. National Institute on Drug Abuse. Drug Facts: Cigarettes and other tobacco products. Revised August 2010. http://www.drugabuse.gov/publications/drugfacts/cigarettes-other-tobacco-products.

20. Centers for Disease Control and Prevention. Epidemiologic notes and reports of illnesses possibly associated with smoking clove cigarettes. *Morbidity and Mortality Weekly Report,* May 1985. http://www.cdc.gov/mmwr.

21. U.S. Department of Health and Human Services. *The health consequences of involuntary exposure to tobacco smoke: A report of the Surgeon General.* Atlanta, GA: U.S. Department of Health and Human Services, 2006. http://www.surgeongeneral.gov/library/reports/secondhandsmoke.

22. American Lung Association. Secondhand smoke. Accessed 2012. http://www.lung.org/stop-smoking/about-smoking/health-effects/secondhand-smoke.html.

23. Centers for Disease Control and Prevention, National Center for Chronic Disease Prevention and Health Promotion. Smoking and tobacco use: Fact sheets. 2009. http://www.cdc.gov/tobacco/data_statistics/fact_sheets/index.htm.

24. Sydor, A. and R. Brown. Molecular Neuropharmacology: A Foundation for Clinical Neuroscience. New York. McGraw-Hill, 2009.

25. Nawrot, P., S. Jordan, J. Eastwood, J. Rotstein, A. Hugenholtz, and M. Feeley. Effects of caffeine on human health. *Food Additives and Contamination* 20:1–30, 2003.

26. National Institute on Drug Abuse. Research Report Series: Anabolic steroid abuse. September 2006. http://www.drugabuse.gov/ResearchReports/Steroids.

27. Medline Plus. Many teen girls use steroids. June 2007. http://www.nlm.nih.gov/medlineplus.

28. Glantz, M., and C. Hartel (Eds.). *Drug Abuse: Origins and Interventions.* Washington, DC: APA Publications, 1999.

29. Maughan, R. Dietary supplements. *Journal of Sports Sciences* 22:95–113, 2004.

30. Powers, S., and S. Dodd. Caffeine and endurance performance: A review. *Sports Medicine* 2:165–174, 1985.

31. Dodd, S., R. Herb, and S. Powers. Caffeine and exercise performance: An update. *Sports Medicine* 15:14–23, 1993.

photo credits

Front matter

v:Kurhan/Shutterstock; vi: F1 Online/Glow Images; vii: Yuri Arcurs/Shutterstock; viii: Pearson Education; ix: Pearson Education; x: Hannamariah/Shutterstock; xi: Blend Images/Alamy Stock Photo; xii: Mike Kemp/Blend Images/Getty Images; xiii: koh sze kiat/Shutterstock; xiv: vario images GmbH & Co.KG/Alamy; xv: Radius Images/Alamy Stock Photo; xvi: Pearson Education

Chapter 1

CO: Val Loh/Getty Images; P. 2: Giantstep Inc/Getty Images; p. 3: DAJ/Getty Images; p. 5: Andy Dean/Fotolia; p. 8: Mixa/Getty Images; p. 9: Monkey Business Images/Shutterstock; p. 10: Top left: H. Mark Weidman Photography/Alamy; p. 10: Bottom: Mark Dadswell/Getty Images; p. 12: Mark Dadswell/Getty Images; p. 16: Stephen Bonk/Fotolia

Chapter 2

CO: meskolo/Fotolia; p. 36: Top right: meskolo/Fotolia; p. 36: Second: JGI/Getty Images; p. 36: Third: Blue Jean Images/Glow Images; p. 36: Fourth: Prudkov/Shutterstock; p. 37: Kurhan/Shutterstock; p. 38: Top left: Kurhan/Shutterstock; p. 38: Bottom right: Dny3d/Shutterstock; p. 38: Bottom left: Alamy; p. 39: Shutterstock; p. 41: Top left: Comstock/Getty Images; p. 41: Top right: Robert Tirey/Alamy; p. 50: Bubbles Photolibrary/Alamy

Chapter 3

CO: Aksonov/Getty Images; p. 54: Paul Matthew Photography/Shutterstcok; p. 56: Top left: Pearson Education; p. 56: Top right: Pearson Education; p. 61: Left: Vasko Miokovic Photography/Getty Images; p. 61: right: F1 Online/Glow Images; p. 64: Jaimie Duplass/Shutterstock; p. 68: babimu/Fotolia; p. 70: David Sacks/Getty Images; p. 80: Pearson Education

Chapter 4

CO: Mike Kemp/Getty Images; p. 93: Andi Berger/Shutterstock; p. 97: Marekuliasz/Shutterstock; p. 100: Pressmaster/Fotolia; p. 101: Yuri Arcurs/Shutterstock; p. 104: Top left: Pearson Education; p. 104: Top right: Pearson Education; p. 104: Bottom left: Pearson Education; p. 104: Bottom right: Pearson Education; p. 105: Top left: Pearson Education; p. 105: Top right: Pearson Education; p. 105: Bottom right: Pearson Education; p. 105: Bottom left: Pearson Education; p. 106: Top left: Pearson Education; p. 106: Top right: Pearson Education; p. 106: Bottom left: Pearson Education; p. 106: Bottom right: Pearson Education; p. 107: Top left: Pearson Education; p. 107: Top right: Pearson Education; p. 107: Bottom left: Pearson Education; p. 107: Bottom right: Pearson Education; p. 108: Top left: Pearson Education; p. 108: Top right: Pearson Education; p. 108: Bottom left: Pearson Education; p. 108: Bottom right: Pearson Education; p. 109: Top left: Pearson Education; p. 109: Top right: Pearson Education; p. 109: Bottom left: Pearson Education; p. 109: Bottom right: Pearson Education; p. 110: Top left: Pearson Education; p. 110: Top right: Pearson Education; p. 114: Top left: Pearson Education; p. 114: Top right: Pearson Education; p. 114: Bottom left: Pearson Education; p. 114: Bottom right: Pearson Education; p. 121: Top left: Pearson Education; p. 121: Top right: Pearson Education; p. 121: Bottom left: Pearson Education; p. 121: Bottom right: Pearson Education; p. 122: Top left: Pearson Education; p. 122: Top right: Pearson Education; p. 124: Pearson Education

Chapter 5

CO: andresr/Getty Images; p. 130: Top: Spike Mafford/Getty Images; p. 130: Bottom: Anna Furman/Shutterstock; p. 132: Koh sze kiat/Shutterstock; p. 134: Top: Pearson Education; p. 134: Bottom: Pearson Education; p. 137: Top left: Pearson Education; p. 137: Top middle: Pearson Education; p. 137: Top right: Pearson Education; p. 137: Bottom: Pearson Education; p. 138: Top: Pearson Education; p. 138: Bottom: Pearson Education; p. 139: Top: Pearson Education; p. 139: Bottom: Pearson Education; p. 140: Top: Pearson Education; p. 140: Middle: Pearson Education; p. 140: Bottom: Pearson Education; p. 141: Top: Pearson Education; p. 141: Bottom: Pearson Education; p. 142: Top: Pearson Education; p. 142: Bottom: Pearson Education; p. 143: Top left: Pearson Education; p. 143: Top right: Pearson Education; p. 143: Bottom left: Pearson Education; p. 143: Bottom right: Pearson Education; p. 144: Top left: Pearson Education; p. 144: Top right: Pearson Education; p. 144: Bottom left: Pearson Education; p. 144: Bottom right: Pearson Education; p. 145: Top left: Pearson Education; p. 145: Top right: Pearson Education; p. 145: Middle left: Pearson Education; p. 145: Middle right: Pearson Education; p. 145: Bottom right: Pearson Education; p. 150: Top: Pearson Education; p. 150: Bottom: Pearson Education

Chapter 6

CO: Christopher Futcher/Getty Images; p. 156: Gregg Adams/Getty Images; p. 158: Top left: Mike Brinson/Getty Images; p. 158: Top right: Jeff Greenberg/PhotoEdit, Inc.; p. 158: Bottom: Tom Mc Nemar/123RF; p. 161: Carolyn Franks/123RF; p. 163: David Gray/Reuters/Landov; p. 167: Right: The Fitness Institute of Texas; p. 167: Left: David Madison/Getty Images; p. 168: David Cooper/The Toronto Star/ZUMAPRESS/Newscom; p. 173: Top left: Pearson Education; p. 173: Top middle: Pearson Education; p. 173: Top right: Pearson Education; p. 173: Bottom left: Pearson Education; p. 173: Bottom middle: Pearson Education; p. 173: Bottom right: Pearson Education; p. 177: left: Pearson Education; p. 177: right: Pearson Education

Chapter 7

CO: SelectStock/Getty Images; p. 187: Tyler Olson/Shutterstock; p. 190: Leland Bobbe/Getty Images; p. 191: Henry Georgi/Getty Images; p.192: Steven Peters/Getty Images; p. 193: Photodisc/Getty Images; p. 196: Top: Betsie Van Der Meer/Getty Images; p. 196: Bottom: Image Source/Getty Images

Chapter 8

CO: michaeljung/Fotolia; p. 213: Hannamariah/Shutterstock; p. 215: lunamarina/Fotolia; p. 218: Yuri Arcurs/Shutterstock; p. 220: Top left: Silkstock/Fotolia; p. 220: Middle left: VikaRayu/Shutterstock; p. 220: Middle right: vitor costa/Shutterstock; p. 220: Bottom left: Ruslan Kuzmenkov/Shutterstock; p. 221: Top left: Norman Chan/Shutterstock; p. 221: Middle left: archana bhartia/Shutterstock; p. 221: Middle right: Barbro Bergfeldt/Shutterstock; p. 221: Bottom right: Alex Staroseltsev/Shutterstock; P. 222: Image Source/Alamy; P. 224 Left: bogonet/Fotolia; p. 224: Right: Viktor1/Shutterstock; p. 225: USDA ChooseMyPlate.gov; p. 229: sai/Fotolia; p. 234: Pearson Education; p. 237: Pascal Broze/AGE footstock; p. 239: Keith Brofsky/Getty Images; p. 240: Alexander Hoffmann/Shutterstock; p. 241 Left: USDA; p. 241 Right: US Food and Drug Administration

glossary

A

1.5-mile run test One of the simplest and most accurate assessments of cardiorespiratory fitness.

accident Event that results in unintended injury, death, or property damage; refers to the event itself, not to its consequences.

acclimatize To undergo physiological adaptations that help the body adjust to environmental extremes.

acquired immunodeficiency syndrome (AIDS) Fatal disease caused by the human immunodeficiency virus (HIV).

acute muscle soreness Muscle discomfort or pain that develops during or immediately following an exercise session that has been too long or too intense.

adaptations Semi permanent changes that occur over time with regular exercise. Adaptations can be reversed when a regular exercise program is stopped for an extended period of time.

adapted sports Sports played solely by people with a disability; also known as *adaptive sports*.

addiction Habitual psychological and physical dependence on a substance or behavior.

adenosine triphosphate (ATP) A high-energy compound that is synthesized and stored in small quantities in muscle and other cells. The breakdown of ATP results in a release of energy that can be used to fuel muscular contraction.

adipose tissue Tissue where fat is stored in the body.

aerobic With oxygen; in cells, pertains to biochemical pathways that use oxygen to produce energy.

aerobic exercise Forms of exercise that primarily use the aerobic energy system and that are designed to improve cardiorespiratory fitness.

air displacement Technique used to assess body composition by estimating body volume based on air displaced when a person sits in a chamber.

alcoholism Disease characterized by an addiction to alcohol and an inability to limit the amount of drinking despite adverse consequences.

allostasis The ability to maintain homeostasis through change.

allostatic load A continual stress level that causes the inability to respond appropriately to stress; leads to compromised health.

alveoli Tiny air sacs in the lungs that are the site of gas exchange.

amino acids The building blocks of protein; 20 different amino acids can be linked in various combinations to create different proteins.

anabolic steroids Synthetic hormones related to the male sex hormone testosterone.

anaerobic Without oxygen; in cells, pertains to biochemical pathways that do not require oxygen to produce energy.

android pattern Pattern of fat distribution characterized by fat stored in the abdominal region; more common in men.

anemia Deficiency of red blood cells and/or hemoglobin that results in decreased oxygen-carrying capacity of the blood.

anorexia nervosa Eating disorder in which a person severely restricts caloric intake because of an intense fear of gaining weight.

antagonist The muscle on the opposite side of a joint.

antioxidants Molecules that neutralize free radicals, preventing them from causing damage to cells.

arrhythmia Irregular heartbeat.

arteries Blood vessels that carry blood away from the heart.

arteriosclerosis Group of diseases characterized by a narrowing, or "hardening," of the arteries.

atherosclerosis Type of arteriosclerosis that results in arterial blockage due to buildup of a fatty deposit (*atherosclerotic plaque*) inside the blood vessel.

autonomic nervous system Branch of the nervous system that controls basic body functions that do not require conscious thought; consists of the parasympathetic and sympathetic branches.

B

bacteria Microorganisms that can cause infectious diseases. STIs caused by bacteria can be cured with antibiotics.

ballistic stretching Type of stretch that involves sudden and forceful bouncing to stretch the muscles.

benign tumor Tumor made up of noncancerous cells.

binge drinking Drinking 5 or more drinks (for men) or 4 or more drinks (for women) within a 2-hour period.

binge eating disorder A compulsive need to gorge on food without purging.

bioelectrical impedance analysis (BIA) Method of assessing body composition by running a low-level electrical current through the body.

biopsy Surgical removal of a tissue sample for laboratory analysis.

blood alcohol concentration (BAC) The concentration of alcohol in the blood measured as a percentage by mass, by mass per volume, or a combination of both. A BAC of 0.20% can mean 2 grams of alcohol per 1000 grams of an individual's blood, or it can mean 0.2 gram of alcohol per 100 milliliters of blood.

body composition The relative amounts of fat and fat-free mass in the body.

body composition The relative amounts of fat and fat-free tissue (muscle, organs, bone) found in the body.

body mass index (BMI) Ratio of body weight (kg) divided by height squared (m2) used to determine whether a person is at a healthy body weight; BMI is related to the percentage of body fat.

Borg Rating of Perceived Exertion (RPE) A subjective way of estimating exercise intensity based on a scale of 6 to 20.

bulimia nervosa Eating disorder that involves overeating (binge eating) followed by vomiting (purging).

burnout Loss of physical, emotional, and mental energy.

C

caffeine Stimulant found in coffee, tea, chocolate, and other foods and beverages.

cancer Disease that involves the uncontrolled growth and spread of abnormal cells; there are more than 100 types that can affect almost every body tissue.

capillaries Thin-walled vessels that permit the exchange of gases (oxygen and carbon dioxide) and nutrients between the blood and tissues.

carbohydrate Macronutrient that is a key energy source.

carbon monoxide Gas produced during the burning of fossil fuels such as gasoline and coal; also present in cigarette smoke.

carcinogen Cancer-causing agent; includes radiation, chemicals, drugs, and other toxic substances.

cardiac output The amount of blood the heart pumps per minute.

cardiorespiratory endurance Measure of the heart's ability to pump oxygen-rich blood to the working muscles during exercise and of the muscles' ability to take up and use the oxygen.

cardiorespiratory endurance The ability to perform aerobic exercises for a prolonged period of time.

cardiovascular disease (CVD) Any disease that affects the heart or blood vessels.

cardiovascular disease (CVD) Disease of the heart and blood vessels.

cartilage Tough connective tissue that forms a pad on the end of long bones such as the femur, tibia, and humerus. Cartilage acts as a shock absorber to cushion the weight of one bone on another and to provide protection from the friction due to joint movement.

chancre A sore that appears at the site of infection in primary-stage syphilis.

chemical dependence Physical and psychological habituation to a substance, such as alcohol or drugs.

chlamydia The most common sexually transmitted infection among heterosexuals in the United States; caused by a bacterial infection within the reproductive organs.

Cholesterol A lipid that is necessary for cell and hormone synthesis. Found naturally in animal foods, but made in adequate amounts in the body.

cocaine Powerful stimulant derived from the leaves of the South American coca plant.

complete proteins Proteins containing all the essential amino acids.

complex carbohydrates Long chains of sugar units linked together to form glycogen, starch, or fiber.

concentric muscle action Action in which the muscle develops tension as it shortens against resistance and/or gravity. Also called positive work.

convection Heat loss by the movement of air or water over the surface of the body.

cool-down A 5- to 15-minute period of low-intensity exercise that immediately follows the primary conditioning period.

coronary heart disease (CHD) Disease that results from atherosclerotic plaque blocking one or more coronary arteries (blood vessels supplying the heart); also called *coronary artery disease.*

cortisol Hormone secreted by the outer layer (cortex) of the adrenal gland.

creeping obesity A slow increase in body weight and percentage of body fat over several years.

cross training The use of a variety of activities for training the cardiorespiratory system.

cryokinetics Rehabilitation technique that incorporates alternating periods of treatment using ice, exercise, and rest.

curl-up test Test used to evaluate abdominal muscle endurance.

cycle ergometer A stationary exercise cycle that provides pedaling resistance so the amount of work can be measured.

D

Daily Values Standard values for nutrient needs used as a reference on food labels; based on a 2,000-calorie/day diet.

dehydration Loss of too much body water, resulting in impaired function.

delayed-onset muscle soreness (DOMS) Muscle discomfort or pain that develops within 24 to 48 hours after an exercise session that is excessive in duration or intensity.

denial Unconscious defense mechanism used to avoid facing painful or difficult circumstances or problems.

dependence A compulsive or chronic need for a substance or behavior.

diabetes Metabolic disorder characterized by high blood glucose levels that is associated with increased risk for cardiovascular disease, kidney disease, nerve dysfunction, and eye damage.

diabetes Metabolic disorder characterized by high blood glucose levels.

distress Negative stress that is harmful to performance.

dual energy X-ray absorptiometry (DXA) Technique for assessing body composition using a low-radiation X-ray; typically used in research or clinical settings and considered a gold-standard measure.

dynamic stretching Stretching that involves moving the joints through the full range of motion to mimic a movement used in a sport or exercise.

dysplasia Abnormal development of cells or tissue.

E

eccentric muscle action Action in which the muscle develops tension as it lengthens while controlling the movement with gravity. Also called negative work.

endocrine system Group of glands and tissues that secrete hormones to regulate body processes.

endorphins Group of hormones released during the stress response.

energy balance The state of consuming a number of calories that is equal to the number expended.

epinephrine Hormone secreted by the inner core (medulla) of the adrenal gland; also called *adrenaline*.

essential amino acids Nine amino acids that cannot be manufactured by the body and must be consumed in the diet.

essential fat Body fat that is necessary for physiological functioning.

eustress Stress that results in improved performance; also called *positive stress*.

evaporation Conversion of water (sweat) to a gas (water vapor); the most important means of releasing heat from the body during exercise.

exercise prescription The individualized amount of exercise that will effectively promote physical fitness for a given person.

exercise Planned, structured, and repetitive bodily movement done to improve or maintain one or more components of fitness.

external locus of control Perception that the events of one's life are outside of his or her control.

F

fascia Dense but thin layer of connective tissue that surrounds the muscle.

fast-twitch fibers Muscle fibers that contract rapidly but fatigue more quickly than slow-twitch fibers. There are two types: type IIa and type IIx.

fats The most common types of lipids found in foods and in your body.

fatty acid Basic structural unit of triglycerides.

fetal alcohol syndrome A cluster of birth defects that may include facial abnormalities and developmental disabilities caused by alcohol consumption during pregnancy.

fiber recruitment Process of involving more muscle fibers to increase muscular force.

fiber Undigestible complex carbohydrate found in whole grains, vegetables, and fruits.

fight-or-flight response Series of physiological reactions that prepare a person to combat a real or perceived threat.

flexibility Ability to move joints freely through their full range of motion.

flexibility The ability to move joints freely through their full range of motion.

free radicals Oxygen molecules that can potentially damage cells.

frequency of exercise The number of times per week that one exercises.

G

general adaptation syndrome Pattern of responses to stress that consists of an alarm stage, a resistance stage, and an exhaustion stage.

ghrelin Hormone that stimulates appetite.

glucose A simple carbohydrate (sugar) that can be used as fuel.

glycemic index Ranking system for carbohydrates based on a food's effect on blood glucose levels.

glycogen Storage form of glucose; stored in the liver and skeletal muscles.

glycolysis Process during which carbohydrates are broken down in cells. Much of the anaerobic ATP production in muscle cells occurs during glycolysis.

Golgi tendon organs Type of proprioceptor found within tendons.

gonorrhea Sexually transmitted infection caused by the *Neisseria gonorrhoeae* bacterium; curable with antibiotics.

gynoid pattern Pattern of fat distribution characterized by fat stored in the hips and thighs; more common in women.

H

heart attack Stoppage of blood flow to the heart, resulting in the death of heart cells; also called *myocardial infarction*.

heart rate reserve (HRR) The difference between the maximal heart rate and resting heart rate.

heart rate The number of heart beats per minute.

heat injury Injury that occurs when the heat load exceeds the body's ability to regulate body temperature. Also called *heat illness*.

hepatitis B virus (HBV) Viral infection that attacks the liver.

herpes General term used to describe infections caused by various types of herpes virus.

high-density lipoprotein (HDL) A combination of protein, fat, and cholesterol in the blood, composed of relatively large amounts of protein. Protects against the fatty plaque accumulation in the coronary arteries that leads to heart disease; also called "good cholesterol."

homeotherm Animal that regulates body temperature to remain close to a set point.

human papillomavirus (HPV) Group of sexually transmitted viruses that can cause genital warts and lead to cervical and other types of cancer.

human papillomavirus (HPV) Sexually transmitted virus that can cause cervical cancer.

humidity The amount of water vapor in the air.

hydrostatic weighing Method of determining body composition that involves weighing an individual on land and in a tank of water.

hyperplasia Increase in the number of muscle fibers.

hypertension High blood pressure.

hypertrophy Increase in muscle fiber size.

hypokinetic disease Disease associated with a lack of exercise.

hypothermia Significant decline in body temperature due to exposure to cold.

I

illicit drugs Illegal drugs or legal substances that are sold illegally.

inclusive sports Sports played by individuals with and without a disability.

incomplete proteins Proteins that are missing one or more of the essential amino acids.

insoluble fiber Fiber that does not dissolve in water; adds bulk and speeds elimination.

intensity of exercise The amount of physiological stress or overload placed on the body during exercise.

internal locus of control Perception that one has control of most of the events of one's life.

interval training Type of training that includes repeated sessions or intervals of relatively intense exercise alternated with lower-intensity periods to rest or recover.

irradiation The use of radiation to kill microorganisms that grow on or in food.

isokinetic Type of exercise that can include concentric or eccentric muscle actions performed at a constant speed using a specialized machine.

isometric Type of exercise in which muscular tension is developed but the body part does not move. Also called static exercise.

isotonic Type of exercise in which there is movement of a body part. Most exercise or sports skills are isotonic exercise. Also called dynamic exercise.

K

kilocalorie Unit of measure used to quantify food energy or the energy expended by the body. Technically, the kilocalorie is the amount of energy necessary to raise the temperature of 1 kilogram of water 1°C. A kilocalorie is often called a *Calorie*.

L

lactic acid By-product of glucose metabolism, produced primarily during intense exercise (greater than 50%–60% of maximal aerobic capacity).

leptin Hormone that depresses appetite.

ligaments Connective tissues within the joint capsule that hold bones together.

lipids Group of insoluble compounds that includes fats and cholesterol.

lipoproteins Combinations of protein, triglycerides, and cholesterol in the blood that have an important role in influencing the risk of heart disease.

low-density lipoprotein (LDL) A combination of protein, fat, and cholesterol in the blood, composed of relatively large amounts of cholesterol. LDLs promote the fatty plaque accumulation in the coronary arteries that leads to heart disease; also called "bad cholesterol."

M

macronutrients Carbohydrates, fats, proteins, and water; necessary for building and maintaining body tissues and providing energy.

maintenance phase The third phase of an exercise program. The goal of this phase is to maintain the increase in strength obtained during the first two phases.

maintenance program Exercising to sustain a desired level of physical fitness.

malignant tumor Tumor made up of cancerous cells.

malnutrition Poor nutrition due to an insufficient or poorly balanced diet or to faulty digestion or utilization of foods.

mammogram X-ray image of the breast used for cancer screening.

marijuana Psychoactive plant mixture (stems, leaves, or seeds) from *Cannabis sativa* or *Cannabis indica*.

meditation Relaxation technique that involves sitting quietly, focusing on a word, image, or the breath, and breathing slowly and rhythmically.

melanoma Less common but more serious type of skin cancer; tends to spread aggressively.

metastasis Spread of cancer cells throughout the body.

micronutrients Vitamins and minerals; they are involved in many body processes, including regulating cell function.

minerals Chemical elements required by the body in small amounts for normal functioning.

motor unit A motor nerve and all of the muscle fibers it controls.

muscle action The shortening of a skeletal muscle (causing movement) or the lengthening of a skeletal muscle (resisting movement).

muscle spindles Type of proprioceptor found within muscle.

muscular endurance Ability of a muscle to generate a submaximal force over and over again.

muscular strength Maximal ability of a muscle to generate force.

N

nervous system The brain, spinal cord, and nerves of the body.

nicotine Addictive and psychoactive substance in tobacco plants.

nonessential amino acids Eleven amino acids that the body can make and are not necessary in the diet.

norepinephrine Hormone secreted by the inner core (medulla) of the adrenal gland.

nutrients Substances in food that are necessary for survival and health.

nutrition The study of nutrients–their digestion, absorption, and metabolism and their effect on health and disease.

O

obese An excessive amount of fat in the body, typically above 25% for men and 35% for women.

omega-3 fatty acid Type of unsaturated fatty acid that lowers blood cholesterol and triglycerides and is found abundantly in some fish.

one-repetition maximum (1 RM) test Measurement of the maximum amount of weight that can be lifted one time.

organic Plant or animal foods that are grown without the use of pesticides, chemical fertilizers, antibiotics, or hormones.

osteoporosis Bone disease in which the mineral content of bone is reduced, and the bone is weakened and at increased risk of fracture.

osteoporosis Condition that involves the loss of bone mass.

overload principle Basic principle of physical conditioning that states that in order to improve physical fitness, the body or specific muscles must be stressed.

overtraining syndrome Phenomenon in which too much exercise and not enough recovery time between workouts result in exercise-related injuries.

overtraining Failure to get enough rest between exercise training sessions.

overweight A weight above the recommended level for health.

ozone Gas produced by a chemical reaction between sunlight and the hydrocarbons emitted from car exhaust.

P

pandemic Illness or infection that occurs over a wide geographic area and affects a high proportion of the population.

parasympathetic branch Division of the autonomic nervous system that is dominant at rest and controls energy conservation and restoration processes.

patellofemoral pain syndrome (PFPS) Common exercise-induced injury, sometimes called "runner's knee," that manifests as pain behind the kneecap (patella).

pelvic inflammatory disease (PID) Inflammatory infection of the lining of the abdominal and pelvic cavity in women.

peptide YY Hormone that depresses appetite.

phospholipid Type of lipid that contains phosphorus and is an important component of cell membranes.

physical activity/exercise (PA/E) Amount of energy expended during any form of physical activity or exercise.

physical activity Movement of the body produced by a skeletal muscle that results in energy expenditure, especially through movement of large muscle groups (i.e., legs).

polyps Growths from mucous membranes; commonly found in the colon and rectum, where they can be indicators of colon cancer.

presbyopia Farsightedness that results from weakening of the eye muscles due to aging.

principle of progression Principle of training that states that overload should be increased gradually.

principle of recuperation The body requires recovery periods between exercise training sessions to adapt to the exercise stress. Therefore, a period of rest is essential for achieving maximal benefit from exercise.

principle of reversibility Loss of fitness due to inactivity.

principle of specificity The effect of exercise training is specific to those muscles involved in the activity.

progressive overload Application of the overload principle to strength and endurance exercise programs.

proprioceptive neuromuscular facilitation (PNF) Series of movements combining stretching with alternating contraction and relaxation of muscles.

proprioceptor Specialized receptor in muscle or tendon that provides feedback to the brain about the position of body parts.

psychoactive drugs Pharmacological agents that alter mood, behavior, and/or cognitive processes.

pubic lice STI caused by a parasitic insect that grips the hair in the pubic area; also called "crabs."

pulmonary circuit Vascular system that circulates blood from the right side of the heart, through the lungs, and back to the left side of the heart.

push-up test Fitness test designed to evaluate endurance of shoulder and arm muscles.

R

range of motion The amount of movement possible at a joint.

responses Changes that occur during exercise to help you meet the demands of the exercise session. These changes return to normal levels shortly after the exercise session.

resting metabolic rate The amount of energy expended during all sedentary activities. Also called *resting energy expenditure*.

RICE Acronym for a treatment protocol for exercise-related injuries; stands for **r**est, **i**ce, **c**ompression, and **e**levation.

S

sarcopenia Loss of skeletal muscle mass that occurs with aging.

saturated fatty acid Type of fatty acid that comes primarily from animal sources and is solid at room temperature.

scabies Infection caused by a parasitic mite that can burrow under the skin between the fingers, on the wrists, under the breasts, and in the pubic area.

secondhand smoke Smoke from the burning end of a cigarette, cigar, or pipe and smoke exhaled by a smoker.

self-efficacy A person's belief in his or her ability to accomplish a specific goal.

set Number of repetitions performed consecutively without resting.

sexually transmitted infections (STIs) A group of more than 25 infections that are spread through sexual contact.

shin splints Term referring to pain associated with injuries to the front of the lower leg.

shoulder flexibility test Fitness test that measures the ability of the shoulder muscles to move through their full range of motion.

sit-and-reach test Fitness test that measures the ability to flex the trunk.

sit-up test Test used to evaluate abdominal and hip muscle endurance.

skinfold test A field test used to estimate body composition; representative samples of subcutaneous fat are measured using calipers to estimate the overall level of body fat.

slow progression phase The second phase of an exercise program. The goal of this phase is to increase muscular strength beyond the starter phase.

slow-twitch fibers Red muscle fibers that contract slowly and are highly resistant to fatigue. These fibers have the capacity to produce large quantities of ATP aerobically. Also known as *type I fibers*.

soluble fiber Viscous fiber that dissolves in water; slows stomach emptying.

specificity of training The concept that the development of muscular strength and endurance, as well as cardiorespiratory endurance, is specific to both the muscle group exercised and the training intensity.

sprain Damage to a ligament that occurs when excessive force is applied to a joint.

stages of change model A framework for understanding how the process of behavior change occurs; includes six stages.

starches Long chains of glucose units; found in foods such as corn, grains, and potatoes.

starter phase The beginning phase of an exercise program. The goal of this phase is to build a base for further physical conditioning.

static stretching Stretching that slowly lengthens a muscle to a point where further movement is limited.

sterol Type of lipid that does not contain fatty acids; cholesterol is the most commonly known sterol.

storage fat Excess fat reserves stored in the body's adipose tissue.

strain Damage to a muscle that can range from a minor separation of fibers to a complete tearing of the muscle.

stress fractures Tiny cracks or breaks in the bone.

stress response Physiological and behavioral changes that occur in reaction to a stressor.

stress State of physical and mental tension in response to an actual or perceived threat or challenge.

stressor Factor that produces stress.

stretch reflex Involuntary contraction of a muscle due to rapid stretching of that muscle.

stroke volume The amount of blood pumped per heartbeat (generally expressed in milliliters).

stroke Brain damage that occurs when the blood supply to the brain is reduced for a prolonged period of time.

subcutaneous fat Fat stored just beneath the skin.

substance abuse Use of illegal drugs, the inappropriate use of legal drugs, and/or the repeated use of drugs to produce pleasure, to alleviate stress, or to alter or avoid reality.

sympathetic branch Division of the autonomic nervous system that is in control when we need to react or respond to challenges; the excitatory branch.

syphilis STI caused by the *Treponema pallidum* bacterium; curable with antibiotics.

systemic circuit Vascular system that circulates blood from the left side of the heart, throughout the body, and back to the right side of the heart.

T

target heart rate (THR) The range of heart rates that corresponds to an exercise intensity of approximately 50%–85% $\cdot$ O$_2$ max. This range results in improvements in aerobic capacity.

ten percent rule The training intensity or duration of exercise should not be increased by more than 10% per week.

tendonitis Inflammation or swelling of a tendon.

tendons Fibrous connective tissue that attaches muscle to bone.

threshold for health benefits The minimum level of physical activity required to achieve some of the health benefits of exercise.

time (duration) of exercise The amount of time invested in performing the primary workout.

tolerance Situation in which a drug/alcohol user requires increasingly larger amounts of the substance to experience the effects.

training threshold The training intensity above which there is an improvement in cardiorespiratory fitness. This intensity is approximately 50% of $\dot{V}O_2$ max.

trans fatty acid Type of fatty acid that increases cholesterol in the blood and is a major contributor to heart disease.

trichomoniasis STI caused by a single-celled protozoan parasite.

triglyceride Form of lipid that is broken down in the body and used to produce energy to power muscle contractions during exercise.

tumor Abnormal growth of tissue; neoplasm.

type of exercise The specific type (mode) of exercise to be performed.

U

unintentional injury Injury resulting from unplanned actions; preferred term for accidental injury.

unsaturated fatty acid Type of fatty acid that comes primarily from plant sources and is liquid at room temperature.

V

Valsalva maneuver Holding the breath during an intense muscle contraction; can reduce blood flow to the brain and cause dizziness and fainting.

veins Blood vessels that transport blood toward the heart.

virus Infectious microorganism that cannot live independently and must invade a host cell to survive.

visceral fat Fat stored around the internal organs.

visualization Relaxation technique that uses appealing mental images to promote relaxation and reduce stress; also called *imagery*.

vitamins Micronutrients that play a key role in many body functions, including the regulation of growth and metabolism; classified as water-soluble or fat-soluble.

VO2 max The maximum amount of oxygen the body can take in and use during exercise.

W

waist-to-hip ratio Ratio of the waist and hip circumferences used to determine the risk for disease associated with the android pattern of obesity.

warm-up Brief (5–15-minute) period of exercise that precedes a workout.

wellness A state of optimal health that encompasses all the dimensions of well-being. Consists of eight major components: physical, emotional, intellectual, spiritual, social, environmental, occupational, and financial wellness.

withdrawal symptoms Symptoms that occur after stopping or reducing the intake of an addictive substance.

index